Loureen Downes, PhD, APRN, FNP-BC
Doctor of Nursing Pra[...]
Director and Pr[...]
School of Nursing, Florida G[...]
Fort Myers, Fl[...]

Lilly Tryon, DNP, APRN, FNP-BC, DipACLM, NBC-HWC, ACSM-EP
Professor
School of Nursing
Southern Adventist University
Collegedale, Tennessee

HEALTH
PROMOTION
and Disease Prevention for Advanced Practice

Integrating Evidence-Based Lifestyle Concepts

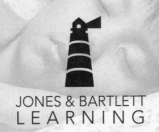

JONES & BARTLETT
LEARNING

World Headquarters
Jones & Bartlett Learning
25 Mall Road
Burlington, MA 01803
978-443-5000
info@jblearning.com
www.jblearning.com

Jones & Bartlett Learning books and products are available through most bookstores and online booksellers. To contact Jones & Bartlett Learning directly, call 800-832-0034, fax 978-443-8000, or visit our website, www.jblearning.com.

Substantial discounts on bulk quantities of Jones & Bartlett Learning publications are available to corporations, professional associations, and other qualified organizations. For details and specific discount information, contact the special sales department at Jones & Bartlett Learning via the above contact information or send an email to specialsales@jblearning.com.

Copyright © 2025 by Jones & Bartlett Learning, LLC, an Ascend Learning Company

All rights reserved. No part of the material protected by this copyright may be reproduced or utilized in any form, electronic or mechanical, including photocopying, recording, or by any information storage and retrieval system, without written permission from the copyright owner.

The content, statements, views, and opinions herein are the sole expression of the respective authors and not that of Jones & Bartlett Learning, LLC. Reference herein to any specific commercial product, process, or service by trade name, trademark, manufacturer, or otherwise does not constitute or imply its endorsement or recommendation by Jones & Bartlett Learning, LLC and such reference shall not be used for advertising or product endorsement purposes. All trademarks displayed are the trademarks of the parties noted herein. *Health Promotion and Disease Prevention for Advanced Practice: Integrating Evidence-Based Lifestyle Concepts* is an independent publication and has not been authorized, sponsored, or otherwise approved by the owners of the trademarks or service marks referenced in this product.

There may be images in this book that feature models; these models do not necessarily endorse, represent, or participate in the activities represented in the images. Any screenshots in this product are for educational and instructive purposes only. Any individuals and scenarios featured in the case studies throughout this product may be real or fictitious but are used for instructional purposes only.

The authors, editor, and publisher have made every effort to provide accurate information. However, they are not responsible for errors, omissions, or for any outcomes related to the use of the contents of this book and take no responsibility for the use of the products and procedures described. Treatments and side effects described in this book may not be applicable to all people; likewise, some people may require a dose or experience a side effect that is not described herein. Drugs and medical devices are discussed that may have limited availability controlled by the Food and Drug Administration (FDA) for use only in a research study or clinical trial. Research, clinical practice, and government regulations often change the accepted standard in this field. When consideration is being given to use of any drug in the clinical setting, the healthcare provider or reader is responsible for determining FDA status of the drug, reading the package insert, and reviewing prescribing information for the most up-to-date recommendations on dose, precautions, and contraindications, and determining the appropriate usage for the product. This is especially important in the case of drugs that are new or seldom used.

24924-8

Production Credits

Vice President, Product Management: Marisa R. Urbano
Vice President, Content Strategy and Implementation: Christine Emerton
Manager, Content Strategy: Donna Gridley
Director, Product Management: Matthew Kane
Product Manager: Tina Chen
Content Strategist: Christina Freitas
Content Coordinator: Samantha Gillespie
Director, Project Management and Content Services: Karen Scott
Manager, Project Manager: Jackie Reynen
Project Manager: Eliza Lewis
Digital Project Specialist: Angela Dooley
Senior Product Marketing Manager: Lindsay White
Content Services Manager: Colleen Lamy

Rights and Permissions Manager: John Rusk
Rights Specialist: Liz Kicaid
Senior Media Development Editor: Troy Liston
Cover Design: Briana Yates
Text Design: Briana Yates
Manufacturing: Wendy Kilborn
Cover Image (Title Page, Part Opener, Chapter Opener):
 © Nuttaphong Sriset/Shutterstock, Hung Chung Chih/
 Shutterstock, StoryTime Studio/Shutterstock, Prostock-studio/
 Shutterstock, Kathleen Gail/Shutterstock, kali9/Getty Images.
Printing and Binding: Sheridan Saline
Cover Printing: Sheridan Saline

Library of Congress Cataloging-in-Publication Data
Names: Downes, Loureen, author. | Tryon, Lilly, author.
Title: Health promotion and disease prevention for advanced practice: integrating evidence-based lifestyle concepts / Loureen Downes and Lilly Tryon.
Description: First edition. | Burlington, MA: Jones & Bartlett Learning, [2025] | Includes bibliographical references and index.
Identifiers: LCCN 2023007032 | ISBN 9781284249248 (paperback)
Subjects: MESH: Health Promotion | Health Behavior | Healthy Lifestyle
Classification: LCC RA418 | NLM WA 590 | DDC 362.1--dc23/eng/20230703
LC record available at https://lccn.loc.gov/2023007032

Printed in the United States of America
28 27 26 25 24   10 9 8 7 6 5 4 3 2 1

Dedication

To the students and providers who will promote health and wellness.

To my supportive husband, William Roger Downes, and our two sons, William Michael Downes and Matthew Downes, the wind beneath my wings, who fuel me to keep on this journey.

–Loureen Downes

I dedicate this book to the memory of my father, Bobby Boles, who taught me, through his life and struggles with lifestyle-related chronic disease, about the need to address lifestyle early and often with my patients and the importance of a whole-person, partnership model of care approach.

–Lilly Tryon

Brief Contents

© Kathleen Gail/Shutterstock; © StoryTime Studio/Shutterstock; © kali9/Getty Images

Contents

PART 1 Principles of Health Promotion   1

CHAPTER 1 Introduction to Health Promotion, Disease Prevention, and Lifestyle Concepts 3

Loureen Downes, PhD, APRN, FNP-BC, DipACLM, FAANP, NBC-HWC

CHAPTER 2 Health Disparities and Determinants of Health 33

Donna M. Hedges, PhD, MSN, MBA, RN, CNE, Terri L. Gibson, DNP, MSN, RN, AMB-BC, DipACLM

© Kathleen Gail/Shutterstock; © StoryTime Studio/Shutterstock; © kali9/Getty Images

PART 2 The Process of Health Promotion 111

PART 3 A-SMART Lifestyle Prescriptions for Health Promotion 265

CHAPTER 11 Adopt Healthy Eating 267

Loureen Downes, PhD, APRN, FNP-BC, DipACLM, FAANP, NBC-HWC, Lilly Tryon, DNP, FNP-BC, DipACLM, NBC-HWC

CHAPTER 12 Stress Less 309

Roberta Christopher, EdD, MSN, ARNP, NE-BC, CAIF, Lila de Tantillo, PhD, MS, APRN, FNP-BC

CHAPTER 13 Move Often 333

Jeff Young, BS, CSCS, ACSM-EIM, Sheila Hautbois, PA-C, MPAS, MPH, CHES®, DipACLM, Nanette Morales, DNP, NP-C, DipACLM

CHAPTER 14 Avoid Alcohol 365

Sara B. Adams, PhD, RN, CNE,
Carol Essenmacher, DNP, PMHCNS-BC

CHAPTER 15 Rest More 383

Josie H. Bidwell, DNP, RN, FNP-C,
DipACLM, Cindy Secrist Rima, DNP,
APRN, ANP-BC, DipACLM,
Lawrence Chan, DO

**CHAPTER 16 Treat Tobacco
Use 399**

Shari Hrabovsky, DEd, MSN, FNP-BC,
Linda Royer, PhD, MPH, MSN, RN

PART 4 **The Practice
of Health
Promotion
for Preventing
and Managing
Chronic
Disease   431**

**CHAPTER 17 Pre-Obesity
and Obesity Prevention
and Management 433**

Loureen Downes, PhD, APRN, FNP-BC,
DipACLM, FAANP, NBC-HWC, Sonya King,
DNP, ARNP, FNP-BC, Rachel Mack, MPAS,
PA-C

CHAPTER 21 Healthy Lifestyle Promotion for the Cancer Continuum 563

Kara Mosesso, MSN, ANP-BC, AOCNP, DipACLM

CHAPTER 22 Health Promotion Interventions for Alzheimer's Disease and Dementia 601

Alicia Craig-Rodriguez, DNP, MBA, APRN, FNP-BC, DipACLM, Carli A. Carnish, DNP, APRN-CNP

CHAPTER 23 The Role of Healthy Lifestyles in Mental Health Promotion 623

Carol Essenmacher, DNP, RN, PMHCNS-BC, Joanne Evans, MEd, RN, PMHCNS-BC, Kelly Freeman, MSN, RN, AGPCNP-BC, DipACLM, Elizabeth Winings, DNP, APRN, PMHNP-BC

Foreword

The United States spends more money on health care than any Western world country yet ranks at the bottom for population health outcomes. One major reason is that only 8% of healthcare spending is invested in wellness and prevention. Further, approximately 60% of Americans have a chronic condition, yet 80% of chronic disease is totally preventable with just a few healthy lifestyle behaviors, such as 150 minutes of physical activity per week, at least five fruits and vegetables per day, no tobacco use, and alcohol in moderation (i.e., no more than one standard size alcoholic beverage per day). If every person in America would engage in these lifestyle behaviors, sleep at least seven hours a night, and practice daily stress reduction, we could nearly wipe out chronic disease. This evidence-based formula is simple but not easy because most people do not change their behaviors unless a crisis happens or their emotions are aroused. To truly motivate people to change their behaviors, we must share evidence plus an emotional story. We also must shift the focus of our health care from being sick/crisis care to wellness and prevention. When I was home alone with my mom at 15 years of age, she sneezed, stroked out, and died right in front of me. As a result, I suffered from terrible posttraumatic stress, depression, and anxiety for a few years. The saddest part of my mom's story is that she had a history of headaches for over a year. With encouragement from my dad, she went for an evaluation with her primary care doctor one week before she died. She was diagnosed with high blood pressure and given a prescription for a blood pressure medication that my dad found in her purse after she died. Her death may have been prevented if she had filled that prescription and taken that medication. That is one of the reasons I am so passionate about wellness, prevention, and motivating people to engage in healthy behaviors. As a result of a dream and my passion, I was able to pitch the concept of being the first chief wellness officer in the nation at a university to the former president of the Ohio State University when I was being recruited, and fortunately, they saw the need. I was appointed to this university-wide wellness position, where my charge is to improve the population health and well-being of faculty, staff, and students. More universities and corporations are now appointing chief wellness officers because they realize there is a wonderful return on and value of investment with this organization-wide leadership role and investment in the well-being of their people.

This book is a greatly needed resource that should be a staple for all health professionals, educators, and learners. It contains essential content to improve population health and well-being through health promotion and healthy lifestyle behaviors. The A-SMART lifestyle prescriptions for health promotion are well organized into the significant lifestyle behaviors that prevent chronic conditions. One of the many strengths of this text is that it is practical and relatable. The chapters on health promotion billing and reimbursement as well as information technology and provider self-care are terrific additions.

© Kathleen Gail/Shutterstock; © StoryTime Studio/Shutterstock; © kali9/Getty Images

Kudos to Loureen Downes and Lilly Tryon on a terrific must-read! More important, everyone needs to put the content from this book into action.

Bernadette Mazurek Melnyk, PhD,
APRN-CNP, FAANP, FNAP, FAAN
Vice President for Health Promotion
University Chief Wellness Officer
Dean and Helene Fuld Health Trust
Professor of Evidence-Based Practice,
College of Nursing

Professor of Pediatrics and Psychiatry,
College of Medicine
Executive Director, Helene Fuld Health Trust
National Institute for EBP
Ohio State University
Editor in Chief, Worldviews on
Evidence-Based Nursing

Preface

Why We Wrote This Book

This textbook emphasizes practical lifestyle approaches to managing and preventing the root causes of the leading chronic diseases in the United States and globally. With laser-like focus, it addresses the tools advanced practice providers (APPs), particularly nurse practitioners and physician assistants, need to contribute to a higher level of care to promote health and prevent diseases. We deemed this book necessary because we could not find a textbook with the advanced lifestyle management content and principles we desired to teach in our graduate-level health promotion courses and to integrate them throughout our curricula.

The evidence is overwhelming that lifestyle-related chronic diseases—such as heart disease, hypertension, strokes, type 2 diabetes, obesity, and multiple types of cancer—are preventable or manageable by lifestyle behaviors. This evidence is further underscored by the integration of lifestyle interventions into many evidence-based guidelines (e.g., American Cancer Society Guideline for Diet and Physical Activity, 2019 ACC/AHA Guideline on the Primary Prevention of Cardiovascular Disease, and Scientific Statement Management of Stage 1 Hypertension, 2021) for the prevention and treatment of lifestyle-related chronic conditions. Yet most APPs lack the preparation to incorporate evidence-based lifestyle intervention into managing patients at risk for or diagnosed with preventable chronic diseases. In clinical practice, patients are often told to change their behavior, such as increasing physical activity, without specific guidance. This book will provide the necessary knowledge, tools, and resources to help the APP to know how to give patients lifestyle-focused prescriptions to improve adherence and health outcomes using specific criteria similar to a medication prescription.

The recent COVID-19 pandemic underscored the devastating effect of chronic diseases on health outcomes. It is now well established that those with the most severe complications and highest mortality due to COVID-19 were disproportionately affected if they had a lifestyle-related chronic condition. Furthermore, the pandemic also highlighted the responsibility of healthcare providers to include lifestyle interventions to prevent chronic diseases. Many providers cite a lack of knowledge, time, and reimbursement as barriers to providing disease prevention and health promotion management to patients with chronic conditions. Therefore, APPs must be prepared to include evidence-informed, cost-effective lifestyle prescriptions using an interprofessional approach to prevent, manage, and treat chronic illnesses. This textbook will fill a gap in knowledge by presenting evidence-based, cutting-edge lifestyle management tactics for chronic diseases, strategies for delivering health promotion in brief encounters, and reimbursement guidelines for health promotion and disease prevention.

Recently, government agencies and organizations have sought to encourage healthcare professionals to be better prepared to provide disease prevention strategies where people live, work, and play and in the clinical setting

© Kathleen Gail/Shutterstock; © StoryTime Studio/Shutterstock; © kali9/Getty Images

to improve health outcomes and provide high-value care. The strength of this textbook lies in the 43 national interprofessional contributors, with expertise in lifestyle medicine, disease prevention, health promotion, and health education garnered over several hundred years of caring for patients in clinical and community settings.

The content in the book is drawn from scientific literature and guidelines from the United States, Canada, and Europe. The science was used to identify practical lifestyle behaviors that can be applied at the personal and population levels to prevent chronic diseases. Additionally, it addresses an approach to health promotion and disease prevention by using environmental, behavioral, and motivational concepts relevant to lifestyle-related chronic diseases.

The topics covered in the text align with competencies that guide the education of APPs, such as population health and person-centered competencies (American Association of Colleges of Nursing, 2021; Competencies for the PA Profession, 2021), and the *Obesity Medicine Education Collaborative Obesity Competencies* (Obesity Medicine Education Collaborative, 2018), as well as national guidelines that include lifestyle intervention as first-line treatment for several chronic conditions such as heart disease, hyperlipidemia, type 2 diabetes, and hypertension.

Organization of the Text

The 23 chapters are organized into four parts. The basic principles used to inform this book are the plethora of evidence that daily habits profoundly affect health outcomes in the short and long term. Each chapter features a research abstract relevant to the topic, a case study with critical thinking questions, a list of evidence-based resources, and a health promotion application activity. Similar concepts may be introduced or addressed in more than one chapter because each chapter was written to stand alone. However, the six foundational lifestyle behaviors of nutrition, stress management, physical activity, alcohol use, sleep, and tobacco cessation are addressed in separate chapters. Also, chapters will address integrating lifestyle behaviors and common lifestyle-related chronic conditions for optimum health outcomes.

Part 1: Principles of Health Promotion

Part I introduces fundamental concepts of promoting health and preventing disease for the individual, population, and provider. Chapter 1 offers practical approaches for assessing lifestyle behaviors and exemplars of lifestyle prescriptions. Chapter 2 addresses health equity and social determinants of health relevant to health promotion. Chapter 3 describes the application of theories and models to health promotion program planning, implementation, and evaluation. Chapter 4 highlights the significance of self-care to provider well-being and is in keeping with the recent national emphasis on the need for providers to care for themselves to prevent burnout and improve resiliency.

Part 2: The Process of Health Promotion

Part 2 further sets the stage for learning about health promotion by discussing the traditional screening procedures across the life spans, such as immunizations and anticipatory guidance (Chapter 5); best practices for patient-centered communication, such as motivational interviewing, to enhance behavior changes (Chapter 6); the utilization of telehealth by the provider and patient to strengthen the practice of lifestyle management (Chapter 7); fundamental prerequisites for reimbursement as well as billing and coding to enhance reimbursement (Chapter 8); assessment of individual and population health needs (Chapter 9); and developing interprofessional community health promotion programs, which may be a valuable resource for scholarly project development (Chapter 10).

Part 3: A-SMART Lifestyle Prescriptions for Health Promotion

Part 3 presents the six evidence-based behaviors to prevent, manage, and treat lifestyle-related chronic diseases. Chapter 11 describes nutrition's role in health, various nutrition assessments, and nutritional prescriptions. Chapter 12 presents the implications of stress across the life span and approaches to stress prevention and management. Chapter 13 focuses on exercise guidelines and practical interventions to promote physical activity. Chapter 14 discusses the health effects of alcohol and evidence-based practice management for alcohol use. Chapter 15 describes the effect of impaired sleep, rest hygiene, and counseling. Chapter 16 presents an overview of tobacco use and the health consequences with theoretical and interprofessional interventions.

Part 4: The Practice of Health Promotion for Preventing and Managing Chronic Disease

Part 4 presents content on managing some of the most common conditions amenable to lifestyle behaviors contributing to significant morbidity, mortality, and disability in the United States. In this section, guidelines and emerging evidence to assess, prevent, manage, or treat pre-obesity and obesity (Chapter 17), type 2 diabetes (Chapter 18), cardiovascular disease (Chapter 19), chronic pain (Chapter 20), some cancers (Chapter 21), Alzheimer's disease and dementia (Chapter 22), and mental health disorders (Chapter 23) are discussed.

In summary, this book is designed to be the primary textbook in a graduate health promotion course or a supplemental text for clinical courses. It serves as a valuable addition to the education of APP students, including those pursuing careers as nurse practitioners and physician assistants. It may also serve as an excellent resource at the point of care for APPs in clinical and community settings. It is alarming that lifestyle behaviors can prevent 80% of chronic diseases, and these diseases account for 85% of health care costs. Unfortunately, most providers do not receive sufficient education on the root causes of these diseases. Though the textbook is not exhaustive, it provides practical guidance for the APP to prevent and promote health and well-being for patients and populations. It will be a valuable addition to any advanced practice curriculum to prepare providers to offer upstream lifestyle behavior solutions to the downstream issues of preventable chronic diseases affecting 6 in 10 adults in the United States. Further, it fills a gap for a health promotion textbook explicitly written for educating APPs.

About the Editors

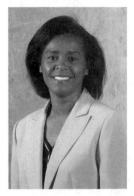

Loureen Downes, PhD, APRN, FNP-BC, DipACLM, FAANP, NBC-HWC, is a Conner Professor in Nursing and Founding Program Director of the Doctor of Nursing Practice Program at Florida Gulf Coast University. She has a Master of Science in Nursing degree from Florida Atlantic University and a doctor of philosophy degree in nursing from the University of Connecticut. As a clinician, Dr. Downes is a board-certified family nurse practitioner, a diplomate of lifestyle medicine, and a health and wellness coach. As a professor, she enjoys teaching nurse practitioner students to use lifestyle as first-line treatment or as an adjunct to traditional treatment regimens. One of her favorite courses to teach is Advanced Health Promotion. Her passion and research interest is to improve dietary habits and physical activity to decrease risk factors for preventable chronic diseases. She frequently contributes to her community and faith-based organization by delivering presentations on preventing and managing chronic diseases through lifestyle behaviors. Her notable research accomplishment includes developing an instrument, the Motivators and Barriers of Healthy Lifestyle Behaviors Scale, used nationally and internationally. Dr. Downes is the author of several peer-reviewed articles and has presented regionally, nationally, and internationally.

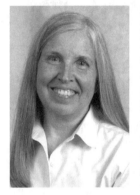

Lilly Tryon, DNP, APRN, FNP-BC, DipACLM, NBC-HWC, ACSM-EP, is a professor at the Southern Adventist University School of Nursing. She has a master's degree in nursing (Drexel University), a doctorate in nursing practice with an emphasis in lifestyle medicine (Southern Adventist University), and holds certifications in lifestyle medicine, health and wellness coaching, plant-based nutrition, and exercise physiology. As a professor, Dr. Tryon focuses on expanding the use of lifestyle medicine in advanced practice nursing. She teaches courses in advanced health promotion, lifestyle medicine, nutrition, culinary medicine, exercise, and health coaching and often uses the analogy of a tour guide (as opposed to a travel agent) to encourage students to go beyond prescribing and coach their patients to take realistic, evidence-based, and sustainable steps for preventing, managing, and reversing chronic disease. Dr. Tryon is a board-certified family nurse practitioner with over 35 years of nursing experience in lifestyle medicine and community health. She practices part-time at LifeMed, a direct primary care and lifestyle medicine practice in Chattanooga, Tennessee, where she focuses on using lifestyle as medicine in addressing the healthcare needs of her patients. She is also a strong advocate of faith-based health ministry and has developed training workshops and materials for using a coaching approach in church health outreach programs.

© Kathleen Gail/Shutterstock; © StoryTime Studio/Shutterstock; © kali9/Getty Images

Acknowledgments

The culmination of this textbook is the result of the collaborative effort of many individuals and organizations that inspired me about lifestyle behaviors and disease outcomes. There are too many who played a part in writing this textbook to mention them all by name. However, I would be remiss if I didn't particularly thank a few individuals for contributing to this book. There are not enough words to express my gratitude to my coeditor, Lilly, for her hard work and countless hours of editing. I appreciate the comments of reviewers of the prospectus for this book, anonymous to us, whose feedback shaped the book's development. I also thank the many contributors for sharing their invaluable expertise and the outstanding editorial team at Jones & Bartlett Learning for their patience and commitment to the project. I recognize Dr. Alexander Powell for his editorial assistance with selected chapters. I also thank my students for inspiring me to write this textbook and Florida Gulf Coast University for allowing me the time to write. I acknowledge my colleagues, friends, and family for their encouragement and support. Special thanks to my mother, Cady Smart, and my second mother, Sheila Williams, who inspired and motivated me through their resilience and strength. Most of all, to God be the glory for his guidance throughout this journey.

Loureen Downes

This text could not have been written without the contributions, assistance, support, and understanding of many. First, the foundation and motivation for my lifelong emphasis on a healthy lifestyle originate from my Lord and Savior, who came that we "may have life and have it more abundantly" (John 10:10). I would like to acknowledge the vision of my coeditor, Loureen, and the countless conversations and interactions that have shaped this book. I am grateful to the American College of Lifestyle Medicine for putting forward lifestyle competencies for healthcare providers and their countless resources and support for the therapeutic use of lifestyle change as the foundation of health and care. I am also deeply indebted to all the contributors whose collective depth of knowledge and experience far exceeds mine. I thank Southern Adventist University for allowing me time to write and my colleagues for supporting this project. The team at Jones & Bartlett Learning has given invaluable direction and assistance to help this book come to life. My students and patients have taught me much about person-centered, evidence-informed, and lifestyle-focused care, and their conversations and stories often came to mind while working on this book. The ongoing love and support received from my family sustained me throughout my work on this book. My husband, Barry, consistently offered much-needed perspective and balance, and my mother, Karen (Boles), always motivated me to see the positive side of everything. Finally, I am grateful to the readers of this text. This is the book I wish I had had when I was a student. I pray it enhances your clinical practice and makes a difference in the health outcomes of your patients.

Lilly Tryon

© Kathleen Gail/Shutterstock; © StoryTime Studio/Shutterstock; © kali9/Getty Images

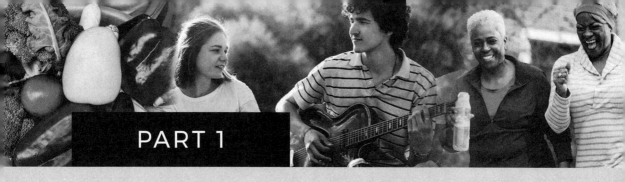

PART 1

Principles of Health Promotion

© Kathleen Gail/Shutterstock; © StoryTime Studio/Shutterstock; © kali9/Getty Images

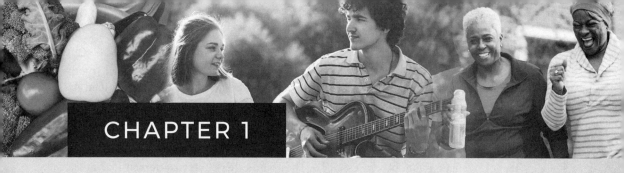

CHAPTER 1

Introduction to Health Promotion, Disease Prevention, and Lifestyle Concepts

Loureen Downes, PhD, APRN, FNP-BC, DipACLM, FAANP, NBC-HWC

The [healthcare provider] of the future will give no medicine but will instruct his patient in the care of the human frame, diet, and the cause and prevention of disease.

Thomas A. Edison

OBJECTIVES

This chapter will enable the reader to:

1. Define lifestyle management and its relationship to lifestyle medicine.
2. Identify the impact of chronic diseases.
3. Determine the economic benefit of lifestyle interventions.
4. Justify a paradigm shift for lifestyle management in practice and education.
5. Assess lifestyle vital signs and risk factors for lifestyle-related chronic diseases.
6. Design a lifestyle management prescription.
7. Using the A-SMART model, apply the lifestyle management strategies to clinical case studies.
8. Synthesize evidence to support improved health outcomes of lifestyle behaviors.

Overview

Worldwide, most morbidity and mortality are caused by the epidemic of chronic diseases, which are preventable by health promotion, disease prevention, and lifestyle behaviors (World Health Organization [WHO], 2021). The reasons for the increase in chronic diseases are multifactorial, including the shift of modern humans from an agrarian society composed of farms and small towns to an industrialized, technological culture. This modern way

© Kathleen Gail/Shutterstock; © StoryTime Studio/Shutterstock; © kali9/Getty Images

of living is associated with increased lifestyle-related disorders, including obesity, cardiovascular disease (CVD), cancer, and type 2 diabetes (T2DM). The modifiable etiology of these and other chronic diseases is attributed to behavioral and environmental determinants, such as the overconsumption of processed foods, inactivity, alcohol consumption, smoking, and chronic stress (Egger et al., 2017). Lifestyle management in mainstream clinical practice is an approach to address these determinants of chronic diseases to improve health outcomes and decrease the chronic disease burden on society.

Lifestyle management, or lifestyle medicine, is the science that works toward integrating health promotion, disease prevention, and healthy lifestyle behaviors into a person's daily choices. It is defined as the use of evidence-informed therapeutic lifestyle prescriptions—eating a whole-food, plant-predominant diet; regular physical activity; restorative sleep; stress management; avoidance of risky substances; and positive social connections—as primary modalities for treatment, prevention, and possibly reversal of chronic diseases (American College of Lifestyle Medicine [ACLM], n.d.). The evidence is overwhelming that health promotion—the process of empowering individuals to increase control over their health through social, environmental, and behavioral interventions—benefits and protects individual health and quality of life by addressing and preventing the root causes of ill health, not just focusing on treatment and cure (WHO, 2016).

Unhealthy lifestyle behaviors are often revealed in patients as increased blood pressure, elevated glucose, hyperlipidemia, and excess weight (WHO, 2021). Tackling these issues is critical to the healthcare sector's battle for better lives for individuals and populations. Advanced practice providers (APPs) are at the forefront of the interprofessional healthcare team to promote health and prevent diseases. Five key lifestyle modification strategies have been identified to decrease mortality from chronic diseases and prolong life span: a healthy diet, regular physical activity, moderate alcohol intake, an ideal weight, and never smoking (Li et al., 2018). These and other strategic interventions are at the core of chronic disease prevention and management.

However, behavior change is a complex process. It requires that the patient be empowered as a partner within an interprofessional healthcare team to strategically assess, evaluate, and implement the tactics needed to slow the rapid increase of chronic diseases. This chapter will outline chronic conditions and their risk factors, the economic impact of chronic diseases and prevention strategies, principles of lifestyle management, considerations for deprescribing, and the application of lifestyle vital signs and lifestyle prescriptions in clinical practice for improved health outcomes.

Impact of Chronic Diseases

Chronic diseases, also known as noncommunicable diseases, are generally defined as illnesses that last at least one year and are caused by multiple factors, including genes, biology, environment, and behavior (WHO, 2021). Chronic diseases impact individuals of all ages, populations, countries, and socioeconomic groups and cause 41 million deaths annually, equaling 71% of all deaths worldwide. Cardiovascular disorders, such as myocardial infarctions and strokes, account for the most frequent chronic disease deaths, with almost 18 million individuals each year, followed by cancers (9.3 million), respiratory diseases (4.1 million), and T2DM (1.5 million). Interestingly, these four groups of diseases are responsible for more than 80% of all chronic disease deaths globally (Hayes & Gillian, 2020).

These chronic diseases significantly impact society, leading to increased cost of health care and impaired quality of life. Furthermore, chronic diseases affect most adults in the United States and are the leading causes of disability and a foremost driver of the rising cost of health care. Sixty percent of American adults have at least one chronic disease, and 40% have two or more (National Center for Chronic Disease Prevention and Health Promotion [NCCDPHP], 2022a). The increase in chronic diseases and the subsequent rise in healthcare costs are unsustainable. APPs armed with evidence-informed lifestyle management skills can change the trajectory of this problem.

Risk Factors for Chronic Diseases

It is well established that a person's risk for developing a chronic disease is associated with multiple factors, including social determinants of health, genes, and lifestyle behaviors (Hayes & Delk, 2018; Hayes & Gillian, 2020). Social determinants of health include where one lives, works, learns, and plays (Hayes & Delk, 2018). Unfortunately, individuals' zip codes can determine more about their health than other factors. Underrepresented individuals—minorities, those of lower socioeconomic status, and people in low-income countries—are more likely to be negatively impacted by social determinants of health (Nugent et al., 2018; WHO, 2021). These factors result in chronic diseases, driving these populations further into poverty due to increased expenditures attributed to healthcare costs. Individuals who experience poverty tend to have decreased education; face systemic barriers, such as limited access to health care; and have increased incidences of chronic diseases and reduced health outcomes (Hayes & Delk, 2018). Therefore, addressing factors related to social determinants

of health is essential to achieving optimal health outcomes.

According to Hayes and Gillian (2020), chronic diseases flourish in certain families. Such a situation is associated with genetics, features inherited from parents, and epigenetics. Epigenetics are environmental and behavioral factors that affect how genes work (Office of Science, 2022). Evidence exists that genes are not the primary determinants of health outcomes. Instead, health outcomes are more likely determined by epigenetics, which dictate the activity of genes. Individuals in the same family have similar living circumstances; therefore, they tend to engage in identical lifestyle behaviors and experience similar social determinants of health that contribute to the risk of developing chronic illnesses (Hayes & Gillian, 2020). Unhealthy behaviors, such as smoking, inadequate dietary intake, and sedentary habits, may be handed down from generation to generation, affecting the risk of developing chronic diseases.

On the other hand, healthy behaviors, such as physical activity and healthy eating, can decrease chronic disease risks even with a genetic tendency toward a particular chronic condition (Office of Science, 2022). Epigenetic modifications are reversible and can change how the body interprets a genetic code. Therefore, epigenetics (environmental and behavioral factors) significantly influence health outcomes more than genes.

The health consequences of lifestyle behaviors, social determinants, and family and medical history of chronic illnesses increase a person's risk of chronic diseases. It cannot be overlooked that chronic diseases may promote other chronic diseases. For example, individuals with chronic conditions are at increased risk of poor mental health, most commonly depression (Hayes & Gillian, 2020). On the other hand, depression increases the risk of chronic diseases. Though social determinants play an essential role in health outcomes, lifestyle behaviors also significantly influence the development of chronic conditions. According to the WHO (2021), four lifestyle risk factors, smoking, unhealthy eating, alcohol use, and sedentary behaviors, contribute substantially to the annual deaths associated with chronic diseases (**Table 1.1**). Other lifestyle patterns, such as chronic stress and insufficient sleep, can also adversely affect health outcomes. APPs must appreciate the relationship among these multiple risk factors to create a multi-factorial approach to alleviating the burden of chronic conditions on individuals and society.

A recent multicohort prospective study by Nyberg et al. (2020) identified the effect of lifestyle behaviors on developing chronic dis-eases. The lifestyle behaviors evaluated in the study included smoking, weight status, phys-ical activity, and alcohol consumption cor-related to chronic diseases, including T2DM, heart disease, cerebrovascular accident, ma-lignancy, asthma, and chronic obstructive pulmonary disease. The results, based on an analytic sample of 116,043 participants with a mean follow-up of 12.6 years, revealed that those with the healthiest lifestyle scores were younger and of higher socioeconomic sta-tus. Furthermore, selected lifestyle behaviors correlated to higher years without chronic

illnesses. The lifestyle factors linked to the most years (about nine years) without chronic diseases were a body mass index (BMI) <25 kg/m^2 and at least two of the follow-ing health behaviors: never smoking, regular physical activity (150 minutes of moderate in-tensity or 75 minutes of vigorous intensity), and moderate alcohol consumption. The re-searchers concluded that the lifestyle factors studied offered an additive effect, rather than a synergistic effect, regarding life span (Nyberg et al., 2020). Therefore, APPs need to encour-age patients to practice more health behaviors for improved health outcomes.

Economic Benefit of Preventing Chronic Diseases

The United States spends twice as much on health care compared to most of the top 10 industrialized countries, including Canada, Australia, New Zealand, and the United King-dom (Tikkanen & Abrams, 2020). In 2020, the overall cost of caring for individuals with chronic diseases in the United States reached $4.1 trillion, equivalent to $12,000 per per-son (Hartman et al., 2021). Although much of the increased cost of health care in 2020 can be attributed to the coronavirus pandemic (Hartman et al., 2021), healthcare costs had increased drastically over the five decades be-fore the pandemic, from 5% in 1960 to 18% in 2019 (Martin et al., 2020). Unfortunately, increased spending has not resulted in overall increased health outcomes. Some measures of a country's health, such as obesity, chronic dis-ease burden, avoidable deaths, suicide rates, and life expectancy, are worse in the United States than in the top 10 most industrialized countries (Tikkanen & Abrams, 2020).

In America, more dollars are used to pro-vide health care for the sick and those with risk factors for chronic diseases compared to interventions that promote prevention and wellness. Only 2.9% of U.S. healthcare

Table 1.1 Annual Chronic Disease Deaths Attributed to Lifestyle Behaviors

Lifestyle	Annual Deaths
Tobacco use, including secondhand smoke	7.2 million deaths
Unhealthy dietary patterns, such as excess sodium intake	4.1 million deaths
Alcohol use, particularly alcohol abuse	>3.3 million deaths
Physical inactivity	1.6 million deaths

Data from World Health Organization. (2021, April 21). *Noncommunicable diseases*. https://www.who.int/news-room/fact-sheets/detail/noncommunicable-diseases

spending advances health and prevention (Martin et al., 2020), whereas 27% of healthcare costs are attributed to five chronic disease risk factors: excess weight, elevated blood pressure, increased blood glucose levels, poor dietary habits, and tobacco use (Bolnick et al., 2020). Nevertheless, there is evidence that innovative health promotion and disease prevention programs can be cost-effective and result in decreased incidences of chronic diseases and reduced cost of health care overall (Edington et al., 2020). Furthermore, risk exposure tends to occur decades before the diagnosis of a condition. As adults age, there are increased incidences of chronic diseases and healthcare spending (Papanicolas et al., 2019). Therefore, Bolnick et al. (2020) indicated that health promotion policy to incentivize healthy lifestyle behaviors should target children and young adults to decrease the risk factors that may eventually lead to chronic diseases if left unchecked.

The benefits of cost-effective chronic disease prevention strategies are determined using various measures, such as cost per quality-adjusted life year (QALY). Public health interventions that cost less than $50,000 per QALY are generally considered cost-effective (NCCDPHP, 2022b). High blood pressure, which contributes to one of the greatest chronic disease expenses and is the leading risk factor for cardiovascular and cerebrovascular disease, provides an excellent example of the cost-effectiveness of health promotion. Individuals with high blood pressure usually require $2,500 more in medical expenses than those without high blood pressure, accounting for $29 billion in prescriptions. Fortunately, there are cost-effective programs for managing hypertension, such as team-based care and self-monitoring. Programs that include team-based care to improve high blood pressure have an average cost of $24,472 per QALY, which is 50% less than the threshold for a cost-effective program (Community Preventative Service Taskforce, 2021). Additionally, when patients are engaged in self-monitoring blood pressure in conjunction with other strategies, the average cost ranges from nearly $3,000 to $11,000 per QALY (Jacob et al., 2017). APPs can engage the interprofessional team and integrate these cost-effective strategies into practice to decrease the disease burden of hypertension on individuals and society.

Another measure of the cost-effectiveness of programs is the return on investment (ROI). Lifestyle wellness and health promotion programs have demonstrated a positive monetary return on investment and improved health outcomes (Edington et al., 2020). For instance, Johnson & Johnson reported that from 2002 to 2008, its employer wellness program yielded nearly $2.00 to $4.00 for every dollar invested (Henke et al., 2011, as cited in Edington et al., 2020). The Centers for Disease Control and Prevention (CDC) identified cost-effective programs for screening risk factors and early identification of several chronic diseases, including breast cancer, diabetes, and tobacco (NCCDPHP, 2023). When these issues are identified and treated early, healthcare costs are decreased, quality of life is improved, and longevity is increased. Most notably, evidence exists that lifestyle change programs, such as the CDC's low-cost National Diabetes Prevention Program, can decrease the risk of T2DM by more than half for those at high risk for T2DM (NCCDPHP, 2022b).

Paradigm Shift and Competencies of Lifestyle Management

The rise in preventable chronic diseases, related conditions, and healthcare costs has created a need for a paradigm shift in health care and health education to address the upstream causes of these diseases. Melnyk (2022) stated that "the time is now for shifting this sick-care paradigm to the absolutely essential wellness and prevention model" (p. 1). APPs are vital to this shift. The expanding lifestyle management field provides the foundational context for APPs to go beyond the traditional approach of "sick" care to "health" care to integrate health promotion interventions and disease prevention into primary care and beyond.

Many professional organizations and governmental agencies, including the American Heart Association, American Diabetes Association, American Cancer Society, and Office of Disease Prevention and Health Promotion, have emphasized lifestyle management principles and practices for preventing or treating health conditions. For instance, the American Cancer Society has developed dietary habits and physical activity guidelines for cancer prevention (Rock et al., 2020). Also, *Healthy People 2030* has identified national goals and objectives to improve Americans health across their life spans, which apply to health promotion, disease prevention, and lifestyle behaviors (Office of Disease Prevention and Health Promotion, n.d.). Examples of *Healthy People 2030* objectives are to increase the number of children, high school students, and adults who get adequate sleep and to reduce motor vehicle accidents due to driving when feeling tired. Providers are encouraged to use sleep health practice guidelines to provide patients with self-care and self-management strategies to treat chronic diseases, improve health outcomes, and decrease healthcare costs.

The paradigm shift also calls for a different approach to patient care, including targeted health promotion and disease prevention interventions (Houlden et al., 2018). According to the WHO (2021), an imperative way to manage chronic diseases is to reduce the risk factors attributed to these conditions using a comprehensive model. Lifestyle management is a comprehensive approach to addressing lifestyle-related chronic diseases.

Additionally, the increased interest in the lifestyle management of diseases is propelled by organizations that promote the education of health professionals, including physicians, nurses, and physician assistants, in lifestyle, health promotion, and disease prevention

principles. Among the many professional organizations is the ACLM, an interprofessional group of health professionals whose mission is to advance evidence-informed lifestyle approaches as a value-based strategy to transform, redefine, and sustain health and health care by treating, reversing, and preventing lifestyle-related chronic diseases (ACLM, n.d.). The ACLM, one of the leaders in lifestyle management, has developed core competencies in lifestyle management for healthcare providers and non-provider healthcare providers (Lianov et al., 2022). The ACLM lifestyle management competencies align with the nurse practitioner (NP) role core competencies (National Organization of Nurse Practitioner Faculties, 2022) and the physician assistant (PA) competencies (Cross-Org Competencies Review Taskforce, 2021). See **Table 1.2** for the mapping of lifestyle management core competencies with selected NP and PA competencies. The educational preparation of APPs provides opportunities for them to become competent in developing innovative lifestyle management principles and techniques in clinical practice.

Background and Role of Lifestyle in Practice

Although lifestyle management is a relatively new subspecialty for health professionals, its practice has existed for centuries (Bodai, 2017). Historical figures, such as Hippocrates (460–370 BC), known as the father of medicine, and Florence Nightingale (1820–1910), the founder of modern nursing, championed concepts of lifestyle management hundreds of years ago. Hippocrates stated, "If we could give every individual the right amount of nourishment and exercise, not too little and not too much, we would have found the safest way to health" (Katz et al., 2018, p. 1452). In 1854, Florence Nightingale addressed the high mortality rate of sick soldiers (Karimi & Alavi, 2015). Nightingale noted a 60% mortality rate from

Table 1.2 Mapping of Lifestyle Management Core Competencies with Selected NP Role Core Competencies and PA Competencies

Common Themes	Lifestyle Medicine Core Competencies[1]	NP Role Core Competencies[2]	PA Competencies[3]
Health promotion	Establish principles of screening, diagnosing, treating and monitoring lifestyle-related diseases and deliver lifestyle medicine-focused anticipatory guidance.	Deliver healthcare services within scope of practice, which includes health promotion, disease prevention, anticipatory guidance, counseling, and disease management.	Employ principles of epidemiology to determine health problems, risk factors, treatment strategies, and disease prevention/health promotion efforts for individuals and populations.
Knowledge and evidence	Determine the evidence that indicates health behaviors are related to key health outcomes.	Apply scientific evidence to improve health outcomes.	■ Apply clinical evidence to diagnose disease. ■ Improve the health of patient populations.
Counseling	Employ motivational interviewing and health coaching approaches.	Apply counseling techniques, such as motivational interviewing, to advance wellness and self-care management.	Counsel, inform, and empower patients and their families to take part in their care and facilitate shared decision-making.
Personal wellness	Create a culture of leadership by developing personal health behaviors.	Establish an environment that fosters self-care and well-being.	Exhibit a commitment to personal wellness and self-care that supports quality patient care.
Collaborative relationship with interprofessional team and stakeholders	Evaluate the evidence for collaborative and chronic care models on improved health behaviors.	Develop a collaborative approach with applicable stakeholders to inform population healthcare needs.	Collaborate with other health professionals to provide effective patient-centered care.

[1]Lianov, L., & Johnson, M. (2010). Physician competencies for prescribing lifestyle medicine. *Journal of the American Medical Association, 304*(2), 202–203. https://doi.org/10.1001/JAMA.2010.903
[2]National Organization of Nurse Practitioner Faculties. (2017). *Advanced practical registered nurse doctoral-level competencies.* https://cdn.ymaws.com/www.nonpf.org/resource/resmgr/competencies/competencies-common-aprn-doctoral-compete.pdf
[3]Cross-Org Competencies Review Taskforce. (2020). *Competencies for the physician assistant profession.* https://paeaonline.org/our-work/current-issues/competencies-for-the-pa-profession

communicable and infectious diseases. Interventions such as clean water and adding fruit to the diet drastically changed the soldiers' health outcomes, decreasing the mortality rates to 2.2%.

As a result of vaccination and antibiotics, communicable and infectious diseases are no longer the leading causes of death worldwide. Chronic diseases have become the leading cause of death globally despite substantial evidence that poor lifestyle behaviors are the root cause of the rise in chronic diseases and healthcare costs. Katz et al. (2018) described several landmark publications that provide historical context to support that modifiable lifestyle behavior was the foremost cause of mortality in the mid-20th century and continues to be so in the 21st century. A publication by McGinnis and Foege (1993) identified tobacco, alcohol, eating habits, and physical activity as the leading causes of death, accounting for 8 out of 10 deaths in the United States. Over a decade later, similar findings were identified by Mokdad et al. (2004), who determined that remarkable increases in mortality were related to tobacco use, physical inactivity, unhealthy dietary patterns, and alcohol consumption.

These findings were extended globally by researchers in Potsdam, Germany, and the United Kingdom. Ford et al. (2009) in Germany determined that 80% of chronic illnesses may be prevented by four factors: never smoking; not being obese; being physically active for more than 210 minutes per week; and eating a healthy diet of fruits, vegetables, whole grains, and low meat intake. In the United Kingdom, Kvaavik et al. (2010) identified four risk factors that decreased life span by 12 years: being active for less than two hours per week, consuming less than three fruits and vegetables per day for less than three days per week, tobacco use, and excessive alcohol consumption. Though the lifestyle behaviors in each study vary slightly, they describe similar behaviors and outcomes. These seminal studies support that health promotion, disease

prevention, and healthy lifestyle behaviors can decrease mortality associated with chronic diseases.

Lifestyle management can occur in a variety of populations and settings. It can be effective in helping individuals, families, and targeted groups in the community and clinical settings to identify and make health behavior changes to prevent chronic illnesses (Egger et al., 2017). The primary care setting is ideal for lifestyle management due to the opportunity for the APP to follow up with patients to monitor progress and health outcome metrics. It may also be implemented in the acute care setting when a patient may be in a state of readiness for behavior change due to an exacerbating chronic disease. Changing well-established behaviors requires patients to partner with their healthcare provider to develop person-centered strategies for sustainable lifestyle changes. The challenge is that this process takes time, knowledge of the science of lifestyle management by the healthcare provider, and patient buy-in.

Although patients are more likely to attempt weight loss and achieve clinically significant weight loss when counseled by a healthcare provider, many who need it do not receive counseling (Pool et al., 2014). According to Zoltick et al. (2021), "practitioners counsel obese patients on weight loss less than half the time" (p. 2). The analysis of data from the National Health and Nutrition Examination Surveys, 1999–2016, indicated that overweight individuals were significantly less likely to be notified of their weight status than those with obesity (Hansen et al., 2020). Furthermore, overweight males were 24% less likely to be informed than females, and Black persons were 19% less likely to be informed than White persons. Also, though nearly two-thirds of young adults aged 20 to 34 and 78% of adults aged 50 to 64 with obesity were notified of their weight status, only about one-fourth of young adults 20 to 34 who were overweight were informed of their weight status. These findings are concerning because addressing overweight status earlier in life may prevent obesity and its comorbidities in early to mid-adulthood. APPs need to communicate weight status and risk factors with patients at all age levels to avert progression to obesity and other chronic diseases.

Evidence shows that most individuals who need lifestyle counseling do not receive it. According to White et al. (2020), "only about 32% of patients receive physical activity counseling from their physician, 28% of smokers reported their provider offered assistance in cessation, and on average less than 1 minute of a patient encounter is spent talking about diet, exercise, or smoking" (p. 271). There are many reasons why providers may not address lifestyle behaviors and provide counseling, including time constraints, lack of knowledge, and insufficient reimbursement (Petrin et al., 2017; Zoltick et al., 2021). These obstacles can be overcome with appropriate training in billing, coding, and innovative practice models, including a value-based reimbursement model, group visits, shared medical appointments, and concierge memberships.

Like any field of concentration, a body of knowledge, skills, and attitudes is required to be competent in health-promoting lifestyle management practices. Therefore, effective lifestyle management also necessitates an adequately educated interprofessional team, including APPs, registered dietitians skilled in comprehensive nutrition counseling, and psychologists for advanced stress management strategies.

Evidence to Support Lifestyle Management

A plethora of scientific evidence exists to support that daily lifestyle behavior significantly impacts short- and long-term health outcomes positively or negatively (Rippe, 2018). The strength of the evidence is underscored by the volume of evidence-based practice

Health Promotion Research Study

Sugar Intake and Sleep Quality in University Students

Background: A study was conducted to investigate the relationship between added sugar intake and sleep quality among university students.

Methodology: One hundred female students (19–25 years old) were randomly selected from a Saudi Arabia university. Students completed the food frequency questionnaire, sleep quality questionnaire, and 24-hour dietary recall.

Results: The results indicated that 83% of participants had poor-quality sleep. There was a significant association between high consumption of added sugars and insufficient sleep quality.

Implications for Advanced Practice: Various factors impact university students' sleep quality, including technological devices, excessive exposure to artificial light, stress students face due to intensive coursework, and the perception that sleep is wasted time. Sleep deprivation is associated with impaired glucose metabolism and elevated blood sugar levels. APPs need to routinely assess sleep quality and provide guidance to individuals for improved sleep.

Reference: Data from Alahmary, S. A., Alduhaylib, S. A., Alkawii, H. A., Olwani, M. M., Shablan, R. A., Ayoub, H. M., Purayidathil, T. S., Abuzaid, O. I., & Khattab, R. Y. (2019). Relationship between added sugar intake and sleep quality among university students: A cross-sectional study. *American Journal of Lifestyle Medicine, 16*(1), 122–129. https://doi.org/10.1177/1559827619870476

guidelines, which include lifestyle behaviors as first-line strategies for the prevention and management of metabolically related conditions (Rippe, 2018). Additionally, there are many randomized controlled trials and various cohort studies that highlight the impact of health behaviors and disease outcomes, including the Nurses' Health Study (NHS) and the Health Professionals Follow-Up Study (HPFS) (Li et al., 2018). The NHS began in 1976 and has contributed extensively to the science of prevention over the past four decades (Colditz et al., 2016). The HPFS began in 1986 and consisted of a sample of men in the health professions as a counterpart to the women's-only NHS (Harvard T. H. Chan School of Public Health, n.d.). The NHS and the HPFS continue to collect data every two years to evaluate similar hypotheses about the relationship between lifestyle behaviors and incidences of illnesses, such as CVD, cancer, and other diseases.

These epidemiological findings are essential to determining disease causality (Colditz et al., 2016). Cohort studies provide a reliable explanation of the cause of illness with less bias than other cause-and-effect designs. **Table 1.3** highlights the NHS's findings

Table 1.3 Important Lifestyle-Related Disease Outcomes from the Nurses' Health Study and Associated Significant Findings

Lifestyle-Related Disease Outcome	Significant Findings
Related to dietary factors:	
T2DM	Increased intake of fruits, vegetables, whole grains, and legumes and decreased red meat, refined sugar, and sugar-sweetened beverages reduce the risk of T2DM.
CVD	Trans fats increase risk.
Breast cancer	Fruits, vegetables, whole grains, low-fat dairy, fish, and chicken lower the risk.
Pancreatic cancer	Fructose and sugar-sweetened soft drinks and low vitamin D increase the risk.
Non-Hodgkin's lymphoma	Trans fats and red meat increase risk.
Cognitive function	Antioxidants, higher nut intake, and Mediterranean diet increase cognitive function.
Related to physical activity:	
T2DM	Sedentary behavior increases risk, and moderate- to high-intensity physical activity decreases the risk of T2DM.
Cardiac disease	Moderate-intensity physical activity decreases cardiac disease risk.
Breast cancer	Moderate to vigorous physical activity >7 hours per week decreases the risk of breast cancer.
Cognitive function	Higher levels of physical activity increase cognitive performance.

Lifestyle-Related Disease Outcome	Significant Findings
Associated with obesity:	
T2DM	Excess weight is the most decisive risk factor for T2DM.
Cardiac disease	Moderate weight gain at age 18 and older increases the risk and mortality from cardiac disease.
Endometrial cancer	Excess weight contributes to 40% of endometrial cancer cases.
Pancreatic cancer	Overweight or inactive women have an increased risk for pancreatic cancer.
Eye disease	Obesity and elevated BMI increase the risk of cataracts.
Related to sleep and shift work:	
T2DM	Too long and too short sleep and decreased sleep quality increase the risk of T2DM.
Cardiac disease	Shift work and not sleeping the optimal 8 hours per day increase risk.

Data from Colditz, G. A., Philpott, S. E., & Hankinson, S. E. (2016). The impact of the Nurses' Health Study on population health: Prevention, translation, and control. *American Journal of Public Health, 106*(9), 1540–1545. https://doi.org/10.2105/AJPH.2016.303343

regarding the association between lifestyle behaviors and chronic diseases. Based on results from the NHS, 8 of 10 heart disease occurrences could be prevented by not smoking, eating a healthy diet, being moderately or vigorously active for a minimum of 30 minutes most days, and limiting alcohol intake to one or fewer drinks per day (Colditz et al., 2016). Additionally, the NHS confirmed increased breast cancer risk even with small amounts of alcohol consumption. Dietary intake was also associated with premenopausal breast cancer: Women who had more consumption of red meat and a lower intake of fiber and fruit as adolescents had higher incidences of breast cancer. Furthermore, the NHS confirmed that excess weight is the strongest predictor of T2DM. Overall, the NHS highlights that lifestyle behaviors can positively or negatively impact the development of chronic diseases such as heart disease, cancer, and T2DM in women.

In another study to analyze cohort data of the NHS (1980–2014) and the HPFS (1986–2014), researchers identified five lifestyle behaviors that could narrow the life-expectancy gap between Americans and individuals in other high-income countries (Li et al., 2018). The five lifestyle factors identified are similar to those previously identified: adhering to a healthy diet, routine physical activity, maintaining BMI within the normal range, moderate alcohol consumption (5 g to 15 g per day for women and 5 g to 30 g per day for men), and never smoking. Overall, those who adhered to the five healthy lifestyle behaviors had lower all-cause, cancer, and CVD mortality than those who did not adhere to the healthy lifestyle behaviors.

Despite the overwhelming evidence that lifestyle practices such as physical activity and healthy eating profoundly affect health outcomes and longevity, only a few Americans adhere to recommended physical activity and dietary guidelines. Seventy-five percent of Americans do not meet the minimum physical activity recommendations (U.S. Department of Health and Human Services, 2018). Also, only 10% of Americans meet the guidelines for vegetable consumption, and only 20% meet the fruit intake recommendations (U.S. Department of Health and Human Services and U.S. Department of Agriculture, 2020). This gap in behaviors related to the recommendations for physical activity and dietary patterns offers an opportunity for APPs to influence the health behaviors of more than 75% of Americans who see a primary care provider annually (Rippe, 2018). The time has come for APPs to integrate the principles of lifestyle management into the daily care of patients to improve health outcomes and decrease the burden of lifestyle-related chronic diseases on the cost of health care. See **Table 1.4** for a sample of guidelines that integrate lifestyle-related health promotion and disease prevention strategies.

Table 1.4 Sample of Guidelines That Integrate Health Promotion and Disease Prevention Strategies

Condition/ Behavior	Organization/ Authors	Guideline	URL
Cancer	American Cancer Society/Rock et al. (2020)	American Cancer Society Guideline for Diet and Physical Activity for Cancer Prevention	https://acsjournals .onlinelibrary.wiley.com/doi /full/10.3322/caac.21591
CVD	American College of Cardiology (ACC) and American Heart Association (AHA)	2019 ACC/AHA Guideline on the Primary Prevention of Cardiovascular Disease	https://doi.org/10.1161 /CIR.0000000000000678
Childhood obesity	American Academy of Pediatrics	Guidelines from the American Academy of Pediatrics for the Prevention and Treatment of Childhood Obesity	https://doi.org/10.1542 /peds.2007-2329C
Diabetes	American Diabetes Association	Standards of Care in Diabetes—2022	https://professional .diabetes.org/content-page /practice-guidelines -resources
Diet	U.S. Department of Health and Human Services and U.S. Department of Agriculture	Dietary Guidelines for Americans, 2020–2025	https://www .dietaryguidelines.gov /resources/2020-2025 -dietary-guidelines-online -materials
Hypertension	Jones et al. (2021)	Scientific Statement of Management of Stage 1 Hypertension, 2021	https://www.ahajournals .org/doi/10.1161 /HYP.0000000000000195
Hypertension	ACC/AHA Taskforce	2017 ACC/AHA/AAPA/ABC/ ACPM/AGS/APhA/ASH/ASPC/ NMA/PCNA Guideline for the Prevention, Detection, Evaluation, and Management of High Blood Pressure in Adults	https://www.ahajournals .org/doi/10.1161 /hyp.0000000000000065

Condition/ Behavior	Organization/ Authors	Guideline	URL
Obesity	Canadian Medical Association	Obesity in Adults: A Clinical Practice Guideline	https://www.cmaj.ca /content/192/31/E875
Obesity	ACC/AHA Task Force on Practice Guidelines and the Obesity Society	Guidelines (2013) for the Management of Overweight and Obesity in Adults	https://onlinelibrary.wiley .com/doi/10.1002/oby.20660
Physical activity	U.S. Department of Health and Human Services	Physical Activity Guidelines for Americans, Second Edition	https://health.gov/sites /default/files/2019-09 /Physical_Activity _Guidelines_2nd_edition.pdf

Health-Promoting Levels of Prevention

The levels of prevention are related to the natural progression of diseases. There are five stages of usual disease progression: underlying, susceptible, subclinical, clinical, and recovery/disability/death (Kisling & Das, 2022). The health promotion prevention levels related to the disease progression stages are primordial, primary, secondary, tertiary, and quaternary (**Table 1.5**). The combination of these approaches not only addresses the upstream etiology to stop the onset of disease by reducing risk factors but also the downstream adverse health outcomes.

Primordial prevention addresses underlying social and environmental risk factors that promote disease onset. In contrast, *primary* prevention interventions avoid the onset of illness or injury by modifying the risk factor, behavior, or environment before the disease occurs. *Secondary* preventive measures lead to early detection and treatment of disease, with the goal of disease reversal or risk factor mitigation to halt disease progression. *Tertiary* prevention aims to rehabilitate an individual with an illness or disability, prevent relapse, and improve quality of life (Kisling & Das, 2022).

Most recently, *quaternary* prevention was added to the scientific literature and is defined as "an action taken to protect individuals (person/patients) from medical interventions that are likely to cause more harm than good" (Kisling & Das, 2021, para. 6). In particular, quaternary prevention should be foremost in APPs' minds for all interventions they recommend to a patient. Health-promoting lifestyle management can be integrated at each level of prevention to enhance patient outcomes and decrease iatrogenic harm.

Lifestyle Vital Signs

Documenting lifestyle behaviors as *lifestyle vital signs* is essential to provide baseline data and monitor progress (Lenz, 2014). Lifestyle vital signs also guide the APP in engaging the patient to take steps to prevent or manage a specific chronic disease. Additionally, documentation of lifestyle vital signs can be useful for referring patients to an interprofessional team of healthcare providers to support healthy lifestyle behaviors.

Adequate documentation of lifestyle behaviors should extend beyond usually recorded tobacco, alcohol, and illicit drug use to include a more comprehensive overview of lifestyle behaviors to prevent or manage chronic diseases. Every patient record should include routinely assessed fundamental lifestyle vital signs, namely, dietary habits, perceived stress, physical activity, alcohol use, sleep habits, and tobacco use. These essential lifestyle vital signs

Table 1.5 Levels of Prevention and Examples

Level of Prevention	Definition	Example	Additional Evidence
Primordial	Prevention of risk factor development	▪ Preventing elevation of blood pressure in normotensive patients ▪ Prenatal education of mothers ▪ Obesity prevention in childhood	Falkner and Lurbe (2020); Lloyd-Jones et al. (2021)
Primary	Prevention of disease or injury before it occurs	▪ Vaccinations ▪ Altering risky behaviors such as poor nutritional intake, tobacco use, and sedentary behaviors	Cho et al. (2020)
Secondary	Preventive measures aimed at early diagnosis and treatment of a condition to prevent more advanced issues from developing and to strive for disease reversal	▪ Blood pressure screening for elevated blood pressure ▪ Screening mammograms for breast cancer detection	Lloyd-Jones et al. (2021)
Tertiary	Preventive measures aimed at rehabilitation of individuals after a significant illness	Cardiac rehabilitation in patients after myocardial infarction or coronary artery bypass	Lloyd-Jones et al. (2021)
Quaternary	Preventive measures to avoid harm secondary to medical interventions	Prevention of adverse outcomes from medical interventions throughout the life span and at each level of prevention	Martins et al. (2018)

Data from Kisling, L. A., & Das, J. M. (2022, May 8). Prevention strategies. *StatPearls*. https://www.ncbi.nlm.nih.gov/books/NBK537222

can be summarized by the acronym A-SMART (adopt healthy eating, stress less, move often, avoid alcohol, rest more, treat tobacco use). Additional lifestyle vital signs may include BMI, waist circumference, and waist-to-hip ratio as objective measures to determine the risk of metabolic disorders or to monitor progress in specific circumstances.

The A-SMART lifestyle vital signs correspond with the lifestyle behavior management strategies or prescriptions represented by the A-SMART lifestyle behaviors model (Downes et al., 2021). The A-SMART model was developed as an evidence-informed approach to assess essential lifestyle behaviors and guide lifestyle counseling to promote overall health and well-being (**Figure 1.1**).

Houlden et al. (2018) outlined a series of questions and strategies for obtaining a lifestyle history. These and other sources were used to inform screening questions for assessing the A-SMART lifestyle vital signs. **Figure 1.2** provides an assessment tool with sample screening questions the APP or a healthcare team member can ask to evaluate essential A-SMART lifestyle vital signs. Scores are assigned to each of the A-SMART vital signs, which can be summed for an overall score. Although the A-SMART vital signs are not yet a validated instrument, the overall score will allow for a quick assessment of the patient's lifestyle habits and monitoring progress. When patients are asked questions about their lifestyle, it conveys that the APP places

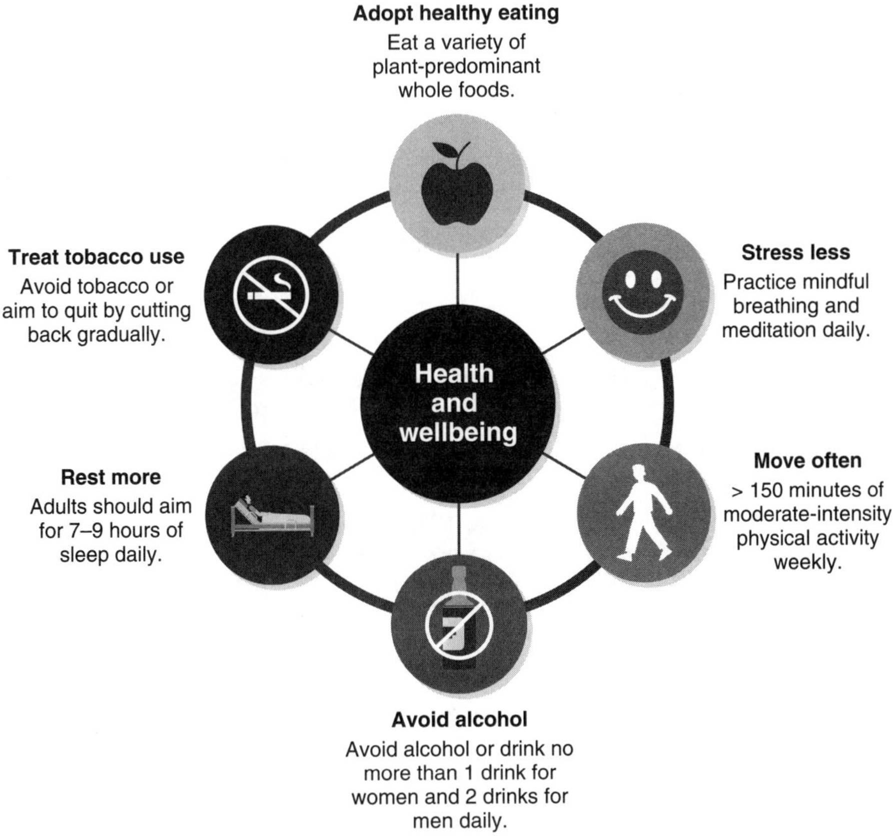

Adopt healthy eating
Eat a variety of
plant-predominant
whole foods.

Stress less
Practice mindful
breathing and
meditation daily.

Treat tobacco use
Avoid tobacco or
aim to quit by cutting
back gradually.

Health
and
wellbeing

Move often
> 150 minutes of
moderate-intensity
physical activity
weekly.

Rest more
Adults should aim
for 7–9 hours of
sleep daily.

Avoid alcohol
Avoid alcohol or drink no
more than 1 drink for
women and 2 drinks for
men daily.

Figure 1.1 A-SMART lifestyle behaviors model.

Slightly adapted from Downes, L., St. Hill, H., & Mays, T. (2021). A-SMART lifestyle behaviors model for health, wellbeing, and immune system enhancement. *The Nurse Practitioner, 46*(9), 31–39. https://doi.org/10.1097/01.NPR.0000769748.45938.10

Lifestyle Vital Sign	Screening Questions	Score

Adopt healthy eating	1. How many days per week do you eat ⩾5 fruits and vegetables?1
	   Score responses: 6–7 days (0 points), 4–5 days (1 point), 2–3 days (2 points), 0–1 day (3 points).
	
	2. How many days per week do you consume sugary foods/drinks?1
	   Score responses: 0–1 day (0 points), 2–3 days (1 point), 4–5 days (2 points), 6–7 days (3 points).
	
	Sum scores for questions 1 and 2. A score of ≥3 indicates a need for further screening, counseling, or referral.	

Figure 1.2 A-SMART lifestyle vital signs assessment.

(continues)

Lifestyle Vital Sign	Screening Questions	Score
Stress less	3. In the past month, how often have you felt your stress level was not manageable?[2] Score responses: Never (0 points), Almost never (1 point), Sometimes (2 points), Fairly often (3 points), Very often (4 points) 4. Do you feel that you have personal support?[2] Score responses: Yes (0 points), No (1 point). *Sum scores for questions 3 and 4. A score of ≥3 indicates a need for further screening, counseling, or referral.*	
Move more	5. On average, how many days a week do you engage in moderate to vigorous physical activity, such as walking?[3] 6. On average, how many minutes do you engage in physical activity at this level?[3] *Multiply responses for questions 6 and 7 for total minutes per week. Score responses: ≥150 minutes of moderate activity or 75 minutes of vigorous activity (0 points), <150 minutes of moderate activity or 75 minutes of vigorous activity (1 point). A score of 1 indicates a need for further screening, counseling, or referral.*	
Avoid alcohol	7. On any single occasion during the past three months, have you had more than five drinks containing alcohol?[4] Score responses: No (0 points), Yes (1 point). *A score of 1 indicates a need for further screening, counseling, or referral.*	
Rest more	8. How many hours do you sleep on a typical night?[2] Score responses: 7–9 hours (0 points), <7 hours or >9 hours (1 point). *A score of 1 indicates a need for further screening, counseling, or referral.*	
Treat tobacco use	9. Do you currently vape or use any form of tobacco? Score responses: No (0 points), Yes (1 point). *A score of 1 indicates a need for further screening, counseling, or referral if ready to quit.*	
TOTAL Score	Sum scores in gray boxes. *Total scores of ≥10 points indicate an overall unhealthy lifestyle vital signs score, with one or more areas needing further screening, counseling, or referral.*	

Figure 1.2 (*continued*)

[1]Powell, H. S., & Greenberg, D. L. (2019, January). Screening for unhealthy diet and exercise habits: The electronic health record and a healthier population. *Preventive Medicine Reports, 14*, 100816. https://doi.org/10.1016/j.pmedr.2019.01.020

[2]Houlden, R. L., Yen, H. H., & Mirrahimi, A. (2018). The lifestyle history: A neglected but essential component of the medical history. *American Journal of Lifestyle Medicine, 12*(5), 404–411. https://doi.org/10.1177/1559827617703045

[3]Exercise is Medicine. (2021). *Physical activity vital sign*. American College of Sports Medicine. www.exerciseismedicine.org/support_page.php/health-care -providers

[4]Taj, N., Devera-Sales, A., & Vinson, D. C. (1998). Screening for problem drinking: Does a single question work? *Journal of Family Practice, 46*(4), 328–335.

[5]Chaput, J. P., Dutil, C., & Sampasa-Kanyinga, H. (2018). Sleeping hours: What is the ideal number and how does age impact this? *Nature and Science of Sleep, 10*, 421–430. https://doi.org/10.2147/NSS.S163071

© Loureen Downes & Lilly Tryon, 2022

importance on personal behavior choices and the role of lifestyle management in decreasing-chronic diseases (Houlden et al., 2018). Ideally, procedures in the clinical setting should include documenting the lifestyle vital signs in the patient medical record at each encounter, similar to other vital signs. The APP should also review the lifestyle vital signs metrics at each encounter for changes to provide relevant lifestyle prevention and management strategies to mitigate risk factors for chronic diseases.

Data from patients with obesity indicate that patients want to discuss lifestyle behaviors with their healthcare provider and are more likely to be successful with behavior change if their healthcare provider offers counseling (Caterson et al., 2019). However, it is essential that the APP use effective strategies to start the conversation, such as seeking permission from the patient to discuss a particular lifestyle behavior. For example, if patients' score for *adopt healthy eating* is greater than three, poor eating habits are indicated. The APP may inform the patients that eating certain foods can lower their risk of heart disease, T2DM, and cancer and then ask the patients, "Would you mind if we discussed ways that you can lower your risk of heart disease?" If the patients do not give permission, the APP should not discuss it at that encounter but should let them know that he or she is available to discuss it at another time if they change their mind. It is essential that conversations about lifestyle occur in a nonjudgmental manner and that patients feel that they are partners with the APP in decisions about their care.

Prescribing Lifestyle Behaviors and Deprescribing Medications

Nearly every evidence-based clinical guideline incorporates lifestyle behaviors as the first-line intervention for chronic diseases such as CVD, hypertension, T2DM, and cancer (Rippe, 2018). However, clinicians are more likely to prescribe a medication with potential side effects than to offer a lifestyle behavior prescription. Medications prescribed for conditions without addressing the lifestyle root causes will have only a Band-Aid effect and may increase the risk of progression of a disease. APPs who collaborate with patients to develop person-centered lifestyle changes as first-line treatment options may avoid adverse medication effects, complications from polypharmacy, disease progression, and unnecessary procedures.

Martinez-Gomez et al. (2018) determined that prescribing healthy lifestyle behaviors and deprescribing medications decrease deaths from all causes and CVD. The study defined polypharmacy as medical management with more than five medications. Six healthy lifestyle behaviors were assessed: not smoking (never or quit >15 years), adopting a nutritious diet, being moderately or very active, being sedentary for seven hours or less per day, and sleep duration of seven to eight hours per day. Those who practiced five to six of the identified healthy lifestyle behaviors were determined to have a healthy lifestyle. Based on this study, it was discovered that even among those with polypharmacy, if they adhered to a healthy lifestyle, they had a 54% less chance of dying from all causes and a 60% less chance of dying from CVD than those who did not practice a healthy lifestyle. This study provides sufficient evidence to support the value of prescribing healthy lifestyle behaviors to decrease mortality.

Deprescribing is the process of decreasing or discontinuing medicines under the guidance of a healthcare provider. Martinez-Gomez et al. (2018) evaluated the effect of replacing medicines with lifestyle behaviors or deprescribing medications while prescribing lifestyle behavior, compared to only deprescribing. The results indicated that replacing medications with lifestyle behaviors was two- to threefold more effective in reducing all causes of mortality than only deprescribing. Further, the number of medications an individual took directly affected death from all causes and CVD. Those who took five or more medicines were twice as likely to die from all causes of CVD than those who took one or no pills. Therefore, APPs should review medications for appropriateness to determine whether deprescribing is warranted. Indeed, a "healthy lifestyle is 'medicine' and may replace medications" (Martinez-Gomez et al., 2018, Discussion section, para. 4). However, the APP should use a person-centered approach to evaluate the risk versus benefits of deprescribing.

There is evidence that those who are on medications who also practice healthy lifestyle behaviors can have substantially decreased incidences of death. Individuals who practiced three or four of the six healthy lifestyle behaviors even while taking two to four medications significantly decreased mortality (Martinez-Gomez et al., 2018). In fact, individuals taking two to four medications and practicing a healthy lifestyle had a 55% lower risk of all-cause mortality and a 53% decreased risk of CVD mortality compared to those with an unhealthy lifestyle. Even those who took one or no medications and practiced unhealthy lifestyles had increased mortality compared to those taking two to four

medicines and practicing a healthy lifestyle. Hence, despite the number of medications a patient takes, practicing healthy lifestyle behaviors is paramount to increasing longevity and decreasing death from all causes, including heart disease, the leading cause of death. Whenever possible, APPs should consider replacing medications with healthy lifestyle prescriptions to reduce the ill effects of polypharmacy and optimize health benefits.

While lifestyle behavior counseling is underutilized, it has been shown that this "advice is more effective in changing behavior when complemented by a written prescription for a lifestyle change" (White et al., 2020, p. 271). The American College of Sports Medicine's (2021) core exercise prescription format, which includes the frequency, intensity, time, and type (FITT) of activity, can be adapted for all lifestyle behaviors. Using the FITT format or the SMART-EST (specific, measurable, attainable, relevant, time-bound, evidence-based, strategic, tailored) format will provide patients with clear, achievable, and quantifiable directions (White et al., 2020). Lifestyle prescriptions are provided in **Table 1.6** as exemplars of the FITT types of prescriptions relevant to the A-SMART behaviors to promote health and well-being.

Table 1.6 Exemplars of A-SMART Lifestyle Behavior Prescriptions

Lifestyle Behavior	Lifestyle Prescription Using FITT
Adopt healthy eating	Example of a FITT prescription to increase vegetable consumption: F: Every day I: Three servings (1/2 cup = 1 serving) T: During lunch and dinner T: Eat a variety of colored vegetables (e.g., spinach, broccoli, cauliflower, carrots, cucumber)
	Example of a FITT prescription for substituting a low-fiber breakfast with a high-fiber breakfast: F: Every day I: Increase fiber to at least 10 g T: During breakfast meal T: Eat a serving of high-fiber breakfast cereal (e.g., oatmeal) with one small apple or 1/2 cup berries and 1/4 cup almonds

Lifestyle Behavior	Lifestyle Prescription Using FITT
Stress less	Example of a FITT prescription for mindful breathing: F: Twice daily I: Focus on breathing deeply T: In the morning before getting out of bed and in the evening before going to sleep T: Inhale deeply through the nose for 4 seconds while expanding the abdomen, hold breath for 7 seconds, then exhale through the mouth for 8 seconds. Repeat 3 times.
Move often	Example of a FITT prescription for low-intensity physical activity: F: Four days a week I: Low intensity, during which you can talk comfortably in full sentences with little to no pause for a breath T: Twenty minutes (may divide into 5- to 10-minute sessions) T: Walk at a leisurely pace before and after work. Example of a FITT prescription for moderate-intensity physical activity: F: Five days a week I: Moderate intensity during which you can talk in short sentences with pauses for a breath T: Thirty minutes each day after dinner T: Walk at a brisk pace
Avoid alcohol	Example of a FITT prescription for a male drinker to limit alcohol: F: Seven days per week I: Limit alcoholic beverages to two or fewer drinks T: Daily T: None recommended. (One drink contains 14 g of pure alcohol. Examples include 12 oz. of regular beer, 5 oz. of wine, or 1.5 oz. of distilled spirits.)
Rest more	Example of a FITT prescription for a shift worker who sleeps during the day: F: Once every 24 hours I: Deep restorative sleep T: 7–8 hours between 8:00 a.m. and 4:00 p.m. T: Daytime sleep, using a light-blocking window covering or an eye mask to block light
Treat tobacco use	Example of a FITT prescription to gradually decrease tobacco use for cessation for a one-pack-per-day smoker: F: Weekly I: Gradual decrease T: Each morning, count out the daily allotment of cigarettes T: Decrease daily tobacco use by 2 cigarettes each week (e.g., 18 cigarettes per day for 1 week, then 16 cigarettes per day for 1 week, and so forth until smoke-free)

Data from Frates, B., Bonnet, J. P., Joseph, R., & Peterson, J. A. (2019). *Lifestyle medicine handbook: An introduction to the powers of healthy habits.* Healthy Living.

Equally important, each lifestyle prescription must fit the patient's unique needs to improve success. Even though the foundational evidence upon which lifestyle management prescriptions are developed is universal, the application of the evidence is exclusive to the patient. Lifestyle management is not a one-size-fits-all prescription. It considers the patient's behavioral, environmental, and social determinants of health and desires (White et al., 2020). Integral to an effective lifestyle prescription is the "sacred bond" between the patient and the provider as they collaborate to attain disease remission and improve health outcomes (Dysinger, 2021, p. 556).

Though examples of lifestyle prescriptions are provided for each A-SMART behavior in Table 1.6, it's important to note that just as medications are prescribed by starting low and going slow, the same principle applies to lifestyle prescriptions. As stated previously, lifestyle behaviors have an additive effect, and the more behaviors practiced, the better the overall health outcome will be. However, when several lifestyle behaviors need to be changed, the lifestyle prescriptions should be introduced gradually to promote adherence and a successful outcome. If patients are required to change several behaviors at once, they may become overwhelmed and discouraged and not adhere to long-term behavior change.

Lifestyle prescriptions can be written and handed to the patient at the conclusion of the encounter and "filled" at home as the patient implements the personalized lifestyle strategies discussed during the visit. Many electronic medical records have customizable prescription templates that can be printed or electronically sent to patients and easily referenced during future encounters (Dysinger, 2021). Lifestyle prescriptions serve as reminders of lifestyle counseling delivered during the visit and may enhance adherence to the behaviors described as first-line treatment in clinical practice guidelines for the prevention and management of metabolically related conditions. Ultimately, the use of lifestyle prescriptions can improve health outcomes, decrease the use of medication, and lower the cost of health care.

Strategies to Enhance Adherence to Lifestyle Management

The success of lifestyle management in preventing and managing chronic diseases will depend on developing an evidence-informed person-centered management plan. Lifestyle vital signs and prescriptions are fundamental components of a lifestyle management approach. There are many behavior change strategies that APPs may utilize when prescribing lifestyle management, such as addressing motivators, barriers, and self-monitoring (Hooker et al., 2018). Too often, healthcare providers give patients behavior change instructions, only to later find out the patient has not followed through. APPs can overcome this phenomenon by proactively assessing facilitators and barriers to lifestyle behaviors and collaboratively developing solutions when prescribing A-SMART lifestyle behaviors by asking patients, "What could get in the way of doing this behavior?" or "What challenges do you anticipate in carrying out this lifestyle prescription?"

Another person-centered approach to individualizing prescriptions and promoting adherence is the Frates MOSS Method™, which stands for motivation, obstacles, strategies, and strengths (Frates et al., 2019). An individual's motivation can be determined by asking open-ended questions, such as "What makes you want to start a particular behavior now?" "What is motivating you to start the behavior?" and "What benefits do you expect to achieve by doing a behavior?" Since obstacles change periodically and may be related to an individual's stage of life, an obstacle for one person could be a motivator for another, underscoring the importance of using a person-centered approach to assess obstacles. For example, caring for children may be an obstacle to one mother's physical activity goals, whereas another mother may find that her children motivate her to be physically active so that she can "be in good shape" to take care of them. Others may not prioritize time for physical activity, focusing all their energy on their children. A key obstacle is not having a distinct motivator for undertaking a particular behavior (Frates et al., 2019).

Strategies are patient-specific tactics developed to overcome obstacles. Examples of strategies that the APP may suggest are the need for social support (e.g., walking groups) and self-monitoring (e.g., using a smartphone app or journal). Strengths are essential to discuss with patients who have previously tried a particular behavior change without success and who may lack confidence. The APP can help patients identify strengths in other areas of their life that may be applied to the desired behavior change. The MOSS Method™ is one of many techniques for determining facilitators and barriers to lifestyle change. In brief, APPs need to evaluate factors that may impact a person's practice of lifestyle behaviors to determine successful person-centered behavior change strategies (Lenz, 2014).

Application of the A-SMART Vital Signs and Prescriptions

The following scenario describes a conventional patient encounter and provides an analysis of opportunities to apply the A-SMART lifestyle vital signs and prescriptions.

Subjective data: M.C. is a 35-year-old cisgender female who comes into the primary care office for the first time with a complaint of fatigue over the past six months. She has no allergies and currently does not take any medications. Her medical history is unremarkable except that both her parents have T2DM. She is single, lives alone, and works the night shift as a store clerk. See the A-SMART lifestyle vital signs relevant to M.C. in **Table 1.7**.

Objective data: M.C.'s vital signs are within normal limits, except her blood pressure is 142/80 mmHg, and her BMI is 31 kg/m². The physical exam is unremarkable.

Assessment: R53.83 Fatigue, other; R03.0 Elevated blood-pressure reading, without diagnosis of hypertension; E66.9 Obesity, unspecified; Z68.31 Body mass index 30–39, adult.

Plan: The APP orders thyroid-stimulating hormone, complete blood count, complete metabolic panel, and hemoglobin A1C. A-SMART vital sign findings are reviewed, and risk factors of obesity, smoking, and sedentary behaviors are discussed. The APP explores which lifestyle behavior the patient is ready to change. The APP and the patient agree to work on increasing sleep hours. Sleep hygiene strategies are provided. Using the MOSS™ approach, the APP identifies motivators, obstacles, strategies, and strengths to improve her sleep. The patient was given a lifestyle prescription to rest more (Table 1.6) and asked to self-monitor by keeping a sleep diary. M.C. was referred to a registered dietitian. A return visit is scheduled in two weeks to review labs, recheck blood pressure, and evaluate sleep progress.

In M.C.'s case, findings from the A-SMART lifestyle vital signs assessment reveal several behaviors that need to be optimized for improved health. This assessment can guide the astute APP to provide additional screening and offer lifestyle counseling. Further discussion

Table 1.7 M.C. Case Study A-SMART Lifestyle Vital Signs Assessment

Lifestyle Vital Sign	Screening Questions	Patient Responses	Score
Adopt healthy eating	1. How many days per week do you eat ≥5 fruits and vegetables? Score responses: 6–7 days (0 points), 4–5 days (1 point), 2–3 days (2 points), 0–1 days (3 points)	"I don't like vegetables, but I eat a banana every day."	3
	2. How many days per week do you consume sugary foods/drinks? Score responses: 0–1 days (0 points), 2–3 days (1 point), 4–5 days (2 points), 6–7 days (3 points)	"I usually have a soda once per day with dinner."	3
	Sum scores for questions 1 and 2.	*A score of ≥3 indicates a need for further screening, counseling, or referral.*	6
	A follow-up dietary screening question is asked: "What do you eat and drink for breakfast, lunch, and dinner, including snacks?"	"I do not eat breakfast except for two cups of coffee; for lunch, I have a burger and fries; for dinner, I have rice, steak, and soda. I don't snack."	
Stress less	3. In the past month, how often have you felt your stress level was not manageable? Score responses: Never (0 points), Almost never (1 point), Sometimes (2 points), Fairly often (3 points), Very often (4 points)	"Almost every day at work, I feel my stress is not manageable."	4
	4. Do you feel that you have personal support? Score responses: Yes (0 points), No (1 point)	"Yes, my faith community provides support."	0
	Sum scores for questions 3 and 4.	*A score of ≥3 indicates a need for further screening, counseling, or referral.*	4
Move often	5. On average, how many days a week do you engage in moderate to vigorous physical activity, such as walking?	"I don't have time to be physically active except at work."	0
	6. On average, how many minutes do you engage in physical activity at this level?		0

Lifestyle Vital Sign	Screening Questions	Patient Responses	Score
	Multiply responses for questions 5 and 6 for total minutes per week. Score responses: ≥150 minutes of moderate activity or 75 minutes of vigorous activity (0 points), <150 minutes of moderate activity or 75 minutes of vigorous activity (1 point).	*Total of 0 minutes per week, which is <150 minutes of moderate activity or 75 minutes of vigorous activity (1 point). A score of 1 indicates a need for further screening, counseling, or referral.*	1
Avoid alcohol	7. On any single occasion during the past three months, have you had more than five drinks containing alcohol? Score responses: No (0 points), Yes (1 point)	"No."	0
Rest more	8. How many hours do you sleep on a typical night? Score responses: 7–9 hours (0 points), <7 hours or >9 hours (1 point)	"I sleep four to five hours." *A score of 1 indicates a need for further screening, counseling, or referral.*	1
Treat tobacco use	9. "Do you currently vape or use any form of tobacco?" Score responses: No (0 points), Yes (1 point)	"Yes, I smoke a pack per day." *A score of 1 indicates a need for further screening, counseling, or referral if ready to quit.*	1
	A follow-up tobacco use screening question is asked: "How long have you been smoking?"	"Fifteen years." *(Note: Fifteen pack-year history of smoking)*	
TOTAL score	Sum scores in gray boxes.	*A score of 13 indicates an overall unhealthy vital signs score with one or more areas needing further screening, counseling, or referral.*	13

with the patient will determine areas in which referrals to other healthcare professionals, such as a dietitian, an exercise specialist, or a mental health professional, might be appropriate. The APP can help the patient prioritize and identify person-centered and evidence-informed lifestyle strategies to improve health outcomes, keeping in mind that behavior changes should be introduced gradually and when the patient is ready. Also, when counseling a patient to make lifestyle changes, it is essential to address personal health goals and identify barriers and facilitators to behavior change.

An APP using a lifestyle lens would also consider the reciprocal nature of the patient's health behaviors and risk factors. For example, poor sleep and other unhealthy lifestyle behaviors contribute to obesity and elevated blood pressure while obesity, in turn, influences sleep and hypertension. Furthermore, health and lifestyle are not linear processes but are interconnected and complex (Egger et al., 2017). An example of linear thinking is "if energy out (basal metabolic rate and calories burned in physical activity) is greater than energy in (calories consumed), it will result

---

Health Promotion Case Study Addressing Lifestyle in an Older Adult Female

Case Description: C.G. is a 67-year-old female diagnosed with heart failure who presented to the primary care clinic for follow-up post-hospitalization one week ago. She reports having shortness of breath after climbing three flights of stairs and swelling in her lower legs. She has a history of T2DM and hypertension. She has lived alone, a widow for 10 years, and can care for herself. She was discharged with insulin, a diuretic, and an antihypertensive.

Vital Signs: Blood pressure 144/90 mmHg left arm, heart rate 90 beats per minute, respiratory rate 20 breaths per minute, temperature 97.9° F.

Physical Exam: The physical exam reveals a well-developed, well-nourished female who appears depressed. She is well kept and appropriately dressed. The exam is unremarkable except for bibasilar crackles and pitting edema in bilateral lower extremities.

Critical Thinking Questions

- What additional subjective data related to lifestyle behaviors do you want to obtain and why?
- What additional lifestyle objective data do you want to assess and why?
- Are there any lifestyle vital signs you would like to obtain and why?
- What lifestyle management strategies would you consider to optimize C.G.'s health outcomes?
- List an intervention for each of the five levels of prevention.
- Write a lifestyle prescription.
- Find research evidence to support lifestyle management of heart failure.

Additional Reading: Razavi, A. C., Monlezun, D. J., Sapin, A., Sarris, L., Schlag, E., Dyer, A., & Harlan, T. (2019). Etiological role of diet in 30-day readmissions for heart failure: Implications for reducing heart failure-associated cost via culinary medicine. *American Journal of Lifestyle Medicine*, *14*(4), 351–360. https://doi.org/10.1177/1559827619861933

---

in weight loss." On the other hand, a systems approach considers the multiple factors that influence health and their interrelatedness (Egger et al., 2017). As in M.C.'s case, inadequate sleep impacts the release of cortisol and other hormones that affect satiety and hunger. Poor sleep can lead to fatigue, fatigue to inactivity, and inactivity to poor eating habits, all of which could subsequently lead to depression, obesity, heart disease, and T2DM. Additionally, poor eating habits, sedentary habits, and substance use can lead to accidents, insomnia, or illnesses that exacerbate the disease cycle. Medications that help control blood pressure, depression, or other health problems may have side effects that lead to weight

gain or other complications. All of these—risk factors, etiology, the condition, and the management—are included in lifestyle management (Egger et al., 2017).

M.C.'s case is a complex interplay of lifestyle, biological, and environmental factors. Without lifestyle management and person-centered behavior change strategies, the outcome will be less than ideal. The takeaway from this case is that biological processes are complex and each behavior contributes to a feedback loop. Even if medications are required, lifestyle management can enhance positive outcomes, reduce the use of drugs, and decrease potential side effects such as weight gain.

Lifestyle Management and Conventional Medicine

Lifestyle management focuses on mitigating the unhealthy lifestyle choices that contribute to disease, whereas conventional medicine treats symptoms and disease (Egger et al., 2017). Hence, in lifestyle management, the patient is actively involved in, rather than passively receiving, care. According to the ACLM (n.d.), lifestyle management should not be viewed as different from conventional medicine but rather as the foundation of conventional practice. Even so, Egger and colleagues' (2017) description of the fundamental differences between lifestyle and conventional management outlined in **Table 1.8** can enlighten the APP.

Lifestyle management does not indicate using only a nonmedical clinical approach. Patient outcomes are enhanced when lifestyle management strategies integrate interventions with conventional medical practices to manage illnesses when warranted. Healthy lifestyle behaviors are integral to optimal chronic disease management and health outcomes. For example, the treatment for uncontrolled

Table 1.8 Differences Between Lifestyle and Conventional Management of Disease

Lifestyle Management	Conventional Management
Treats lifestyle behavior/environmental causes.	Treats individual risk factors.
Patient is engaged as a partner in care and required to make significant lifestyle behavior changes.	Patient is less likely to be engaged in care and is not required to make significant lifestyle behavior changes.
Treatment is often long term.	Treatment is usually short term.
Accountability is also on individuals as partners in their care.	Accountability is on the clinician only.
Emphasis is on amending health behavior/ environment, and medication is secondary.	Medication is usually the endpoint of care.
Emphasis is on motivation and agreement.	Emphasis is on diagnosis and prescription.
Focus is on primordial, primary, secondary, and tertiary prevention.	Objective is disease management.
Much consideration of the environment.	Less consideration of the environment.

Data from Egger, G., Binns, A., Rossner, S., & Sagner, M. (2017). *Lifestyle medicine: Lifestyle, the environment, and preventive medicine in health and disease* (3rd ed.). Elsevier.

Health Promotion Activity: Review the Nurses' Health Study in the Context of Lifestyle

Review the findings of the 40-year-long longitudinal Nurses' Health Study (NHS) at https://nurseshealthstudy.org. Describe the NHS results that pertain to the association of lifestyle behaviors and environmental factors and their relationship to various chronic diseases.

hypertension may include lifestyle behaviors such as increased physical activity, decreased sodium intake, and antihypertensive medications. The evidence-informed practice involves using lifestyle management to consider ecological determinants of disease and modify behavior while using conventional management to adjust medications.

Summary

Globally, lifestyle-related chronic diseases pose a significant burden on society. In the United States, CVD, cancers, and T2DM are the leading causes of morbidity and mortality. The primary risk factors for these common disorders are poor lifestyle behaviors, including unhealthy eating patterns, chronic stress, inactivity, alcohol consumption, lack of adequate sleep, tobacco use, and social determinants of health. These risk factors increase the cost of health care, with the United States spending more on health care than most industrialized countries but with lower longevity and worse healthcare outcomes. The good news is that most lifestyle-related chronic diseases can be prevented by integrating the six strategies of the A-SMART model into daily practice. In fact, 80% of lifestyle-related chronic conditions would not exist if individuals would eat a healthy dietary pattern of predominately plant sources, achieve a BMI within the normal range, be physically active, and not smoke. Also, lifestyle behavior interventions tend to be cost effective compared to conventional treatment strategies.

Further, even when individuals have a genetic predisposition or already have a chronic illness, if they practice healthy behaviors, their health outcomes and longevity may increase compared to those who do not practice healthy behaviors. Epigenetic changes are reversible with positive lifestyle behavior changes. It is well known that healthy lifestyle behaviors can decrease incidences of chronic diseases, reverse disease progression, and promote longevity.

Although most Americans do not practice recommended dietary and physical activity habits for optimum health outcomes, only a few receive advice on these and other lifestyle behaviors from a health professional. Still, there is evidence that those who receive lifestyle counseling are more likely to make lifestyle change. Providers face many barriers to implementing lifestyle behaviors in practice. However, with adequate training in the core competencies of lifestyle medicine and the relevant advanced practice registered nurse (APRN) and PA health promotion and disease prevention competencies, APPs will be better prepared to provide lifestyle management in practice. APPs owe it to their patients to provide the lifestyle counseling they need. APPs must seek to overcome barriers to integrating lifestyle management into their practice by participating in educational opportunities, seeking out effective ways of coding and billing, and relying on the interprofessional team by referring patients to other healthcare team members when warranted. **Table 1.9** list a sample of evidence-based resources to enhance and support lifestyle management assessment and application.

APPs who use effective lifestyle management strategies can promote healthy behaviors that decrease incidences of the leading causes of illness, disability, and death in the United States. These tactics require that APPs assess and evaluate lifestyle vital signs and develop person-centered prescriptions considering personal, environmental, and social barriers. APPs must collaborate with patients to create distinctive health behavior strategies and include written instructions using a lifestyle prescription model that provides clear, measurable, and attainable action steps. The overarching goal of lifestyle management is to promote health, decrease incidences of preventable chronic diseases, and decrease the economic burden of chronic diseases on society by integrating evidence-informed lifestyle as medicine in mainstream practice.

TABLE 1.9	Evidence-Based Resources for Health Promotion, Disease Prevention, and Lifestyle Concepts

Resource	URL
American College of Lifestyle Medicine	https://www.lifestylemedicine.org
American Institute for Cancer Research	https://www.aicr.org/cancer-prevention
Dietary Guidelines for Americans	https://www.dietaryguidelines.gov
Epigenetics	https://learn.genetics.utah.edu/content/epigenetics
Healthy People 2030	https://health.gov/healthypeople
Tracking Network for Lifestyle Risk Factor Data	https://www.cdc.gov/nceh/tracking/topics/LifestyleRiskFactors.htm
Physical Activity Guidelines	https://health.gov/our-work/physical-activity/current-guidelines
Physicians Committee for Responsible Medicine	https://www.pcrm.org
The Plantrician Project	https://plantricianproject.org
Institute of Lifestyle Medicine	https://www.instituteoflifestylemedicine.org
True Health Initiative	https://www.truehealthinitiative.org
Video: Lifestyle Medicine	https://vimeo.com/134629158 https://vimeo.com/281875215
Video: Heart Disease	https://vimeo.com/136965421
Video: Type 2 Diabetes	https://vimeo.com/137208481

Acronyms

ACC/AHA: American College of Cardiology and American Heart Association

ACLM: American College of Lifestyle Medicine

APP: advanced practice provider

APRN: advanced practice registered nurse

A-SMART: adopt healthy eating, stress less, move often, avoid alcohol, rest more, treat tobacco use

BMI: body mass index

CDC: Centers for Disease Control and Prevention

CVD: cardiovascular disease

FITT: frequency, intensity, time, type

HPFS: Health Professionals Follow-Up Study

MOSS: motivation, obstacles, strategies, strengths

NCCDPHP: National Center for Chronic Disease Prevention and Health Promotion

NHS: Nurses' Health Study

NONPF: National Organization of Nurse Practitioner Faculties

NP: nurse practitioner

PA: physician assistant

QALY: quality-adjusted life year
ROI: return on investment
SMART-EST: specific, measurable, attainable, relevant, time-bound, evidence-based, strategic, tailored

T2DM: type 2 diabetes
WHO: World Health Organization

References

Alahmary, S. A., Alduhaylib, S. A., Alkawii, H. A., Olwani, M. M., Shablan, R. A., Ayoub, H. M., Purayidathil, T. S., Abuzaid, O. I., & Khattab, R. Y. (2019). Relationship between added sugar intake and sleep quality among university students: A cross-sectional study. *American Journal of Lifestyle Medicine, 16*(1), 122–129. https://doi.org/10.1177/1559827619870476

American College of Lifestyle Medicine. (n.d.). *What is lifestyle medicine?* Retrieved September 30, 2022, from https://www.lifestylemedicine.org

American College of Sports Medicine. (2021). General principles of exercise prescription. In *ACSM's guidelines for exercise testing and prescription* (11th ed., pp. 126–129). Wolters Kluwer.

Bodai, B. (2017). Lifestyle medicine: A brief review of its dramatic impact on health and survival. *The Permanente Journal, 22*, 17–25. https://doi.org/10.7812/TPP/17-025

Bolnick, H. J., Bui, A. L., Bulchis, A., Chen, C., Chapin, A., Lomsadze, L., Mokdad, A. H., Millard, F., & Dieleman, J. L. (2020). Health-care spending attributable to modifiable risk factors in the USA: An economic attribution analysis. *The Lancet Public Health, 5*(10), e525–e535. https://doi.org/10.1016/S2468-2667(20)30203-6

Caterson, I. D., Alfadda, A. A., Auerbach, P., Coutinho, W., Cuevas, A., Dicker, D., Hughes, C., Iwabu, M., Kang, J. H., Nawar, R., Reynoso, R., Rhee, N., Rigas, G., Salvador, J., Sbraccia, P., Vázquez-Velázquez, V., & Halford, J. C. G. (2019). Gaps to bridge: Misalignment between perception, reality and actions in obesity. *Diabetes, Obesity and Metabolism, 21*(8), 1914–1924. https://doi.org/10.1111/dom.13752

Chaput, J. P., Dutil, C., & Sampasa-Kanyinga, H. (2018). Sleeping hours: What is the ideal number and how does age impact this? *Nature and Science of Sleep, 10*, 421–430. https://doi.org/10.2147/NSS.S163071

Cho, L., Davis, M., Elgendy, I., Epps, K., Lindley, K. J., Mehta, P. K., Michos, E. D., Minissian, M., Pepine, C., Vaccarino, V., & Volgman, A. S. (2020). Summary of updated recommendations for primary prevention of cardiovascular disease in women: JACC state-of-the-art review. *Journal of the American College of Cardiology, 75*(20), 2602–2618. https://doi.org/10.1016/J.JACC.2020.03.060

Colditz, G. A., Philpott, S. E., & Hankinson, S. E. (2016). The impact of the Nurses' Health Study on population health: Prevention, translation, and control. *American Journal of Public Health, 106*(9), 1540–1545. https://doi.org/10.2105/AJPH.2016.303343

Community Preventative Service Taskforce. (2021). *Heart disease and stroke prevention: Team-based care to improve blood pressure control.* https://www.thecommunityguide.org/resources/one-pager-team-based-care-improve-blood-pressure-control

Cross-Org Competencies Review Taskforce. (2021). *Competencies for the PA profession.* https://www.aapa.org/download/90503

Downes, L., St. Hill, H., & Mays, T. (2021). A-SMART lifestyle behaviors model for health, wellbeing, and immune system enhancement. *The Nurse Practitioner, 46*(9), 31–39. https://doi.org/10.1097/01.NPR.0000769748.45938.10

Dysinger, W. S. (2021). Lifestyle medicine prescriptions. *American Journal of Lifestyle Medicine, 15*(5), 555. https://doi.org/10.1177/15598276211006627

Edington, D. W., Burton, W. N., & Schultz, A. B. (2020). Health and economics of lifestyle medicine strategies. *American Journal of Lifestyle Medicine, 14*(3), 274. https://doi.org/10.1177/1559827620905782

Egger, G., Binns, A., Rossner, S., & Sagner, M. (2017). *Lifestyle medicine: Lifestyle, the environment, and preventative medicine in health and disease* (3rd ed.). Elsevier.

Exercise is Medicine. (2021). *Physical activity vital sign.* American College of Sports Medicine. www.exercisetismedicine.org/support_page.php/health-care-providers

Falkner, B., & Lurbe, E. (2020). Primordial prevention of high blood pressure in childhood: An opportunity not to be missed. *Hypertension, 75*(5), 1142–1150. https://doi.org/10.1161/HYPERTENSIONAHA.119.14059

Ford, E. S., Bergman, M. M., Kroger, J., Schienkiewita, A., Weikert, C., & Boeing, H. (2009). Healthy living is the best revenge. *Archives of Internal Medicine, 169*(15), 1355–1362. https://doi.org/10.1001/archinternmed.2009.237

Frates, B., Bonnet, J. P., Joseph, R., & Peterson, J. A. (2019). *Lifestyle medicine handbook: An introduction to the powers of healthy habits.* Healthy Learning.

Hansen, A. R., Rustin, C., Opoku, S. T., Shevatekar, G., Jones, J., & Zhang, J. (2020). Trends in US adults with overweight and obesity reporting being notified by doctors about body weight status, 1999–2016. *Nutrition, Metabolism and Cardiovascular*

Diseases, *30*(4), 608–615. https://doi.org/10.1016/j .numecd.2020.01.002

Hartman, M., Martin, A. B., Washington, B., Catlin, A., & The National Health Expenditure Accounts Team. (2021). National health care spending in 2020: Growth driven by federal spending in response to COVID-19 pandemic. *Health Affairs*, *41*(1). https:// doi.org/10.1377/hlthaff.2021.01763

Harvard T. H. Chan School of Public Health. (n.d.). *Health Professionals Follow-Up Study*. Retrieved September 30, 2022, from https://sites.sph.harvard.edu/hpfs

Hayes, T. O., & Delk, R. (2018, September 4). Understanding the social determinants of health. *American Action Forum*, 1–9. https://www.americanactionforum .org/research/understanding-the-social-determinants -of-health

Hayes, T. O., & Gillian, S. (2020). *Background: Understanding the connections between chronic disease and individual-level risk factors*. American Action Forum. https:// www.americanactionforum.org/research/background -understanding-the-connections-between-chronic -disease-and-individual-level-risk-factors

Hooker, S. A., Punjabi, A., Justesen, K., Boyle, L., & Sherman, M. D. (2018). Encouraging health behavior change: Eight evidence-based strategies. *Family Practice Management*, *25*(2), 31–36.

Houlden, R. L., Yen, H. H., & Mirrahimi, A. (2018). The lifestyle history: A neglected but essential component of the medical history. *American Journal of Lifestyle Medicine*, *12*(5), 404–411. https://doi .org/10.1177/1559827617703045

Jacob, V., Chattopadhyay, S. K., Proia, K. K., Hopkins, D. P., Reynolds, J., Thota, A. B., Jones, C. D., Lackland, D. T., Rask, K. J., Pronk, N. P., Clymer, J. M., & Goetzel, R. Z. (2017). Economics of self-measured blood pressure monitoring: A community guide systematic review. *American Journal of Preventive Medicine*, *53*(3), e105–e113. https://doi.org/10.1016/j .amepre.2017.03.002

Karimi, H., & Alavi, N. M. (2015). Florence Nightingale: The mother of nursing. *Nursing and Midwifery Studies*, *4*(2), 29475.

Katz, D. L., Frates, E. P., Bonnet, J. P., Gupta, S. K., Vartiainen, E., & Carmona, R. H. (2018). Lifestyle as medicine: The case for a true health initiative. *American Journal of Health Promotion*, *32*(6), 1452– 1458. https://doi.org/10.1177/0890117117705949

Kisling, L. A., & Das, J. M. (2022). Prevention strategies. *StatPearls*, 1–4. https://www.ncbi.nlm.nih.gov/books /NBK537222

Kvaavik, E., Batty, D., Ursin, G., Huxley, R., & Gale, C. R. (2010). Influence of individual and combined health behaviors on total and cause-specific mortality in men and women. *Archives of Internal Medicine*, *170*(8), 711–718. https://doi.org/10.1001 /archinternmed.2010.303

Lenz, T. L. (2014). Documenting lifestyle medicine activities. *American Journal of Lifestyle Medicine*, *8*(4), 242– 243. https://doi.org/10.1177/1559827614529071

Li, Y., Pan, A., Wang, D. D., Liu, X., Dhana, K., Franco, O. H., Kaptoge, S., Di Angelantonio, E., Stampfer, M., Willett, W. C., & Hu, F. B. (2018). Impact of healthy lifestyle factors on life expectancies in the US population. *Circulation*, *138*(4), 345–355. https://doi .org/10.1161/CIRCULATIONAHA.117.032047

Lianov, L. S., Adamson, K., Kelly, J. H., Matthews, S., Palma, M., & Rea, B. L. (2022). Lifestyle medicine core competencies: 2022 update. *American Journal of Lifestyle Medicine*, *16*(6), 734–739. https://doi.org /10.1177/15598276221121580

Lianov, L., & Johnson, M. (2010). Physician competencies for prescribing lifestyle medicine. *Journal of the American Medical Association*, *304*(2), 202–203. https://doi .org/10.1001/JAMA.2010.903

Lloyd-Jones, D. M., Albert, M. A., & Elkind, M. (2021). The American Heart Association's focus on primordial prevention. *Circulation*, *144*, E233–E235. https://doi .org/10.1161/CIRCULATIONAHA.121.057125

Martin, A. B., Hartman, M., Lassman, D., & Catlin, A. (2020). National health care spending in 2019: Steady growth for the fourth consecutive year. *Health Affairs*, *40*(1), 14–24. https://doi.org/10.1377 /hlthaff.2020.02022

Martinez-Gomez, D., Guallar-Castillon, P., Higueras-Fresnillo, S., Banegas, J. R., Sadarangani, K. P., & Rodriguez-Artalejo, F. (2018). A healthy lifestyle attenuates the effect of polypharmacy on total and cardiovascular mortality: A national prospective cohort study. *Scientific Reports*, *8*(1). https://doi.org/10.1038 /S41598-018-30840-9

Martins, C., Godycki-Cwirko, M., Heleno, B., & Brodersen, J. (2018). Quaternary prevention: Reviewing the concept. *The European Journal of General Practice*, *24*(1), 106–111. https://doi.org/10.1080/13814788.2017.1422177

McGinnis, J. M., & Foege, W. H. (1993). Actual causes of death in the United States. *Journal of the American Medical Association*, *270*(18), 2207–2212. https://doi .org/10.1001/JAMA.1993.03510180077038

Melnyk, B. M. (2022). Moving from sick care to well care: A paradigm shift is needed to reduce cardiovascular disease and improve hypertension control. *Worldviews on Evidence-Based Nursing*, *19*(1), 4–5. https://doi .org/10.1111/WVN.12552

Mokdad, A. H., Marks, J. S., Stroup, D. F., & Gerberding, J. L. (2004). Actual causes of death in the United States, 2000. *Journal of the American Medical Association*, *291*(10), 1238–1245. https://doi .org/10.1001/jama.291.10.1238

National Center for Chronic Disease Prevention and Health Promotion. (2022a, July 21). *About chronic diseases*. Centers for Disease Control and Prevention. https://www.cdc.gov/chronicdisease/about/index.htm

National Center for Chronic Disease Prevention and Health Promotion (NCCDPH). (2022b, December 21). *Health and economic benefits of diabetes interventions.* Centers for Disease Control and Prevention. https://www.cdc.gov/chronicdisease/programs-impact/pop/diabetes.htm

National Center for Chronic Disease Prevention and Health Promotion. (2023, March 14). *Health and economic benefits of chronic disease interventions.* Centers for Disease Control and Prevention. https://www.cdc.gov/chronicdisease/programs-impact/pop/index.htm

National Organization of Nurse Practitioner Faculties. (2017). *Advanced Practical Registered Nurse Doctoral-Level Competencies.* https://cdn.ymaws.com/www.nonpf.org/resource/resmgr/competencies/common-aprn-doctoral-compete.pdf

National Organization of Nurse Practitioner Faculties. (2022). *Nurse practitioner role core competencies.* https://www.nonpf.org/resource/resmgr/competencies/nonpf_np_role_core_competenc.pdf

Nugent, R., Bertram, M. Y., Jan, S., Niessen, L. W., Sassi, F., Jamison, D. T., Pier, E. G., & Beaglehole, R. (2018). Investing in non-communicable disease prevention and management to advance the Sustainable Development Goals. *Lancet, 391*(0134), 2029–2035. https://doi.org/10.1016/S0140-6736(18)30667-6

Nyberg, S. T., Singh-Manoux, A., Pentti, J., Madsen, I. E. H., Sabia, S., Alfredsson, L., Bjorner, J. B., Borritz, M., Burr, H., Goldberg, M., Heikkilä, K., Jokela, M., Knutsson, A., Lallukka, T., Lindbohm, J. V., Nielsen, M. L., Nordin, M., Oksanen, T., Pejtersen, J. H., . . . Kivimäki, M. (2020). Association of healthy lifestyle with years lived without major chronic diseases. *JAMA Internal Medicine, 180*(5), 760–768. https://doi.org/10.1001/jamainternmed.2020.0618

Office of Disease Prevention and Health Promotion. (n.d.). *Sleep: Healthy People 2030.* U.S. Department of Health and Human Services. Retrieved June 12, 2022, from https://health.gov/healthypeople/objectives-and-data/browse-objectives/sleep

Office of Science. (2022, August 15). *What is epigenetics?* Centers for Disease Control and Prevention, Office of Genomics and Precision Health. https://www.cdc.gov/genomics/disease/epigenetics.htm

Papanicolas, I., Woskie, L. R., Orlander, D., Orav, E. J., & Jha, A. K. (2019). The relationship between health spending and social spending in high-income countries: How does the US compare? *Health Affairs, 38*(9), 1–9. https://doi.org/10.1377/hlthaff.2018.05187

Petrin, C., Kahan, S., Turner, M., Gallagher, C., & Dietz, W. H. (2017). Current attitudes and practices of obesity counselling by health care providers. *Obesity Research & Clinical Practice, 11*(3), 352–359. https://doi.org/10.1016/J.ORCP.2016.08.005

Pool, A. C., Kraschnewski, J. L., Cover, L. A., Lehman, E. B., Stuckey, H. L., Hwang, K. O., Pollak, K. I., & Sciamanna, C. N. (2014). The impact of physician weight discussion on weight loss in US adults. *Obesity Research & Clinical Practice, 8*(2), e131–e139. https://doi.org/10.1016/j.orcp.2013.03.003

Powell, H. S., & Greenberg, D. L. (2019, January). Screening for unhealthy diet and exercise habits: The electronic health record and a healthier population. *Preventive Medicine Reports, 14,* 100816. https://doi.org/10.1016/j.pmedr.2019.01.020

Rippe, J. M. (2018). Lifestyle medicine: The health promoting power of daily habits and practices. *American Journal of Lifestyle Medicine, 12*(6), 499–512. https://doi.org/10.1177/1559827618785554

Rock, C. L., Thomson, C., Gansler, T., Gapstur, S. M., McCullough, M. L., Patel, A. V., Andrews, K. S., Bandera, E. V., Spees, C. K., Robien, K., Hartman, S., Sullivan, K., Grant, B. L., Hamilton, K. K., Kushi, L. H., Caan, B. J., Kibbe, D., Black, J. D., Wiedt, T. L., . . . Doyle, C. (2020). American Cancer Society guideline for diet and physical activity for cancer prevention. *CA: A Cancer Journal for Clinicians, 70*(4), 245–271. https://doi.org/10.3322/caac.21591

Taj, N., Devera-Sales, A., & Vinson, D. C. (1998). Screening for problem drinking: Does a single question work? *Journal of Family Practice, 46*(4), 328–335.

Tikkanen, R., & Abrams, M. K. (2020). *U.S. health care from a global perspective, 2019: Higher spending, worse outcomes?* The Commonwealth Fund. https://www.commonwealthfund.org/publications/issue-briefs/2020/jan/us-health-care-global-perspective-2019

U.S. Department of Health and Human Services. (2018). *Physical activity guidelines for Americans.* https://health.gov/our-work/physical-activity/current-guidelines

U.S. Department of Health and Human Services and U.S. Department of Agriculture. (2020). *Dietary guidelines for Americans: 2020–2025.* https://www.dietaryguidelines.gov/sites/default/files/2020-12/Dietary_Guidelines_for_Americans_2020-2025.pdf

White, N. D., Bautista, V., Lenz, T., & Cosimano, A. (2020). Using the SMART-EST goals in lifestyle medicine prescription. *American Journal of Lifestyle Medicine, 14*(3), 271–273. https://doi.org/10.1177/1559827620590775

World Health Organization. (2016, August 20). *Health promotion.* https://www.who.int/news-room/questions-and-answers/item/health-promotion

World Health Organization. (2021, April 21). *Noncommunicable diseases.* https://www.who.int/news-room/fact-sheets/detail/noncommunicable-diseases

Zoltick, D., Scribani, M. B., Krupa, N., Kern, M., Vaccaro, E., & Jenkins, P. (2021). Healthy lifestyle counseling by healthcare practitioners: A time to event analysis. *Journal of Primary Care and Community Health, 12.* https://doi.org/10.1177/21501327211024427

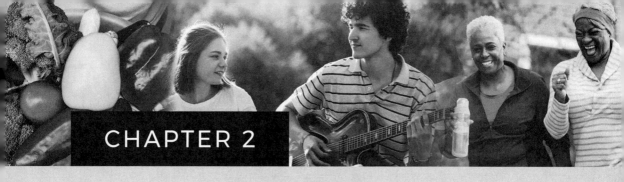

Health Disparities and Determinants of Health

Donna M. Hedges, PhD, MSN, MBA, RN, CNE
Terri L. Gibson, DNP, MSN, RN, AMB-BC, DipACLM

It is more important to know what sort of person has a disease than to know what sort of disease a person has.

Hippocrates

OBJECTIVES

This chapter will enable the reader to:

1. Distinguish among health disparity, healthcare disparity, and health equity.
2. Explain the role of culture, race, and ethnicity in health disparity.
3. Summarize the relationship between social determinants of health and health disparity.
4. Articulate the advocacy role of the advanced practice provider in appraising policy recommendations to decrease health disparities.
5. Reflect on personal biases and perspectives that influence the provision of equitable care.
6. Appraise tools and resources to enhance clinicians' ability to effectively assess and address social determinants of health in patient care.

Overview

This chapter will provide an overview of health disparities and the social determinants of health (SDOH) and is designed to enable advanced practice providers (APPs) to differentiate among health disparities, healthcare disparities, and health inequity and to understand their relationship with SDOH. Concepts such as social justice and bias are explored to empower APPs to create change through their practices, one patient at a time. National and global resources are included to assist APPs in developing a deeper understanding and integration of strategies to mitigate the effects of disparities and SDOH. Activities within the chapter will provide the opportunity to appraise personal biases toward populations experiencing health disparities, expand knowledge, and design quality improvement

© Kathleen Gail/Shutterstock; © StoryTime Studio/Shutterstock; © kali9/Getty Images

and research initiatives related to the SDOH relevant to practice.

Healthcare delivery is a complex adaptive system influenced by various factors ranging from regulatory and political to financial and operational. Given this complexity, APPs are challenged to understand, navigate, and overcome barriers to care and health promotion resources. The existence of health disparities, health inequities, and SDOH further complicates the ability of all individuals to receive quality care regardless of racial, ethnic, gender orientation, and socioeconomic status. Current events within communities across the nation have increased focus on SDOH, ethnicity, race, and health inequity. APPs are often faced with the implications of disparity and SDOH within the communities they serve. In exploring health disparities and SDOH, it is crucial to understand the concept of social justice as a foundation for health equity.

Concept of Social Justice

Foundational to understanding health disparities and SDOH is the concept of social justice. The United Nations (2006) published the proceedings from the International Forum for Social Development, which identified six inequalities related to the concept of social justice: (a) distribution of income; (b) distribution of assets; (c) distribution of opportunities for work and employment; (d) distribution for civic and political participation; (e) distribution of access to knowledge; and (f) distribution of health services, social security, and the provision of a safe environment. This seminal work sought to set the foundation for social justice on the global level. In this way, the United Nations aligned the concept of social justice with distributive justice, which requires equality of rights, equality of opportunities, and equality

in living conditions. Strategies to reduce the effects of SDOH are rooted in mitigating inequalities related to economics, education, health care, and the environment.

Social justice in health care is inextricably intertwined with the concept of justice applied to disparities and the elements of SDOH. In the context of health and wellness, social justice is defined as the existence of an equitable distribution of health services regardless of race or ethnicity and as the foundation of public health (Matwick & Woodgate, 2017; Stronks et al., 2016). These definitions establish that all individuals are equal and have value. Given this, all individuals have a right to access healthcare resources to be healthy and productive members of society. Yet health disparities and health inequity conflict with the concept of social justice. As APPs provide care to diverse populations, the injustice of health inequalities must be evaluated along with SDOH, such as income, employment, and education. With this knowledge, APPs can begin to explore disparities in health and health care.

Disparities in Health and Health Care

Disparities in health coverage, chronic health conditions, mental health, and mortality result from long-standing systematic inequality in economics, housing, and healthcare systems (Carratala & Maxwell, 2020). APPs are often the primary healthcare providers in healthcare settings throughout all socioeconomic levels in diverse racial, ethnic, and rural populations. Over the past two decades, the role of APPs has evolved in terms of responsibility and scope of practice. Given this, APPs need to differentiate among health disparities, healthcare disparities, and health inequities to understand their influence on the health and well-being of populations.

Health Disparity

According to the Centers for Disease Control and Prevention (CDC), health disparities can be defined as "preventable differences in the incidence of disease, injury, violence, or opportunities to achieve optimal health that are experienced by socially disadvantaged populations" (CDC, 2020, para. 1). These health disparities exist across the life span. Health disparities refer to differences among specific population groups and present as barriers to attaining an individual's complete state of health and well-being. Health disparities are manifested by worse health outcomes associated with disadvantaged racial and ethnic groups and any socioeconomically disadvantaged population (Braveman, 2014). Additionally, health disparities are also linked to demographics, such as age, gender, disability status, and gender orientation (Ndugga & Artiga, 2021).

Healthy People 2030 (HP2030) provides a more comprehensive definition that includes health disparity among groups experiencing greater social or economic obstacles to health based on mental health and cognitive, sensory, or physical disability (Office of Disease Prevention and Health Promotion [ODPHP], n.d.-c). The concept of social disadvantage is fundamental to understanding health disparities and refers to individuals' social position, which is often beyond their control. Social disadvantage can result from racial or ethnic prejudice or cultural bias in employment, housing, and health care. Individuals with low levels of financial income, education, and employment status have the most adverse health status compared to those with a higher level of these social factors (Braveman, 2014; Braveman et al., 2011).

Healthcare Disparities

Healthcare disparities are differences in access to or availability of healthcare services and facilities as well as variations in the incidence of disease and disabilities in vulnerable populations (Agency for Healthcare Research and Quality, 2018). Healthcare disparity refers to healthcare systems and is manifested by a lower healthcare quality for racial and ethnic minorities. Minorities, the aged, and those living in poverty are less likely to receive routine medical care and more likely to face higher morbidity and mortality rates than nonminorities (American Medical Association, n.d.). Bias, stereotyping, and prejudice contribute to racial and ethnic disparities in health care and health systems.

Health Inequity

Health equity refers to the degree to which everyone has the opportunity to attain full health potential, and "no one is disadvantaged from achieving this potential because of social position or any other socially defined circumstance" (National Academies of Medicine [NAM], 2017, p. 31). Conversely, health inequity, which is avoidable, unnecessary, and unjust, exists when there are differences in the health and well-being of groups and communities with unequal status in society (NAM, 2017; Whitehead, 1992). Health inequities result from an unequal distribution of resources leading to detrimental social, economic, and environmental conditions that are demonstrated by incidence and prevalence, mortality, and disease burden (National Institutes of Health, 2017). The *burden of disease* concept was developed by the World Health Organization (WHO) to reflect morbidity and mortality related to diseases, injuries, and risk factors as estimated by the number of years of life lost and the number of years of life with a disability. By assessing the burden of disease, APPs and leaders of national and global healthcare organizations can advocate for and formulate effective healthcare policies based on meaningful health information.

As healthcare providers, healthcare leaders, legislators, and the global community grapple with the implications of health disparities, Braveman et al. (2011) offer guiding principles to inform the way forward:

- All individuals should be afforded dignity and be valued equally.
- Health, as an essential human right, provides the ability to fully participate in society.
- All individuals should have the ability to maintain their health status without discrimination and inequality.
- The prosperity and advancement of a society depend on the health of its citizens.
- Healthcare disparities leading to poor health outcomes present a barrier to overcoming social disadvantage.
- Resources required to maintain a healthy life should be distributed equitably.
- Collaboration between the healthcare sector and governmental agencies is necessary to reduce the adverse health outcomes related to health disparities and SDOH.

Poor health outcomes and the effects of advancing chronic diseases inhibit an individual's ability to pursue the benefits of employment, education, social interaction, and participating as a productive member of society. The absence of health incurs individual physical and psychological costs, increases societal and personal healthcare expenditures, and taxes available healthcare resources. APPs can make a positive impact toward reducing health disparities by viewing and treating patients with dignity and respect; understanding the experiences of children and their families; and promoting every individual's potential for well-being, which includes actively engaging individuals in the process of improving their own well-being. The path toward healthcare equity relies on collaboration between healthcare providers and legislators to advocate for

and enact health policies that reduce the barriers to accessing health care. The role of the APP in patient and health policy advocacy is presented later in this chapter.

Relevance to APPs

With these definitions and guiding principles in mind, APPs can think critically about the scope of the issues associated with health and healthcare disparities. APPs are uniquely positioned to assume an active role in advocating for vulnerable populations. Comfort in discussing SDOH with patients and their families is essential for all APPs. Such discussions are integral to person-centered care and provide crucial information for after-care teaching and identification of appropriate healthcare resources. Expanding the awareness of APPs to the detrimental effects of health disparities and the critical need for health equity will assist in developing strategies designed to mitigate health disparities in their community of care. Furthermore, through interprofessional collaboration, APPs can have a positive influence on achieving the Robert Wood Johnson Foundation's national health outcomes of optimal health and well-being regardless of socioeconomic and geographic considerations; equitable access to affordable, high-quality care; the inclusion of all individuals; and decreased healthcare spending (Plough, 2015).

Understanding the foundational concept of social justice, the nature and implications of health disparities, and how these relate to patient care can assist APPs in developing their professional practice and providing comprehensive care to all patient populations. The following section provides the intersection of culture, race, and ethnicity in relation to health disparities. It is essential to understand and acknowledge the past to be able to change the future. It is equally important to understand how an individual's heritage and social factors serve as obstructions to social justice and equity in health care.

Health Disparities: A Historical Perspective

The earliest correlation between socioeconomic and environmental factors and health outcomes was identified three centuries ago when Ramazzini observed a high incidence of breast cancer in Catholic nuns (Gibbons, 2005). In 1775, an association was made between occupation and the incidence of cancer. In 1840, differences were noted in mortality rates based on poverty level and lifestyle factors within poor working-class groups. Evidence that the focus of medicine needed to shift from changing the individual to changing society was identified in 1849, specifically that implementing strategies to improve schools and working conditions would decrease disparities in mortality rates among populations (Gibbons, 2005).

Gibbons (2005) relates that investigation into the effects of socioeconomic and environmental factors on the incidence of disease and death in Europe continued throughout the 20th century, revealing an increased incidence of disparity in infant mortality over 40 years between 1910 and 1950. With evidence of health disparities increasing, the British government formed the Working Group on Inequities in Health in 1977, leading to the publication of the Black Report in 1980. The Black Report served as the first systematic study to raise awareness of the complexity of health disparity and called for changes to improve living conditions for the poor and disadvantaged. Since 1985, the U.S. Department of Health and Human Services has coordinated several initiatives to reduce or eliminate health disparities. These initiatives sought to address factors contributing to health disparities, such as socioeconomic, lifestyle behaviors, social environment, and access to health promotion and disease prevention services within racial and ethnic populations. Despite these efforts, disparities continue to exist. To better understand health and healthcare disparities, it is essential to understand the influence of culture, race, and ethnicity on health outcomes. The following section utilizes research data to illustrate how these factors can disadvantage individuals, communities, and populations.

Role of Culture, Race, and Ethnicity in Health Disparities

The implications of health disparities and culture, race, and ethnicity can be examined in the context of existing data associated with comorbid disease and with past and current public health concerns. Significant episodes of widespread disease highlight ongoing barriers to healthcare services access where people live, work, play, and pray. For example, in a study of 4,518 short-term and critical access hospitals across 50 states, low-income communities have far fewer intensive care unit beds per capita than wealthier communities (Kanter et al., 2020). In another study, Wang and colleagues (2021) explored health disparities and the economic burdens of cancer associated with poor nutrition. The study findings demonstrated that poor nutrition significantly contributed to disparities in health among racial and ethnic minorities and socioeconomically disadvantaged groups (Wang et al., 2021). **Table 2.1** provides race and ethnicity data related to health coverage, chronic health conditions, mental health, and leading cause of death (Carratala & Maxwell, 2020).

Factors such as racism, discrimination, disadvantages in economics and education, and access to quality health care are underlying causes for disparities in chronic disease incidence rates. According to the Kaiser Family Foundation, people of color demonstrate significantly lower levels across various health status measures and are at risk of being uninsured (Ndugga & Artiga, 2021). For example, the impact of social

Table 2.1 Race and Ethnic Health Disparities* in the United States, 2017–2018

Race/Ethnicity	Health Coverage	Chronic Health Conditions	Mental Health	Leading Cause of Death
African Americans and Black Americans	■ 10.6% were uninsured compared with 5.9% of non-Hispanic Whites. ■ 89.4% had coverage compared with 93.7% of White Americans. ■ 12.1% under age 65 had no coverage.	■ 13.8% reported having fair or poor health compared with 8.3% of non-Hispanic Whites. ■ 80% of African American women are overweight or obese compared with 64.8% of White Americans. ■ 12.6% of African American children had asthma compared with 7.7% of non-Hispanic White children. ■ 42% of African American adults over age 20 had hypertension compared with 28.7% of non-Hispanic White adults.	■ 8.7% of adults received mental health services compared with 18.6% of non-Hispanic White adults.	■ Heart disease, cancer, and accidents. ■ Highest mortality rate for all cancers combined compared to any other group. ■ Twice the national average of 5.8 infant deaths per 1,000 live births. ■ 11.4 men and 2.8 women per 100,000 die by suicide.
Hispanic Americans or Latinx Americans	■ 16.1% were uninsured compared with 5.9% non-Hispanic Whites. ■ 83.9% of Hispanics had coverage compared with 93.7% non-Hispanic Whites. Of these, 39.5% had government health coverage. ■ 20.1% under age 65 had no coverage. ■ 7.7% of children had no coverage compared with 4.1% non-Hispanic White, 4.0% non-Hispanic Black, and 3.8% non-Hispanic Asian.	■ 10% reported fair or poor health compared with 8.3% non-Hispanic Whites. ■ 21.5% over age 20 were diagnosed with diabetes compared with 13% of Whites over age 20. ■ 25% with hypertension. ■ Women were 40% more likely to have cervical cancer and 20% higher mortality than non-Hispanic Whites.	■ 8.8% of adults received mental health services compared to 18.6% non-Hispanic White adults. ■ 6.8% received prescription medication compared with 15.4% non-Hispanic Whites. ■ 4.6% of adults reported serious psychological distress. ■ 40% higher number of female adolescent suicide attempts than non-Hispanic White adolescent females.	■ Cancer, heart disease, accidents. ■ Life expectancy of 81.9 years is longer than that of non-Hispanic Whites. ■ 40% higher Puerto Rican infant mortality compared to non-Hispanic Whites. ■ 5.1 infant deaths per 1,000 live births.

Asian Americans	■ 7.3% were uninsured. ■ 92.7% had coverage, with 29.6% government coverage.	■ Tuberculosis is 35 times higher. ■ Lower incidence of overall cancer but twice the incidence of liver and inflammatory bowel disease cancer. ■ Twice as likely for chronic hepatitis B and eight times more likely to die from hepatitis B. ■ 40% more likely for diabetes and 80% more likely for end-stage renal disease.	■ 2.1% reported serious psychological distress, with 6.3% receiving mental health services. ■ 3.6% received prescription medications.	■ Cancer, stroke, heart disease, accidents, and diabetes. ■ 3.8 infant deaths per 1,000 live births. ■ Suicide is the leading cause of death for ages 15 to 24.
Native Hawaiian or other Pacific Islander Americans	■ 8.3% were uninsured; 66.9% had private coverage compared with 75.4% of White Americans. ■ 33.5% with government coverage.	■ Higher rates of smoking, alcohol consumption, and obesity compared with other populations. ■ Higher tuberculosis rate than other populations. ■ 10% more likely to be diagnosed with coronary heart disease than non-Hispanic Whites. ■ 80% more likely to be obese than non-Hispanic Whites.	■ 6.9% of adults reported a major depressive episode in the previous year. ■ 21.1% of adults reported any form of mental illness. ■ 10.9% received mental health services. ■ 6.3% received prescription medication.	■ The highest mortality rate for all types of cancer in the United States. ■ Cancer, heart disease, accidents, stroke, diabetes. ■ 7.6 infant deaths per 1,000 live births in the population.
American Indians and Alaska Natives	■ 14.9% were uninsured.	■ 17.4% reported failing to poor health. ■ HIV infection is twice as high compared with non-Hispanic Whites. ■ Three times more likely to have diabetes with 2.5 times the mortality rate. ■ Adolescents are 30% more likely to be obese. ■ Highest cigarette smoking rates among all racial/ethnic populations in the United States.	■ 4.5% reported serious psychological distress. ■ 14.1% received mental health services. ■ 11.6% received prescription medications.	■ Heart disease, cancer, and accidents. ■ Chronic liver disease was the 4th leading cause of death. ■ Lung cancer was the leading cause of cancer-related deaths. ■ 9.2 infant deaths per 1,000 live births in this population. ■ Suicide was the 2nd leading cause of death in ages 10 to 34.

*As compared with non-Hispanic Whites

Data from Carratala, S., & Maxwell, C. (2020, May 7). *Health disparities by race and ethnicity.* Center for American Progress. https://www.americanprogress.org/article/health-disparities-race-ethnicity

disparities relative to cardiovascular disease was investigated in a study conducted by Abdalla et al. (2020). This cross-sectional study of 44,986 participants, aged 20 years and older, examined how the burden of cardiovascular disease differed between individuals with higher and those with lower socioeconomic status. The findings demonstrated that the incidence of cardiovascular disease decreased at a faster rate in individuals with higher socioeconomic resources. In addition to comorbid diseases, epidemics and pandemics, such as tuberculosis, malaria, and HIV and AIDS, provide excellent examples of how culture, race, and ethnicity can exacerbate barriers, such as access to care, diagnosis, and treatment.

Significant public health threats such as these expose vulnerabilities within healthcare systems regarding the availability of equipment, therapeutic medical supplies, and adequate numbers of healthcare professionals. Additionally, public health monitoring and tracking within populations can be complicated by the lack of availability of trained personnel and the willingness and ability of individuals to seek medical attention. Challenges also exist regarding the timely development of therapeutic modalities that can either eradicate or mitigate the spread and potentially debilitating effects of widespread disease. To illustrate this, the following section examines the impact of the COVID-19 pandemic on racial and ethnic communities.

COVID-19 Pandemic

The consequences of COVID-19 have focused renewed attention on long-standing racial and ethnic disparities in health and health care, income, employment, and living conditions (Robichaux & Sauerland, 2021). Data reported by race and ethnicity demonstrated a higher incidence of COVID-19 cases and significantly higher mortality rates within the African American and Latino populations (Hooper et al., 2020; Selden & Berdahl, 2020). For example, in New York City, African American, Asian, and Hispanic communities comprised 8 out of 10 zip codes with the highest deaths (Peretz et al., 2020).

A disparity exists in the prevalence of comorbidities or preexisting conditions among racial and ethnic groups. In a study conducted by Selden and Berdahl (2020) relative to the COVID-19 pandemic, health data were analyzed across racial and ethnic groups to examine the impact of risk for infection and the influence of employment and household composition on individual health. The findings from the study demonstrated that COVID-19 health risk factors alone did not exclusively explain the disparity in COVID-19 morbidity and mortality among minority populations (Selden & Berdahl, 2020). The findings from the data analysis suggest that employment and household composition may contribute to the disparity seen in COVID-19 infection. It was noted that African Americans and Hispanics were less likely to practice social distancing or to work from home and were more likely to work in food-related and healthcare jobs, which increased the likelihood of exposure to COVID-19. The study also examined the effect of poverty, lack of insurance, and access to health care. Psychological stress related to these disparities was shown to correlate with the development of comorbidities (Selden & Berdahl, 2020). Study findings supported that the differences in COVID-19 morbidity and mortality may be more strongly supported by the effects of social determinants of health in comparison to factors related to comorbidities (Selden & Berdahl, 2020).

The shift away from face-to-face medical appointments to telemedicine further complicated the access to timely medical care by racial and ethnic populations. The implementation of telemedicine required significant financial resources and personnel, making the transition to telemedicine prohibitive for vulnerable communities (Weigel et al., 2020). The lack of reliable internet access and service in low-income and rural communities exacerbated health inequities and left many individuals without the means to be evaluated and treated for COVID-19. Further work is needed to assess inequities within vulnerable communities, employ strategies to mitigate these inequities, and strengthen community-based resources (Sundar, 2020).

COVID-19 and other health crises focus attention on the persistent effects of unresolved health disparities on national and global levels (Cassoobhoy et al., 2021). The impact of COVID-19 will have a long-lasting effect on disadvantaged communities in terms of food insecurity, accessibility to in-person health services, and rates of employment and financial recovery (Peretz et al., 2020). Since threats to global health such as COVID-19 will continue to present challenges, targeted health policy and deployment of more equitable resources to communities that lack essential infrastructure and resources are needed to mitigate health disparities (Cassoobhoy et al., 2021).

APPs play an integral role in advocating for populations subject to health disparities and increasing health promotion services within disadvantaged communities. Associating health disparities to the SDOH is critical to addressing the myriad health issues that challenge racial and ethnic populations within the APP's scope of care. An overview of the SDOH and HP2030 and a summary table of resources are presented in the next section.

Social Determinants of Health

From a holistic standpoint, APPs are aware that individuals cannot be treated in isolation from their environment and family of origin. The focus placed on social determinants by

various national and global health agencies validates the critical importance of the environment in health promotion and disease prevention (ODPHP, n.d.-b). Therefore, it is essential to recognize the relationship between environmental factors and the nature of health disparities. The concept of epigenetics and the development of acute and chronic diseases is briefly explained as a foundation for understanding the importance of the SDOH.

Role of Epigenetics

To appreciate the influence of SDOH and well-being, APPs first need to understand the emerging information on epigenetics. Environmental factors such as lack of food availability, pollution, abuse, lack of access to health care, and socioeconomic stressors (i.e., employment, education level, and exposure to crime and violence) can result in genetic changes that lead to chronic health conditions within minority populations (Mancilla et al., 2020). These genetic changes result from biological stress and can have implications throughout the life span (Mancilla et al., 2020). The National Academies of Sciences, Engineering, and Medicine (NASEM, 2016) published evidence suggesting that parents' inability to provide a safe, stable, and nurturing environment is particularly detrimental to brain development during the first five years of life. Furthermore, studies demonstrate that toxic stress in childhood correlates to midlife and late-life conditions, such as addiction and substance abuse, metabolic disorders, cardiovascular disease, cancer, and Alzheimer's disease (Mancilla et al., 2020).

Environmental stress can negatively affect childhood development and result in social, emotional, and behavioral problems (Halfon et al., 2017). It is noted that physical and psychological stress during pregnancy can lead to preeclampsia, preterm birth, and gestational diabetes. Additionally, effects of toxic environmental stress on early child-hood include fetal alcohol spectrum disorder, developmental disorders, behavioral health problems, and asthma (Mancilla et al., 2020). Children living in poverty often experience chronic stress resulting from parent incarceration, neighborhood and domestic violence and substance abuse, discrimination related to social and economic status, and housing and food insecurity (Halfon et al., 2017).

APPs must advocate for interventions designed to increase access to education and health care for children to reduce the negative effects of SDOH. Additionally, APPs must screen, assess, and advocate for children and families. Screening children for SDOH must be followed by an evaluation to determine whether social needs are met. APPs must be knowledgeable about SDOH and must incorporate screening for social needs into the history and physical assessments for all patients to identify factors that present challenges to health promotion and well-being (O'Gurek & Henke, 2018).

Screening for Social Needs

Screening for environmental stressors and SDOH is a critical part of the APP's initial and ongoing physical and psychosocial assessment of patient populations. SDOH, such as food insecurity, safety, and housing, can significantly impact a patient's health and well-being. Social needs screening is the responsibility of all healthcare providers and is an essential part of the patient's plan of care (American Hospital Association [AHA], 2019; O'Gurek & Henke, 2018). **Table 2.2** provides examples of screening tools to assist APPs in identifying and mitigating SDOH. While screening for social needs is an integral part of the patient's plan of care, there are barriers to obtaining this essential information. Inadequately meeting social needs negatively influences patients' ability to attend provider visits, contributing further to lack of healthcare access and poor outcomes (Fiori et al., 2020).

Barriers to Social Needs Screening

As APPs implement social needs screening, it would not be unusual to encounter barriers to effective identification of patient social needs. The AHA (2019) investigated the integration of routine screening for social needs in patient care and identified the following clinician barriers:

- Discomfort in engaging in conversations about social needs
- Insufficient time for collecting social needs information

Table 2.2 Screening Tools for Social Needs

Agency	Tool	URL
American Academy of Family Physicians	Social Needs Screening Tool	https://www.aafp.org/dam/AAFP /documents/patient_care/everyone _project/hops19-physician-form-sdoh.pdf
American Hospital Association	Screening for Social Needs: Guiding Care Teams to Engage Patients (See page 15 for links to assessment tools and resources.)	https://www.aha.org/toolkitsmethodology /2019-06-05-screening-social-needs -guiding-care-teams-engage-patients
National Association of Community Health Centers	Protocol for Responding to and Assessing Patients' Assets, Risks, and Experiences	https://prapare.org

- Lack of systems to document and track social needs data
- Perceived lack of efficacy to address social needs

The reasons cited for patient reluctance to discuss social needs include shame, fear, stigma, trauma, power dynamics, and social and cultural norms (AHA, 2019). Approaching patients with a caring, nonjudgmental attitude can serve as the foundation for therapeutic relationships between APPs and patients and their families.

In a cross-sectional study of 768 nurses in three hospitals, researchers explored the knowledge, perceived self-efficacy, and intended behaviors relative to integrating SDOH into clinical practice (Phillips et al., 2020). Fifty percent of the nurses were comfortable addressing access to care issues compared to the other SDOH factors. Barriers to the discussion of SDOH included lack of time to address specific needs and lack of awareness of internal and external resources. These findings demonstrate that more nurses need to address SDOH concerns, not just those in public health–related roles. Furthermore, education and support for interventions to address the needs of patients are necessary, including consideration of increased collaboration within the interprofessional healthcare team. It is likely that many clinicians have completed prior health education without adequate knowledge of SDOH and the implications these factors have on personal health and well-being. Attention to these concepts can aid APPs in partnering with the patient to deliver a more holistic approach to health care.

Strategies for Effective Social Needs Screening

The AHA (2019) recommends specific approaches that can enhance the APP's ability to perform effective screening (**Table 2.3**). APPs must promote trust, collaboration, support, and partnership with community groups to address issues relative to diverse populations. Active listening and empathic inquiry are primary ways for APPs to listen effectively to patient concerns and respond nonjudgmentally. The use of motivational interviewing, in which APPs empower patients to take control of their health, can result in lifestyle behavior change. APPs must also understand that patients may have a history of coping mechanisms that enable them to manage traumatic experiences. By valuing patients and their life experiences, APPs can convey dignity, support, and cultural competence within the APP and patient relationship (AHA, 2019). As APPs become aware of the factors that influence health and learn how to screen for risk factors, they can instruct patients on how to identify and access necessary resources.

APPs must view themselves as partners in healthcare delivery. Partnering with patients encourages them to become active participants in their care. In choosing their path to wellness, patients are more likely to be engaged and successful. It is also important for APPs to see the value in an interprofessional approach to conducting social history assessments, providing advice as needed, and being knowledgeable about resources so that appropriate referrals can be given (Andermann, 2018). See **Table 2.4** for additional strategic considerations for social needs screenings.

Developing professional awareness *and* identifying community referral resources are critical to caring for children and families who are especially at risk due to social determinants (Francis et al., 2018). Strategies to promote family health, mitigate environmental stressors, and promote child welfare and self-esteem can reduce epigenetic changes that result in illness throughout the life span (Mancilla et al., 2020). With this understanding of how factors beyond an individual's control can affect growth and development, the focus of this chapter will shift to a more in-depth discussion of the SDOH.

Table 2.3 Approaches for Effective Social Needs Screening

Approach	Description
Cultural competency: The ability to interact effectively with people from different cultures.	Cultural competency training helps care team members increase their sensitivity to cultural diversity, reduce language barriers, and build an understanding of life experiences that shape a person's identity.
Motivational interviewing: Counseling method that helps people resolve challenges and find the internal motivation to change their behavior.	Motivational interviewing empowers patients to take control of their health and behaviors by setting goals based on their wishes and current circumstances.
Active listening: Technique in which the listener fully concentrates on, understands, responds to, and remembers what is said.	Active listening teaches providers how to properly listen to what patients are saying, identify any underlying hesitance, and in return ask open-ended questions related to their challenges.
Empathetic inquiry: A technique that integrates motivational interviewing and trauma-informed care to facilitate collaboration and emotional support.	Empathetic inquiry allows care team members to connect with patients, increase relatability, and suggest nonjudgmental approaches to improve health.
Asset-based: An approach to care that focuses on the individual's strengths and potential.	Recognize that, alongside having needs, patients and communities have many assets that can be leveraged to address their social needs. An asset-based approach allows the provider–patient conversation to be reframed from a focus on deficits to connecting with the strengths, interests, and areas the patient finds meaningful. At the community level, an asset-based approach helps identify, partner with, and leverage resourceful organizations such as schools, community-based or faith-based organizations, government, local businesses, and people in the community to collectively build on existing resources and form new community connections.
Trauma-informed: A framework that involves understanding and responding to behaviors/actions and needs resulting from trauma.	Trauma-informed care is a holistic approach to treating a patient where it is assumed that each individual has a history of trauma and coping mechanisms. Integrate trauma-sensitive questions and practices to increase resiliency and to support personalized patient care.

© Used with permission of American Hospital Association.

Table 2.4 Strategic Considerations for Social Needs Screenings

Screening Step	Strategic Considerations
Engage community stakeholders	■ Gain insight into what questions should be asked. ■ Identify any community sensitivities or perceived barriers to asking questions. ■ Identify community advocates to support social needs screening processes beyond the clinical settings. ■ Build relationships with community members and organizations to identify existing community resources to address social needs challenges.

Screening Step	Strategic Considerations
Create a safe space for conducting screenings	■ Consult with community stakeholders about options for where to screen. ■ Allow adequate time to discuss social needs. ■ If in person, make sure the space is quiet and private.
Get buy-in from the patients	■ Explain the purpose of social needs screening and its value for tailored or personalized patient care. ■ Ask permission to ask sensitive questions. ■ Recognize patients' autonomy. ■ Recognize the sensitivity of the questions being asked and ensure confidentiality. ■ Be transparent. Clarify that they are not being singled out or discriminated against. ■ Communicate the possibility of connecting them to resources. ■ Show support and respect at all times.
Learn from the patients	■ Identify patients' priorities. ■ Recognize the trade-offs they need to make for their health. ■ Learn how patients perceive their social needs. ■ Inquire about their language preference. ■ Practice empathy by putting yourself in patients' shoes.
Train clinicians and care team members	■ Educate staff about various social needs and data on the community served. ■ Encourage relationship building with patients. ■ Bring in resources to acquire knowledge on cultural competency, motivational interviewing, and trauma-informed care, as seen in Table 2.3.
Apply cultural competency skills	■ Note any stigma or cultural concerns. ■ Withhold judgment. ■ Express empathy and respect. ■ Note any cultural attitudes or beliefs that might impact screening. ■ Develop screening tools, questionnaires, and other forms of educational material in multiple languages to reduce language barriers and increase better understanding.
Identify individual and community strengths and assets	■ Reframe deficits as assets. ■ Promote self-efficacy. ■ Identify patients' individual strengths.
Develop effective documentation processes	■ Standardize a screening tool and a place, such as the electronic health record, to record answers. ■ Account for screening answers in future encounters to avoid having similar conversations multiple times.
Develop actionable next steps	■ Create a workflow plan for when a patient is screened positive. ■ Partner with community organizations to identify existing resources. ■ Equip clinicians and care teams with referral sources.
Scale the screening process	■ How can the organization screen everyone? Who might need extra attention? ■ Work with other internal departments and physician practices to streamline approaches and data collection. ■ Use insights and data from screening to develop community initiatives.

© Used with permission of American Hospital Association.

Health Promotion Case Study Assessing SDOH

Case Description: J.A. is a 78-year-old retired farmer. Most of his life was spent on the farm taking care of cattle and keeping the farm equipment in working order. He quit smoking 10 years ago after a two-pack-per-day habit that began at the age of 14. Approximately four years ago, J.A. had sinus surgery to correct problems resulting from a facial injury. Unfortunately, he experienced postoperative complications causing him to lose vision in his right eye, and he now complains of cataract symptoms in his left eye. His wife of 35 years will not allow him to drive their vehicle after J.A. had two accidents that totaled their previous vehicles. She is a lifelong smoker who recently quit smoking a few months ago after her healthcare provider convinced her that smoking was causing her abdominal aortic aneurysm to grow and that surgical repair was needed. The couple lives in a very rural community, with a population of 700, and in a house they own. Food and medical resources are located about 30 minutes away from their community.

Critical Thinking Questions

1. What SDOH factors are relevant to J.A. and his wife's health and social history?
2. Based on your knowledge of the SDOH, what questions and assessments would be pertinent if J.A. presented to the APP for a medical office visit?
3. What priority concerns need to be addressed?
   a. What is J.A.'s primary concern?
   b. What would be your priority concern?
   c. What assumptions or biases do you have about J.A. prior to talking with him?
4. What are the potential actions to consider?
   a. Physical care
   b. Social or environmental needs
   c. Education
   d. Illness prevention or mitigation of health complications
   e. Other

SDOH and HP2030

SDOH are the nonmedical conditions largely beyond a person's control and are associated with where people are born, develop, live, work, and age (WHO, 2010). These include economic stability, education quality and access, healthcare access and quality, neighborhood and built environment, and social and community context. **Table 2.5** provides descriptions of the SDOH.

The effects of SDOH were identified as early as 1983 when the United States published *Health, United States, 1983*, which determined that significant disparities in health existed between minority Americans compared to the general population. In the 1990s,

it became apparent that concerted efforts to eliminate racial and ethnic disparities were inseparable and foundational to the provision of quality health care (Burton et al., 2020). The effort to eliminate racial and ethnic health disparities led to the Healthy People Initiative (ODPHP, n.d.-a). The initiative began in 1979 with the landmark report *Healthy People: The Surgeon General's Report on Health Promotion and Disease Prevention*. The first set of measurable 10-year health objectives designed to improve health and promote well-being were published in 1990. *Healthy People 1990* was followed by *Healthy People 2000, 2010, 2020, and 2030*.

HP2030 builds on the previous decades of work and includes Leading Health Indicators,

Table 2.5 SDOH Descriptions

SDOH	Description
Economic stability	Recent statistics highlight the 1 in 10 poverty rates for people living in the United States. HP2030 emphasizes the need to focus on helping more people attain economic stability to afford adequate housing, healthy foods, and health care. Interventions include assisting people in securing and keeping a job through career counseling, childcare support, and policy activities that support funding for necessities and education.
Education quality and access	The level of education attained directly influences health and longevity. Therefore, HP2030 focuses on improving educational opportunities for children and adolescents. Certain populations of children are at increased risk of being less likely to graduate from high school and go to college, including low-income families; those with disabilities; and those experiencing discrimination, including bullying.
Healthcare access and quality	Approximately 1 in 10 people in the United States do not have health insurance, and many do not receive needed healthcare services (ODPHP, n.d.-e). Because many individuals cannot afford health services and medications, interventions should include support for increasing insurance coverage and promoting access to care for those living too far away from healthcare providers.
Neighborhood and built environment	The study of environmental effects on the genetic expression of disease is known as epigenetics (Mancilla et al., 2020). Where people live, including their house and neighborhood, influences their health. The role of the environment, such as neighborhoods prone to violence, poor air quality, and unsafe water and building materials, places the inhabitants at risk regarding safety and health measures. Interventions are needed at the local, state, and federal levels, including attention to policy changes.
Social and community context	Relationships and connectedness to others are essential factors in personal well-being. How individuals interact with family, friends, neighbors, social groups, and coworkers influences health and well-being. Some individuals and population groups are more at risk for challenges beyond their control, including personal safety, uncivil behaviors, loneliness, and abandonment. Purpose in life, spiritual care, and participation in faith communities must also be considered necessary for addressing the whole person (Neathery, 2018).

which identify the high-priority objectives focused on health promotion throughout the life span (ODPHP, n.d.-d). These determinants represent five main categories of social needs that result in unequal and avoidable differences in health status within and between communities and populations (**Figure 2.1**). Unmet social and environmental needs adversely affect the health of individuals and populations, leading to a higher incidence of morbidity and mortality (Andermann, 2016; Kreuter et al., 2021; Lathrop, 2020).

There is significant alignment between the SDOH and the key issues identified by the CDC and HP2030 (**Table 2.6**). Evidence suggests that the Healthy People Initiative has resulted in significant health-related progress, including reducing death rates for heart disease and cancer, infant and maternal mortality, and risk factors contributing to other chronic diseases.

There is a need for continued efforts to collaborate with public and private sector organizations to research and address health

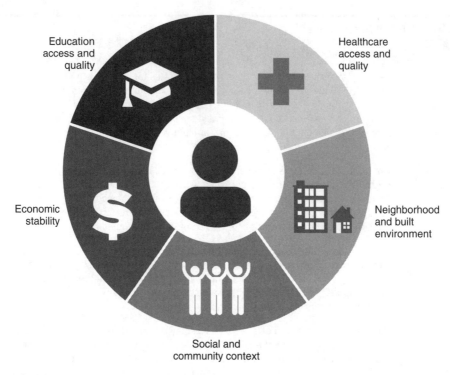

Figure 2.1 Social determinants of health.

Reproduced from Healthy People 2030, U.S. Department of Health and Human Services, Office of Disease Prevention and Health Promotion. https://health.gov/healthypeople/objectives-and-data/social-determinants-health

Table 2.6 Alignment of SDOH, HP2030, and the CDC

SDOH[1]	HP2030 Goal[1]	CDC[2]
Economic stability	Help people earn steady incomes that allow them to meet their health needs.	▪ Link between financial resources: income, cost of living, socioeconomic status, and health. ▪ Key issues: poverty, employment, food security, and housing stability.
Education access and quality	Increase education opportunities and help children and adolescents do well in school.	▪ Connection among education, health, and well-being. ▪ Key issues: high school graduation, enrollment in higher education, general education attainment, and early childhood education and development.
Healthcare access and quality	Increase access to comprehensive, high-quality healthcare services.	▪ Connection between access to and understanding of health services and an individual's health. ▪ Key issues: access to health care, primary care, health insurance coverage, and health literacy.

SDOH[1]	HP2030 Goal[1]	CDC[2]
Neighborhood and environment	Create neighborhoods and environments that promote health and safety.	■ Connection between where people live—housing, neighborhood, and environment—and their health and well-being. ■ Key issues: quality of housing, access to transportation, availability of healthy foods, air and water quality, and neighborhood crime and violence.
Social and community context	Increase social and community support.	■ Connection among the characteristics of the contexts within which people live, learn, work, and play and their health and well-being. ■ Key issues: community cohesion, civic preparation, discrimination, conditions in the workplace, and incarceration.

[1]Office of Disease Prevention and Health Promotion. (n.d.-f). *Healthy People 2030: Social determinants of health.* Retrieved February 20, 2023, from https://health.gov/healthypeople/priority-areas/social-determinants-health

[2]Centers for Disease Control and Prevention. (2023, April 7). *CDC Research on SDOH.* https://www.cdc.gov/publichealthgateway/sdoh/research.html
Data from Office of Disease Prevention and Health Promotion. (n.d.-d). *Healthy People 2030: Leading health indicators.* Retrieved February 20, 2023, from https://health.gov/healthypeople/objectives-and-data/leading-health-indicators

promotion practices for all people and communities (Chandra et al., 2017; NASEM, 2021). The achievable goals and objectives from HP2030 serve as a guide for improving the health of individuals, communities, and stakeholders. Multiple organizations are actively engaged in addressing societal needs and providing quality resources. **Table 2.7** summarizes these organizations, their missions, and their contributions.

Presence of Implicit Bias

Research suggests that healthcare provider behaviors and attitudes contribute to health disparities (Hall et al., 2015). Additionally, the presence of implicit bias can negatively influence the quality of relationships between APPs and patients, treatment decisions and compliance with treatments, and the quality of patient outcomes (Hall et al., 2015). Bias is the positive or negative evaluation of something or someone. Implicit bias occurs when the person is unaware of their bias (Gopal et al., 2021). As APPs seek to build rapport and trust relationships with patients, it is critical to reflect on personal biases that impede supportive patient relationships.

In the classic work of Freire (2007), conditions for effective resolution of population concerns include the need for successful dialogue and collaboration with all individuals. Successful dialogue and collaboration require profound love for the world and people, humility, faith in people, hope that there will be positive results from engagement efforts, and critical thinking about the complex process of the anticipated transformation (Freire, 2007). Collaborative dialogue between APPs and patients serves as the basis for formulating a person-centered plan of care. However, implicit bias can act as an obstruction to establishing effective APP and patient relationships and can be detrimental to patient outcomes.

Efforts designed to educate or address policies for community health improvement must

Table 2.7 Organizations That Address SDOH

Organization	History, Mission, Role	Contribution and Accomplishments
American Hospital Association	Advancing health in America from a hospital organization and health system perspective.	Utilizes current research to inform organizations about the current healthcare climate and includes resources to guide planning and implementation.
Centers for Disease Control and Prevention	The nation's health protection agency and engages in protecting Americans from health and safety threats, domestic and foreign.	This robust organization provides a wealth of data, resources, and connections to organizations that support the "health security of our nation."
County Health Rankings	Progress from the past 10 years indicates summary findings: (a) Gaps in life expectancy remain. (b) The past affects the present. (c) There is work to be done. (d) Even the healthiest counties can do better. (e) Child poverty remains a formidable barrier to the health of our nation today. (f) The racial opportunity gap persists.	The emphasis is to provide an understanding that where people live influences their health.
HP2030	A national initiative that has existed since 1979 and focuses on promoting health and reducing disease prevalence through the development of objectives related to current evidence and trends.	The goals and specific objectives are updated every decade. The fifth rendition of this monitoring platform is currently published.
Institute for Health Improvement	Uses improvement science to assist with the development of initiatives to improve and sustain better health outcomes globally.	Key areas of focus: ■ Pursuing safe and high-quality care ■ Improving the health of populations ■ Building the capacity to improve ■ Innovating and sparking action
National Academies of Sciences, Engineering, and Medicine	A private, nonprofit organization of the country's leading researchers.	*Consensus Study Report, 2019.* Many additional resources and publications as well.
Robert Wood Johnson Foundation	Began collaborations in 2013 to develop a holistic, integrated approach to address population health and well-being (Chandra et al., 2017).	The culture of health measures align with the County Health Rankings model (University of Wisconsin Population Health Institute, 2022).

Organization	History, Mission, Role	Contribution and Accomplishments
U.S. Department of Health and Human Services (HHS) National Committee on Vital and Health Statistics (NCVHS)	The mission of HHS is to enhance the health and well-being of Americans. The NCVHS focuses on community health improvement.	The framework provides community leaders a "blueprint of key" areas to address for improvement processes.
Center for Community Health and Development at the University of Kansas	The mission is "to promote community health and development by connecting people, ideas, and resources."	Free online resources are provided to assist with assessment and integration of actions designed to promote healthy community development.
World Health Organization	Continues to be invested in addressing SDOH and health equity.	The organization collaborates with many other experts to provide evidence and updates regarding initiatives in progress.

incorporate the perspective of those toward whom the program is directed, including their participation in planning and implementation. APPs must pause to consider their personal views on disparities, equity, and vulnerable populations and the tendency to assign blame and think in terms of distinguishing among the color of people's skin, their accent, and their background (Marcelin et al., 2019).

Approaching the provision of care while keeping an attitude of unconditional positive regard is critical to patient care. Seeking to view the situation from the individual's lived experience can inform the APP and stimulate various resources to deliver optimal care. One strategy to assist APPs in seeing situations from the patients' view is to consider the concept of cultural humility. Cultural humility involves learning about patients from a cultural context, recognizing the existence of a power imbalance within the APP and patient relationship, and suspending judgment (Foronda et al., 2016; Miyagawa, 2020). Lifelong learning and critical self-reflection, which lead to exploring cultural beliefs, values, and preferences with all patients, are integral to developing cultural humility (Foronda et al., 2016).

APPs convey cultural humility by actively listening to patient concerns, being aware of their nonverbal communication (i.e., body language), recognizing their lack of knowledge, and being willing to ask for clarification or help (Foronda et al., 2016). The American Speech-Language-Hearing Association (2021) provides a tool that APPs can use to assess their cultural humility (**Table 2.8**).

Challenges to Addressing Bias

Despite increased attention to implicit bias and the need to develop cultural humility, challenges to mitigating implicit bias remain. One challenge is that implicit bias is beyond the APP's conscious awareness yet still influences behaviors and attitudes toward patients (FitzGerald & Hurst, 2017). Examples of implicit bias include longer wait times for ethnic and racial patients, basing treatment options on patient characteristics, ordering fewer or more diagnostic procedures, and condescending tone and body language (Hall et al., 2015). The following research

TABLE 2.8	Evidence-Based Resources for SDOH	
Organization	**Resource**	**URL**
Agency for Healthcare Research and Quality	Studies, tools, and resources to address SDOH	https://www.ahrq.gov/sdoh/index.html
American Academy of Family Physicians	Links to AAFP initiatives, resources, and policies on SDOH	https://www.aafp.org/news/media-center/kits/social-determinants-of-health.html
American Academy of Family Physicians	Social Needs Screening Tool	https://geriatrictoolkit.missouri.edu/Social-Needs-Screening-Tool-AAFP.pdf
American Hospital Association	Information on SDOH and links to other initiatives	https://www.aha.org/social-determinants-health/populationcommunity-health/community-partnerships
American Hospital Association	The Screening for Social Needs: Guiding Care Teams to Engage Patients document is helpful for integrating screening for social needs, including skill-building tools.	https://www.aha.org/toolkits methodology/2019-06-05-screening-social-needs-guiding-care-teams-engage-patients
American Speech-Language-Hearing Association	Cultural Competence Check-In Self-Reflection tool	https://www.asha.org/siteassets/uploadedfiles/multicultural/self-reflection-checklist.pdf
Center for Community Health and Development at the University of Kansas	The Community Tool Box website includes action models and resources for teaching, learning, implementation, and evaluation related to promoting healthier communities.	https://ctb.ku.edu/en/table-of-contents/overview/models-for-community-health-and-development/social-determinants-of-health/main
Centers for Disease Control and Prevention	Data, tools for action, programs, and policy with specific attention to SDOH and well-being	https://www.cdc.gov/social determinants/index.htm
Centers for Disease Control and Prevention	Resources for SDOH and dementia	https://www.cdc.gov/aging/disparities/index.htm
County Health Rankings and Roadmaps	Provides county-level statistics designed to quantify the health and wellness status of U.S. communities	https://www.countyhealth rankings.org
Healthy People 2030	Data-driven national objectives to address SDOH and improve health and well-being (see Table 2.6 for broad goals related to each SDOH category).	https://health.gov/healthy people/objectives-and-data/social-determinants-health

Organization	Resource	URL
Institute for Healthcare Improvement	Education and resources to empower and support local change agents, including white papers on key topics, video messages, and certificate programs	http://www.ihi.org/Engage /Initiatives/100MillionHealthier Lives/Pages/default.aspx
Institute for Health Metrics and Evaluation	Global health research for improving health policy and practice	https://www.healthdata.org
Millbank Foundation	Public charity focused on improving the lives of people with disabilities	https://milbankfoundation.net
National Academies of Sciences, Engineering, and Medicine	*Integrating Social Care into the Delivery of Health Care: Moving Upstream to Improve the Nation's Health*	https://www.national academies.org/our-work /integrating-social-needs-care -into-the-delivery-of-health -care-to-improve-the-nations -health
National Committee on Vital and Health Statistics	*Measurement Framework for Community Health and Well-Being, V4* provides a benchmark for best practices and multisectoral indicators for communities.	https://ncvhs.hhs.gov/wp -content/uploads/2018/03 /NCVHS-Measurement -Framework-V4-Jan-12-2017 -for-posting-FINAL.pdf
National Committee for Quality Assurance	*SDOH Resource Guide*	https://www.ncqa.org/wp -content/uploads/2020/10 /20201009_SDOH-Resource _Guide.pdf
Neighborhood Atlas	The Neighborhood Atlas makes SDOH metrics available for research, program planning, and policy development.	https://www.neighborhoodatlas .medicine.wisc.edu
Office of Minority Health	Policies and initiatives to improve SDOH in racial and ethnic minority populations	https://www.minorityhealth .hhs.gov
Robert Wood Johnson Foundation	Developed a framework for action, four primary action areas, and 10 principles to build a culture of health	https://www.rwjf.org/en /cultureofhealth.html
Well Being in the Nation (WIN) Network	Measures, policies, investments, and infrastructure to improve health and well-being in the nation	https://winnetwork.org
World Health Organization	*Integrating Equity, Gender, Human Rights and Social Determinants into the Work of WHO: Roadmap for Action*	https://www.who.int/publications /m/item/integrating-equity --gender--human-rights-and -social-determinants-into-the -work-of-who--roamap-for -action-(2014-2019)

Health Promotion Research Study

Evaluating Racial Bias in Health Care

Background: Research suggests that 11% to 20% of Black adult patients experienced discrimination in health care in 2019 and healthcare bias resulted in decreased levels of trust in healthcare providers and follow-up with treatment plans (Stepanikova & Oats, 2017).

Methodology: To explore biased language in health care, Sun and colleagues (2022) conducted a study to investigate the presence of racism and bias in patients' medical records. The study included 40,113 history and physical notes from 18,459 adult patients and utilized machine learning to detect the use of negative patient descriptors varied by patient race or ethnicity (Sun et al., 2022). Ethnic groups represented in the study were White (29.7%), Black (60.6%), Hispanic or Latino (6.2%), and Other (3.5%). The mean age was 47.4, and 56.0% were female.

Results: Approximately 8% of the medical records included one or more negative descriptors, such as "refused," "not adherent," "not compliant," and "agitated" (Sun et al., 2022, p. 5). Black patients had a 2.54 times greater likelihood of being described by negative descriptors after the researchers adjusted for sociodemographic and health characteristics.

Implications for Advanced Practice: APPs must reflect upon the use of negative descriptors when interacting with patients and when documenting in the patients' medical record. Implicit bias on the part of APPs can result in a lack of patient trust, decreased willingness to follow treatment plans, failure to return for follow-up healthcare visits, and worsening healthcare status.

References: Sun, M., Oliwa, T., Peek, M. E., & Tung, E. L. (2022). Negative patient descriptors: Documenting racial bias in the electronic health record. *Health Affairs, 41*(2), 1–9. https://doilorg /10.1377/hlthaff.2021.01423

Data from Stepanikova, I., & Oates, G. (2017). Perceived discrimination and privilege in health care: The role of socioeconomic status and race. *American Journal of Preventive Medicine, 52*(1 Suppl. 1), S86–S94. https://doi.org/doi:10.1016/j.amepre.2016.09.024

---

study illustrates how implicit bias can result in the use of negative patient descriptors and reflect racial bias in the electronic health record.

Another challenge in mitigating implicit bias is the lack of diversity of healthcare providers compared to the increasing diversity of the patient population they serve. This incongruency in diversity can result in unconscious bias, which leads to stereotyping and prejudice. This can negatively influence healthcare provider behavior, patient–provider interactions, and decision-making and perpetuates healthcare disparities (Marcelin et al., 2019). As a result, implicit bias can affect treatment decisions, compliance with treatment, and

patient health outcomes. Developing cultural humility can assist APPs when caring for patients who represent cultures different from their own and thereby enable APPs to mitigate cultural differences when establishing a person-centered plan of care.

APPs as Advocates

As APPs become more knowledgeable about the challenges patients experience due to SDOH and implicit bias of healthcare providers, they can use this knowledge to advocate for patients, influence health policy development, and mitigate the effects of healthcare inequity. Advocacy for patients and effective health policy align with the concept of social justice in health care and places APPs at the forefront of mitigating health disparities and inequities within the communities they serve.

Advocacy for patients includes ensuring respect for their autonomy and right to self-determination, promoting communication between patients and healthcare providers, and facilitating access to needed resources. Gerber (2018) listed four steps of advocacy when providing care for diverse patients: (a) assessment, which necessitates therapeutic conversations to understand patient values and unique needs; (b) patient goal identification, accomplished through discussions about related organizational policies and options for care while empowering and facilitating patient decision-making; (c) implementation of the advocacy plan through support of the patient, including assisting with care coordination; and (d) evaluating the results of advocacy efforts.

On a broader level, advocacy also includes promoting public health policy and health programs that break the cycle of poor health by targeting SDOH (Williams et al., 2018). Advocacy for health policy requires that APPs become knowledgeable about existing health policies, policies that are in development, and power and privilege imbalances that place ethnic and racial populations at a disadvantage (Robichaux & Sauerland, 2021). This knowledge, combined with their healthcare skills, experience, and expertise, equip APPs to serve as advocates for legislation, healthcare regulations, and health policy decisions on the local, state, and national levels. Through contact with legislators and decision-makers, APPs can educate about crucial public health issues and address the needs of underrepresented individuals and populations. In this way, APPs are critical to the education, activation, and implementation phases of health policy development (American Public Health Association, n.d.).

Interprofessional Approach to SDOH

The concepts of health equity and disparities and the determinants of health are complex, and addressing the effects of SDOH on populations requires collaboration, knowledge, and expertise within the healthcare disciplines. An interprofessional approach that integrates lifestyle interventions is necessary to effectively support patients in well-being and prevention of chronic disease and to address health disparities across populations (Cassoobhoy et al., 2021). The American College of Lifestyle Medicine convened an interprofessional team tasked to explore strategies and solutions to mitigate SDOH. This collaborative work took place in 2020 at the Health Disparities Summit and resulted in four recommendations: (a) educate clinicians and promote minority clinician representation to expand physician and APP knowledge of lifestyle medicine; (b) empower patients to self-advocate by providing peer-to-peer education and educational materials and resource programs to increase health literacy; (c) build community engagement through collaboration between local government agencies, healthcare and religious organizations, and other community services; and (d) advocate for policy change that facilitates empowering individuals and communities to achieve health equity (Cassoobhoy et al., 2021). The APP can play an integral role in fostering interprofessional collaboration and leading healthcare initiatives reflected in these four recommendations.

Interprofessional education is for developing collaborative care teams designed to meet the complex needs of diverse populations. In 2010, the WHO published the *Framework for Action on Interprofessional Education & Collaborative Practice*, which identified increased collaboration through interprofessional education to reduce fragmentation within the healthcare system and improve health outcomes. One year earlier, the Interprofessional

Education Collaborative (IPEC) was formed by six national associations of schools of health professionals representing dentistry, nursing, medicine, osteopathic medicine, pharmacy, and public health. The IPEC's *Core Competencies for Interprofessional Collaborative Practice* was published in 2011 and updated in 2016. These competencies were established to provide guidance for interprofessional collaborative practice and curriculum development throughout health profession schools (IPEC, 2016).

Nursing accreditation and practice standards also support interprofessional education and collaborative practice. In 2011, the Institute of Medicine published *The Future of Nursing Report: Leading Change, Advancing Health*, which called for nurses to function at their full scope of practice and identified the critical need for interprofessional education (Institute of Medicine, 2011). The NASEM (2021) followed with *The Future of Nursing 2020–2030: Charting a Path to Achieve Health Equity* in 2021, which highlighted the nurse's role in addressing SDOH and health equity and improving the nation's health and well-being. That same year, the American Association of Colleges of Nursing (AACN, 2021) published *The Essentials: Core Competencies for Professional Nursing Education. The Essentials* provides a new model for nursing practice that includes 10 domains, two of which pertain to population health and

interprofessional partnerships. While these reports are specific to nursing, the content and recommendations are applicable to all APPs. After all, the responsibility to address health and healthcare disparities, health inequity, and SDOH does not rest on any one healthcare discipline.

Considering the significant impact that SDOH, health and healthcare disparities, and health inequity have on patients' well-being, it is not surprising that the health professions acknowledge the need for an interprofessional educational focus and collaborative approach to meeting the needs of vulnerable populations. Given the importance of health disparities and SDOH, clinicians must understand the wide variety of determinants of health and work together to implement effective interventions at the individual, population group, and community levels (AACN, 2021).

Summary

This chapter provides foundational knowledge designed to assist APPs in addressing the effects of SDOH within the populations they serve. SDOH are conditions largely beyond an individual's control and are influenced by socioeconomics, educational levels, and availability and access to resources such as employment and health care. Health disparities

---

Health Promotion Activity: Assessing SDOH

Assess the social determinants in the community you serve. You may start with a disparity in health, such as a life expectancy difference between groups, and consider what social determinants influence them.

1. Of the five SDOH (see Figure 2.1), which one has the most negative effect on health in your community? Is this SDOH long-standing or the result of recent changes within the community?
2. Investigate and list the available community resources designed to address this SDOH. Do you believe these resources are adequate?
3. Based on your investigation and assessment of community resources, how can you incorporate screening for this SDOH into your practice?
4. As an APP, what advocacy opportunities can you identify to help mitigate the negative effects of this SDOH within your patient population?

are preventable differences in the incidence of diseases within populations while healthcare disparities relate to differences in access to healthcare services. Health and healthcare disparities can result in lower healthcare quality and increased chronic health conditions. Without adequate access to healthcare resources, vulnerable populations face higher incidences of comorbidities and mortality. These disparities serve as major obstructions to health promotion and conflict with the concept of social justice.

Dynamics within families and the communities in which they live can have negative developmental and health consequences throughout the life span. The study of epigenetics reveals how toxic stress levels can alter the brain development and health status of children from birth to five years of age. Epigenetic changes can also be responsible for the incidence of cognitive health issues in older adults. Through effective social needs screening, APPs can detect factors that impact a patient's well-being, identify educational needs, and provide relevant community resources to address SDOH and assist patients in making healthier lifestyle decisions.

The concepts of implicit bias, self-reflection, and cultural humility are integral to the development of trust within APP and patient relationships. Taking the time to learn how individuals' cultural beliefs may influence their healthcare decisions conveys respect for the patients and assists APPs in establishing a person-centered plan of care. Self-reflection allows APPs to consider their own values and cultural beliefs as they interact with individuals from a culture different from their own. Actively listening, aligning words and body language, and demonstrating a willingness to ask for clarification can reduce the risk of stereotyping and prejudice on the part of APPs.

Racial and ethnic disparities continue to exist in health care despite the efforts of national and global organizations to address disparities through health system improvements and health policy development. To effectively promote health equity, APPs must collaborate with interprofessional teams and healthcare, governmental, and social service agencies to remove barriers to health care. APPs are uniquely positioned to significantly influence the health and well-being of the populations they serve through advocacy, knowledge, expertise, and dedication to promoting health equity and reducing health disparities. Various organizations and websites are identified in Table 2.8 and throughout this chapter to provide additional resources for APPs as they seek to further develop knowledge and skills to address SDOH and identify advocacy opportunities.

Acronyms

AACN: American Association of Colleges of Nursing

AHA: American Hospital Association

APP: advanced practice provider

CDC: Centers for Disease Control and Prevention

HP2030: *Healthy People 2030*

IPEC: Interprofessional Education Collaborative

NAM: National Academies of Medicine

NASEM: National Academies of Sciences, Engineering, and Medicine

ODPHP: Office of Disease Prevention and Health Promotion

SDOH: social determinants of health

WHO: World Health Organization

References

Abdalla, S. M., Yu, S., & Galea, S. (2020). Trends in cardiovascular disease prevalence by income level in the United States. *JAMA Network Open, 3*(9), 1–14. https://doi.org/10.1001/jamanetworkopen.2020.18150

Agency for Healthcare Research and Quality. (2018). *2018 National healthcare quality and disparities report.* https://www.ahrq.gov/research/findings/nhqrdr/nhqdr18/index.html

American Association of Colleges of Nursing (2021). *The essentials: Core competencies for professional nursing education.* https://www.aacnnursing.org/Portals/42/AcademicNursing/pdf/Essentials-2021.pdf

American Hospital Association. (2019). *Screening for social needs: Guiding care teams to engage patients.* https://www.aha.org/system/files/media/file/2019/09/screening-for-social-needs-tool-value-initiative-rev-9-26-2019.pdf

American Medical Association. (n.d.). *Reducing disparities in health care.* Retrieved May 15, 2022, from https://www.ama-assn.org/delivering-care/patient-support-advocacy/reducing-disparities-health-care

American Public Health Association. (n.d.). *The power of advocacy.* Retrieved September 30, 2022, from https://www.apha.org/-/media/Files/PDF/advocacy/Power_of_Advocacy.ashx

American Speech-Language-Hearing Association. (2021). *Cultural competence check-in: Self-reflection.* https://www.asha.org/siteassets/uploadedfiles/multicultural/self-reflection-checklist.pdf

Andermann, A. (2016). Taking action on the social determinants of health in clinical practice: A framework for health professionals. *Canadian Medical Association Journal, 188*(17–18), E475–E482. https://doi.org/10.1503/cmaj.160177

Andermann, A. (2018). Screening for social determinants of health in clinical care: Moving from the margins to mainstream. *Public Health Reviews, 39*(19), 1–17. https://doi.org/10.1186/s40985-018-0094-7

Braveman, P. (2014). What are health disparities and health equity? We need to be clear. *Public Health Reports, 129*(2), 5–8. https://doi.org/10.1177/00333549141291S203

Braveman, P. A., Kumanyika, S., Fielding, J., LaVeist, T., Borrell, L. N., Manderscheid, R., & Troutman, A. (2011). Health disparities and health equity: The issue is justice. *American Journal of Public Health, 101*(Suppl. 1), S149–S155. https://doi.org/10.2105/AJPH.2010.300062

Burton, E. C., Bennett, D. H., & Burton, L. M. (2020). COVID-19: Health disparities and social determinants of health. *International Social Work, 63*(6), 771–776. https://doi.org/10.1177/0020872820944985

Carratala, S., & Maxwell, C. (2020, May 7). *Health disparities by race and ethnicity.* Center for American Progress. https://www.americanprogress.org/issues/race/reports/2020/05/07/484742/health-disparities-race-ethnicity

Cassoobhoy, A., Sardana, J. J., Benigas, S., Tips, J., & Kee, A. (2021). Building health equity: Action steps from the American College of Lifestyle Medicine's Health Disparities Solutions Summit (HDSS) 2020. *American Journal of Lifestyle Medicine, 16*(1), 61–75. https://doi.org/ https://doi.org/10.1177/15598276211052248

Centers for Disease Control and Prevention (CDC). (2020). *Health disparities.* https://www.cdc.gov/healthyyouth/disparities/index.htm

Centers for Disease Control and Prevention. (2023, April 7). *CDC Research on SDOH.* https://www.cdc.gov/publichealthgateway/sdoh/research.html

Chandra, A., Acosta, J. D., Carman, K. G., Dubowitz, T., Leviton, L., Martin, L. T., Miller, C., Nelson, C., Orleans, T., Tait, M., Truijillo, M. D., Towe, V. L., Yeung, D., & Plough, A. L. (2017). Building a national culture of health: Background, action framework, measures, and next steps. *Rand Health Quarterly, 6*(2), 3.

Fiori, K. P., Heller, C. G., Rehm, C. D., Parsons, A., Flattau, A., Braganza, S., Lue, K., Luaria, M., & Racine, A. (2020). Unmet social needs and no-show visits in primary care in a US northeastern urban health system, 2018–2019. *American Journal of Public Health, 110*(52), S242–S250. https://doi.org/10.2105/AJPH.2020.305717

FitzGerald, C., & Hurst, S. (2017). Implicit bias in healthcare professionals: A systematic review. *BMC Medical Ethics, 18*(19). https://doi.org/10.1186/s12910-017-0179-8

Foronda, C., Reinholdt, M. M., & Ousman, K. (2016). Cultural humility: A concept analysis. *Journal of Transcultural Nursing, 27*(3), 210–217. https://doi.org/10.1177/1043659615592677

Francis, L., DePriest, K., Wilson, M., & Gross, D. (2018). Child poverty, toxic stress, and social determinants of health: Screening and care coordination. *Online Journal of Issues in Nursing, 23*(3), 2. https://doi.org/10.3912/OJIN.Vol23No03Man02

Freire, P. (2007). *Pedagogy of the oppressed.* Continuum.

Gerber, L. (2018). Understanding the nurse's role as a patient advocate. *Nursing, 48*(4), 55–58. https://doi.org/10.1097/01.NURSE.0000531007.02224.65

Gibbons, M. C. (2005). A historical overview of health disparities and the potential of eHealth solutions. *Journal of Medical Internet Research, 7*(5), e50–e56. https://doi.org/10.2196/jmir.7.5.e50

Gopal, D. P., Chetty, U., O'Donnell, P., Gajria, C., & Blackadder-Weinstein, J. (2021). Implicit bias in healthcare: Clinical practice, research and decision making. *Future Healthcare Journal, 8*(1), 40–48. https://doi.org/10.7861/fhj.2020-0233

Halfon, N., Larson, K., Son, J., Lu, M., & Bethell, C. (2017). Income inequality and the differential effect of adverse childhood experiences in US children. *Academic Pediatrics, 17*(7), S70–S78. https://doi.org/10.1016/j.acap.2016.11.007

Hall, W. J., Chapman, M. V., Lee, K. M., Merino, Y. M., Thomas, T. W., Payne, B. K., Eng, E., Day, S. H., & Coyne-Beasley, T. (2015). Implicit racial/ethnic bias among health care professionals and its influence on health care outcomes: A systematic review. *American Journal of Public Health, 105*(12), e60–e76. https://doi.org/10.2105/AJPH.2015.302903

Hooper, M. W., Napoles, A. M., & Perez-Stable, E. J. (2020). COVID-19 and racial/ethnic disparities. *JAMA, 323*(24), 2466–2467. https://doi.org/10.1001/jama.2020.8598

Institute of Medicine. (2011). *The future of nursing: Leading change, advancing health.* National Academies Press. https://doi.org/10.17226/12956

Interprofessional Education Collaborative. (2016). *Core competencies for interprofessional collaborative practice: 2016 update.* https://www.ipecollaborative.org/ipec-core-competencies

Kanter, G. P., Segal, A. G., & Groeneveld, P. W. (2020). Income disparities in access to critical care services. *Health Affairs, 39*(8), 1362–1367. https://doi.org/10.1377/hlthaff.2020.00581

Kreuter, M. W., Thompson, T., McQueen, A., & Garg, R. (2021). Addressing social needs in health care settings: Evidence, challenges, and opportunities for public health. *Annual Review of Public Health, 42,* 329–344. https://doi.org/10.1146/annurev-publhealth-090419-102204

Lathrop, B. (2020). Moving toward health equity by addressing social determinants of health. *Nursing for Women's Health, 24*(1), 36–44. https://doi.org/10.1016/j.nwh.2019.11.003

Mancilla, V. J., Peeri, N. C., Silzer, T., Basha, R., Felini, M., Jones, H. P., Phillips, N., Tao, M., Thyagarajan, S., & Vishwanatha, J. K. (2020). Understanding the interplay between health disparities and epigenomics. *Frontiers in Genetics, 11*(903), 1–14. https://doi.org/10.3389/fgene.2020.00903

Marcelin, J. R., Siraj, D. S., Victor, R., Kotadia, S., & Maldonado, Y. A. (2019). The impact of unconscious bias in healthcare: How to recognize and mitigate it. *Journal of Infectious Diseases, 220* (Suppl. 2), S62–S73. https://doi.org/10.1093/infdis/jiz214

Matwick, A. L., & Woodgate, R. L. (2017). Social justice: A concept analysis. *Public Health Nursing, 34*(2), 176–184. https://doi.org/10.1111/phn.12288

Miyagawa, L. A. (2020, March 16). *Practicing cultural humility when serving immigrant and refugee communities.* https://ethnomed.org/resource/practicing-cultural-humility-when-serving-immigrant-and-refugee-communities

National Academies of Medicine. (2017). *Communities in action: Pathways to equity.* National Academies Press. https://doi.org/10.17226/24624

National Academies of Sciences, Engineering, and Medicine. (2016). *Parenting matters: Supporting parents of children ages 0–8.* National Academies Press. https://doi.org/10.17226/21868

National Academies of Sciences, Engineering, and Medicine. (2021). *The future of nursing 2020–2030: Charting a path to achieve health equity.* National Academies Press. https://doi.org/10.17226/25982

National Institutes of Health. (2017). *Health disparities.* http://www.nhlbi.nih.gov/health/educational/healthdisp

Ndugga, N., & Artiga, S. (2021, May 11). *Disparities in health and health care: Five key questions and answers.* Kaiser Family Foundation. https://www.kff.org/racial-equity-and-health-policy/issue-brief/disparities-in-health-and-health-care-five-key-questions-and-answers

Neathery, M. (2018). Treatment and spiritual care in mental health: Recovery as a journey, not a destination. *Journal of Christian Nursing, 35*(2), 86–93. https://doi.org/10.1097/CNJ.0000000000000475

Office of Disease Prevention and Health Promotion. (n.d.-a). *Disparities.* Retrieved September 30, 2022, from https://www.healthypeople.gov/2020/about/foundation-health-measures/Disparities

Office of Disease Prevention and Health Promotion. (n.d.-b). *Environmental health.* Retrieved September 30, 2022, from https://health.gov/healthypeople/objectives-and-data/browse-objectives/environmental-health

Office of Disease Prevention and Health Promotion. (n.d.-c). *Health equity in Healthy People 2030.* Retrieved September 30, 2022, from https://health.gov/healthypeople/priority-areas/health-equity-healthy-people-2030

Office of Disease Prevention and Health Promotion. (n.d.-d). *Healthy People 2030: Leading health indicators.* Retrieved September 30, 2022, from https://health.gov/healthypeople/objectives-and-data/leading-health-indicators

Office of Disease Prevention and Health Promotion. (n.d.-e). *Increase the proportion of people with health insurance—AHS-01.* Retrieved September 30, 2022, from https://health.gov/healthypeople/objectives-and-data/browse-objectives/health-care-access-and-quality/increase-proportion-people-health-insurance-ahs-01

Office of Disease Prevention and Health Promotion. (n.d.-f). *Healthy People 2030: Social determinants of health.* Retrieved February 20, 2023, from https://health.gov/healthypeople/priority-areas/social-determinants-health

O'Gurek, D. T., & Henke, C. (2018). A practical approach to screening for social determinants of health. *American Academy of Family Physicians, 25*(3), 7–12.

Peretz, P. J., Ismal, N., & Matiz, L. A. (2020). Community health workers and COVID-19: Addressing social determinants of health in times of crisis and beyond.

New England Journal of Medicine, *383*(19), e108. https://doi.org/10.1056/NEJMp2022641

Phillips, J., Richard, A., Mayer, K. M., Shilkatis, M., Fogg, L. F., & Vondracek, H. (2020). Integrating the social determinants of health into nursing practice: Nurses' perspectives. *Journal of Nursing Scholarship*, *52*(5), 497–505. https://doi.org/ 10.1111/jnu.12584

Plough, A. L. (2015). Building a culture of health: A critical role for public health services and systems research. *American Journal of Public Health*, *105*(S2), S150–S152. https://doi.org/ 10.2105/AJPH.2014.302410

Robichaux, C., & Sauerland, J. (2021). The social determinants of health, COVID-19, and structural competence. *Online Journal of Issues in Nursing*, *26*(2). https://doi.org/10.3912/OJIN.Vol26No02PPT67

Selden, T. M., & Berdahl, T. A. (2020). COVID-19 and racial/ethnic risk disparities in health risk, employment, and household composition. *Health Affairs*, *39*(9), 1624–1632. https://doi.org/10.1377/hlthaff.2020.00897

Stepanikova, I., & Oates, G. (2017). Perceived discrimination and privilege in health care: The role of socioeconomic status and race. *American Journal of Preventive Medicine*, *52*(1 Suppl. 1), S86–S94. https://doi.org/10.1016/j.amepre.2016.09.024

Stronks, K., Toebes, B., Hendriks, A., Ikram, U., & Venkatapuram, D. (2016). *Social justice and human rights as a framework for addressing social determinants of health: Final report to the Task Group on Equity, Equality, and Human Rights*. World Health Organization. https://apps.who.int/iris/handle/10665/350401

Sun, M., Oliwa, T., Peek, M. E., & Tung, E. L. (2022). Negative patient descriptors: Documenting racial bias in the electronic health record. *Health Affairs*, *41*(2), 1–9. https://doi.org/10.1377/hlthaff.2021.01423

Sundar, K. R. (2020). A patient with COVID-19 is left behind as care goes viral. *Health Affairs*, *39*(8), 1453–1455. https://doi.org/10.1377/hlthaff.2020.00447

United Nations. (2006). *Social justice in an open world: The role of the United Nations*. https://www.un.org/esa/socdev/documents/ifsd/SocialJustice.pdf

University of Wisconsin Population Health Institute. (2022). *2022 County health rankings national findings report*. https://www.countyhealthrankings.org/reports/2022-county-health-rankings-national-findings-report

Wang, L., Du, M., Cudhea, F., Griecci, C., Michaud, D. S., Mozaffarian, D., & Zhang, F. F. (2021). Disparities in health and economic burdens of cancer attributable to suboptimal diet in the United States, 2015–2018. *American Journal of Public Health*, *111*(11), 2008–2018. https://doi.org/ 10.2105/AJPH.2021.306475

Weigel, G., Ramaswamy, A., Sobel, L., Salganicoff, A., Cubanski, J., & Freed, M. (2020, May 11). *Opportunities and barriers for telemedicine in the U.S. during the COVID-19 emergency and beyond*. https://www.kff.org/womens-health-policy/issue-brief/opportunities-and-barriers-for-telemedicine-in-the-u-s-during-the-covid-19-emergency-and-beyond

Whitehead, M. (1992). The concepts and principles of equity and health. *International Journal of Health Services*, *22*(3), 429–445. https://doi.org/10.2190/986L-LHQ6-2VTE-YRRN

Williams, S. D., Phillips, J. M., & Koyama, K. (2018). Nurse advocacy: Adopting a health in all policies approach. *Online Journal of Issues in Nursing*, *23*(3). https://doi.org/10.3912/OJIN.Vol23No03Man01

World Health Organization. (2010). *A conceptual framework for action on the social determinants of health*. https://www.who.int/publications/i/item/9789241500852

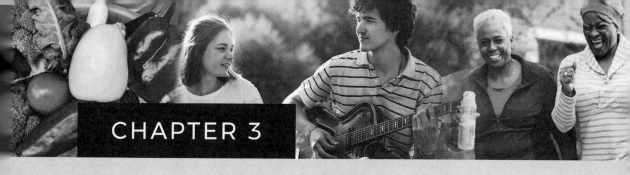

CHAPTER 3

Theoretical Approaches to Health Promotion and Disease Prevention

Cindy Farris, PhD, MSN, MPH, BSN, CNE
Megan Amaya, PhD, CHES, NBC-HWC

Nothing is more practical than a good theory.

Kurt Lewin (1951, p. 169)

OBJECTIVES

This chapter will enable the reader to:

1. Examine how theories and models inform health promotion and disease prevention in advanced practice.
2. Describe characteristics and concepts of select health behavior, healthcare, nursing, and program planning theories and models relevant to health promotion.
3. Discuss the application of select theories and models and implications for promoting individual and population health in advanced practice.
4. Consider factors for selecting appropriate theories to design health promotion interventions for patients or populations.

Overview

A theory presents a systematic way of understanding events or situations (Rural Health Information Hub, n.d.) and can inform the development of health promotion and disease prevention strategies and programs. Health behavior theories and models draw upon various disciplines, such as psychology, sociology, anthropology, consumer behavior, and marketing. These theories and models give clinicians and planners tools for moving beyond intuition to design and evaluate health behavior and health promotion interventions based on an understanding of behavior. A good theory can help one step back, consider

© Kathleen Gail/Shutterstock; © StoryTime Studio/Shutterstock; © kali9/Getty Images

the larger picture, and develop measurable program objectives (Sharma & Romas, 2012). Theories become useful when filled with practical topics, goals, and solutions. Models may draw on several theories to help understand a particular problem in a specific setting or context.

According to Rimer and Glanz (2005), theory provides a road map for studying problems developing appropriate interventions and evaluating their effectiveness. Advanced practice providers (APPs) can use theory and strategic planning models to identify the most relevant target audiences, develop and manage health programs, and increase effectiveness and efficiency through meaningful evaluation (Sharma & Romas, 2012). Health promotion theory thus plays a critical role throughout the program planning process. Using theory as a foundation for program planning and development is consistent with the continued emphasis on using evidence-informed interventions in public health, behavioral health, medicine, and nursing. Program planning, implementation, and evaluation based on theory are more likely to succeed than those developed without the benefit of a theoretical perspective (Rimer & Glanz, 2005).

APPs will often find it necessary to motivate patients to take ownership of their health and wellness. When used in clinical practice, theories and models help APPs understand possible approaches for supporting healthy lifestyle behavior change. Theory guides interactions with patients, informs the comprehensiveness of the assessment and questions asked, impacts the strategies chosen for fostering and supporting change, and influences methods for evaluating patient outcomes.

Multiple health promotion theories exist due to varied health problems, behaviors, populations, cultures, and contexts for health promotion (Rimer & Glanz, 2005). This chapter will examine several health promotion and behavior change theories and their implications for advanced practice. Also addressed are considerations for selecting appropriate theories when designing health promotion interventions. The more APPs can implement strategies grounded in evidence-informed theories, the more significant the improvement in patient and population health outcomes.

Prevailing Health Behavior Theories and Models

There is no all-encompassing theory or model related to health behavior change. Commonly used theories and models for understanding health behavior include the theory of reasoned action, theory of planned behavior, social cognitive theory, self-determination theory, social-ecological model, health belief model, and transtheoretical model (see **Table 3.1** for a summary of these health behavior theories and models). These theories and models help to explain why people behave in specific ways regarding their health practices. They also suggest practical ways to influence health behavior change.

Theory of Reasoned Action and Theory of Planned Behavior

The theory of reasoned action (TRA) (Fishbein & Ajzen, 1975) and the associated theory of planned behavior (TPB) (Ajzen, 1985) explore the relationships between a behavior and the beliefs, attitudes, and intentions related to the behavior. The TRA and TPB assume that *behavioral intention* is the most important determinant of behavior. According to the TRA, behavioral intention is influenced by a person's *attitude* toward performing a behavior and *subjective norm*, their belief about whether individuals who are significant to them approve or disapprove of the behavior (**Figure 3.1**). The

Table 3.1 Health Behavior Theories and Models

Theory/Model	Author(s)	Key Constructs	Practical Application
Health belief model (HBM)	Leventhal, Kegeles, Hockbaum, and Rosenstock, 1950s	■ Perceived susceptibility ■ Perceived severity ■ Perceived benefits ■ Perceived barriers ■ Cue to action ■ Self-efficacy	■ Helps patients develop an accurate perception of their own risk and vulnerability ■ Provides education ■ Discusses barriers and challenges and ways to overcome them ■ Identifies cues that may trigger behavior change ■ Discusses confidence in the ability to participate in healthy behavior
Self-determination theory (SDT)	Deci and Ryan (1985)	■ Motivation ■ Autonomy ■ Competence ■ Relatedness	■ Supports patients' need for autonomy, competence, and relatedness by using open-ended questions, affirmations, reflections, and summaries
Social cognitive theory (SCT)	Bandura (1986)	■ Reciprocal determinism ■ Behavioral capability ■ Expectations ■ Self-efficacy ■ Observational learning ■ Reinforcements	■ Works with patients to set goals, behavior contracts, monitoring, and reinforcement
Social–ecological model (SEM)	Bronfenbrenner (1977)	■ Intrapersonal factors ■ Interpersonal processes and primary groups ■ Institutional factors ■ Community factors ■ Public policy	■ Influences knowledge, beliefs, and attitudes ■ Influences social connections ■ Partners to facilitate healthy change in the physical environment ■ Influences initiatives or policies ■ Champions policies at the local or state level
■ Theory of reasoned action (TRA) ■ Theory of planned behavior (TPB)	Fishbein and Ajzen (1975); Ajzen (1985)	■ Behavioral intention ■ Attitude ■ Subjective norm ■ Perceived behavioral control	■ Understands attitudes and beliefs as well as influencers ■ Offers solutions that resonate with values
Transtheoretical model (TTM)	Prochaska and DiClemente (1983)	■ Precontemplation ■ Contemplation ■ Preparation ■ Action ■ Maintenance	■ Includes education ■ Utilizes motivational interviewing ■ Emphasizes the benefits ■ Helps patients set behavior goals ■ Provides support and reinforcement

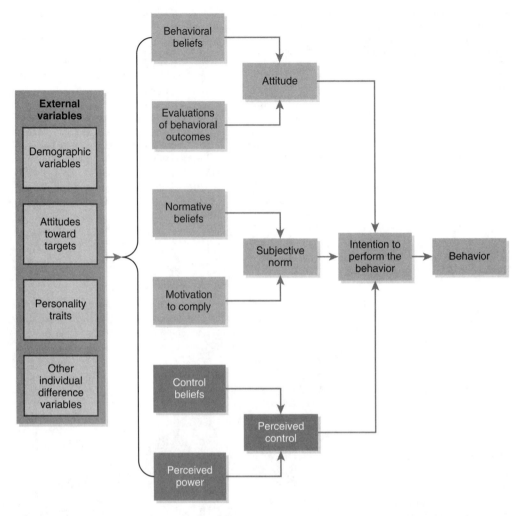

Figure 3.1 Theory of reasoned action and theory of planned behavior.

White boxes show the theory of reasoned action; the entire figure shows the theory of planned behavior.

Amalathas, T., Brande, S., Catalano, J., & Lucano, I. G. (n.d.). *Models and mechanisms of public health*. https://courses.lumenlearning.com/suny-buffalo-environmentalhealth/chapter/measurement-and
-application-of-constructs/ [CC LICENSED CONTENT, ORIGINAL. Authored by: Tereka Amalathas, Spencer Brande, Joe Catalano, Isaac G Lucano. Located at: https://courses.lumenlearning.com/suny-buffalo-
environmentalhealth/. License info: https://creativecommons.org/licenses/by-nc-sa/4.0/]

TPB differs from the TRA in that it includes one additional construct, *perceived behavioral control*. This construct has to do with individuals' belief that they can control a particular behavior. This construct was added to account for situations in which people's behavior, or behavioral intention, is influenced by factors beyond their control.

Implications for Practice

The TRA and TPB have been frequently used as a framework and predictive mechanism of applied research on sexual behavior, especially in the prevention of sexually transmitted diseases. A 2018 study examining the prediction of condom use in 18- to 25-year-olds found that the TRA and TPB predicted that participants with the intention to use a condom were more likely to do so (Gomes & Nunes, 2018). The investigation used a cross-sectional survey design measuring intrapersonal variables (attitude toward condoms), perceived behavioral control (sexual risk behavior beliefs), sexual satisfaction and sexual self-esteem, subjective norm (perception of the pressure a partner exerted to use or not use condoms), interpersonal variables (parental communication about sex), and situational variables (alcohol use, social). A confirmatory analysis found that the model was predictive of behavior. By understanding patients' attitudes, beliefs, and what influences their decisions, APPs can offer solutions that resonate with the patients' belief system and, ultimately, have a better chance of influencing them to make healthy decisions.

Social Cognitive Theory

The social cognitive theory (SCT) (Bandura, 1986) describes a dynamic, ongoing process of learning that occurs within a social context. SCT evolved from Bandura's research on the social learning theory, which asserts that people learn not only from their own experiences but also by observing the actions of others and the benefits of those actions. Bandura updated the social learning theory, adding the construct of self-efficacy and renaming it SCT. SCT integrates concepts and processes from cognitive, behaviorist, and emotional models of behavior change. The theory accounts for specifics of behavior, the influence of individual experiences, actions of others, and environmental factors on health behavior.

Key constructs of SCT include the following:

1. *Reciprocal determinism*: Interactions and influences among behavior, personal factors, and the environment. Bandura theorized that a person's behavior influences and is influenced by personal factors and the social environment.

2. *Behavioral capability*: To perform a behavior, one must know what and how to do it.

3. *Outcome expectations*: The results an individual anticipates from taking action. Outcome expectations can be health related (e.g., weight loss) or non–health related (e.g., affirmation from others).

4. *Self-efficacy*: Belief in one's own capacity to execute behaviors necessary to produce specific performance attainments (Bandura, 1977, 1986, 1997). If individuals have a sense of self-efficacy, they can change behaviors even when faced with obstacles. If they do not feel they can exercise control over their health behavior, they are not motivated to act or persist through challenges. Bandura considered self-efficacy the most important personal factor in behavior change. There are four sources of efficacy (Bandura, 1977, 1986, 1997):

   • *Mastery experiences*: Experience one gains when taking on a new challenge and is successful. One of the best ways to learn a new skill or improve one's performance is by practicing.

   • *Vicarious experiences*: Observing other people completing a task or behavior successfully.

   • *Verbal persuasion*: Receiving positive verbal feedback while undertaking a complex task persuades individuals to believe they have the skills and capabilities to succeed.

   • *Physiological state*: Individual's emotional, physical, and psychological well-being can influence how they feel about their abilities in a particular situation. For example, if someone has an injury, he or she might find it harder to perform specific exercises.

5. *Observational learning*, or modeling: The process whereby individuals learn through the experiences of others rather than through their own experience.

6. *Reinforcements*: Responses to behavior will affect whether one will repeat it. Positive reinforcements (rewards) increase a person's likelihood of repeating the behavior. Negative reinforcements may make repeated behavior more likely by motivating the person to eliminate a negative stimulus (e.g., when drivers put the key in the car's ignition, the beeping alarm reminds them to fasten their seat belt). Reinforcements can be internal or external. Internal rewards are psychological outcomes, such as the feeling of accomplishment or a positive emotional reaction. External rewards (e.g., token incentives) can encourage continued participation in multiple-session programs. However, they are generally ineffective for sustaining long-term change because they do not bolster a person's desire or commitment to change.

Implications for Practice

The SCT is used in many health promotion interventions. The research shows that self-efficacy and goal setting are the strongest determinants of physical activity and healthy eating (Anderson-Bill et al., 2011; Bagherniya et al., 2018; Doerksen & McAuley, 2014; Stacy et al., 2016; Young et al., 2014). Strategies for successful behavior change include setting incremental goals (e.g., exercising for 10 minutes each day), behavioral contracting (a formal contract with specified goals and rewards), and monitoring and reinforcement (feedback from self-monitoring or record keeping). APPs can discuss these components with their patients to facilitate successful behavior change.

Self-Determination Theory

The SDT (Deci & Ryan, 1985) represents a broad framework for studying human motivation. SDT posits that the extent to which an individual's environment nurtures and meets three primary psychological needs (autonomy, competence, relatedness), self-regulation of behavior can occur (Moore et al., 2016; **Figure 3.2**). Conditions supporting the individual's experience of autonomy, competence, and relatedness are argued to foster motivation and engagement for activities, including enhanced performance, persistence, and creativity. Additionally, self-determination proposes that the degree to which any of these three psychological needs is unsupported or thwarted within a social context will have a robust detrimental impact on wellness in that setting.

Implications for Practice

A person experiencing high, autonomous motivation is more likely to have more remarkable persistence, flexibility and creativity, interest and enjoyment; better health; and a higher quality of close personal relationships (Ryan, 2013). In a study by Martin et al. (2017), college students who believed that their APPs supported their autonomy in pursuing exercise had stronger perceived confidence than students who viewed their healthcare practitioner as less supportive of autonomy. Students also exhibited more mindfulness behavior. When working with patients, APPs can employ open-ended questions to spark patients' thoughts about their motivation, strengths, and opportunities. This approach supports their need for autonomy, competency, and relatedness and can lead to an unexpected intrinsic motivation and self-determination to change behavior. One health coaching model that health professionals can use is Miller and Rollick's (2012) OARS model:

- *Open-ended questions*: Asking open-ended questions gives APPs insight into the patients' experiences, thoughts, beliefs, and feelings and helps to build a trusting, professional relationship.

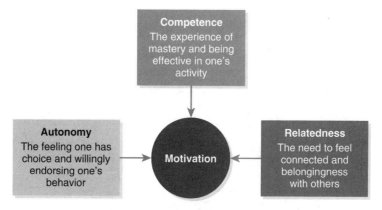

Figure 3.2 Self-determination theory.

Reproduced with permssion from Ryan, R., & Deci, R. (n.d.). *Self-determination theory.* Behavior Institute. https://www.besci.org/models/self-determination -theory

- *Affirmations*: Affirming the patients' responses develops rapport and affirms their strengths, thereby allowing APPs to build on the patients' level of self-efficacy and encourage them to take responsibility for their own decisions.
- *Reflections:* Offering reflections conveys to the patients that they have been heard. Reflections are not limited to patients' words but also include their emotions and behavior.
- *Summaries:* Summarizing the conversation demonstrates that APPs understand the patients' goals and provides an opportunity to check the patients' understanding of the key elements of the plan developed together.

Social-Ecological Model

The SEM helps APPs understand the range of factors affecting behavior and the interplay among individuals, relationships, communities, and societal factors (**Figure 3.3**). The principles of this model are consistent with SCT concepts, which suggest that creating an environment conducive to change is essential for making it easier to adopt healthy behaviors (Office of Behavioral and Social Sciences Research, 2016). The tenets of the SEM recognize that individuals are embedded within larger social systems, and they describe the interactive characteristics of individuals and environments that underlie health outcomes. Building on the multilevel framework of the ecological systems theory, developed by Bronfenbrenner (1977), McLeroy et al. (1988) emphasized five levels of influence specific to health behavior: intrapersonal factors, interpersonal processes and primary groups, organizational factors, community factors, and public policy. They also posited the idea that behaviors both shape and are shaped by the social environment.

Many community settings use the multilevel strategies of the SEM to address whole-community health issues (Wold & Mittlemark, 2018). Within health promotion, ecological approaches have been used as foundations for program planning and evaluation as well as to better understand determinants of health behaviors (Glasgow et al., 1999; Green & Kreuter, 1999).

Implications for Practice

A program guided by the SEM might include intervention strategies at the following levels:

- *Individual*: Influencing patient knowledge, skill, and attitudes for health behavior

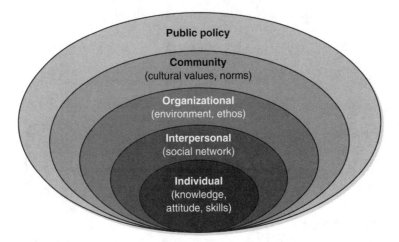

Figure 3.3 Social–ecological model.

Alghzawi, H. M., & Ghanem, F. K. (2021). Social ecological model and underage drinking: A theoretical review and evaluation. *Psychology, 12*(5), 817–828. https://doi.org/ 10.4236/psych.2021.125050

change through screening, patient education, or coaching. For example, APPs might screen for tobacco use and educate about the serious health consequences of smoking. Knowledge is not enough, but it creates awareness and helps to stimulate attitude toward behavior change.

- *Interpersonal*: Facilitating change by influencing the patients' social connections (e.g., family, friends, community) or using health champions and patient navigators to support and encourage them with behavior change. Using the smoking example, APPs might explore with patients who they can enlist in their social network to support the behavior change.
- *Organizational*: Facilitating change by influencing social institutions, such as workplaces, places of worship, or educational institutions, to develop health promotion initiatives or policies. An example could be promoting a smoke-free workplace policy to discourage smoking or sponsoring a smoking cessation class at a local church.

- *Community*: Becoming involved with community leaders and coalitions to impact community development and leverage resources and services for health promotion. For example, APPs could partner with a community advocacy group to facilitate healthy change in the physical environment, such as tobacco-free policies and ordinances.
- *Public policy*: Becoming involved at the legislative and regulatory level to influence change in areas such as policy, laws, and taxes. APPs may champion policies at the local or state level that promote and support healthy behaviors, such as state-wide laws prohibiting tobacco use in public spaces.

APPs do not need to be involved at all levels of the SEM. Instead, they may decide where their greatest impact can be and focus their energy and efforts on that specific level.

Health Belief Model

The health belief model (HBM; Rosenstock, 1974), one of the first health behavior theories, was developed by U.S. Public Health Service psychologists to understand why so few people adopted disease prevention strategies or participated in screening tests for the early detection of disease. Later uses of the HBM were for patients' responses to symptoms and compliance with medical treatments and for developing health policy.

Major concepts of the HBM include (a) *perceived susceptibility* to a condition, illness, or disease and *perceived severity* (e.g., death, disability, impact on others) and (b) *perceived benefits* and *perceived barriers* to preventive or treatment strategies. If a person perceives little threat of the condition or its severity or perceives little benefits or significant barriers to change, successful behavior change is unlikely. Additional concepts in this theory include *self-efficacy* and *cues to action*, stimuli needed to trigger the decision to accept a recommended health action. Cues can be internal (e.g., chest pains, wheezing) or external (e.g., advice from others, illness of a family member, newspaper article; **Figure 3.4**).

In a recent randomized controlled trial, the HBM was used to impact women's knowledge and perceived beliefs about the warning signs of cancer (Sharifikia et al., 2019). The intervention group received educational content focused on the warning signs of cancers, highly ranked cancers in the population, risk factors, and healthy lifestyle behaviors. The control group received the educational material after the posttest and completion of the study. All the HBM constructs significantly increased in the intervention group compared to the control group.

Implications for Practice

Using type 2 diabetes as an example, APPs can consider implementing various strategies based on the model's constructs.

- *Perceived susceptibility*: Help patients perceive their risk and vulnerability to developing diabetes by relating risk factors or screening for abnormal glucose levels.
- *Perceived severity*: Provide education about the consequences of diabetes.
- *Perceived benefits*: Offer education about how to take action and what the potential positive benefits will be if they do so.

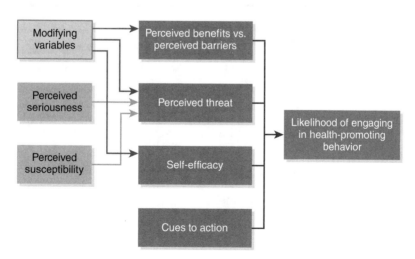

Figure 3.4 Health belief model.

Reproduced with permission from Levanthal, H., Kegeles, S. S., Hockbaum, G., & Rosenstock, I. (n.d.). *Health Belief Model*. Behavior Institute. https://www.besci.org/models/health-belief-model

- *Perceived barriers*: Discuss ways to overcome barriers and offer reassurance and assistance.
- *Cues to action*: Identify cues that may trigger behavior change (e.g., physical symptoms, diabetes in a family member).
- *Self-efficacy*: Discuss the patients' confidence in their ability to participate in a healthy behavior (e.g., exercise) to lower the risk of developing diabetes and help them to set goals for change.

Transtheoretical Model

The TTM, developed by Prochaska and DiClemente (1983), evolved out of studies comparing the experiences of smokers who quit on their own with those of smokers receiving professional treatment. The TTM's basic premise is that behavior change is a process, not an event. As individuals attempt to change a behavior, they move through five stages called the stages of change (Prochaska & Velicer, 1997; **Table 3.2**). It is important to note that how individuals pass through the stages

may vary, depending on the type of behavior change. For example, individuals trying to give up smoking may experience the stages differently from those seeking to improve their dietary habits. People do not systematically progress from one stage to the next, ultimately "graduating" from the behavior change process. Instead, they may enter the change process at any stage, relapse to an earlier stage, and begin the change process again.

Implications for Practice

In the clinical setting, APPs can work with patients to gauge their readiness to change and provide vital information for the patients to consider for behavior change. This process can be individualized based on the patients' current knowledge and stage.

- *Patients in precontemplation*: This stage provides an opportunity for increasing awareness and providing education. Share important information about a health condition and associated preventive behaviors.

Table 3.2 The TTM Stages of Change

Stage of Change	Description of Stage
Precontemplation	The individuals do not intend to take action in the foreseeable future, usually measured as the next six months.
Contemplation	The individuals intend to take action in the next six months. They are more aware of the pros of changing but are also aware of the cons. Weighing the costs and benefits of changing can produce ambivalence that can cause them to remain in this stage for long periods.
Preparation	The individuals intend to take action in the immediate future, usually measured as the next month. They have a plan of action, such as joining a gym, consulting a counselor, talking to their provider, or relying on a self-change approach.
Action	The individuals have made specific behavior changes within the past six months.
Maintenance	The individuals have maintained behavior change for six or more months and are working to prevent relapse. Those in maintenance grow increasingly confident that they can continue their new behavior.

Health Promotion Research Study

Applying the Chronic Care Model

Background: Vulnerable populations, such as the uninsured, should have access to chronic care management programs. Using the chronic care model (CCM) framework, effective clinical and self-management outcomes were developed for those with high-risk diabetes.

Methodology: A pilot program using the CCM framework was implemented to determine its effectiveness in improving clinical and self-management outcomes of high-risk patients with diabetes attending a free clinic for the uninsured. A pre-/postintervention design with an intentionally small sample size was planned for this pilot study. The inclusion criteria were active patients diagnosed with type 2 diabetes and a sustained hemoglobin A1C above 9 mg/dL. The exclusion criteria included patients without telephone access or who had a documented history of noncompliance regarding their health regimen. From a sample of 28 potential participants, 19 consented to participate, with 13 completing the pilot program.

Results: A comparison of baseline and posttest findings showed a statistically significant reduction in hemoglobin A1C but only a downward trend in blood pressure, triglycerides, and low-density lipoprotein (LDL) levels. All patients had documented self-management goals and reported high satisfaction with the program.

Implications for Advanced Practice: Practice implications include developing community relationships that can be essential for finding volunteer providers and case managers, free or low-cost medications, and access to community resources that will support the self-management efforts of patients. Educating community and political leaders on the social burden of chronic illness in the uninsured population may stimulate action to expand resources to promote self-management. Seeking opportunities for grant funding or partnerships to expand the use of health technology in underresourced clinics could positively impact serving the needs of this vulnerable population.

Reference: Data from Tillman, P. (2020). Applying the chronic care model in a free clinic. *Journal for Nurse Practitioners, 16*, e117ee121. https://doi.org/10.1016/j.nurpra.2020.05.016

- *Patients in contemplation*: Use motivational interviewing techniques to emphasize the benefits of making the change, increase motivation, and resolve ambivalence to change.
- *Patients in the preparation stage*: Continue emphasizing the benefits of making the desired change and help them set behavioral goals.
- *Patients in the action stage*: Provide support and reinforcement of the behavior change choice, including goal setting. Anticipate barriers and potential solutions.
- *Patients in the maintenance stage*: Continue to provide support and reinforcement if necessary.

Healthcare and Nursing Theories and Models for Health Promotion

APPs are charged with assisting their patients in achieving optimal health. Theoretical frameworks are useful for APPs to consider addressing behavioral changes, especially those strategies needed in health promotion and disease prevention. Although most health promotion theories can be relevant to aspects noted in primary care settings (Thomas et al., 2014), examples of theories and models developed from the unique perspective of health care and nursing include Nightingale's environmental theory, transcultural nursing theory, goal attainment theory, 5As framework, Pender's health promotion model, self-care model/self-care deficit theory, interaction model of client health behavior, and chronic care model. See **Table 3.3** for a summary of these theories and models.

Nightingale's Environmental Theory

During the Crimean War in the 1850s, Florence Nightingale was concerned with the environmental surroundings of the military patients (Rector & Stanley, 2022). Nightingale believed

Table 3.3 Select Healthcare and Nursing Theories and Models for Health Promotion

Theory/Model	Author(s)	Key Constructs	Practical Application
5As	Fiore et al. (2000); Glasgow et al. (2001)	■ Assess, advise, agree, assist, arrange	Completes a thorough assessment with patient and family input to enhance success.
Chronic care model (CCM)	MacColl Center for Health Care Innovation; Wagner (1998)	■ Health system ■ Self-management support ■ Delivery system design ■ Decision support ■ Clinical information systems ■ More applicable for ambulatory settings	■ Provides effective chronic disease management and affordable access to health care. ■ Shares knowledge of resources. ■ Advocates for health policy changes. ■ Emphasizes the development of self-care management skills and a thorough, effective plan of care that includes all parties.
Environment theory	Nightingale (1860)	■ Clean water, pure air, sufficient food supplies, cleanliness, sufficient light, and efficient drainage are important components directly related to the client's overall recovery. ■ Built community (social determinants of health)	Utilizes a holistic approach to assess the clients' home and work environment as factors impeding positive health outcomes.
Theory of goal attainment	King (as cited in George, 2002a)	■ Nurse and patient must work together in communicating information, setting goals, and then taking action to achieve those goals. ■ Mutual trust is key.	Collaborates with clients and families to set realistic goals with input from all parties.

Theory/Model	Author(s)	Key Constructs	Practical Application
Health promotion model (HPM)	Pender (2011)	■ Individual characteristics and experiences, behavior-specific cognitions and affect, and behavioral outcomes lead to motivation to change behavior. ■ Direct and indirect effects on the likelihood of engaging in health-promoting behaviors.	Assess the desire to change behavior and what and where the clients and families are in the process.
Interaction model of client health behavior (IMCHB)	Cox (1982, 2003)	■ Model is holistic and patient focused. ■ The client should have personal responsibility and control over the health promotion effort.	Involve patients and families in the decision for a change in health promotion, or behavior will not change.
Self-care model	Orem (2001)	■ Fully compensatory system ■ Partially compensatory system ■ Supportive-educative system	Assess self-management of the health problem and what stage the patients and families are in.
Transcultural theory	Leininger (as cited in George, 2002b)	■ Cultural beliefs affect health promotion and client behavior.	APPs need to address cultural health beliefs and health practices during the assessment.

that clean water, pure air, sufficient food supplies, cleanliness, sufficient light, and efficient drainage were essential components directly related to the patients' overall recovery. Her theory focuses on preventive care and control of the environment, which is imperative to enhancing the health outcomes of populations served by healthcare providers (Rector & Stanley, 2022). The application of Nightingale's environmental theory is very apparent in today's concerns about social determinants of health and designing healthy communities. The built community, an aspect of the social determinants of health, refers to all aspects of the human environment. Poor housing, lack of parks, and increased pollution are examples of how the built community can contribute to health issues (Jackson, 2012; **Figure 3.5**).

Implications for Practice

Nightingale's environmental theory is a patient-care theory based on the individual rather than on the nursing process. Environmental factors can affect the patient, thus interfering with patient health outcomes (Nursing Theory, 2020). Gilbert (2020) noted the importance of Nightingale's theory on contemporary infection control methods, which create

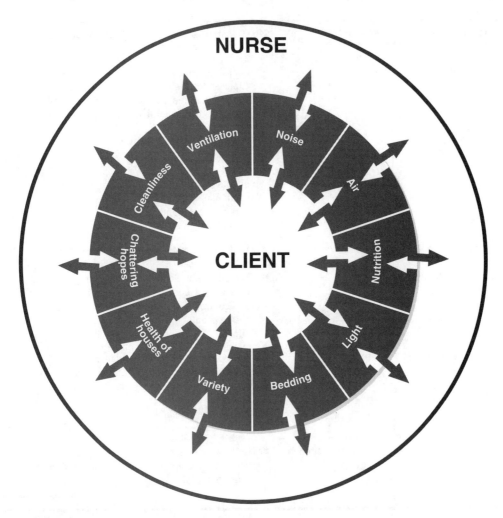

Figure 3.5 Nightingale's environmental theory.

Reproduced with permission from Nurseslabs. Gonzalo, A. (2023, January 12). *Florence Nightingale: Environmental theory.* https://nurseslabs.com/florence-nightingales-environmental-theory

a safe environment for effective healing and well-being that promotes healthy outcomes. APPs must be attuned to outside environmental factors that allow for the management of the patients' physical, psychological, nutritional, and overall well-being. A thorough assessment of environmental factors should be paramount during the patient assessment to provide a more holistic approach to improving health outcomes. APPs must also thoroughly assess the built community's possible impact on the health of their patients, families, and community.

Transcultural Nursing Theory

Culture is an important factor when discussing the health of the individual. Some patients have cultural health beliefs that could influence their understanding and adoption of proposed health promotion behaviors. For example, Asian/Pacific Islanders have a strong sense of family, and the oldest male in the family makes healthcare decisions. Hispanic populations rely on family and religion when making decisions that affect their health

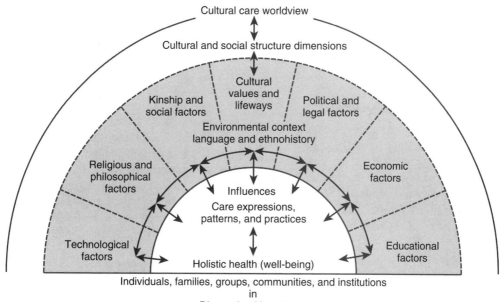

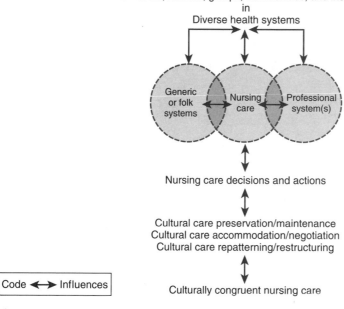

Figure 3.6 Leininger's sunrise model.

Data from Leininger, M. M. (1991). *Culture, care, diversity, and universality: A theory of nursing.* National League for Nursing Press.

(EuroMed Info, 2021). APPs must be culturally sensitive and competent to address health promotion concepts with their patients.

Leininger's transcultural nursing theory addresses the extent that culture can affect the behaviors of individuals, families, communities, and populations (George, 2002b). The sunrise model of Leininger's theory depicts the contexts (political, legal, economic, educational, cultural beliefs, kinship, and technological) through which patients develop culture and social structure and demonstrates the interrelations of the concepts of the theory (**Figure 3.6**). Understanding these factors fosters a therapeutic relationship between patients and APPs, influences patient care, and enables culturally congruent health promotion for patients from diverse backgrounds and ethnicities (George, 2002b).

Implications for Practice

APPs must examine cultural health beliefs and practices to provide a thorough approach to effective health outcomes. Additionally, many components of Leininger's model can be utilized as diversity and cultural differences arise in their practice settings. Chiatti (2019) used components of the sunrise model in collecting comprehensive data related to cultural aspects of life, health, and caring in Ethiopian immigrants who now reside in the United States. This qualitative ethnonursing research method enabled participants to express their meaning of care based on their cultural perspectives. Participants perceived healthcare providers who did not ask about culture, language preference, dietary practices, and family dynamics as not caring. This perception could jeopardize the patients' willingness to have further healthcare encounters and potentially negatively affect health outcomes.

Goal Attainment Theory

King's theory of goal attainment is based on the premise that APPs and clients must work together to identify a problem, communicate information, set goals, and then take actions to attain mutually agreed-upon health goals (George, 2022a). APPs must develop a trusting and effective relationship with their patients. The desired health outcome will not be achieved without establishing goals for health promotion through mutual development. Using the nursing process to achieve these goals is an emphasis in George's (2002a) model.

Implications for Practice

A practical application of King's theory of goal attainment to advanced practice is the research on APP and client interactions. Interactions such as disturbances, mutual goal setting, and transactions were observed. Interestingly, it was noted that *disturbances*, or health issues, identified during clinical encounters were essential in the progression toward goal attainment (Silva & Ferreira, 2016). Elements such as social exchange, symptom reporting, role explanation, and information around clinical processes strengthened the relationship and led to a greater degree of participation by the patients in goal attainment. APPs should reflect on their practice, embrace disturbances in the clinical encounter, and attend to these as opportunities for mutual goal setting (DeLeon-Demare et al., 2015; Silva & Ferreira, 2016).

5As Framework

Developed for tobacco cessation and widely adopted as a strategy for counseling a broad range of behaviors and health conditions, the 5As can provide a framework for the APP (Fiore et al., 2000; Glasgow et al., 2001). Using the 5As makes it possible to seek reimbursement from Medicare for obesity prevention and treatment (American Academy of Physician Assistants, 2014). Following are the 5As (Dowling, 2018):

- *Assess*: Ask about and assess behavioral health risks and factors affecting the choice of behavior change goals.
- *Advise*: Give clear, specific, and personalized behavior change advice, including information about personal health harms and benefits.
- *Agree*: Collaboratively select appropriate goals and strategies based on the patients' interest and willingness to change the behavior.
- *Assist*: Counsel the patients to achieve goals by acquiring the skills, confidence, and social and environmental support for behavior change. This step might be supplemented with adjunctive medical treatments when appropriate.
- *Arrange*: Schedule follow-up to provide ongoing help and support and adjust the plan as needed. This step may also include referral to intensive or specialized treatment.

Implications for Practice

Once a patient who needs health behavior change is identified, APPs can use the 5As to aid the patients as well as include a complete health history focusing on cause and associated risk factors. For example, for patients needing obesity management, APPs may ask them how they feel about their current weight in the assess step. During the advise step, APPs may request that patients keep a two-week food diary. In the agree phase, the patients and APPs agree to the desired outcome, such as losing 20 pounds in six months. During the assist step, the patients and APPs collaboratively set reasonable, specific short-term goals, and the APPs provide resources and ideas to further support the patients. In the arrange step, the APPs and patients establish a follow-up plan, such as sending in the food diary after two weeks or making a follow-up appointment in one month to gauge success.

Pender's Health Promotion Model

Pender's health promotion model (HPM) is one of the most widely used models for health promotion. This model describes the multidimensional nature of persons as they interact within their environment to pursue health, which is defined as a positive dynamic state directed at increasing patients' well-being rather than the absence of disease (Pender, 2011). Pender's model focuses on three areas: individual characteristics and experiences, behavior-specific cognitions and affect, and behavioral outcomes. The HPM notes that each person has unique personal features, experiences, and attitudes that affect motivation and subsequent actions toward health behavior change (Pender et al., 2015).

The major constructs of the HPM include the following:

1. *Individual characteristics and experiences* that influence health behavior, such as biological (e.g., age, body mass index, aerobic capacity), psychological (e.g., self-esteem, motivation, anxieties), and sociocultural (e.g., ethnicity, education, socioeconomic status) factors. Additionally, an individual's prior behavior, such as the frequency of similar behavior in the past, and positive or negative experiences with change, impact the likelihood of engaging in health-promoting behaviors.

2. *Behavior-specific cognition and affect* encompasses individuals' thinking about health behavior change, such as perceived benefits of action, perceived barriers to action, and perceived self-efficacy. *Activity-related affect* is the emotional response (positive or negative) to a behavior. Behaviors associated with positive affect are more likely to be repeated or maintained long term. Conversely, behaviors associated with negative affect are likely to be avoided. *Interpersonal influences*, such as the behaviors, beliefs, or attitudes of others, can influence behavior change. People are more likely to change a behavior if it is socially reinforced (e.g., social norms, modeling, positive support). *Situational influences*, such as a safe or toxic environment, can also facilitate or impede health behavior.

3. *Behavioral outcome* is the desired behavioral outcome and the endpoint in the HPM because these behaviors result in improved health, enhanced functional ability, and better quality of life at all stages of development. Within the behavioral outcome, there is a *commitment to a plan of action*, which is the concept of intention and identification of a planned strategy leading to the implementation of healthy behavior. However, *competing demands* that cannot be avoided and *competing preferences* that are not resisted have the potential to derail the plan (Pender, 2011; Pender et al., 2015).

Implications for Practice

The HPM can assist APPs in assessing and counseling patients on healthy lifestyles. It can also be a valuable framework for health education. Mansouri et al. (2020) used the HPM and the HBM in comparing the sexual function scores of females with type 2 diabetes. The study noted that utilizing an educational program based on both models had significant effects on the sexual function of females with type 2 diabetes. Using two models focused on health beliefs and, ultimately, the concept of health promotion provided a more comprehensive approach.

Self-Care Model/Self-Care Deficit Theory

Patients are more apt to change and maintain health behaviors if they take ownership of their behavior. In the theory of self-care, Orem (2001) focused on the performance of activities that individuals initiate on their own accord to maintain life, health, and well-being. Self-care requisites were noted that were critical to life processes and the maintenance of functioning, such as food, air, water, elimination, rest, social interaction, and safety. These requisites are similar to the components in Nightingale's environmental theory and Maslow's hierarchy of needs (Maslow, 1943). Orem believed that to stay alive, humans must engage in communication and connection with their environment and themselves and act deliberately to identify needs and make informed decisions.

Orem's model is composed of three interrelated theories: (a) the theory of self-care, which is further classified into wholly compensatory, partially compensatory, and supportive-educative; (b) the self-care deficit theory; and (c) the theory of nursing systems (Orem, 2001). A wholly compensatory system must provide total care because the patient cannot do self-care. A partially compensatory system allows the provider and patient to work together to accomplish appropriate and effective care. A supportive-educative system is where the practitioner would reinforce self-care aspects (Orem, 2001). The system patients are in depends on the illness and their need for assistance. APPs play a pivotal role in helping the patients with the self-care deficit theory. Orem identified five methods of helping: acting for and doing for others, guiding others, supporting others, providing an environment promoting personal development to meet future demands, and teaching others (Orem, 2001). Although Orem's self-care model was mainly focused on individuals, it can also be helpful in larger contexts, such as vulnerable populations.

Implications for Practice

Yip (2021) provided a practice update for APPs regarding the application of Orem's self-care deficit nursing theory. Research into the use of Orem's theory has been mostly limited to investigating the specific aspects of the theory rather than how the construct is practiced. The case study approach observed an APP who worked in an asthma clinic. A comparison was made between the case management of the APP and components of Orem's theory across four key operations: diagnostic, prescriptive, treatment, and case management. Even though there were strengths and limitations, the conclusion was that Orem's theory provided an effective framework in primary care settings for improving health outcomes by allowing the APP to foster the patient's ability to undertake self-care in chronic disease management.

Interaction Model of Client Health Behavior

The interaction model of client health behavior (IMCHB), developed by Cox (1982), is a person-centered and holistic health behavior model that is most useful in situations where the patient is personally responsible and has power and control over the health problem or health promotion effort. APPs must realize that individual patients have unique characteristics, knowledge, and personal responsibilities that affect their health behavior.

The IMCHB has three major elements:

1. *Client singularity* describes the unique intrapersonal and contextual configuration of the patient based on background variables (demographics, social influence, previous healthcare experience, and environmental resources) and dynamic variables (affective response to a health concern or issue, intrinsic motivation, and cognitive appraisal).

2. *Client–professional interaction* is the extent to which APPs attend to patients' singularity and tailor the intervention approach to that singularity. Components include emotional support, provision of health information, decision control, and professional or technical competencies.

3. *Health outcome* is concerned with health behavior or health state that is behaviorally related. Components include utilization of healthcare services, clinical health status indicators, the severity of healthcare problems, adherence to the recommended care regimen, and satisfaction with care (Cox, 1982; Kim et al., 2020; **Figure 3.7**).

Implications for Practice

Morales (2011) used the IMCHB to identify determinants of sedentary behavior in first-year college students. The study provided information on the modifiable determinants of sedentary behavior for use in intervention development to reduce or prevent overweight and obesity in this unique population. One of the best components of the IMCHB is acknowledging individuals' singular identity and the right to select health behaviors for their health promotion (Kim et al., 2020). APPs who take the time to understand the uniqueness of each patient and collaborate with the patient to develop individualized health promotion approaches can achieve positive health outcomes.

Chronic Care Model

The chronic care model (CCM) is an evidence-informed framework developed to prevent

and manage chronic disease (Holstein, 2018). Since noncommunicable diseases, also known as chronic diseases, account for 74% of deaths worldwide (World Health Organization, 2020), APPs must work effectively with populations with one or more chronic conditions. The CCM identifies the essential elements of a healthcare system that encourage high-quality chronic disease care (**Figure 3.8**). These elements include the community, health system, self-management support, delivery system design, decision support, and clinical information systems. The CCM has been used to improve ambulatory care and guide clinical quality initiatives in the United States (Wagner, 1998). The model can be applied to various chronic illnesses, healthcare situations, and target populations, making it very useful in all settings.

The CCM emphasizes the role of patients and their relationship with APPs to achieve optimal health outcomes. Evaluation of the use of the CCM is centered around increasing providers' expertise and skill, educating and supporting patients through patient-oriented interventions, and making better use of registry-based information systems (Renders et al., 2000). The key to effective health promotion and improving health outcomes in chronic diseases will be congruent chronic care management through continuity of care.

Implications for Practice

Holstein (2018) noted the importance of quality improvement in primary care to decrease the chronic disease burden. The emphasis should be on providing effective chronic disease management and affordable access to health care to improve the quality of life for individuals who are chronically ill. APPs can be change agents for the chronically ill by utilizing concepts in the CCM during provider–patient encounters. Other strategies include emphasizing self-care management skills; developing a thorough, effective plan of care that includes all parties; sharing knowledge of local, state, and

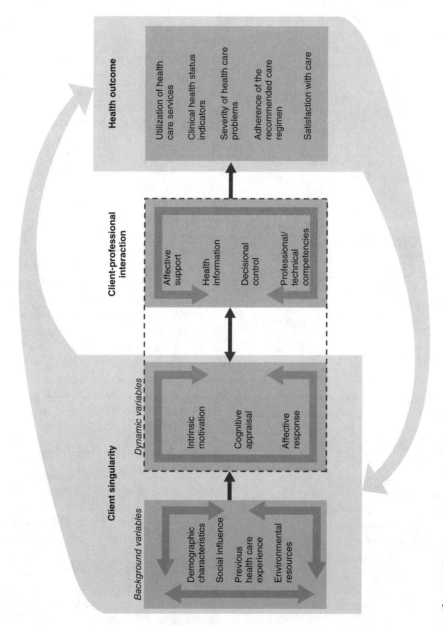

Figure 3.7 Interaction model of client behavior.

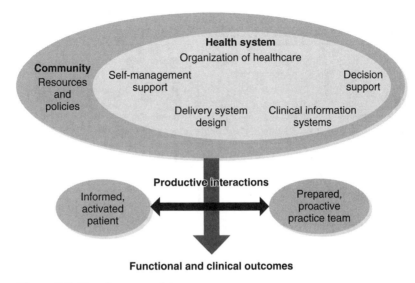

Figure 3.8 Chronic care model.

national resources; and leading health policy changes to reduce gaps in care for this vulnerable population.

Theories and Models for Program Planning

Theories and models can also guide the planning of community health promotion programs and their adoption by target populations. Examples include the PRECEDE-PROCEED model, the vulnerable populations model, and the diffusion of innovation theory (**Table 3.4**).

PRECEDE-PROCEED Model

The PRECEDE-PROCEED model, developed by Green (1974) and Green and Kreuter (1991), is a logic model that provides a road map for designing health education and health promotion programs. The model encourages APPs and planners to view individual health and health behavior within a broader socioecological context. Planners are guided

through a process that starts with the desired outcome (quality of life) and works backward to identify a mix of strategies for achieving objectives (**Figure 3.9**).

Because the model views health behavior as being influenced by both individual and environmental forces, it has two distinct components: an educational diagnosis (PRECEDE) and an ecological diagnosis (PROCEED). PRECEDE is an acronym for predisposing, reinforcing, enabling constructs in educational/environmental diagnosis and evaluation. This component posits that an educational diagnosis is needed to design a health promotion intervention, just as a medical diagnosis is necessary to design a treatment plan. PROCEED stands for policy, regulatory, and organizational constructs in educational and environmental development. Together, these two components of the model help APPs plan programs that exemplify an ecological perspective.

The PRECEDE-PROCEED model has eight phases (Green & Kreuter, 1999). The first four phases make up the PRECEDE

Health Promotion Case Study Applying Theoretical Concepts in Clinical Practice

Case Description: B.T., a 30-year-old African American woman who wants to lose weight and feel healthier, is seen at the clinic. She states that she would like to have more energy during the day. Hypertension is prominent in her family history. Her father had a mild heart attack and three heart stents by age 50. Upon assessment, her blood pressure is 138/90 mmHg. Height is 5'3" and weight is 192 lb. B.T. states that her stress level is high. She says that she occasionally has headaches and has no time to consider exercising. She is unable to get a job even though she has a college education. Her husband works full-time, making minimum wage. They have two children under the age of three. She is a nonsmoker.

Critical Thinking Questions

- Apply the theoretical concepts of Pender's HPM to B.T.
  - What are some of the individual characteristics and experiences that have influenced B.T.'s desire to lose weight?
  - What are B.T.'s perceived benefits of action, perceived barriers to action, perceived self-efficacy, and activity-related affect?
  - Are there any interpersonal or situational influences that may facilitate or impede her health behavior change?
  - What competing demands and/or preferences have the potential to derail her efforts?
- Apply the TTM to B.T.'s readiness to change.
  - Identify the stage of change that B.T. appears to be in and your rationale.
  - List some appropriate health promotion strategies for her stage.
- Apply the HBM to B.T.'s situation.
  - How can the HBM guide a conversation with B.T. to better understand her beliefs about change? What questions might you ask?
  - What cues to action might B.T. have already experienced to trigger her decision to lose weight? What additional cues to action can you offer as her provider?
  - Identify one or two strategies you could use to build her self-efficacy.
- Evaluate the usefulness of these health behavior theories to B.T.'s case. What insights did you gain?

Table 3.4 Select Theories and Models for Program Planning

Theory/Model	Author(s)	Key Constructs	Practical Application
Diffusion of innovation theory	Rogers (2003)	■ Awareness of the need for an innovation ■ Decision to adopt (or reject) the innovation ■ Initial use of the innovation to test it ■ Continued use of the innovation	■ Address attitudes, knowledge, and perception of behavior. ■ Design effective health education and health promotion programs.

Theory/Model	Author(s)	Key Constructs	Practical Application
PRECEDE-PROCEED model	Green (1974); Green and Kreuter (1991)	The first four steps include: 1. Social assessment 2. Epidemiological assessment 3. Educational and ecological assessment 4. Administrative and policy assessment The last four comprise: 5. Implementation 6. Process evaluation 7. Impact evaluation 8. Outcome evaluation	■ Examine predisposing, reinforcing, and enabling factors. ■ Identify strategies and best practices to design the intervention. ■ Consider administrative, regulation, and policy issues. ■ Evaluate efforts, including procedures, immediate impact, and longer-term outcomes.
Vulnerable populations conceptual model (VPCM)	Leight (2003)	■ Resource availability ■ Relative risk ■ Health status	■ Identify resource availability, relative risk, and health status.

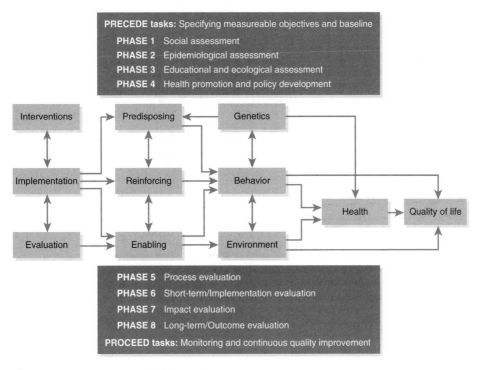

Figure 3.9 PRECEDE-PROCEED model.

component. These phases are diagnostic, addressing both educational and environmental issues, and include social assessment, epidemiological assessment, behavioral and environmental assessment, educational and ecological assessment, and administrative and policy assessment. To conduct a *social assessment*, the planner may use multiple data collection activities (e.g., key informant interviews, focus groups, participant observation, surveys) to understand the community's perceived needs and priorities. The *epidemiological assessment* may include secondary data analysis or original data collection to prioritize the community's health needs and establish program goals and objectives. In phase 3, the *educational and ecological assessment*, factors that affect the health problem are identified. The three types of influencing factors include the following:

1. *Predisposing factors* motivate or provide a reason for behavior; they include knowledge, attitudes, cultural beliefs, and readiness to change.
2. *Enabling factors* enable persons to act on their predispositions; these factors include available resources, supportive policies, assistance, and services.
3. *Reinforcing factors* come into play after a behavior has been initiated; they encourage repetition or persistence of behaviors by providing continuing rewards or incentives. Social support, praise, reassurance, and symptom relief might all be considered reinforcing factors.

In phase 4, *administrative and policy assessment*, planners design the action plan to address the health issues. Strategies reflect information gathered in previous steps, the availability of needed resources, and organizational policies and regulations that could affect program implementation.

The last four phases of the model make up the PROCEED component and include program implementation, process evaluation, impact evaluation, and outcome evaluation of the health promotion program. Before *implementation* begins, APPs should develop plans for evaluating the intervention's *process*, *impact*, and *outcome*.

The PRECEDE-PROCEED model for health program planning and evaluation is widely taught and used in health promotion, with over 1,000 published applications (Porter, 2015). Numerous studies have supported the PRECEDE-PROCEED model's positive impact on the effectiveness of health promotion programs. Some of these studies include preventive behaviors for type 2 diabetes mellitus in high-risk individuals (Moshki et al., 2017), health promotion options for breast cancer survivors (Tramm et al., 2012), a fitness-emphasized physical activity and heart-healthy nutrition education program for elementary school children (Slawta & DeNeui, 2009), and an internet-based weight management program for young adults (Kattelmann et al., 2014), among others.

Implications for Practice

While most APPs will not use the PRECEDE-PROCEED model in a clinical setting, the model is beneficial to those working in the community setting. Community healthcare workers may focus, for example, on reducing rates of cardiovascular disease in a particular population or setting (e.g., neighborhood) by increasing physical activity levels. The team, involving community members, would examine the predisposing, reinforcing, and enabling factors, then identify strategies and best practices to design the intervention as well as administrative, regulation, and policy issues that may influence the implementation of the intervention. After implementation, the final three phases include evaluating the efforts, including procedures, immediate impact, and longer-term outcomes. During implementation and evaluation, the APP and team should be prepared to revisit the PRECEDE portion of the model to determine gaps between the plan and reality. If there is a gap, it may be warranted to go back to PRECEDE and adjust where needed to ensure that the intervention will bring about the desired outcome.

Vulnerable Populations Conceptual Model

Vulnerable populations lack sufficient community resources, leading to increased morbidity, poorer health outcomes, and increased mortality. The vulnerable populations conceptual model (VPCM) demonstrates how relative risk and resource availability affect the health status of vulnerable populations (Albarran & Nyamathi, 2011; **Figure 3.10**). *Relative risk* addresses the likelihood of exposure to risk factors and is reflected in lifestyle behaviors, choices, and exposure to stressful events. *Resource availability* speaks to socioeconomic and environmental resources, such as income, jobs, education, housing, availability of health

care, quality of health care, and family and community patterns, which are components of the social determinants of health. Health status is noted as morbidity and mortality (Leight, 2003). Like the PRECEDE-PROCEED model, the VPCM offers a lens for APPs to identify needs and design effective health promotion strategies.

Implications for Practice

Vulnerable groups often experience inequalities in health care. Rawlett (2011) used both the HBM and the VPCM in a medically underserved rural population. This focus population is affected by a lack of community resources, increased risk factors, and poor health outcomes. The HBM focused on the individuals' perceptions and the likelihood of taking action while the VPCM focused on resource availability, relative risk, and health status. Both frameworks were systematically

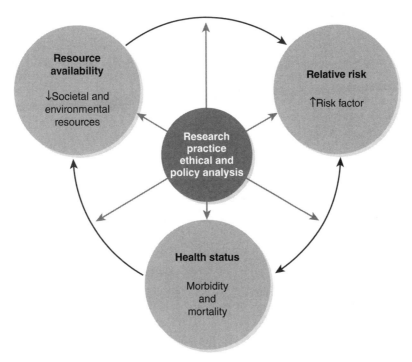

Figure 3.10 Vulnerable populations conceptual model.

evaluated by established criteria. The VPCM was considered a better fit to explore the hypothesis that there is a relationship among access to health care, use of health promotion services, and disease states in susceptible populations.

APPs can use the concepts of the VPCM when assessing the health status of patients and certain populations. Albarran and Nyamathi (2011) used the VPCM to evaluate the vulnerable population of migrant workers living in the United States. They noted that migrant workers are compromised by many factors that increase their risk of contracting HIV, including limited access to health services, multiple sexual partners, lower use of condoms, and improper injection practices. Lack of resources positively affects relative risk, which in turn influences health status and vice versa. The theory-informed APP will assess both the relative risk for disease and the availability of resources.

Diffusion of Innovations Theory

The diffusion of innovations (DOI) theory, developed by Rogers in the 1960s, explains how an *innovation* (e.g., a new idea, an object, or a practice) is adopted by an individual, organization, or community (Rogers, 2003). The innovation is *diffused* (disseminated) through communication in the social system (e.g., family, community, population). The result of this diffusion is that people adopt the innovation as part of a social system. *Adopters* are people who do something different from what they have done previously (e.g., purchase or use a new product or perform a new behavior). The key to adoption is to perceive the idea, behavior, or product as new or relevant (Boston University Medical Campus, n.d.; Rimer & Glanz, 2005).

Implications for Practice

There are five established adopter categories in the DOI theory. When promoting an innovation, the APP can use different strategies to appeal to the different adopter categories.

1. *Innovators* want to be the first to try the innovation. They are very willing to take risks and are often the first to develop new ideas. Very little, if anything, needs to be done to appeal to this population.
2. *Early adopters* represent opinion leaders. They enjoy leadership roles, embrace change opportunities, and are aware of the need to change. Strategies to appeal to this population include how-to manuals and information sheets on implementation. They do not need the information to convince them to change.
3. *Early majority* people are rarely leaders, but they adopt new ideas before the average person. They typically need to see evidence that the innovation works before they are willing to embrace it. Strategies to appeal to this population include success stories and proof of the innovation's effectiveness.
4. *Late majority* people are skeptical of change and will only adopt an innovation after the majority has tried it. Strategies to appeal to this population include information on how many others have tried and successfully adopted the innovation.
5. *Laggards* are bound by tradition and very conservative. They are very skeptical of change and are the most challenging group to bring on board. Strategies to appeal to this population include statistics, fear appeals, and pressure from other adopter groups.

The stages by which a person adopts innovation and whereby diffusion is accomplished include awareness, decision to adopt or reject, initial use, and continued use. The most successful health behavior or health program adoption results from understanding the target population and the factors influencing their adoption rate (Boston University Medical Campus, n.d.; Rimer & Glanz, 2005). While most of the general population tends to fall in the middle categories, it is still necessary to understand the characteristics of the target populations to understand how adoption will fall.

Mohammadi et al. (2018) analyzed the adoption of evidence-based practice (EBP) relating to change in behavior. The EBP adoption was influenced by various factors, such as individual innovation, attitude, knowledge, and perceived EBP attributes. Among these factors, attitude had the most significant effect on EBP adoption. APPs could use these findings to identify factors that will influence EBP adoption of modifiable behaviors as well as the proper design of effective health education and health promotion.

Selecting Theories for Health Promotion Interventions

The preceding discussion of various health promotion theories illustrates how each theory or model looks at health behavior and health promotion practice differently. Some theories focus on the individual and offer perspectives for understanding why someone does or does not adopt certain behaviors. Other theories look at larger issues impacting health and behavior, such as social contexts and policies. Each provides a different lens for viewing the problem or situation. At times, multiple theories are needed to address complex health issues.

In the same way that one wouldn't choose a telephoto lens for taking a close-up photo, APPs need to be able to select appropriate theories to inform health promotion interventions. Rimer and Glanz (2005) note that effective practice is informed by theories that are matched to the patient or situation. Therefore, the first task for the APP isn't to choose a theory but to thoroughly assess the behavior, patient, health problem, target population, or environment.

Furthermore, the situation and setting are important when choosing a health promotion theory. Different theories are more effective for informing interventions for individuals, organizations, or communities. For example, when needing to promote healthy behavior at the individual level (e.g., helping a patient to adopt healthier eating patterns), the TTM would be useful for assessing patient readiness to change, the HBM would help the APP in identifying the patient's barriers to change, and the 5As would guide the APP's conversation with the patient. APPs involved in health promotion at an organizational level (e.g., developing a workplace policy allowing flextime to attend health programs or a school counseling program to address teen alcoholism) or community level (e.g., building a coalition to address an inner-city food desert or developing an initiative to access to mental health services for veterans) might find the PRECEDE-PROCEED model or the VPCM more relevant for guiding the health promotion process.

Health Promotion Activity: Reflection on Theory in Practice

Review the following qualitative study using Leininger's theory with Ethiopian immigrants.

Abstract

- **Introduction:** The purposes of this mini-study were to identify and describe the culture care beliefs and practices of Ethiopian immigrants in the mid-Atlantic region of the United States and advance the science of transcultural nursing.
- **Methodology:** Leininger's theory of culture care diversity and universality guided the research and was the framework for the design of this qualitative ethnonursing mini-study. Data were collected from 15 participants through in-depth interviews.
- **Results:** Five themes and 14 care patterns emerged from the data, including preserving cultural heritage, supporting family and friends, the importance of religion and prayer, valuing freedom, cultural caring, and therapeutic communication.

Discussion: Participants valued health care and medical technology in the United States. They wanted nurses to inquire about their culture, language preference, food and dietary practices, and family dynamics. The nurses' perceived lack of caring and unavailability of interpreters in healthcare settings negatively affected access to care.

- **Implications for Practice:** Based on the research of Ethiopian immigrants' culture care beliefs and practices, nursing implications related to culturally congruent care preferences were contextualized. Participants expressed satisfaction with some aspects of health care in the United States, including nurses' knowledge and advanced healthcare technology. However, their dissatisfaction with nurses' perceived lack of caring and the absence of interpreters in outpatient healthcare settings was of particular concern. A negative relationship between immigrants and healthcare providers may cause these patients to avoid future healthcare activities, further exacerbating disparities in receiving quality care.

Reflection Questions
- What changes in your practice can provide more culturally competent care to improve health outcomes for different cultures and ethnicities?
- How will you incorporate theories and models into improving health outcomes for your clients?

Reference: Data from Chiatti, B. (2019). Culture care beliefs and practices of Ethiopian immigrants. *Journal of Transcultural Nursing, 30*(4), 340–349. https://doi.org/10.1177/1043659618817589

Summary

Health promotion theories and models are evidence-informed approaches to promoting successful healthy lifestyle behavior change in patients. Whether used in clinical or community-based settings, theory helps APPs understand behavior and design effective health promotion programs and services to support healthy lifestyle behavior change in patients and improve population health outcomes. See **Table 3.5** for additional health promotion theory evidence-based resources.

Select health behavior, healthcare, nursing, and program planning theories and models, as well as practice considerations and

TABLE 3.5	Evidence-Based Resources for Health Promotion Theory
Resources	**URL**
Glanz, K., Rimer, B. K., & Viswanath, K. (2008). *Health behavior and health education* (4th ed.). Jossey-Bass.	https://www.academia.edu/6487965/HEALTH_BEHAVIOR_AND_HEALTH_EDUCATION_Theory_Research_and_Practice_4TH_EDITION
Social and Behavioral Theories, e-Source Behavioral and Social Sciences Research, National Institutes of Health	https://obssr.od.nih.gov/sites/obssr/files/Social-and-Behavioral-Theories.pdf
Theory at a Glance, National Institutes of Health, National Cancer Institute	https://cancercontrol.cancer.gov/sites/default/files/2020-06/theory.pdf
Nursing Theories & Models, Nursology	https://nursology.net/nurse-theories
Rural Health Promotion and Disease Prevention Toolkit, Rural Health Information Hub	https://www.ruralhealthinfo.org/toolkits/health-promotion/1/introduction

implications, were presented in this chapter. However, there are many more from which APPs can choose when considering and addressing the multiple factors that impact health and health behavior. APPs are encouraged to do a thorough assessment before selecting an appropriate theory and implementing health promotion interventions for patients and populations. Being a partner with their patients through these processes can be invaluable for achieving healthier patients, families, and communities.

Acronyms

5As: assess, advise, agree, assist, arrange
APP: advanced practice provider
CCM: chronic care model
DOI: diffusion of innovations
EBP: evidence-based practice
HBM: health belief model
HPM: health promotion model
IMCHB: interaction model of client health behavior
OARS: open-ended questions, affirmations, reflections, summaries
PRECEDE: predisposing, reinforcing, enabling constructs in educational/environmental diagnosis and evaluation

PROCEED: policy, regulatory, and organizational constructs in educational and environmental development
SCT: social cognitive theory
SDT: self-determination theory
SEM: social–ecological model
TPB: theory of planned behavior
TRA: theory of reasoned action
TTM: transtheoretical model
VPCM: vulnerable populations conceptual model

References

Ajzen, I. (1985). From intentions to actions: A theory of planned behavior. In J. Kuhl & J. Beckmann (Eds.), *Action control: From cognition to behavior* (pp. 11–39). Springer-Verlag.

Albarran, C., & Nyamathi, A. (2011). HIV and Mexican migrant workers in the United States: A review applying the vulnerable populations conceptual model. *Journal of the Association of Nurses in AIDS Care, 22*(3), 174–185. https://doi.org/10.1016/j.jana.2010.08.001

American Academy of Physician Assistants. (2014). *Statement of the American Academy of Physician Assistants for the hearing record of the Senate Finance Committee on chronic illness: Addressing patients' unmet needs.* https://www.aapa.org/wp-content/uploads/2017/01/AAPA_Statement_Finance_Com_Hearing_Record_7-15-14.pdf

Anderson-Bill, E., Winett, R. A., & Wojcik, J. R. (2011). Social cognitive determinants of nutrition and physical activity among web-health users enrolling in an online intervention: The influence of social support, self-efficacy, outcome expectations, and self-regulation. *Journal of Medical Internet Research, 13*(1), e28. https://doi.org/10.2196/jmir.1551

Bagherniya, M., Firoozeh, M. D., Sharma, M., Maracy, M. R., Birgani, R. A., Ranjbar, G., Taghipour, A., Safraian, M., & Keshavarz, S. A. (2018). Assessment of the efficacy of physical activity level and lifestyle behavior interventions applying social cognitive theory for overweight and obese girl adolescents. *Journal of Research in Health Sciences, 18*(2), e00409.

Bandura, A. (1977). Self-efficacy: Toward a unifying theory of behavioral change. *Psychological Review, 84*(2), 191–215. https://doi.org/10.1037/0033-295X.84.2.191

Bandura, A. (1986). *Social foundations of thought and action: A social cognitive theory.* Prentice Hall.

Bandura, A. (1997). *Self-efficacy: The exercise of control.* W. H. Freeman.

Boston University Medical Campus. (n.d.). *Diffusion of innovation theory.* Retrieved September 30, 2022, from https://sphweb.bumc.bu.edu/otlt/mphmodules/sb/behavioralchangetheories/behavioralhangetheories4.html

Bronfenbrenner, U. (1977). Toward an experimental ecology of human development. *American Psychologist, 32*(7), 513–531. https://doi.org/10.1037/0003-066X.32.7.513

Chiatti, B. D. (2019). Culture care beliefs and practices of Ethiopian immigrants. *Journal of Transcultural Nursing*, *30*(4), 340–349. https://doi.org/10.1177/104365 9618817589

Cox, C. L. (1982). An interaction model of client health behavior: Theoretical prescription for nursing. *Advances in Nursing Science*, *5*(1), 41–56. https://doi.org/10.1097/00012272-198210000-00007

Cox, C. L. (2003). Online exclusive: A model of health behavior to guide studies of childhood cancer survivors. *Oncology Nursing Forum*, *30*(5), E92–E99. https://doi.org/10.1188/03.ONF.E92-E99

Deci, E. L., & Ryan, R. M. (1985). *Intrinsic motivation and self-determination in human behavior.* Plenum.

DeLeon-Demare, K., MacDonald, J., Gregory, D., Katz, A., & Halas, G. (2015). Articulating nurse practitioner practice using King's theory of goal attainment. *Journal of the American Association of Nurse Practitioners*, *27*, 631–636. https://doi.org/10.1002/2327-6924.12218

Doerksen, S., & McAuley, E. (2014). Social cognitive determinants of dietary behavior change in university employees. *Frontiers in Public Health*, *23*(2). https://doi.org/10.3389/fpubh.2014.00023

Dowling, R. (2018, December 25). Reimbursement for obesity counseling. *Journal of Medical Economics*, *95*(24), 22.

EuroMed Info. (2021). *How culture influences health beliefs.* https://www.euromedinfo.eu/how-culture-influences-health-beliefs.html

Fiore, M. C., Bailey, W. C., Cohen, S. J., Dorfman, S. F., Goldstein, M. G., & Gritz, E. R. (2000). *Treating tobacco use and dependence: Clinical practice guideline.* Department of Health and Human Services.

Fishbein, M., & Ajzen, I. (1975). *Belief, attitude, intention, and behavior: An introduction to theory and research.* Addison-Wesley.

George, J. B. (2002a). Systems framework and theory of goal attainment: Imogen M. King. In J. B. George (Ed.), *Nursing theories: The base for professional nursing practice* (5th ed., pp. 241–261). Pearson Education.

George, J. B. (2002b). Theory of culture care diversity and universality: Madeleine M. Leininger. In J. B. George (Ed.), *Nursing theories: The base for professional nursing practice* (5th ed., pp. 489–518). Pearson Education.

Gilbert, H. (2020). Florence Nightingale's environmental theory and its influence on contemporary infection control. *Collegian*, *27*, 626–623. https://doi.org/10.1016/j.colegn.2020.09.006

Glasgow, R. E., Eakin, E. G., Fisher, E. B., Bacak, S. J., & Brownson, R. C. (2001). Physician advice and support for physical activity: Results from a national survey. *American Journal of Preventive Medicine*, *21*, 189–196. https://doi.org/10.1016/s0749-3797(01)00350-6

Glasgow, R. E., Vogt, T. M., & Boles, S. M. (1999). Evaluating the public health impact of health promotion interventions: The RE-AIM framework. *American Journal of Public Health*, *89*(9), 1322–1377. https://doi.org/10.2105/ajph.89.9.1322

Gomes, A., & Nunes, M. (2018). Predicting condom use: A comparison of the theory of reasoned action, the theory of planned behavior and an extended model of TPB. *Psicologia: Teoria E Pesquisa*, *33*.

Green, L. W. (1974). Toward cost-benefit evaluations of health education: Some concepts, methods, and examples. *Health Education Monographs*, *2*(S1), 34–64. https://doi.org/ 10.1177/10901981740020S106

Green, L. W., & Kreuter, M. W. (1991). *Health promotion planning: An educational and environmental approach* (2nd ed.). Mayfield.

Green, L. W., & Kreuter, M. W. (1999). *Health promotion planning: An educational and environmental approach* (3rd ed.). Mayfield.

Holstein, B. A. (2018). Managing chronic disease in affordable primary care. *Journal for Nurse Practitioners*, *14*(8), 496–501. https://doi.org/10.1016/j.nurpra.2018.03.007

Jackson, R. (2012). *Designing healthy communities.* Jossey-Bass.

Kattelmann, K. K., White, A. A., Greene, G. W., Byrd-Bredbenner, C., Hoerr, S. L., Horacek, T. M., Kidd, T., Colby, S., Phillips, B. W., Koenings, M. M., Brown, O. N., Olfert, M. D., Shelnutt, K. P., & Morrell, J. S. (2014). Development of young adults eating and active for health (YEAH) internet-based intervention via a community-based participatory research model. *Journal of Nutrition Education & Behavior*, *46*(2), S10–S25.

Kim, Y., Lee, H., & Ryu, G. W. (2020). Theoretical evaluation of Cox's interaction model of client health behavior for health promotion in adult women. *Korean Journal of Women Health Nursing*, *26*(2), 121–130. https://doi.org/10.4069/kjwhn.2020.06.13

Leight, S. (2003). The application of a vulnerable populations conceptual model to rural health. *Public Health Nursing*, *20*(6), 440–448. https://doi.org/10.1046/j.1525-1446.2003.20604.x

Lewin, K. (1943). Psychology and the process of group living. *Journal of Social Psychology*, *17*(1), 113–131. https://doi.org/10.1080/00224545.1943.9712269

Mansouri, A., Shahramian, I., Salehi, H., Kord, N., Khosravi, F., & Heidari, A. (2020). Effect of sexual health education based on health belief and Pender health promotion models on the sexual function of females with type II diabetes. *Journal of Diabetes Nursing*, *8*(1), 992–1001.

Martin, J. J., Byrd, B., Wooster, S., & Kulik, N. (2017). Self-determination theory: The role of the health care professional in promoting mindfulness and perceived competence. *Journal of Applied Behavior Research*, *22*, e12072. https://doi.org/10.1111/jabr.12072

Maslow, A. H. (1943). A theory of human motivation. *Psychological Review*, *50*(4), 370–396. https://doi.org/10.1037/h0054346

McLeroy, K. R., Bibeau, D., Steckler, A., & Glanz, K. (1988). An ecological perspective on health promotion programs. *Health Education Quarterly, 15*(4), 351–377. https://doi.org/ 10.1177/109019818801500401

Miller, W. R., & Rollnick, S. (2012). *Motivational interviewing: Helping people change.* Guilford Press.

Mohammadi, M., Poursaberi, R., & Salahshoor, M. (2018). Evaluating the adoption of evidence-based practice using Rogers's diffusion of innovation theory: A model testing study. *Health Promotion Perspectives, 8*(1), 25–32. https://doi.org/10.15171/hpp .2018.03

Moore, M., Jackson, E., & Tschannen-Moran, B. (2016). *Coaching psychology manual* (2nd ed.). Wolters Kluwer.

Morales, M. (2011). Determinants of sedentary behavior in college freshman students using the interaction model of client health behavior. (UMI Number: 3455131). [Doctoral dissertation, University of Virginia]. ProQuest Dissertations and Theses Global.

Moshki, M., Dehnoalian, A., & Alami, A. (2017). Effect of precede–proceed model on preventive behaviors for type 2 diabetes mellitus in high-risk individuals. *Clinical Nursing Research, 26*(2), 241–253. https://doi.org /10.1177/1054773815621026

Nightingale, F. (1860). *Notes on nursing: What it is and what it is not.* William Carter. https://www.google.com/books /edition/Notes_on_Nursing/1pREAQAAMAAJ?hl =en&gbpv=1&printsec=frontcover

Nursing Theory. (2020). *Nightingale's environment theory.* https://nursing-theory.org/theories-and-models /nightingale-environment-theory.php

Office of Behavioral and Social Sciences Research. (2016). *Social and behavioral theories.* National Institutes of Health, Department of Health and Human Services. https://obssr.od.nih.gov/sites/obssr/files/Social -and-Behavioral-Theories.pdf

Orem, D. (2001). *Nursing: Concepts of practice* (6th ed.). Lippincott Williams & Wilkins.

Pender, N. (2011). *The health promotion model manual.* https://deepblue.lib.umich.edu/bitstream/handle /2027.42/85350/HEALTH_PROMOTION_MANUAL _Rev_5-2011.pdf

Pender, N. J., Murdaugh, C. L., & Parsons, M. A. (2015). *Health promotion in nursing practice* (7th ed.). Prentice Hall.

Porter, C. M. (2015). Revisiting PRECEDE-PROCEED: A leading model for ecological and ethical health promotion. *Health Education Journal, 75*(6), 753–764. https://doi.org/10.1177/0017896915619645

Prochaska, J. O., & DiClemente, C. C. (1983). Stages and processes of self-change of smoking: Toward an integrative model of change. *Journal of Consulting and Clinical Psychology, 51*(3), 390–395. https://doi.org /10.1037/0022-006X.51.3.390

Prochaska, J. O., & Velicer, W. F. (1997). The transtheoretical model of health behavior change. *American Journal of Health Promotion, 12*(1), 38–48. https://doi .org/10.4278/0890-1171-12.1.38

Rawlett, K. (2011). Analytical evaluation of the health belief model and the vulnerable populations conceptual model applied to a medically underserved rural population. *International Journal of Applied Science and Technology, 1*(2), 15–21.

Rector, C., & Stanley, M. (2022). *Community and public health nursing: Promoting the public's health* (10th ed.). Wolters Kluwer.

Renders, C. M., Valk, G. D., Griffin, S. J., Wagner, E., van Eijk, J. T., & Assendelft, W. J. J. (2000). Interventions to improve management of diabetes mellitus in primary care, outpatient and community settings. *Cochrane Database of Systematic Reviews.* https://doi .org/10.1002/14651858.CD001481

Rimer, B. K., & Glanz, K. (2005). *Theory at a glance: A guide for health promotion practice* (2nd ed.). U.S. Department of Health and Human Services, National Institutes of Health, National Cancer Institute. https:// cancercontrol.cancer.gov/sites/default/files/2020-06 /theory.pdf

Rogers, E. M. (2003). *Diffusion of innovations* (5th ed.). Free Press.

Rosenstock, I. (1974). Historical origins of the health belief model. *Health Education & Behavior, 2*(4), 328–335. https://doi.org/10.1177/109019817400200403

Rural Health Information Hub. (n.d.). *Defining health promotion and disease prevention.* Retrieved March 1, 2022, from https://www.ruralhealthinfo.org/toolkits /health-promotion/1/definition

Ryan, R. (2013). *On motivating oneself and others: Research and interventions using self-determination theory* [Conference presentation]. Coaching in Leadership and Healthcare Conference 2013, Harvard/McLean Medical School, Cambridge, MA.

Sharifikia, I., Rohani, C., Estebsari, F., Matbouei, M., Salmani, F., & Hossein-Nejad, A. (2019). Health belief model-based intervention on women's knowledge and perceived beliefs about warning signs of cancer. *Asia Pacific Journal of Oncology in Nursing, 6*(4), 431–439. https://doi.org/10.4103/apjon.apjon _32_19

Sharma, M., & Romas, J. A. (2012). *Theoretical foundations of health education and health promotion* (2nd ed.). SAGE.

Silva, R. N., & Ferreira, M. D. (2016). Users' participation in nursing care: An element of the theory of goal attainment. *Contemporary Nurse, 52*(1), 74–84. https:// doi.org/10.1080/10376178.2016.1172493

Slawta, J. N., & DeNeui, D. (2009). Be a fit kid: Nutrition and physical activity for the fourth grade. *Health Promotion Practice, 11*(4), 522–529. https://doi.org /10.1177/1524839908328992

Stacy, F. G., James, E. L., & Lubans, D. R. (2016). Social cognitive theory mediators of physical activity in a lifestyle program for cancer survivors and carers: Findings from the ENRICH randomized controlled trial. *International Journal of Behavioral Nutrition and Physical Activity*, 13(49). https://doi.org/10.1186/s12966-016-0372-z

Thomas, J. J., Hart, A. M., & Burman, M. E. (2014). Improving health promotion and disease prevention in NP-delivered primary care. *Journal for Nurse Practitioners*, 10(4), 221–228. https://doi.org/10.1016/j.nurpra.2014.01.013

Tillman, P. (2020). Applying the chronic care model in a free clinic. *Journal for Nurse Practitioners*, 16, e117ee121. https://doi.org/10.1016/j.nurpra.2020.05.016

Tramm, R., McCarthy, A., & Yates, P. (2012). Using the PRECEDE–PROCEED model of health program planning in breast cancer nursing research. *Journal of Advanced Nursing*, 68(8), 1870–1880. https://doi.org/10.1111/j.1365-2648.2011.05888.x

Wagner, E. H. (1998). Chronic disease management: What will it take to improve care for chronic illness? *Effective Clinical Practice*, 1(1), 2–4.

Wold, B., & Mittlemark, M. B. (2018). Health-promotion research over three decades: The social-ecological model and challenges in implementation of interventions. *Scandinavian Journal of Public Health*, 46(Suppl. 20), 20–26. https://doi.org/10.1177/1403494817743893

World Health Organization. (2020). *Cause of death, by noncommunicable diseases*. https://data.worldbank.org/indicator/SH.DTH.NCOM.ZS

Yip, J. Y. C. (2021). Theory-based advanced nursing practice: A practice update on the application of Orem's self-care deficit nursing theory. *SAGE Open Nursing*, 7, 1–7. https://doi.org/10.1177/23779608211011993

Young, M. D., Plotnikoff, R. C., Collins, C. E., Callister, R., & Morgan, P. J. (2014). Social cognitive theory and physical activity: A systematic review and meta-analysis. *Obesity Review*, 15(12), 983–995. https://doi.org/10.1111/obr.12225

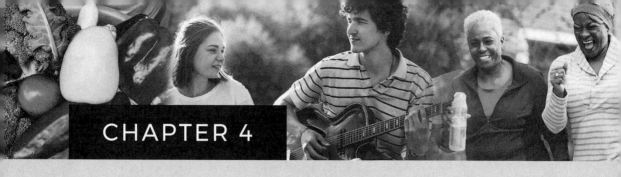

CHAPTER 4

Provider Self-Care and Modeling of Healthy Lifestyle Behaviors

Elizabeth Click, DNP, ND, RN, CWP
Jennifer Drost, PA-C, MS
Gia Merlo, MD, MBA

Rest and self-care are so important. When you take time to replenish your spirit, it allows you to serve others from the overflow. You cannot serve from an empty vessel.

Eleanor Brownn, author

OBJECTIVES

This chapter will enable the reader to:

1. Describe the potential impact of provider self-care on patient health.
2. Summarize the healthy lifestyle behaviors that comprise comprehensive self-care.
3. Evaluate the benefits associated with the inclusion of self-care content within advanced practice provider educational programs.
4. Identify the health benefits associated with self-care practice at work.
5. Discuss four main barriers that limit advanced practice provider self-care behaviors.
6. Initiate healthy lifestyle behaviors in advanced practice providers' lives.

Overview

This chapter describes why self-care is critical for advanced practice provider (APP) well-being. Key lifestyle medicine self-care pillars are discussed as well as the numerous positive professional and personal outcomes of such practice. Organizations such as workplaces and higher education institutions serve an important purpose in encouraging APP self-care. After reading this chapter, current and future APPs should be motivated to incorporate healthy lifestyle behaviors into their own lives.

© Kathleen Gail/Shutterstock; © StoryTime Studio/Shutterstock; © kali9/Getty Images

Importance of Self-Care

Lack of self-care practice within their own lives presents a barrier for APPs addressing lifestyle behaviors with their patients (Clark & Hauser, 2016). Helping future clinicians learn about self-care and practice skills to enhance their health would remove that barrier. The success of such self-care education integration efforts on students' well-being has been documented (Clark & Pelicci, 2011). Offering in-depth education on the lifestyle behaviors that prevent chronic conditions, as well as those that will improve health once a chronic condition is present, is essential for all APPs and academic institutions (Click, 2015). In-depth education needs to be available for future clinicians so that they have the necessary tools to maintain their own health as well as to educate and support patients in practicing healthy behaviors (While, 2014).

While self-care educational initiatives have been and continue to be implemented in educational institutions, often the ability of the individual APP to maintain satisfaction from work becomes challenging. This breakdown, often leading to burnout, is a topic that has received significant press in popular and academic literature since the COVID-19 pandemic started. Clinician burnout is not a new concept. It was reported in the literature in the 1970s and has continued to gain prominence as being the clinician symptoms that encompass emotional exhaustion, depersonalization, and decreased accomplishment from work (Merlo & Rippe, 2021). APP burnout has been addressed in the literature as having multiple contributing factors, including the changing landscape of the U.S. healthcare system, system pressure of increased job demands, technology changes, scarcity of resources, and struggles with maintaining work–life balance (National Academies of Sciences, Engineering, and Medicine, 2019b). These issues often lead to decreased satisfaction with work,

loss of connection with patients, and overall disconnection from the aspects of work that clinicians find rewarding.

The published literature focuses on physicians and nurses, with limited data available for other types of APPs. Therefore, the nursing literature will be described with a note that further research is ongoing for other APPs and will be welcomed to understand the phenomena better. A study found that about 63% of hospital nurses report burnout (BusinessWire, 2017). The American Nurses Foundation launched a national initiative for nurses in 2020 to target nurses' well-being (ANA Enterprise, n.d.). The website has free tools and apps to support nurses' mental health. The literature suggests that nurses reporting symptoms of burnout are also reporting overlap or causation from what has historically been termed *moral distress* (Hiler et al., 2018). Moral distress was defined by Jameton (1984) as knowing the right thing to do in a given situation but being unable to do so secondary to rules or culture (e.g., organizational or institutional). In 2017, the American Nurses Association (ANA) furthered the conversation by publishing a call to action to explore moral resilience as necessary to a culture of ethical practice (ANA, 2017). Compassion fatigue is described as exhaustion from working with victims of trauma and is reported to increase the incidence of burnout among APPs (Zeidner et al., 2013).

While researchers are further refining the definitions, measuring the numbers affected, attempting to understand the causes, and conducting studies on outcomes, the statistics on the effects on the healthcare system are compelling. Indeed, the prevalence and factors associated with burnout lead many nurses to consider leaving the field, as noted by a large national sample survey reported in the *Journal of the American Medical Association* (Shah et al., 2021). Overall, this survey and other emerging literature highlight the importance of nurses implementing strategies to alleviate burnout at a system and an individual level. While system reforms may be needed and long overdue, this chapter outlines a few of the individual interventions and organizational initiatives that may be useful to foster APPs' self-care.

Definition of Self-Care

Self-care is defined by the World Health Organization (n.d.) as "the ability of individuals, families, and communities to promote health, prevent disease, maintain health, and to cope with illness and disability with or without the support of a healthcare provider." Therefore, self-care encompasses everything APPs do to foster personal well-being. The majority of self-care practices fall into the evidence-informed A-SMART (adopt healthy eating, stress less, move often, avoid alcohol,

rest more, treat tobacco use) lifestyle prescriptions (see **Table 4.1**).

Personalization of self-care practices is encouraged. While engaging in all of the behaviors mentioned in Table 4.1 is important, if there is still significant stress, the APP might consider adding more tools to a self-care tool kit in the areas that need reinforcement. For example, effective ways to improve resilience may include learning to incorporate (clinically appropriate) humor into interactions with others or perhaps setting boundaries in relationships (Mills et al., 2018).

It is also important to explore what self-care means to APPs and whether they consider it a priority in their life. Because of the time-intensive requirements of providing health care as well as the harmful belief that clinicians must prioritize others' well-being before their own, many clinicians fail to recognize the importance of self-care (Mills et al., 2017). This chapter emphasizes that the self is

Table 4.1 A-SMART Lifestyle Prescriptions

A-SMART Prescription	Short Definition	Specific Examples of Incorporating A-SMART Prescriptions Into Daily Life
Adopt healthy eating	Eating a whole-food, plant-based diet with minimal salt, oil, and sugar	Eat a lunch of lentil soup, collard greens, and fresh berries.
Stress less	Building resilience through life purpose, positive relationships, and healthy coping strategies	Meditate for 10 minutes each night before bed (check YouTube for free, guided options).
Move often	Exercising at least 150 minutes per week at a moderate intensity	Walk briskly for 30 minutes before work.
Avoid alcohol	Minimizing potentially disease-promoting substances, such as alcohol and drugs	In social situations, swap out alcohol for a glass of sparkling water.
Rest more	Incorporating good sleep hygiene habits	Power off all electronics an hour before sleep.
Treat tobacco use	Stopping the use of tobacco products or vaping	Swap out at least one smoking break with 5 minutes of deep-breathing exercises.

the most critical patient to care for since self-care is crucial to being an effective healthcare provider.

APP Self-Care

Health care is an exceptionally trying occupation with some of the highest rates of stress and suicide (Agerbo et al., 2007). Additionally, as discussed earlier in this chapter, burnout is a challenge most healthcare professionals will face at some point in their careers (Kapu et al., 2019). By learning and practicing self-care, APPs can prepare themselves to be resilient and ready for any challenge. Traditionally, the culture of health care has not given precedence to teaching or encouraging clinicians to care for themselves; however, healthcare leaders argue that this model is outdated and must be reexamined. For example, in 2019, the Mayo Clinic published recommendations in a paper titled "Healing the Professional Culture of Medicine" to address the lack of teaching or encouraging self-care among clinicians and suggested the need to focus more attention and resources on clinician well-being (Shanafelt et al., 2019). While clinicians may experience higher levels of stress than other employees, they are similar to other employees in that healthier employees, particularly those who practice self-care, are more productive and use fewer healthcare resources than those who do not. Additionally, clinicians should not wait until they are working to implement self-care practices; healthcare students who practice self-care report improved overall satisfaction with their lives, including less stress, less negative emotions, increased positive affect, and greater self-compassion (Ayala et al., 2018).

Impact on Patient Outcomes

Research focused on APPs and their lifestyle choices suggests that most are not healthy role models (Ross et al., 2019). Furthermore, while most APPs feel they should counsel patients on healthy lifestyle modifications, only 1 in 10 are competent to do so (Parker et al., 2011). In the same way that APPs are less likely to counsel about healthy behaviors that they do not follow themselves, abundant evidence suggests that they are more likely to counsel about healthy behaviors when they engage in these behaviors themselves. For example, physically active healthcare clinicians provide better patient counseling regarding physical activity (Binns et al., 2007; Buchholz & Purath, 2007; Frank et al., 2008; Howe et al., 2010; Lobelo et al., 2009).

Patients are also more likely to follow clinicians' advice when the healthcare provider is a healthy role model (Frank et al., 2000). Given that 80% of chronic diseases may be preventable or treatable with lifestyle modification (World Health Organization, 2005), clinicians' habits may have more impact on our patients than we realize (Eller et al., 2016). Similarly, when clinicians are stressed and not taking good care of themselves, they may be causing harm to patients because clinician–patient relationships (and therefore the amount they can influence patients positively) may be negatively affected by provider stress (Zeb et al., 2021).

Perhaps more worrisome than APPs being proficient in lifestyle counseling is that some healthcare professionals do not feel it is their responsibility as clinicians to be healthy role models (Blake et al., 2011). Studies indicate that clinicians do not teach behaviors they do not engage in themselves. For example, if clinicians smoke cigarettes, they are unlikely to counsel patients to quit smoking (Tong et al., 2010). Similarly, if clinicians exercise but do not engage in any other healthy behaviors, they tend to only counsel patients about exercise (Livaudais et al., 2005). Thus, it is incumbent upon APPs to engage in self-care not just for their personal well-being but also for the well-being of their patients (Scales & Buman, 2016). Thankfully, there are published, peer-reviewed best practices and evidence-informed guidelines to learn basic lifestyle medicine competencies (Lianov & Johnson, 2010).

Institutional Impact

Enhanced productivity, improved retention, reduced turnover, and decreased absenteeism are just a few of the benefits organizations may experience when self-care practices, such as nutritious meals, stress management, physical activity, sleep hygiene, and substance avoidance, are implemented by APPs. There is an association between healthy lifestyle self-care practices and absenteeism (Virtanen et al., 2018) and presenteeism (Chang et al., 2015). Energized individuals taking good care of themselves are more likely to focus on necessary work and have the energy and commitment required to complete projects. That type of wellness orientation by APPs may also lead to positive health effects for patients.

Similar to the literature on burnout, the impact of provider self-care has been most frequently studied within nursing and physician populations. The meaning and definition of self-care practice among palliative care nurses and physicians were studied by Mills et al. (2018). Within hospitals, nurses participating in their institution's wellness program improved their resilience (Neville & Cole, 2013) and enhanced their well-being while decreasing their likelihood of chronic disease development related to lifestyle behaviors (Sorrell, 2015). Mujika et al. (2017) reported that personal experience in managing healthy lifestyle behaviors affects the type of patient education and support nurses provide. For example, Spanish nurses' smoking status was found to impact patient behavior change support. The opportunity to promote well-being and self-care within the healthcare professions, such as nursing, has never been more vital (Johnston & Click, 2017), yet

further exploration of this effect by researchers is necessary.

Physicians are the second most frequently studied professional population when examining well-being and self-care. Wallace et al. (2009) explored the impact of physician wellness and noted that physician well-being influences how quality healthcare systems function. If that same influence applies to all APPs, then improving APP well-being is critical for all healthcare system operations and to address the state of chronic health issues within the United States. The United States spends 90% of the $3.8 trillion healthcare budget on chronic health conditions, and that expense continues to rise (Centers for Disease Control and Prevention, 2023). Excellent opportunities exist to enhance the health and well-being of APPs by encouraging their own self-care behaviors and the healthy lifestyle behaviors of their patients. Those efforts may ultimately positively affect health in the United States while decreasing the rising healthcare expenses.

The power of organizational leaders to mold the daily lifestyle behaviors of others within their organization is another important consideration. Seeing leaders take the time for physical activity during the workday, eating nutritious meals and snacks, and taking relaxation breaks to enhance energy available for work provides a model upon which APPs may base their own self-care practice. When leaders acknowledge the importance of self-care in contributing to successful goal completion and engage in healthy self-care practices, they create a pathway for others in their organization to do the same (Ross et al., 2017). Without that type of role modeling in place, it can be challenging for clinicians to take the time and devote effort to the healthy practices that sustain their well-being and that of the organization. This type of leader support provides a critical foundation for healthy organizational functioning and encourages ongoing self-care practices. Addressing why self-care and well-being are essential for individuals and organizations to operationalize in their lives will help APPs understand the importance of those efforts within their organization (Johnston & Click, 2017).

Professional Organizational Support for APP Self-Care

Daily practice of healthy lifestyle behaviors leads to numerous organizational benefits. The *Healthy People 2030* guidelines (Mager & Moore, 2020) offer public health goals for the United States to improve health and well-being and prevent disease. The ANA's *Healthy Nurse, Healthy Nation* challenge (ANA, n.d.) also identifies essential health goals for the nation and provides additional information regarding desired goals for the nursing profession. The guidelines note that when APPs practice self-care activities, their health can be better, and their positive impact on patients can be greater. The ANA (n.d.) acknowledges wellness and self-care's power to positively impact nursing practice and encourages other organizations to foster that orientation within nurses.

It also suggests that nurses may be more attuned to patients' wellness needs if they have spent time focusing on their own well-being beforehand (Strout, 2012).

The information available on the importance of self-care and well-being for physicians has grown over the past 20 years (Yester, 2019) and was affirmed in the "Oath to Self-Care and Well-Being" (Panda et al., 2020). Not only is self-care critical for ongoing physician well-being, but it also impacts leadership effectiveness (Shanafelt et al., 2020). The American Academy of Physician Associates (2021) acknowledged the prevalence of burnout among practitioners and provided prevention and support resources for clinicians. Continuous enhancement of health and well-being for APPs is critical as work to address the nation's health needs progresses.

Educational Support for APP Self-Care

Positive outcomes have been achieved by organizations that encourage provider self-care; however, some have questioned whether that

---

Health Promotion Research Study

Provider Self-Care in the Clinical Environment

Background: Intensive care unit (ICU) nurses experience some of the highest levels of burnout because of excessive workloads, end-of-life concerns, prolonged care, and ethical dilemmas.

Methodology: Self-care and mindfulness wellness program activities were incorporated into an ICU to support staff, alleviate stress, and promote staff resilience.

Results: The power of micro-restorative practices in the clinical environment to decrease stressors associated with patient care was highlighted. The importance of leadership, organizational support, and barrier reduction was emphasized to facilitate stress and burnout reduction.

Implications for Advanced Practice: Incorporating specific self-care strategies and activities within the workplace can potentially improve the stress levels of ICU healthcare staff.

Reference: Data from Alvarez, C., & Mulligan, P. (2020). Replenish at work: An integrative program to decrease stress and promote a culture of wellness in the intensive care unit. *Critical Care Nursing Clinics of North America, 32,* 369–381. https://doi.org/10.1016/j.cnc.2020.05.001

emphasis should start earlier via integration of self-care content within higher education curriculum (Click, 2015; National Academies of Sciences, Engineering, and Medicine, 2019a). If clinicians learn about the importance of self-care and practice self-care while in school, the transfer of those practices to the professional clinical environment may be more likely.

Integration of self-care content within nursing school curricula has been advocated (Click, 2015; Stark et al., 2012) and is effective (Ashcraft & Gatto, 2018; Brown & Barr, 2019; Green, 2019). Silva et al. (2020) issued a call for undergraduate and graduate nursing education to include health promotion and self-care topics within curricula to strengthen daily lifestyle behaviors. However, few published articles describe the curricular details of current efforts within nursing and other healthcare provider educational programs. The fact that some authors have questioned the fit of self-care within nursing practice raises additional questions regarding the status of this content within curricula (Whitehead, 2011).

Differing perspectives exist regarding the focus on self-care within provider educational programs. On the one hand, the absence of depth in wellness and prevention content within health education curricula is noted (Clark & Hauser, 2016). However, the evidence is strong concerning healthy lifestyle behavior practices improving health (Riegel et al., 2017). Other studies have found that nurses have the competencies required to address disease prevention for their patients (Kemppainen et al., 2012). Identification of the best educational practices to encourage provider self-care and address patients' well-being needs is necessary.

Research conducted in the past 15 years has focused on a wide variety of well-being behaviors practiced by students and APPs. Recently, an eHealth intervention (Tsai &

Liu, 2015) and mind-body self-care module (Drew et al., 2016) have been described. Gardner et al. (2006) found that stress management, sleep hygiene, and physical activity were the healthy behaviors of most interest and need for nursing students. Clark and Pelicci (2011) describe the development and outcomes of *Life Balance and Stress Management Course*, an online self-care course, focused on helping nursing students evaluate their beliefs, assumptions, and behaviors to enhance their self-care and better manage the stressors associated with being a student. Outcomes of the *Life Balance and Stress Management Course* indicated that students developed transformative ways to cope with stress, such as journaling, developing supportive relationships, and paying attention to their bodies. Journaling is a tool that can facilitate self-care efforts (Lauterbach & Hentz, 2005). Blake et al. (2011) found that "positive begets positive," meaning that physically active student nurses tended to also engage in other healthy lifestyle behaviors. However, the need for earlier curricular emphasis on healthy lifestyle behaviors was highlighted. Lobelo and Garcia de Quevedo (2016) advocated for the inclusion of detailed assessment and evaluation of lifestyle medicine and health promotion in healthcare professions curricula. There is an urgent need for new methods to facilitate student implementation of curricular self-care knowledge within their lives.

While examples of self-care and wellness content integration within the curriculum exist, gaps within this educational focus are present. More curricular development is required to ensure that future APPs know how to take care of themselves and use those healthy practices to enhance the well-being needs of their patients. Integrating behavior change work more extensively within courses is necessary to encourage healthy lifestyle behaviors practiced by clinicians (Stanuelewicz et al., 2020).

Future Implications for Education

To increase the likelihood that future healthcare professionals practice what they preach, educational programs should continue to incorporate practice-based well-being content that facilitates lifestyle behavior change for students (Johnston & Click, 2017). Integrating work from the National Wellness Institute (2021), American College of Lifestyle Medicine (2021), Health Enhancement Research Organization (2021), and Wellness Council of America (2021) into APP curricula may strengthen the ability of future APPs to take care of themselves. Additionally, APPs can enhance their own health by applying the content from other chapters in this book into their lives. Increased self-care practices may positively impact the health of those who APPs serve (Weaver et al., 2018). Boorman (2009) suggested that nursing students need specific help transferring their knowledge in school to their regular lifestyle practices. There is a disconnect between what nursing students know and how they live their lives, which is significant enough to warrant the implementation of more educational courses focused on healthy lifestyle practices. It is quite probable that other APPs may also benefit from the inclusion of healthy self-care practices within their educational programs.

Within the professional realm, an emphasis on prevention rather than on health promotion within curricula may be a barrier preventing widespread focus on self-care (Beaudet et al., 2011). A focus on individual and clinical approaches within education rather than on larger population health initiatives may also contribute to this situation. Beaudet et al. (2011) posited that increased attention to population-based health promotion education is needed for nurses to be better prepared to offer wellness support to patients and themselves. Expanding the breadth and depth of curricular content focused on population health may serve as an additional method to increase the likelihood of self-care practices by APPs (American Association of Colleges of Nursing, 2021).

Workplace Wellness Programs Support APP Self-Care

While corporations have offered wellness programs and services for decades, similar efforts within hospitals, clinics, and healthcare systems are newer if they exist at all. Fortunately, a growing body of evidence supports a focus on well-being within healthcare environments (Brand et al., 2017; Mills et al., 2018). The need for employee wellness programs that target nurses was highlighted by McElligott et al. (2009). McElligott and colleagues (2010) found that nurses older than 40 years of age benefited from the structure of a workplace wellness program to encourage healthy lifestyle behavior practice and overall well-being. Increasing the availability of specific workplace wellness initiatives will provide opportunities to integrate self-care within APPs' lives, leading to a greater likelihood of long-term practice. Through the creation of workplace wellness programs, where APPs work, new opportunities to encourage regular wellness and self-care practices will arise.

A culture of health, hospital manager support, and education were key organizational best practices identified by Kemppainen et al. (2012). Implementing environmental changes that encourage a culture of health and well-being is a critical first step. For example, offering more nutritious foods in the cafeteria and vending machines and offering those foods at discounted prices encourage healthier eating. Placing signs by stairwells may encourage people to use the stairs rather than the elevators. Reinforcing the importance of managers practicing self-care to enhance their health while promoting similar practices by the clinicians reporting to them is also a crucial organizational workplace wellness effort (Ross et al., 2019).

Creating professional development and educational opportunities that move beyond clinical services to health promotion and population health management will facilitate the change necessary to see the broader practice of health promotion activities by APPs. Physical activity, stress management, nutrition, weight management, and tobacco cessation are key lifestyle behaviors featured in workplace wellness programs (Johnston & Click, 2017). Targeting those lifestyle behaviors that most significantly impact chronic health conditions will positively affect health within workplace populations. Implementation of specific programs in those key workplace wellness program categories can occur in a variety of ways. Some organizations provide incentives for walking or biking to work. Occasionally, community programs and tax credits support those options. Offering physical activity program initiatives within the school and work environments is an important way to encourage improved fitness. Fitness competitions may motivate healthcare professionals to increase physical activity levels (Boorman, 2009). McElligott et al. (2009) discussed the possibility of developing fitness centers and creating relaxation rooms to provide healthy behavior practice areas for clinicians.

Offering multisession stress management programs focused on meditation, mindfulness, and relaxation helps provide skills practice that transfers easily into daily life. Discussing mental health and the importance of counseling support during times of need is critical for APPs. Normalizing clinician participation in counseling can improve clinician mental health and provide a solid foundation to better address patients' mental well-being needs. When space is available, devoting several rooms for quiet and relaxation provides an environmental nudge toward mental self-care.

While education about basic nutrition guidelines should be included within provider curricula, healthcare systems can encourage better nutritional health through various other opportunities. Serving nutritious food in cafeterias, offering nutrition education sessions by registered dieticians, providing subsidies for participation in supervised weight management programs, and identifying healthy catering options are additional efforts that organizations can implement to encourage better nutritional health for APPs.

Tobacco use is a necessary behavior to curtail. Many hospitals now ask their clinicians to be tobacco-free and offer cessation programs, hotlines, and additional cessation support. Those programmatic efforts will lead to the most significant impact on healthcare costs over time (Centers for Disease Control and Prevention, 2022).

Offering wellness development opportunities at work, to engage in self-care behaviors daily, is a strategy that would encourage APPs to take better care of themselves. This concentrated effort and comprehensive focus broadly impact APPs' self-care efforts and significantly positively impact patient health and well-being.

The system of APP self-care role modeling is portrayed in **Figure 4.1**. When APPs integrate the A-SMART lifestyle behaviors into their own lives, they will enhance their own health while serving as role models and guides for their patients. When workplaces, health systems, and higher education support and facilitate the development of healthy lifestyles for healthcare professionals, they serve as important support systems and advocates for the well-being of all.

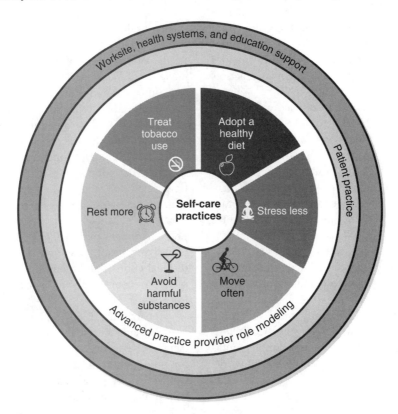

Figure 4.1 APP self-care role modeling system.

Barriers Preventing Implementation of Self-Care Strategies

A complex web of personal and organizational factors presents potential barriers to implementing organizational self-care and general individual well-being strategies. Belief in one's ability to achieve health through lifestyle behaviors may be an issue within the personal realm. The past practice of unhealthy behaviors may cause some clinicians to doubt their ability to support their patients' similar efforts. For example, although healthcare professionals play an essential role in encouraging ideal weight management for patients, nurses' lack of self-confidence may prevent them from fully actualizing that potential role (Zhu et al., 2013). Lack of skills and training and low self-efficacy were found to impact healthcare provider counseling for physical activity efforts (Hebert et al., 2012; Lobelo & Garcia de Quevedo, 2016). Internal conflicts can arise for clinicians engaged in unhealthy behaviors when trying to help patients correct those same behaviors. Duaso et al. (2014) identified internal conflict as an issue when studying the outcomes of physician smokers who were counseling patients to cease tobacco use. Mills et al. (2018) highlighted that workplace culture might be a barrier if self-care practice is not encouraged. Integrating self-care and health promotion management for patients within curriculums may be one promising strategy to reduce the personal barriers of self-efficacy and internal conflict.

Health Promotion Case Study Provider Self-Care

Case Description: H.Z. is a 41-year-old female who presented to her APP two months ago with fatigue, a sense of dread about going to work, and a new diagnosis of type 2 diabetes.

- Social history: APP who works clinically full-time. Married with two children and is the primary caretaker for several aging relatives.

Lifestyle Vital Signs

- Adopt healthy eating: Most of her meals are fast food, eaten in her car.
- Stress less: She admits high stress due to work and caregiving responsibilities. She has also limited her social activities to be present at her children's soccer practices and games.
- Move often: She no longer has time for exercise.
- Avoid alcohol: She feels anxious before bed, so she typically has a glass or two of wine to "try to unwind."
- Rest more: In recent years, she has cut back on sleep to accommodate her busy schedule.
- Treat tobacco: She is a nonsmoker.

The APP suggested that she invest time for self-care and used motivational interviewing to collaborate on a wellness plan. H.Z. committed to the plan and returned to the APP for follow-up. She has regained her sense of purpose and no longer has fatigue. She has effectively reversed her type 2 diabetes by adopting the following self-care strategies:

- She swapped out fast food for a whole-food, plant-based diet that she and her family plan and batch prepare together on Sunday afternoons.
- She walks briskly around the perimeter of the soccer field during her children's practices and games.
- She delegated some of the responsibilities she had taken on for her aging relatives to her siblings, nieces, and nephews.
- She and her family agreed to have electronics off and lights out by 10:00 p.m.
- She meditates for 5 minutes, using an app, each evening instead of drinking alcohol.
- She and her husband agreed that they would have a "date night" every other Friday and she would have a "friend night" every other Saturday.
- She swapped out her nightly glass of wine for a glass of sparkling water.

H.Z. notes that she "knew" all these strategies but had difficulty implementing them until she saw physical evidence (elevated HbA1C) of her declining health.

Critical Thinking Questions

1. How might you start the conversation about self-care with a patient, particularly one who is a healthcare provider?
2. Why might self-care be more difficult for healthcare providers than others?
3. What resources might you offer a patient who recognizes the need for self-care?

Addressing additional barriers beyond the dearth of educational offerings may increase APPs' likelihood of healthy lifestyle practices. Barriers such as time, expense, and fatigue are just a few that make it challenging to practice healthy lifestyle behaviors. Time is a universal personal and organizational barrier to self-care integration and practice. APPs work within busy organizations that strive to meet broad goals. Creating change within an organization so that APPs have time to focus on self-care while at work is necessary.

For APPs, expense issues may create additional barriers to self-care integration both within the workday and within individuals' lives. Financial resources may not be available within organizations to develop self-care–focused workplace programs. Creating budget lines for the health and well-being of clinicians sends a strong message to all clinicians and staff that the organization realizes the benefit and value of investing in its people. When organizations further prioritize these efforts by allowing clinicians and staff to spend part of their workday engaged in self-care and well-being endeavors, the likelihood of seeing positive lifestyle role models at work will increase.

The final significant barrier to self-care integration at work is fatigue. Increasing demands at work frequently lead to more time spent at work. More reports of provider burnout have been shared in the recent past (Bradley & Chahar, 2020; Panagioti et al., 2018) as clinicians work harder and longer. Finding the motivation and drive to focus on well-being is challenging when experiencing fatigue and exhaustion. Emphasizing work–life balance and encouraging adequate self-care (e.g., rest, nutrition, activity, stress management, sleep) are critical success strategies in preventing fatigue and removing that barrier to well-being.

For APPs, addressing these barriers to self-care practice within the workplace and individually is critical. A sound, comprehensive plan will proactively consider these issues and integrate strategies to avoid having these barriers cause issues with self-care practice. **Table 4.2** provides links to online evidence-based resources to support provider self-care.

Summary

Encouraging provider self-care is an important step toward greater well-being. When APPs learn about the A-SMART lifestyle behaviors (adopt healthy eating, stress less, move often, avoid alcohol, rest more, treat tobacco use) in school and are encouraged to incorporate those behaviors into their own lives, their health will be stronger. As more workplaces and health systems realize the importance of self-care for their employees, there will be support at work for ongoing self-care practices. The impact of those healthy lifestyle behaviors will improve APP well-being and will also encourage similar practices for patients through patient education and provider role modeling. The positive effect on patient self-care is also important to highlight.

Envision a future where APPs learn to care for their health during their professional education. Professionals entering the workplace would be prepared to maintain

---

Health Promotion Activity: Improving Self-Care Practices

As you reflect on the barriers that may be present in self-care practices, write a 500- to 1,000-word narrative focusing on the following:

- What are the self-care practices in your life that are not being addressed?
- What are the potential barriers to completing your self-care practices?
- Based on the chapter, what are potential strategies you can initiate to improve the self-care practices you identified?

Activity: After completing the reflection, take 20 minutes to begin one of the identified self-care practices today.

TABLE 4.2	Evidence-Based Resources for Provider Self-Care

Resource	URL
Addressing Health Worker Burnout	https://www.hhs.gov/sites/default/files/health-worker-wellbeing-advisory.pdf
American Nurses Association's *Healthy Nurse, Healthy Nation* Challenge	https://www.healthynursehealthynation.org
American College of Lifestyle Medicine	https://www.lifestylemedicine.org
Health Enhancement Research Organization	https://hero-health.org
Wellness Council of America	https://www.welcoa.org
National Wellness Institute	https://nationalwellness.org
NutritionFacts.org	https://nutritionfacts.org
Provider self-care toolkit	https://www.ptsd.va.gov/professional/treat/care/toolkits/provider/index.asp
Resource Compendium for Health Care Worker Well-Being	https://nam.edu/compendium-of-key-resources-for-improving-clinician-well-being
Well-Being Initiative	https://www.nursingworld.org/practice-policy/work-environment/health-safety/disaster-preparedness/coronavirus/what-you-need-to-know/the-well-being-initiative

their well-being while also focusing on the well-being needs of their patients. In this future reality, APPs would be provided opportunities and support to ensure better patient health and achieve population health.

Moving from an emphasis on a neutral health state to a state of high-level wellness (Travis & Ryan, 2004) will help APPs use the power of lifestyle behavior practice to significantly impact their health and their patients' well-being. Now is the time for APPs to tap into the power of wellness and self-care to manifest better health for themselves and their patients.

Acronyms

ANA: American Nurses Association
APP: advanced practice provider

A-SMART: adopt healthy eating, stress less, move often, avoid alcohol, rest more, treat tobacco use
ICU: intensive care unit

References

Agerbo, E., Gunnell, D., Bonde, J. P., Mortensen, P. B., & Nordentoft, M. (2007). Suicide and occupation: The impact of socio-economic, demographic and psychiatric differences. *Psychological Medicine, 37*(8), 1131–1140. https://doi.org/10.1017/S0033291707000487

American Academy of Physician Associates. (2021). *PA burnout.* https://www.aapa.org/career-central/pa-burnout

American Association of Colleges of Nursing. (2021). *Commission on Collegiate Nursing Education.* https://www.aacnnursing.org/CCNE

American College of Lifestyle Medicine. (2021). *What is lifestyle medicine?* https://www.lifestylemedicine.org

American Nurses Association. (n.d.). *Healthy nurse, healthy nation challenge.* Retrieved January 18, 2021, from https://www.healthynursehealthynation.org

American Nurses Association. (2017). *A call to action: Exploring moral resilience toward a culture of ethical practice.* https://bit.ly/2J7B34w

ANA Enterprise. (n.d.). *The well-being initiative.* Retrieved May 18, 2021, from https://www.nursingworld.org/practice-policy/work-environment/health-safety/disaster-preparedness/coronavirus/what-you-need-to-know/the-well-being-initiative

Ashcraft, P. F., & Gatto, S. L. (2018). Curricular interventions to promote self-care in pre-licensure nursing students. *Nurse Educator, 43*(3), 140–144. https://doi.org/10.1097/NNE.0000000000000450

Ayala, E. E., Winseman, J. S., Johnsen, R. D., & Mason, H. R. C. (2018). U.S. medical students who engage in self-care report less stress and higher quality of life. *BMC Medical Education, 18*(1), 189. https://doi.org/10.1186/s12909-018-1296-x

Beaudet, N., Richard, L., Gendron, S., & Boisvert, N. (2011). Advancing population-based health promotion and prevention practice in community health nursing. *Advances in Nursing Science, 34*(4), E1–E12. https://doi.org/10.1097/ANS0b013e3182300d9a

Binns, H. J., Mueller, M. M., & Ariza, A. J. (2007). Healthy and fit for prevention: The influence of clinician health and fitness on promotion of healthy lifestyles during health supervision visits. *Clinical Pediatrics, 46*(9), 780–786. https://doi.org/10.1177/0009922807303229

Blake, J., Malik, S., Mo, P. K. J., & Pisano, C. (2011). "Do as say, but not as I do": Are next generation nurses role models for health? *Perspectives in Public Health, 131*(5), 231–239. https://doi.org/10.1177/1757913911402547

Boorman, S. (2009, November). *The NHS health and well-being final report.* https://webarchive.nationalarchives.gov.uk/ukgwa/20130124052412/http:/www.dh.gov.uk/prod_consum_dh/groups/dh_digitalassets/documents/digitalasset/dh_108907.pdf

Bradley, M., & Chahar, P. (2020, June 23). *Burnout of healthcare clinicians during COVID-19.* https://www.ccjm.org/content/ccjom/early/2020/07/01/ccjm.87a.ccc051.full.pdf

Brand, S. L., Coon, J. T., Fleming, L. E., Carroll, E., Bethel, A., & Wyatt, K. (2017). Whole-system approaches to improving the health and well-being of healthcare workers: A systematic review. *PLOS One, 12*(12), 1–26. https://doi.org/10.1371/journal.pone.0188418

Brown, C. J., & Barr, B. (2019). Student experience of self-care in an online master of science in nursing course. *Nursing Education Perspectives, 40*(3), 168–170. https://doi.org/10.1097/01.NEP.0000000000000402

Buchholz, S. W., & Purath, J. (2007). Physical activity and physical fitness counseling patterns of adult nurse practitioners. *Journal of the American Academy of Nurse Practitioners, 19*(2), 86–92. https://doi.org/10.1111/j.1745-7599.2006.00197.x

BusinessWire. (2017, January 9). *The employee burnout crisis: Study reveals big workplace challenge in 2017.* https://www.businesswire.com/news/home/20170109005377/en/The-Employee-Burnout-Crisis-Study-Reveals-Big-Workplace-Challenge-in-2017

Centers for Disease Control and Prevention. (2022, August 3). *Burden of cigarette use in the U.S.* https://www.cdc.gov/tobacco/campaign/tips/resources/data/cigarette-smoking-in-united-states.html

Centers for Disease Control and Prevention. (2023, March 23). *Health and economic costs of chronic diseases.* https://www.cdc.gov/chronicdisease/about/costs/index.htm

Chang, Y., Su, C., Chen, R., Yeh, C., Huang, P., Chen, C., & Chu, M. (2015). Association between organization culture, health status, and presenteeism. *Journal of Occupational Environmental Medicine, 57*(7), 765–771. https://doi.org/10.1097/JOM.0000000000000439

Clark, C. A., & Hauser, M. E. (2016). Lifestyle medicine: A primary care perspective. *Journal of Graduate Medical Education, 8*(5), 665–667. https://doi.org/10.4300/JGME-D-15-00804.1

Clark, C. S., & Pelicci, G. (2011). An integral nursing education: A stress management and life balance course. *International Journal for Human Caring, 15*(1), 13–22. https://doi.org/10.20467/1091-5710.15.1.13

Click, E. R. (2015). Self-care. In M. J. Smith, R. Carpenter, & J. J. Fitzpatrick (Eds.), *Encyclopedia of Nursing Education* (pp. 20–21). Springer.

Drew, B. L., Motter, T., Ratchneewan, R., Goliat, L. M., Sharpnack, P. A., Govoni, A. L., Bozeman, M. C., & Rababah, J. (2016). Care for the caregiver: Evaluation of mind-body self-care for accelerated nursing students. *Holistic Nursing Practice, 30*(3), 148–154. https://doi.org/10.1097/HNP.0000000000000140

Duaso, M. J., McDermott, M. S., Mujika, A., Purssell, E., & While, A. (2014). Do doctors' smoking habits influence their smoking cessation practices? A systematic review and meta-analysis. *Addiction, 109,* 1811–1823. https://doi.org/10.1111/add.12680

Eller, L. S., Lev, E. L., Yuan, C., & Watkins, A. V. (2016). Describing self-care self-efficacy: Definition, measurement, outcomes, and implications. *International Journal of Nursing Knowledge, 29*(1), 38–48. https://doi.org/10.1111/2047-3095.12143

Frank, E., Breyan, J., & Elon, L. (2000). Physician disclosure of healthy personal behaviors improves credibility and ability to motivate. *Archives of Family Medicine, 9*(3), 287–290. https://doi.org/10.1001/archfami.9.3.287

Frank, E., Tong, E., Lobelo, F., Carrera, J., & Duperly, J. (2008). Physical activity levels and counseling practices of U.S. medical students. *Medicine & Science in Sports & Exercise, 40*(3), 413–421. https://doi.org/10.1249/MSS.0b013e31815ff399

Gardner, E. A., Deloney, L. A., & Grando, V. T. (2006). Nursing student descriptions that suggest changes for the classroom and reveal improvements needed in study skills and self-care. *Journal of Professional Nursing, 23*(2), 98–104. https://doi.org/10.1016/j.profnurs.2006.07.006

Green, C. (2019). Teaching accelerated nursing students' self-care: A pilot project. *Nursing Open, 7*(1), 225–234. https://doi.org/10.1002/nop2.384

Health Enhancement Research Organization. (2021). *Research studies.* https://hero-health.org/research/hero-research-studies

Hebert, E. T., Caughy, M. O., & Shuval, K. (2012). Primary care clinicians' perceptions of physical activity counselling in a clinical setting: A systematic review. *British Journal of Sports Medicine, 46,* 625–631. https://doi.org/10.1136/bjsports-2011-090734

Hiler, C. A., Hickman, R. L., Jr., Reimer, A. P., & Wilson, K. (2018). Predictors of moral distress in a US sample of critical care nurses. *American Journal of Critical Care, 27*(1), 59–66. https://doi.org/10.4037/ajcc2018968

Howe, M., Leidel, A., Krishnan, S. M., Weber, A., Rubenfire, M., & Jackson, E. A. (2010). Patient-related diet and exercise counseling: Do clinicians' own lifestyle habits matter? *Preventive Cardiology, 13*(4), 180–185. https://doi.org/10.1111/j.1751-7141.2010.00079.x

Jameton, A. (1984). *Nursing practice: The ethical issues.* Prentice Hall.

Johnston, J., & Click, E. R. (2017). Wellness. In J. J. Fitzpatrick (Ed.), *Encyclopedia of Nursing Research* (4th ed., pp. 787–788). Springer.

Kapu, A. N., Card, E. B., Jackson, H., Kleinpell, R., Kendall, J., Lupear, B. K., LeBar, K., Dietrich, M. S., Araya, W. A., Delle, J., Payne, K., Ford, J., & Dubree, M. (2019). Assessing and addressing practitioner burnout: Results from an advanced practice registered nurse health and well-being study. *Journal of the American Association of Nurse Practitioners, 33*(1), 38–48. https://doi.org/10.1097/JXX.0000000000000324

Kemppainen, V., Tossavainen, K., & Turunen, H. (2012). Nurses' role in health promotion practice: An integrative review. *Health Promotion International, 28*(4), 490–501. https://doi.org/0.1093/heapro/das034

Lauterbach, S. S., & Hentz, P. B. (2005). Journaling to learn: A strategy in nursing education for developing the nurse as person and person as nurse. *International Journal for Human Caring, 9*(1), 29–35. https://doi.org/10.20467/1091-5710.9.1.30

Lianov, L., & Johnson, M. (2010). Physician competencies for prescribing lifestyle medicine. *Journal of the American Medical Association, 304*(2), 202–203. https://doi.org/10.1001/jama.2010.903

Livaudais, J. C., Kaplan, C. P., Haas, J. S., Pérez-Stable, E. J., Stewart, S., & Des Jarlais, G. (2005). Lifestyle behavior counseling for women patients among a sample of California physicians. *Journal of Women's Health, 14*(6), 485–495. https://doi.org/10.1089/jwh.2005.14.485

Lobelo, F., Duperly, J., & Frank, E. (2009). Physical activity habits of doctors and medical students influence their counselling practices. *British Journal of Sports Medicine, 43*(2), 89–92. https://doi.org/10.1136/bjsm.2008.055426

Lobelo, F., & Garcia de Quevedo, I. (2016). The evidence in support of physicians and health care clinicians as physical activity role models. *American Journal of Lifestyle Medicine, 10*(1), 36–52. https://doi.org/0.1177/1559827613520120

Mager, N. D., & Moore, T. S. (2020). *Healthy people 2030:* Roadmap for public health for the next decade. *American Journal of Pharmaceutical Education, 84*(11), 8462. https://doi.org/10.5688/ajpe8462

McElligott, D., Capitulo, K., Morris, D., & Click, E. (2010). The effect of a holistic program on health-promoting behaviors in hospital registered nurses. *Journal of Holistic Nursing, 28*(3), 175–183. https://doi.org/10.1177/0898010110368860

McElligott, D., Siemers, S., Thomas, L., & Kohn, N. (2009). Health promotion in nurses: Is there a healthy nurse in the house? *Applied Nursing Research, 22,* 211–215. https://doi.org/10.1016/j.apnr.2007.07.005

Merlo, G., & Rippe, J. (2021). Physician burnout: A lifestyle medicine perspective. *American Journal of Lifestyle Medicine, 15*(2), 148–157. https://dpo/prg/10.1177/1559827620980420

Mills, J., Wand, T., & Fraser, J. A. (2017). Palliative care professionals' care and compassion for self and others: A narrative review. *International Journal of Palliative Nursing, 23*(5), 219–229. https://doi.org/10.12968/ijpn.2017.23.5.219

Mills, J., Wand, T., & Fraser, J. A. (2018). Exploring the meaning and practice of self-care among palliative care nurses and doctors: A qualitative study. *BMC Palliative Care, 17*(1), 63. https://doi.org/10.1186/s12904-018-0318-0

Mujika, A., Arantzamendi, M., Lopez-Dicastillo, O., & Forbes, A. (2017). Health professionals' personal behaviors hindering health promotion: A study of nurses who smoke. *Journal of Advanced Nursing, 73*, 2633–2640. https://doi.org/10.1111/jan.13343

National Academies of Sciences, Engineering, and Medicine. (2019a). *A design thinking, systems approach to well-being within education and practice: Proceedings of a workshop.* National Academies Press. https://doi.org/10.17226/25151

National Academies of Sciences, Engineering, and Medicine. (2019b). *Taking action against clinician burnout: A systems approach to professional well-being.* National Academies Press. https://doi.org/10.17226/25521

National Wellness Institute. (2021). *Six dimensions of wellness.* https://nationalwellness.org/resources/six-dimensions-of-wellness

Neville, K., & Cole, D. (2013). The relationships among health promotion behaviors, compassion fatigue, burnout, and compassion satisfaction in nurses practicing in a community medical center. *Journal of Nursing Administration, 43*(6), 348–354. https://doi.org/10.1097/NNA.0b013e3182942c23

Panagioti, M., Geraghty, K., Johnson, J., Zhou, A., Panagopoulou, E., Chew-Graham, C., Peters, D., Hodkinson, A., Riley, R., & Esmail, A. (2018). Association between physician burnout and patient safety, professionalism, and patient satisfaction: A systematic review and meta-analysis. *Journal of the American Medical Association, 178*(10), 1317–1331. https://doi.org/10.1001/jamainternmed.2018.3713

Panda, M., O'Brien, K. E., & Lo, M. C. (2020). Oath to self-care and well-being. *American Journal of Medicine, 133*(2), 249–252. https://doi.org/10.1016/j.amjmed.2019.10.001

Parker, W., Steyn, N., Levitt, N., & Lombard, C. (2011). They think they know but do they? Misalignment of perceptions of lifestyle modification knowledge among health professionals. *Public Health Nutrition, 14*(8), 1429–1438. https://doi.org/10.1017/S1368980009993272

Riegel, P., Moser, D. K., Buck, H. G., Dickson, V. V., Dunbar, S. B., Lee, C. S., Lennie, T. A., Lindenfeld, J., Mitchell, J. E., Treat-Jacobson, D. J., & Webber, D. E. (2017). Self-care for the prevention and management of cardiovascular disease and stroke: A scientific statement for healthcare professionals from the American Heart Association. *Journal of the American Heart Association, 6*(9), 1–27. https://doi.org/10.1161/JAHA.117.006997

Ross, A., Bevans, M., Brooks, A. T., Gibbons, S., & Wallen, G. R. (2017). Nurses and health-promoting behaviors: Knowledge may not translate into self-care. *AORN Journal, 105*(3), 267–275. https://doi.org/10.1016/j.aorn.2016.12.018

Ross, A., Yang, L., Wehrien, L., Perez, A., Farmer, N., & Bevans, M. (2019). Nurses and health-promoting self-care: Do we practice what we preach? *Journal of Nursing Management, 27*(3), 599–608. https://doi.org/10.1111/jonm.12718

Scales, R., & Buman, M. (2016). Paradigms in lifestyle medicine and wellness. In J. A. K. Mechanick & R. A. Kushner (Eds.), *Lifestyle medicine: A manual for clinical practice* (pp. 29–40). Springer.

Shah, M. K., Gandrakota, N., Cimiotti, J. P., Ghose, N., Moore, M., & Ali, M. K. (2021). Prevalence of and factors associated with nurse burnout in the US. *JAMA Network Open, 4*(2), e2036469. https://doi.org/10.1001/jamanetworkopen.2020.36469

Shanafelt, T. D., Makowski, M. W., Wang, H., Bohman, R., Leonard, M., Marrington, R. A., Minor, L., & Trockel, M. (2020). Association of burnout, professional fulfillment, and self-care practices of physician leaders with their independently rated leadership effectiveness. *Journal of the American Medical Association, 3*(6), 1–11. https://doi.org/10.1001/jamanetowrkopen.2020.7961

Shanafelt, T. D., Schein, E., Minor, L. B., Trockel, M., Schein, P., & Kirch, D. (2019). Healing the professional culture of medicine. *Mayo Clinic Proceedings, 94*(8), 1556–1566. https://doi.org/10.1016/j.mayocp.2019.03.026

Silva, E. J., Jr., Balsanelli, A. P., & Neves, V. R. (2020). Care of the self in the daily living of nurses: An integrative review. *Brazilian Nursing Journal, 73*(2), e20180668. https://dx.doi.org/10.1590/0034-7167-2018-0668

Sorrell, J. (2015). Ethics: Employer-sponsored wellness programs for nurses: The ethics of carrots and sticks. *Online Journal of Issues in Nursing, 20*(1). https:///dx.doi.org/ 10.3912/OJIN.Vol20No01EthCol01

Stanuelewicz, N., Knox, E., Narayanasamy, M., Shiyji, N., Khunti, K., & Blake, H. (2020). Effectiveness of lifestyle health promotion interventions for nurses: A systematic review. *International Journal of Environmental Research and Public Health, 17*(17). https://doi.org/10.3390/ijerph17010017

Stark, M. A., Hoekstra, T., Hazel, D. L., & Barton, B. (2012). Caring for self and others: Increasing health care students' healthy behaviors. *Work, 42*(3), 393–401. https://doi.org/10.3233/WOR-2012-1428

Strout, K. (2012). Wellness promotion and the Institute of Medicine's future of nursing report. *Holistic Nursing Practice, 26*(3), 129–136. https://doi.org/10.1097/HNP.0b013e31824ef581

Tong, E. K., Strouse, R., Hall, J., Kovac, M., & Schroeder, S. A. (2010). National survey of U.S. health professionals' smoking prevalence, cessation practices, and beliefs. *Nicotine & Tobacco Research, 12*(7), 724–733. https://doi.org/10.1093/ntr/ntq071

Travis, J., & Ryan, R. S. (2004). *The wellness workbook.* Celestial Arts.

Tsai, Y. C., & Liu, C. H. (2015). An eHealth education intervention to promote healthy lifestyles among

nurses. *Nursing Outlook, 63*(3), 245–254. https://doi
.org/10.1016/j.outlook.2014.11.005

Virtanen, M., Ervasti, J., Head, J., Oksanen, T., Salo, P.,
Pentti, J., Kouvonen, A., Väänänen, A., Suominen, S.,
Koskenvuo, M., Vahtera, J., Elovainio, M., Zins, M.,
Goldberg, M., & Kivimäki, M. (2018). Lifestyle factors and risk of sickness absence from work: A multicohort study. *The Lancet, 3*(11), E545–E554. https://
doi.org/10.1016/S2468-2667(18)30201-9

Wallace, J. E., Lemaire, J. B., & Ghali, W. A. (2009).
Physician wellness: A missing quality indicator. *The
Lancet, 374,* 1714–1721. https://doi.org/10.1016
/S0140-6736(09)61424-0

Weaver, G. M., Mendenhall, B. N., Hunnicutt, D.,
Picarella, R., Leffelman, B., Perko, M., & Bibeau, D. L.
(2018). Performance against WELCOA's worksite
health promotion benchmarks across years among
selected US organizations. *American Journal of
Health Promotion, 32*(4), 1010–1020. https://doi
.org/10.1177/0890117116679305

Wellness Council of America. (2021). *Workplace wellness
certifications, trainings, and resources.* https://www
.welcoa.org

While, A. (2014). Are nurses fit for their public health
role? *International Journal of Nursing Studies, 51,*
1191–1194. https://doi.org/10.1016/j.ijnurstu.2014
.01.008

Whitehead, D. (2011). Health promotion in nursing: A Derrid-
ean discourse analysis. *Health Promotion International,
26,* 117–127. https://doi.org/10.1093/heapro/daq073

World Health Organization. (n.d.). *What do we mean
by self-care?* Retrieved January 24, 2022, from
https://www.who.int/reproductivehealth/self-care
-interventions/definitions/en

World Health Organization. (2005). *Preventing chronic
diseases: A vital investment.* https://apps.who.int/iris
/handle/10665/43328

Yester, M. (2019). Work-life balance, burnout, and physician wellness. *The Health Care Manager, 38*(3), 239–246.
https://doi.org/10.1097/HCM.00000000000000277

Zeb, H., Arif, I., & Younas, A. (2021). Mindful self-care practice
of nurses in acute care: A multisite cross-sectional survey.
Western Journal of Nursing Research. Advance online publication. https://doi.org/10.1177/01939459211004591

Zeidner, M., Hadar, D., Matthews, G., & Roberts, R. D.
(2013). Personal factors related to compassion fatigue
in health professionals. *Anxiety, Stress & Coping, 26*(6),
595–609. https://doi.org/10.1080/10615806.2013.7
77045

Zhu, D. Q., Norman, I. J., & While, A. (2013). Nurses' self-
efficacy and practices relating to weight management
of adult patients: A path analysis. *International Journal
of Behavioral Nutrition and Physical Activity, 10*(131),
1–11. https://doi.org/10.1186/1479-5868-10-131

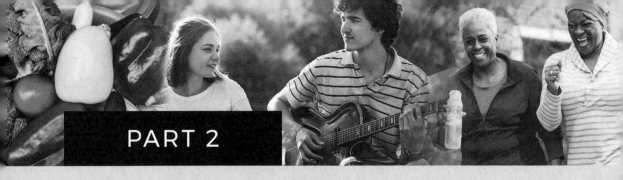

PART 2

The Process of Health Promotion

© Kathleen Gail/Shutterstock; © StoryTime Studio/Shutterstock; © kali9/Getty Images

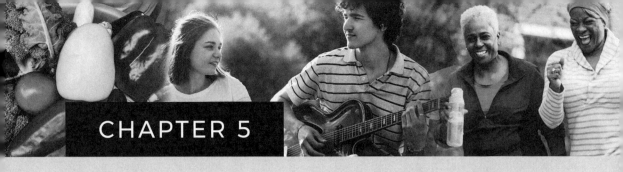

CHAPTER 5

Health Promotion Across the Life Span

Mary Ann Dugan, DNP, APRN, FNP-BC

The greatest medicine of all is to teach people how not to need it.

Hippocrates

OBJECTIVES

This chapter will enable the reader to:

1. Recognize common health needs of individuals across the life span and age-specific health issues that may affect lifelong health.
2. Discuss recommended preventive services for all populations and specific key considerations for average-risk patients across the life span.
3. Incorporate national guidelines into health promotion efforts and patient well-being.
4. Look for opportunities to address primordial, primary, secondary, and tertiary prevention strategies at every patient visit.
5. Deliver the four significant types of clinical preventive care—immunizations, screenings, lifestyle changes/behavioral counseling, and chemoprevention—when addressing the health promotion needs of patients and populations.

Overview

This chapter aims to discuss the prevention of healthcare needs of individuals across the life span. Advanced practice providers (APPs) are well positioned to help patients prevent acute and chronic diseases before their onset. Maximizing best health practices has been a hallmark of health promotion for years. The U.S. Preventive Services Task Force (USPSTF) is a group of national experts who make evidence-informed recommendations and strive to offer clinician resources for disease prevention and preventive services for all patients.

Although the annual wellness exam has become the conventional slated time to identify and discuss health promotion goals that

© Kathleen Gail/Shutterstock; © StoryTime Studio/Shutterstock; © kali9/Getty Images

guide many preventive health services, APPs should look for opportunities to address primordial, primary, secondary, and tertiary prevention strategies at every patient visit. Incorporating health promotion strategies and preventive efforts into each visit will enhance well-being and help sustain health. Additionally, interprofessional collaboration can augment the delivery of preventive health services (Fowler et al., 2020).

Fletcher (2022) describes four significant types of clinical preventive care applicable across the life span: immunizations, screenings, lifestyle changes and behavioral counseling, and chemoprevention. These four types of care are used as a framework for addressing the health promotion needs of each population in this chapter.

Immunizations

Immunizations are recommended across the life span and are an essential component of the annual wellness exam for all patients. Immunizations have yielded an enormous effect on longevity and quality of life, decreasing complications or severity of communicable diseases and mitigating economic burden (Jameson et al., 2018). COVID-19 and influenza vaccinations are recommended for children, adolescents, and adults (Division of Viral Diseases [DVD], 2022b; Fletcher, 2022). Additional immunization considerations for each of these populations will be discussed throughout the chapter.

The Centers for Disease Control and Prevention (CDC) recommends that all individuals six months and older, including pregnant women, receive an influenza vaccination before each fall season (National Center for Immunization and Respiratory Diseases [NCIRD], n.d.-c). This recommendation has rare exceptions, and several vaccine options are available each year. Patients with high-risk medical conditions, who are under two years old or over 65 years old,

or who are immunocompromised are especially vulnerable to influenza (NCIRD, n.d.-b).

The literature and guidelines regarding COVID-19 continue to evolve. Currently, COVID-19 vaccinations are recommended for children, adolescents, pregnant women, and adults. Coronavirus disease, also known as infectious COVID-19, is caused by the SARS-CoV-2 virus, and it resulted in a worldwide pandemic in 2020. Most individuals infected with COVID-19 will have mild or moderate symptoms, but some will become critically ill and possibly die. Older persons; immunocompromised individuals; and those with obesity and obesity-related diseases such as cardiovascular disease, respiratory disease, diabetes, and cancer are particularly vulnerable to serious consequences of COVID-19. At this time, experts recommend minimizing the risk of a COVID-19 infection by maintaining a six-foot distance from people not in the same household, wearing properly fitted face masks, frequently washing hands, choosing well-ventilated spaces or opening windows, and vaccination (DVD, 2022a; World Health Organization [WHO], n.d.).

Screenings

The USPSTF is a team of national experts who collaborate in providing guidance in prevention and evidence-informed medicine. Their goal is to improve the health of people across the life span by making recommendations about clinical preventive care, including screenings, counseling services, and preventive medications (USPSTF, n.d.-a). These USPSTF recommendations are integrated throughout this chapter.

Healthy People 2030 sets national goals for improving health for persons across the life span. This group aims to attain health and well-being through measurable goals grounded in evidence-informed policies and programs. *Healthy People 2030* goals aim to prevent disease, disability, injury, and premature death. Furthermore, goals include eliminating health disparities, attaining health equality, and procuring health literacy to improve the health of all persons across the lifespan (Office of Disease Prevention and Health Promotion [ODPHP], (n.d.-a).

Lifestyle Changes and Behavioral Counseling

Noncommunicable diseases, such as diabetes, heart disease, and cancer, are now the leading cause of death worldwide (WHO, 2021). These diseases are primarily driven by modifiable behaviors (e.g., unhealthy diet, tobacco use, physical inactivity) and metabolic risk factors (e.g., overweight/obesity, elevated blood pressure, hyperglycemia), making lifestyle and behavioral counseling a key health promotion strategy in preventive care. The A-SMART (adopt healthy eating, stress less, move often, avoid alcohol, rest more, treat tobacco use) lifestyle behaviors are integrated throughout the patient population sections of this chapter.

Chemoprevention

Chemoprevention, or chemoprophylaxis, is the administration of medications, vitamins, or other agents to reduce the risk of or prevent disease or infection (Merriam-Webster, n.d.-a; National Cancer Institute [NCI], n.d.-a; Woolf et al., 2008). Simply stated, chemoprevention is "the use of drugs to prevent disease" (Fletcher, 2022, para. 10). Some dietary foods may also be protective and beneficial for health maintenance, health promotion, and prevention of chronic diseases, including cancer (Hernández-Ledesma & Hsieh, 2017). For example, epidemiological evidence has shown that consuming certain foods may prevent up to 35% of cancer occurrences.

Specific Health Promotion Considerations by Age Group

General health promotion recommendations for all populations are summarized in **Table 5.1**. However, each age and stage of development has unique health problems and health promotion needs. Grades A and B recommendations for individuals at average risk for disease are discussed in the following sections and summarized in **Table 5.2**. A full discussion of health promotion and disease prevention interventions for people who are at high risk of developing a disease or who already have a disease is beyond the scope of this chapter.

Pregnant Women and Prenatal Development

One of the key strategies for promoting a healthy birth and maintaining the pregnant woman's health is early and regular prenatal care (National Institutes of Health [NIH], n.d.). Customarily, checkups with a provider occur once monthly during weeks 4 to 28, twice monthly during weeks 28 to 36, and weekly during weeks 36 to birth. Depending on individual risk factors, more frequent visits may be required (NIH, n.d.). Chronic conditions such as heart disease, diabetes, and obesity can precipitate a higher risk of pregnancy complications and infertility (American College of Obstetricians and Gynecologists [ACOG], 2017; National Center for Chronic Disease Prevention and Health Promotion [NCCDPHP], n.d.-c; NIH, n.d.). A select example is poor control of diabetes, which may compound the risk for congenital disabilities.

Delivery before 37 weeks of pregnancy is defined as preterm birth and occurs in 10% of births in the United States. Preterm birth infants tend to have lifelong consequences,

Table 5.1 Recommended Considerations for All Populations

Recommendation	Population	Reference	Comments
COVID-19 vaccination	Children ≥5 years, adolescents, adults, pregnant women	DVD (2022b)	Continues to evolve through pandemic
Influenza vaccination	Everyone 6 months and older	NCIRD (n.d.-c)	Preference in fall
Seat belt use	All ages	National Safety Council (n.d.)	Motor vehicle accident (MVA) is the leading cause of death for ages 1–24 years.
HIV testing at least once yearly if having unsafe sex or sharing injection equipment	All ages	Division of STD Prevention (DSTDP, n.d.-a)	
Throat and rectal STD testing	All who have had oral or anal sex	DSTDP (n.d.-a)	
Depression screening	Adolescents and adults (affects 8% of persons ≥12 years in the U.S.)	USPSTF (2016c, 2016d, 2019c)	Patient Health Questionaire-2 (PHQ-2) accepted as initial screening for all ages. PHQ-2 and PHQ-9 are commonly used and validated screening tools.
Obesity screening	All ages	Jameson et al. (2018)	Body mass index (BMI)

such as chronic lung disease, vision problems, and developmental delays (e.g., cerebral palsy). Maternal chronic conditions such as hypertension and diabetes significantly increase the risk of preterm birth. Pregnant adolescents also have a higher risk of premature births (NCCDPHP, n.d.-e), and some lack prenatal care associated with this risk (Debiec et al., 2010). African American women are 50% more likely than White women to have a preterm birth. Subsequently, Black infant death rates are two times higher than those for White infants (NCCDPHP, n.d.-e). Lack of prenatal care for all women carries a seven times greater risk of premature birth (Debiec et al., 2010). APPs can help improve preconception health care during pregnancy and balance risk with evidence-based findings to leverage the best plan for a healthy pregnancy and delivery.

Immunizations

Several vaccines are recommended before, during, or after pregnancy to keep pregnant women and their babies safe and healthy (Kerr et al., 2017; National Center on Birth Defects and Developmental Disabilities [NCBDDD], n.d.). Antibodies that pregnant women produce in response to a vaccine protect them and their babies upon delivery. Live vaccines, such as measles, mumps, and rubella (MMR), should be given to women at least one month prior to pregnancy (Division of Healthcare Quality Promotion [DHQP], n.d.).

Table 5.2 Health Promotion Key Considerations for Average-Risk Patients

Population	Disease Prevention	Recommendation	Schedule
Pregnant women	Alcohol risk to unborn child	Inquire about unhealthy alcohol use/misuse	Throughout pregnancy
	Asymptomatic bacteriuria	Urine culture	12–16 weeks of gestation or at the first prenatal visit
	Chlamydia, gonorrhea	Nucleic acid amplification test, urine or cervical swab	At-risk pregnant women starting early in pregnancy (DSTDP, n.d.-a)
	Depression	PHQ-2, PHQ-9, or Edinburgh Postnatal Depression Scale	During the perinatal period and the 6- to 12-week postpartum period (Maurer et al., 2018)
	Diabetes	Oral glucose tolerance test	6–12 weeks after delivery for women who have had gestational diabetes (ACOG, n.d.-a)
	Gestational diabetes	Oral glucose challenge test and oral glucose tolerance test	All asymptomatic pregnant women after 24 weeks of gestation
	HBV, hepatitis C (HCV)	HBV panel, HCV antibody test	At the first prenatal visit
	HIV	Reactive immunoassay or rapid HIV test followed by confirmatory test	All pregnant women
	Preeclampsia	Blood pressure	Throughout pregnancy
	Rh(D) incompatibility	Rh(D) blood typing and antibody testing	At the first prenatal visit and repeated for all unsensitized Rh(D)-negative women at 24–28 weeks of gestation unless the biological father is known to be Rh(D)-negative
	Syphilis	Venereal disease research laboratory (VDRL) test or rapid plasma reagin (RPR) test	Early in pregnancy (DSTDP, n.d.-a)
	Unhealthy drug use/misuse	Prenatal risk overview	During pregnancy and postpartum

(continues)

Table 5.2 **Health Promotion Key Considerations for Average-Risk Patients**   (*continued*)

Population	Disease Prevention	Recommendation	Schedule
Infants	Immunization schedule	Variable	DVD (2002b), NCIRD (2022b)
Children	Amblyopia	Visual acuity and ocular alignment tests	Children aged 3–5 years should be screened at least once
	Dyslipidemia	Cholesterol level	Children and adolescents once between ages 9–11 and again between ages 17–21 (Arnett et al., 2019)
	Immunization schedule	Variable	DVD (2022b), NCIRD (n.d.-b, 2022b)
	Obesity	Age- and sex-specific BMI in the 95th percentile or greater	All children and adolescents aged ≥6 years
Adolescents	Depression	PHQ for adolescents, Beck Depression Inventory	Adolescents aged 12–18 years. Opportunistic screening may be appropriate due to infrequent healthcare visits.
	HIV	Reactive immunoassay or rapid HIV test followed by confirmatory test	All adolescents from age 13 should be tested at least once (DSTDP, n.d.-b).
	Immunization schedule	Variable	DVD (2022b), NCIRD (n.d.-b, 2022b)
	Obesity	Age- and sex-specific BMI in the 95th percentile or greater	All children and adolescents aged ≥6 years
Women	Breast cancer	Mammogram with or without clinical breast examination	Women aged 50–75 years, every 2 years American Cancer Society (n.d.) recommends that women aged 40–44 years should be given the option to start annual screening if they choose and women aged 45–54 years, every year; women aged ≥55 years can switch to screening every other year or continue yearly.

Population	Disease Prevention	Recommendation	Schedule
	Cervical cancer	High-risk HPV (hrHPV), Pap smear	For women aged 21–29 years, Pap smear alone every 3 years; for women aged 30–65 years, Pap smear alone every 3 years or Pap smear with hrHPV every 5 years or hrHPV alone every 5 years
	Chlamydia, gonorrhea	Nucleic acid amplification test	Every year for sexually active women <25 years old; every year for sexually active women >25 years old with risk factors such as new or multiple sex partners or a sex partner who has an STD (DSTDP, n.d.-b)
	Intimate partner violence	Humiliation, Afraid, Rape, Kick (HARK); Hurt/Insult/Threaten/Scream (HITS); Extended Hurt/Insult/Threaten/Scream (E-HITS); Partner Violence Screen (PVS); and Woman Abuse Screening Tool (WAST)	Annually
Men	AAA	Ultrasound Once in men aged 65–75 years who have ever smoked or who have a family history of AAA	USPSTF (2019b)
	HCV	Anti-HCV antibody testing followed by polymerase chain reaction (PCR) test	At least once yearly for sexually active gay, bisexual, and other men who have sex with men living with HIV (DSTDP, n.d.-b)
	STDs: syphilis, chlamydia, gonorrhea, HIV	VDRL or RPR, nucleic acid amplification test on urine or cervical swab, reactive immunoassay or rapid HIV test followed by confirmatory test	At least once yearly for all sexually active gay, bisexual, and other men who have sex with men; increase to every 3–6 months if multiple or anonymous partners (DSTDP, n.d.-b)

(continues)

Table 5.2 **Health Promotion Key Considerations for Average-Risk Patients**   (*continued*)

Population	Disease Prevention	Recommendation	Schedule
Adult men and women	Cardiovascular disease	Blood pressure, cholesterol, 10-year atherosclerotic cardiovascular disease (ASCVD) risk calculator	All adults aged 40–75 years, routinely assess cardiovascular risk factors; for adults without known ASCVD and low-density lipoprotein (LDL) 70–189 mg/dL, calculate 10-year risk of ASCVD (Arnett et al., 2019)
	Colorectal cancer	Fecal occult blood testing (gFOBT), fecal immunochemical test (FIT), stool DNA, sigmoidoscopy, colonoscopy	Aged 45–49 years (Grade B) and aged 50–75 years (Grade A): gFOBT or FIT every year or stool DNA-FIT every 1 to 3 years or computed tomography colonography every 5 years or flexible sigmoidoscopy every 5 years or flexible sigmoidoscopy every 10 years + annual FIT or colonoscopy screening every 10 years
	Depression	PHQ-2, PHQ-9, Hospital Anxiety and Depression Scales	All adults who have not been screened previously
	HCV	Anti-HCV antibody followed by confirmatory PCR test	All adults aged 18–79 years at least once
	HIV	Reactive immunoassay or rapid HIV test followed by confirmatory test	All adults aged 18–64 years at least once (DSTDP, n.d.-b)
	Hypertension	Blood pressure	Adults aged 18–39 years, every 3-5 years; adults ≥40 years, every year
	Immunization schedule	Variable	DVD (2022b), NCIRD (n.d.-b, 2022a)
	Prediabetes and T2DM	Fasting blood glucose, hemoglobin A1C, oral glucose tolerance test	Adults aged 35–70 years who have overweight or obesity, every 3 years
	Unhealthy alcohol use/misuse	Alcohol Use Disorders Identification Test–Consumption (AUDIT-C), Single Alcohol Screening Question (SASQ)	All adults aged 18 years and older

Population	Disease Prevention	Recommendation	Schedule
	Unhealthy drug use/misuse	National Institute on Drug Abuse (NIDA) Quick Screen; Alcohol, Smoking and Substance Involvement Screening Test (ASSIST)	All adults aged 18 years and older
Older adults	Cardiovascular disease	Blood pressure, cholesterol, 10-year ASCVD risk calculator	All adults aged 40–75 years, routinely assess cardiovascular risk factors; for adults without known ASCVD and LDL 70–189 mg/dL, calculate 10-year risk of ASCVD (Arnett et al., 2019)
	Depression	PHQ-2, PHQ-9, Cornell Scale for Depression in Dementia, Geriatric Depression Scale (Maurer et al., 2018)	All adults who have not been screened previously
	Fall risk	Assess history of falls, gait, mobility, and functional limitations	Adults aged ≥65 years
	Functional assessment	Katz Index for ADLs, Lawton Scale for IADLs	Adults aged ≥65 years (Reuben & Leonard, 2022)
	Immunization schedule	Variable	DVD (2022b), NCIRD (n.d.-b, 2022a)
	Mild cognitive impairment	Montreal Cognitive Assessment (MoCA)	Nasreddine et al. (2005)
	Osteoporosis	Dual-energy X-ray absorptiometry (DEXA) scan	Women aged ≥65 years
	Prediabetes and T2DM	Fasting blood glucose, hemoglobin A1C, oral glucose tolerance test	Adults aged 35–70 years who have overweight or obesity, every 3 years
	Unhealthy alcohol use/misuse	AUDIT-C, SASQ	All adults aged 18 years and older
	Unhealthy drug use/misuse	NIDA Quick Screen; ASSIST	All adults aged 18 years and older

Unless otherwise indicated, recommendations from the U.S. Preventive Services Task Force. (n.d. -b). *A & B recommendations.* Retrieved June 25, 2022, from https://www.uspreventiveservicestaskforce.org/uspstf/recommendation-topics/uspstf-and-b-recommendations

Influenza. The CDC recommends that women receive an inactivated influenza vaccine during every pregnancy (DHQP, n.d.).

Tdap. Tetanus, diphtheria, and pertussis (Tdap) vaccines are also recommended during every pregnancy (DHQP, n.d.). Tdap is preferred in the early third trimester (27–36 weeks) of each pregnancy to prevent life-threatening complications from pertussis (whooping cough) in newborns.

COVID-19. The COVID-19 vaccine series and booster shot are recommended for women who are pregnant, breastfeeding, and trying to become pregnant. Evidence-based literature continues to mount, indicating that the COVID-19 vaccine is safe and effective during pregnancy. There is no evidence that COVID-19 vaccines cause fertility problems in women or men (DVD, 2022a).

Screening

Diabetes. Health promotion strategies for prenatal risk factors, gestational diabetes, and postpartum care are necessary to mitigate the **risks** associated with diabetic conditions. The USPSTF (2021b) recommends that all asymptomatic pregnant women be screened for gestational diabetes mellitus after the 24th week of gestation. ACOG (n.d.-a) advocates for oral glucose tolerance testing in postpartum weeks 6 to 12.

Tobacco Use. The USPSTF (2021d) advises that all providers screen for tobacco use and provide behavioral interventions for those who use tobacco (Grade A recommendation).

Sexually Transmitted Diseases (STDs). The USPSTF recommends that all pregnant women should be screened for syphilis, hepatitis B virus (HBV) infection (at first prenatal visit), and human immunodeficiency virus (HIV) as Grade A recommendations (Lee et al., 2016; USPSTF, 2018).

Down Syndrome. The prenatal period should include screening for Down syndrome, also known as trisomy 21, in the fetus of an older pregnant female (Fletcher, 2022).

Anemia. Anemia is the most common ailment during pregnancy (Szweda & Jóźwik, 2016). However, the USPSTF (2015) found inadequate evidence to support that APPs or other healthcare providers should be screening for anemia in asymptomatic pregnant patients.

Infection. Urinary tract infections (UTIs) are the second most common ailment during pregnancy. UTIs can occur in up to 10% of all pregnant women (Szweda & Jóźwik, 2016). The USPSTF (2019a) recommends screening all pregnant women for asymptomatic bacteriuria via urine culture (Grade B recommendation).

Lifestyle Counseling

Adopting healthy behaviors before and during pregnancy helps to prevent not only congenital disabilities but also other harmful consequences such as prematurity or low birth weight infants. Examples of healthy behaviors for prenatal planning and pregnancy include the following:

- Refraining from smoking and avoiding exposure to secondhand smoke, to decrease risk of preterm birth, low birth weight, cleft lip, cleft palate, and infant death.
- Not using marijuana or other illegal drugs, to reduce risk of preterm birth, low birth weight, and congenital disabilities.
- Avoiding alcohol to prevent miscarriage, stillbirth, fetal alcohol syndrome, and numerous lifelong disabilities for the child.
- Preventing infections, which can give rise to severe illness, congenital disabilities, and lifelong disabilities such as hearing loss or learning problems.
- Avoid overheating and fever to decrease the risk of neural tube defects.

APPs can also help prenatal women prevent and control chronic diseases before and during pregnancy to increase the chances of a healthy pregnancy and delivery. For example, obesity is a red flag for cardiac complications during pregnancy and a modifiable risk factor that should be addressed in the preconception period. APPs perform an important role in providing lifestyle counseling and resources for adopting healthy lifestyle behaviors.

Weight. In addition to the aforementioned examples of healthy behaviors, pregnant women should optimize a healthy weight because a BMI ≥30 kg/m^2 sets the stage for complications. Increasing caloric intake for pregnant women should be incremental, with an additional 340 calories per day starting in the second trimester and a little more in the third trimester (ACOG, n.d.-c). Women carrying twins are advised to consume 600 additional calories daily, and those carrying triplets should consume an additional 900 extra calories daily.

Iron-Rich Foods. ACOG (n.d.-c) advises pregnant women to include iron-rich foods in their diets, such as organ meats, red meat, and shellfish, and healthier plant sources of iron, such as beans, lentils, dark leafy greens, and fortified breakfast cereals. In addition, pregnant women should eat foods rich in vitamin C, such as oranges, grapefruit, strawberries, broccoli, and peppers, to help the body absorb iron.

Cardiovascular Risks. A study of 790 pregnancies found that 23% of women with obesity (BMI ≥30 kg/m²) had a cardiac event during their pregnancy versus 14% of women with normal body weight. The researchers also found increased cardiac events such as death/arrest, heart failure, arrhythmias, myocardial infarction, stroke, thromboembolic events, and aortic dissection. Preeclampsia was more common in obese women than in those with a normal weight (Pfaller et al., 2021). Low-dose

aspirin (81 mg daily) should be prescribed as a precautionary medication after 12 weeks of gestation in those at high risk for preeclampsia (USPSTF, n.d.-c).

Tobacco Use. Smoking during pregnancy is associated with 5% to 8% of preterm births and 5% to 7% of preterm birth-related deaths. Additionally, 20% of newborns have a low birth weight due to mothers who smoked during pregnancy. Secondhand smoke exposure is directly linked to preterm births, low birth weight newborns, and sudden infant death syndrome (SIDS) (NCCDPHP, n.d.-e). There are several strategies for improvement, such as comprehensive laws for smoke-free environments, increases in tobacco prices, mass media campaigns, and free services to help quit.

Physical Activity. Both pregnant and postpartum women should aim to do moderate-intensity aerobic exercise for 150 minutes per week (Piercy et al., 2018). Regular exercise during pregnancy enhances the well-being of the fetus and pregnant mother by reducing back pain, alleviating constipation, fostering healthy weight gain, and strengthening heart and blood vessels. Regular exercise may decrease the risk of gestational diabetes, preeclampsia, and cesarean delivery and reduce joint stress. Benefits of exercise during postpartum include helping to lose pregnancy weight, a decreased risk for deep vein thrombosis, and improved mood (ACOG, n.d.-b).

Breastfeeding. The USPSTF (2016b) recommends providing breastfeeding interventions during pregnancy and after birth. Breastfeeding has substantial benefits for the postpartum mother, such as making the weight loss process much more manageable (ACOG, n.d.-d). Additionally, breastfeeding prompts the release of oxytocin, which causes the uterus to contract and, subsequently, may decrease the amount of postpartum bleeding. Breastfeeding also lowers rates of type 2 diabetes (T2DM), high blood pressure, and breast and ovarian cancers.

Birth Spacing. Preterm births are prevalent for women with close pregnancies (NCCDPHP, n.d.-e). DeFranco et al. (2014) designed a population-based retrospective cohort study on over 454,000 live births ≥20 weeks and found that insufficient birth spacing is analogous to decreased gestational age for all births. APPs and other healthcare providers should counsel patients that the ideal spacing between delivery and a successive pregnancy is 18 months to 5 years (ACOG, 2017).

Chemoprevention

Folic Acid. Any woman who is planning to become pregnant is advised to take 400 mcg to 800 mcg of folic acid daily to prevent neural tube defects, anencephaly, and spina bifida (ACOG, 2017; Kerr et al., 2017; NCBDDD, n.d.; Office of Dietary Supplements, 2021; Scholl & Johnson, 2000; USPSTF, 2017a). Furthermore, folate deficiency while pregnant has been associated with preterm deliveries, low birth weight infants, and fetal growth retardation (Scholl & Johnson, 2000).

Iron. Iron supplementation and treatment of iron deficiency anemia in pregnant women are implied to improve maternal and infant health outcomes. Nevertheless, there is inadequate evidence to support routine iron supplementation during pregnancy for maternal health or birth outcomes (USPSTF, 2015). ACOG (n.d.-c) advises that women who are not pregnant need 18 mg of iron per day, and pregnant women need to increase iron intake to 27 mg per day. This increased amount of iron is found in most prenatal vitamins. ACOG recommends that pregnant women take a prenatal vitamin every day and eat a healthy diet.

Other clinical preventive service recommendations for pregnant women and prenatal development are listed in Table 5.2.

Pediatrics

The American Academy of Pediatrics (AAP) *Bright Futures Guidelines for Health Supervision of Infants, Children, and Adolescents* provides essential underpinnings for each pediatric visit (Hagan et al., 2017). These include (a) observation of the parent–child interactions as well as developmental monitoring; (b) physical examination, screening/risk assessment, and immunization; and (c) anticipatory guidance. The AAP (n.d.-a) recommends the following schedule for well-child visits: 1 month, 2 months, 4 months, 6 months, 9 months, 12 months, 15 months, 18 months, 24 months, 30 months, and then yearly from 3 to 21 years of age. A compendium of preventive pediatric healthcare recommendations is included in **Table 5.3**.

Immunizations

Vaccines prevent approximately 2.5 million deaths annually for children under five years of age (NCRID, n.d.-a). Visit schedules in childhood are predominantly guided by childhood immunizations to prevent 15 different diseases. Each visit should review whether the child is up to date on their immunizations. Meningococcal vaccinations and the human papillomavirus (HPV) series are recommended during adolescence (Fletcher, 2022; NCIRD, n.d.-a). In the United States, nearly one-quarter of meningococcal disease cases are among adolescents and young adults 11 to 24 years of age. Resources for pediatric vaccine schedules can be found in Table 5.3.

Screening

Infancy (Newborn Through 11 Months). Each year millions of newborns are screened for genetic, endocrine, and metabolic disorders that may affect their long-term health or survival. Newborns are also tested for hearing loss and critical congenital heart defects before being discharged from the hospital or birthing

TABLE 5.3	Evidence-Based Resources: Health Promotion Across the Life Span

Organization	Resource	URL
American Academy of Family Practice	Bright Futures Guidelines	https://www.aap.org/en/practice-management/bright-futures
	KidsDoc Symptom Checker	https://www.healthychildren.org/English/tips-tools/symptom-checker/Pages/default.aspx
	LGBTQ Health Toolkit	https://www.aafp.org/family-physician/patient-care/care-resources/lbgtq.html
	Recommendations for Preventive Pediatric Health Care table	https://downloads.aap.org/AAP/PDF/periodicity_schedule.pdf
	AAP Schedule of Well-Child Care Visits	https://healthychildren.org/English/family-life/health-management/Pages/Well-Child-Care-A-Check-Up-for-Success.aspx
American Cancer Society	Guidelines for the Early Detection of Cancer	https://www.cancer.org/healthy/find-cancer-early/american-cancer-society-guidelines-for-the-early-detection-of-cancer.html
American Thoracic Society	Guidelines for Initiating Pharmacologic Treatment in Tobacco-Dependent Adults	https://www.atsjournals.org/doi/pdf/10.1164/rccm.202005-1982ST
Centers for Disease Control and Prevention	BMI Percentile Calculator for Child and Teen	https://www.cdc.gov/healthyweight/bmi/calculator.html
	Adult BMI Calculator	https://www.cdc.gov/healthyweight/assessing/bmi/adult_BMI/English_bmi_calculator/bmi_calculator.html
	HEADS UP to Health Care Providers (Concussion Information and Online Training)	https://www.cdc.gov/headsup/providers/index.html
	Immunization Schedules (Website)	https://www.cdc.gov/vaccines/schedules/index.html
	Immunization Schedules (App)	https://www.cdc.gov/vaccines/schedules/hcp/schedule-app.html
	LGBT Youth Resources and Health Services	https://www.cdc.gov/lgbthealth/health-services.htm
	STD Treatment Guide (Website)	https://www.cdc.gov/std/default.htm

(continues)

TABLE 5.3	Evidence-Based Resources: Health Promotion Across the Life Span	*(continued)*

Organization	Resource	URL
	STD Treatment Guide (App)	https://www.cdc.gov/std/treatment-guidelines/provider-resources.htm#MobileApp
Immunization Action Coalition	Q&A About Vaccine Administration	https://www.immunize.org/askexperts/administering-vaccines.asp
Medical Home Portal	Screening for Eating Disorders	https://www.medicalhomeportal.org/clinical-practice/screening-and-prevention/screening-for-eating-disorders#d1240769e422
National Center for Chronic Disease Prevention and Health Promotion (NCCDPHP)	Information on NCCDPHP activities and divisions	https://www.cdc.gov/chronicdisease/resources/publications/aag.htm
National Eating Disorders Association	Support for those with eating disorders	https://www.nationaleatingdisorders.org
National Safety Council	Child Passenger Safety	https://www.nsc.org/road-safety/safety-topics/child-passenger-safety
Office on Women's Health	Stages of Pregnancy	https://www.womenshealth.gov/pregnancy/youre-pregnant-now-what/stages-pregnancy
U.S. Department of Agriculture and Department of Health and Human Services	Dietary Guidelines for Americans, 2020–2025	https://www.dietaryguidelines.gov/sites/default/files/2020-12/Dietary_Guidelines_for_Americans_2020-2025.pdf
U.S. Department of Health and Human Services	Aging	https://www.hhs.gov/aging/index.html
	Healthy People 2030 Objectives and Data	https://health.gov/healthypeople/objectives-and-data
	Office of Minority Health	https://www.minorityhealth.hhs.gov
	Office on Women's Health	https://www.womenshealth.gov
	Physical Activity Guidelines for Americans, 2nd Edition	https://health.gov/sites/default/files/2019-09/Physical_Activity_Guidelines_2nd_edition.pdf
U.S. Health Resources and Services Administration	LGBTQIA+ Glossary of Terms for Health Care Teams	https://www.lgbtqiahealtheducation.org/wp-content/uploads/2020/10/Glossary-2020.08.30.pdf
U.S. Preventive Services Task Force	Recommendation Topics	https://www.uspreventiveservicestaskforce.org/uspstf/recommendation-topics

center (CDC, n.d.-c). Ocular antibiotic prophylaxis is administered to all newborns to prevent gonococcal ophthalmia neonatorum (Fletcher, 2022).

Newborn behavior and care should be addressed during visits as well as other social determinants of health risks, such as food security, intimate partner violence, and sibling and family relationships (Hagan et al., 2017). Assessing secondhand smoke exposure is also recommended since secondhand smoke increases the risk of impaired lung function and lung and ear infections in infants (NCCDPHP, n.d.-e).

Early Childhood (1 Through 4 Years). The AAP recommends a complete physical examination at two years old that includes plotting height, weight, and BMI and assessing visual acuity, abdominal masses, skin abnormalities, and language development (Hagan et al., 2017). Screening for autism spectrum disorder (18–24 months) and lead should also be considered. Additionally, the AAP has recommended selective blood pressure screening for all children beginning at three years of age (Hagan et al., 2017).

Vision. All three- to five-year-old children should be screened at least once for vision abnormalities to detect amblyopia or its associated risk factors. Potential risk factors may include strabismus or refractive errors. Providers should also consider risk factors such as first-degree relative family history, prematurity, low birth weight, low parental education levels, and maternal smoking or substance abuse during pregnancy (USPSTF, 2017c).

Obesity. Twenty percent of children and adolescents in the United States are obese (Hales et al., 2017). The staggering obesity rate for children ages two to five years is 13.9% and continues to climb with age (National Center for Health Statistics [NCHS], 2017). Styne et al. (2017) recommend individualized genetic testing when obesity is present before five years old, particularly in patients with excessive hyperphagia, family history of exorbitant

obesity, or other clinical indications of a genetic obesity syndrome. One goal of *Healthy People 2030* is an emphasis on helping people sustain physical exercise and subsequently maintain a healthy weight (ODPHP, n.d.-d).

Middle Childhood (5 Through 10 Years). The five- and six-year-old visits should include screening for hearing, oral health, and vision and, in select cases, anemia, lead, dyslipidemia, and tuberculosis (Hagan et al., 2017). Social determinants of health risk factors may include family, neighborhood, or after-school care. The AAP (n.d.-a) also advises an annual sports physical or activity participation physical as an adjunct to the annual exam. Key considerations for children at seven to eight years of age include analyzing the child's weight, nutrition, and physical activity. Dyslipidemia screening should occur once between 9 and 11 years of age (Hagan et al., 2017).

Obesity. The prevalence of obesity in children aged 6 to 11 years in the United States is 18.4% (NCHS, 2017). Children who have obesity are positioned to have obesity in adulthood (NCCDPHP, n.d.-d). Children with both parents who are obese are 10 to 12 times more likely to be obese themselves (Bahreynian et al., 2017; Reilly et al., 2005; Whitaker et al., 2010). The USPSTF (2017b) recommends that providers screen for obesity in children six years and older and refer as needed for comprehensive, intensive behavioral interventions to achieve a healthy weight (Grade B recommendation).

Adolescence (11 Through 21 Years). Recommended screenings for adolescents include height, weight, BMI, blood pressure, vision and hearing, high cholesterol, anemia, tuberculosis, depression, drug and alcohol use, cervical abnormalities (in females), HBV, HIV, chlamydia, and gonorrhea (Office of Population Affairs, n.d.).

Obesity. The USPSTF (2017b) recommends screening for obesity in adolescents. Adolescents aged 12 to 19 years have obesity rates of 22.2% (NCCDPHP, n.d.-b). One contributing factor is that only 25% of adolescents get the recommended 60 minutes per day of moderate to vigorous physical activity (NCCDPHP, n.d.-d; Piercy et al., 2018).

Eating Disorders. Eating disorders are a group of mental illnesses that affect up to 5% of the population, adversely affecting individuals and their families through multifaceted psychological and physical impairments. The main types of eating disorders are anorexia nervosa, bulimia nervosa, binge-eating disorder, and other specified feeding or eating disorders. These can affect physical, psychological, and social function and cause severe health consequences. The physical consequences of eating disorders, such as weight loss and purging behaviors, are significant and sometimes fatal. Eating disorders may affect all ages, from 5 to 80 years old, and all genders, with females being twice as likely to have an eating disorder (American Psychiatric Association [APA], n.d.-a; Deloitte Access Economics, 2020). Nine percent of the U.S. population will have an eating disorder at some point in their lifetime (Deloitte Access Economics, 2020). Eating disorders most often develop in adolescence and young adulthood between the ages of 12 and 35 (APA, n.d.-a). Unfortunately, society has historically labeled eating disorders as only occurring in thin, White females, especially those who are affluent. Subsequently, those of higher weight, racial and ethnic minorities, socioeconomically disadvantaged, and males may be overlooked and lack proper screening and treatment (Sonneville & Lipson, 2018).

Hornberger and colleagues (2021) at the AAP developed a compendium of screening resources for eating disorders, such as the National Eating Disorders Association (NEDA) Eating Disorder Screening Tool, Eating Attitudes Test (EAT-26), Eating Disorder Screen for Primary Care (ESP), and the Sick-Control-One stone-Fat-Food (SCOFF) Questionnaire. Two key pearls were also highlighted as part of this resource: (a) Malnutrition can arise in a patient of any weight, and (b) emphasis was placed on screening for suicidality (AAP, n.d.-a).

Adverse Childhood Experiences (ACEs).
ACEs are traumatic incidents that occur to children under 18 years old (National Child Traumatic Stress Network, 2019). Examples of ACEs include exposure to violence, abuse, and direct or indirect neglect in the home or community. Children's surroundings can erode their sense of safety and stability. Substance use, mental health problems, and unreliability are examples of environmental pitfalls that may lead to poor health and well-being (Division of Violence Prevention, n.d.). ACEs are also a catalyst for substance use, mental health issues, and chronic illnesses in adulthood. Merrick et al. (2018) found that almost 62% of adult respondents had at least one ACE and almost 25% reported three or more ACEs.

Gender Identity Issues. Gender dysphoria refers to psychological distress related to a difference between individuals' experienced or expressed gender and their assigned gender at birth (APA, n.d.-b). Various terms are used to describe these differences, including lesbian, gay, bisexual, transgender, queer/questioning (one's sexual or gender identity), intersex, and asexual/aromatic/agender. These terms are abbreviated as LGBTQIA in *Merriam-Webster* dictionary (n.d.-b). A complete list of LGBTQIA+ terms can be found in Table 5.3. It is important to recognize that terms and definitions vary across communities and continue to evolve. The AAP (n.d.-b) notes that gender identity may become more apparent as gender characteristics percolate throughout puberty and as youths develop romantic interests. While this is true for some, others have reported gender dysphoria as early as preschool.

One of the *Healthy People 2030* goals is to ameliorate the health, safety, and well-being of the LGBT population by gathering population-level data to improve health promotion care for this population (ODPHP, n.d.-b). LGBT adolescents are a priority due to a higher risk of being bullied, having suicidal ideation, and using illegal drugs. Reducing these risks and STDs is a primary *Healthy People 2030* goal. Klein et al. (2018) advise that provider visits are sensitive and should be custom fit to transgender and gender-diverse individuals. Preventive visits should include identifying and treating mental health diagnoses but avoiding the presumption that they are related to gender identity. Preventive services should be grounded in each individual patient's current anatomy, medication profile, and behaviors.

Lifestyle Counseling (Anticipatory Guidance)

Infancy (Newborn Through 11 Months). Anticipatory guidance, parent and infant interaction, and safe environments should be addressed at each visit (Hagan et al., 2017). The AAP advises a discussion with parents about circumcision benefits and risks, nutrition and feeding guidance, correct installation of a rear-facing car seat in the back seat, placement of babies on their back to sleep, pet risks, installation of smoke and carbon monoxide detectors, and safe storage of firearms in the home. Cord care includes air-drying and keeping diapers below the naval. Parents should be advised never to hit or shake the newborn. Tap water temperature should be set at less than 120 degrees Fahrenheit. Parents should also be counseled about avoiding heatstroke and never leaving a child alone in the car or the bathtub. Education regarding frequent handwashing should be included (Hagan et al., 2017).

Breastfeeding and Diet. The U.S. Department of Agriculture and the U.S. Department of Health and Human Services (USDA & HHS, 2020) recommend exclusive human milk breastfeeding until an infant is at least six months old and continued breastfeeding to 12 months or longer. ACOG endorses many benefits of breastfeeding for the newborn, such as the right amount of nutrients for growth and development; easier digestion than formula

milk, with less gas or constipation; and a lower risk of SIDS. Breast milk also contains antibodies that minimize the risk of ear and respiratory infections, diarrhea, and allergies (ACOG, n.d.-d). An alternative to breastfeeding is to provide an iron-fortified formula. Solid foods can be initiated at six months of age and gradually increased. Moreover, providers should encourage a diet from all food groups without added sugar or high sodium through the toddler years.

Sudden Infant Death. Each year, approximately 3,400 infant deaths are due to sleep-related causes such as accidental suffocation or strangulation (NCCDPHP, n.d.-e). When sleeping, infants should be placed on their back on a firm mattress covered with a fitted sheet in a safe crib free of pillows, loose bedding, and soft objects. Placing awake infants on their abdomen with supervision for "tummy time" is appropriate beginning at two months.

Dental Care. The USPSTF (2021c) advises that primary care providers prescribe fluoride supplementation starting at six months old for those who have a water supply with insufficient fluoride. At the start of primary tooth eruption, dental healthcare providers should apply fluoride varnish to the primary teeth of all infants and children. Fluoride supplementation and varnish are both Grade B recommendations. The AAP advises a dentist evaluation by 12 months or after the first tooth eruption and to brush teeth twice daily with a soft toothbrush and a small amount of fluoridated toothpaste (Hagan et al., 2017).

Early Childhood (One Through Four Years). Anticipatory guidance should include temperament and behavior, children's expressive behaviors, toilet training, and preschool plans. Television and digital media should be limited to one hour per day. Sunscreen use should be strongly advised as well as a protective hat and clothing (Hagan et al., 2017).

Middle Childhood (5 Through 10 Years). The five- to six-year-old child is at a landmark age when children typically prepare to enter school and leave home or separate from parents or other caregivers. Entering school gives rise to new learning, expectations, friends, after-school care and activities, and parent–teacher connections. Anticipatory guidance should include bedtime routines, healthy breakfast, exploration of the new school, a safe home, aftercare, and an individualized educational plan for children with identified disabilities (Hagan et al., 2017). Other safety considerations and areas for advisement are car, outdoor, water, home, and firearm safety.

APPs should offer anticipatory guidance for the seven- to eight-year-old child regarding dental care, including visiting the dentist twice yearly, wearing a mouth guard during sports, and supplementing with fluoride as appropriate. Safety is a priority and should include discussions about seat belt use, water, sun protection, and firearm safety. Safety with adults is also a chief consideration and should consist of a discussion about rules for not keeping secrets from parents and safeguarding private parts (Hagan et al., 2017).

Nine and 10-year-old children are establishing social and emotional competence. They are demonstrating independent decision-making skills. Caring and supportive relationships with family members, older adults, and peers continue to evolve. Provider guidance should include developmental considerations, mental health, pubertal onset, personal hygiene, and sexual safety (Hagan et al., 2017).

Diet and Exercise. The AAP advises helping children choose healthy eating patterns by offering a regular breakfast, encouraging consumption of fruits and vegetables, and providing healthy food options. Additional recommendations include caregivers being role models for healthy eating patterns and eating together as a family (Hagan et al., 2017). HHS and AAPs recommend that children and adolescents engage in 60 minutes or more of physical activity daily (AAP, n.d.-a; Piercy et al., 2018).

Adolescence (11 Through 21 Years). In early adolescence, children may show interest in managing their health. APPs may opt to do the beginning of the visit with both parents and children and then spend some time alone with the children to provide an atmosphere of full disclosure and to foster self-management (Hagan et al., 2017). Providers should help parents and their early adolescent children navigate risk reduction such as preventing pregnancy and sexually transmitted infections; driving safely and using seat belts; avoiding using tobacco, e-cigarettes, alcohol, and drugs; and preventing acoustic trauma (Hagan et al., 2017). Anticipatory guidance for the 15- to 17-year-old should include first addressing any concerns of the adolescents and parents. Additionally, the Bright Futures Adolescence Expert Panel has prioritized key talking points in this age group to include risks such as interpersonal violence; connectedness with family, peers, and community; school performance; nonviolent coping with stress and conflicts; personal care; and emotional well-being (Hagan et al., 2017).

Sleep. Sleep is recognized as an inherent part of good health. Adolescents aged 13 to 18 need 8 to 10 hours of sleep each night (NCCDPHP, n.d.-d; Piercy et al., 2018). Sleep deprivation in the adolescent may cause negative effects such as being more moody or irritable or problems with cognition such as attention, memory, decision-making, or decreased creativity and innovation. Studies have shown that adolescents who are sleep deprived tend to have poorer grades in school, to fall asleep in school, and to be absent. Teenagers have the greatest risk for falling asleep at the wheel while driving (Nationwide Children's Hospital, n.d.).

Tobacco Use. Young persons may use tobacco by smoking cigarettes or e-cigarettes or vaping. In the United States, 9 of 10 adult smokers admit to smoking their first cigarette prior to 18 years old, and 31 of every 100 high school adolescents presently use tobacco. Nicotine preps the brain for addiction and has negative neurobiological effects on learning, memory, and attention (NCCDPHP, n.d.-d; Yuan et al., 2015). The USPSTF (2020) recommends lifestyle counseling for adolescents to prevent the initiation of tobacco use.

Chemoprevention

Despite their widespread use, routine use of vitamins or minerals is not needed for healthy children who are growing and consuming a variety of foods and who have adequate exposure to sunlight. Vitamin D supplementation may be required for children who drink nondairy milk or drink little or no cow's milk (AAP, n.d.-c; Duryea, 2022).

Health Promotion Case Study Female College Student

Case Description: A.L. is an 18-year-old freshman who presents to a local clinic to talk about birth control options. She has recently become sexually active with her boyfriend of three months. She states that he is her first "real" boyfriend but reports five total male lifetime partners, all of whom have been at college this semester. She comes from a strict Catholic family in which premarital sexual relationships are forbidden.

- Allergies: No known drug allergies.
- Medications: Daily multivitamin when she remembers to take it; no over-the-counter meds.
- Medical history: Seasonal allergies; reports she is "healthy."
- Vaccines: Health records indicate that she signed a waiver for the meningitis vaccine due to lack of insurance but now has coverage through a college health plan. Her parents refused the HPV vaccine from their primary care provider years ago, presuming it may encourage promiscuous behaviors. All other immunizations are up to date.
- Social history: Lives in dormitory.
- Vitals: 98.1° F, heart rate 82 beats per minute, respiratory rate 18 beats per minute, blood pressure 120/78 mmHg right arm, BMI 29 kg/m^2.
- Physical exam: The patient is a well-dressed, well-nourished female who appears nervous and occasionally avoids eye contact. The exam is unremarkable.

Critical Thinking Questions

- What additional subjective data related to health promotion and screening are important to derive and why?
- Are there any considerations for the vital signs you would like to address?
- What is your plan to support a healthy lifestyle?
- What health maintenance areas need to be addressed?
- When will you have her follow up?
- Please support your assessments and plan with a rationale.

Additional Reading: Paladine, H. L., Ekanadham, H., & Diaz, D. C. (2021, February 15). Health maintenance for women of reproductive age. *American Family Physician, 103*(4), 209–217. https://www.aafp.org/afp/2021/0215/p209.html

---

Centers for Disease Control and Prevention. (2021). *Sexually transmitted diseases (STDs)*. https://www.cdc.gov/std/default.htm

Adults

In 2017, the life expectancy of a person born in the United States was 78.6 years, with a male average of 76.1 and a female average of 81.1 (NCHS, 2018). The emergence of COVID-19 has ameliorated efforts to improve life expectancy. COVID-19 has reduced approximations of life expectancy at birth by roughly 1.5 years to 77.3 years for the general population. COVID-19 deaths in 2021 suggest a continued decline in life expectancy compared with prepandemic projections (Andrasfay & Goldman, 2021; Arias et al., 2021). Although adults are less likely to receive preventive care than children, 83.4% of adults see a healthcare provider annually for health concerns (NCHS, 2020a, 2021). APPs can utilize these problem-focused visits as opportunities to provide clinical preventive services to improve health outcomes, life expectancy, and quality of life.

Immunizations

The detriment for unvaccinated adults yields consequences such as chronic illnesses, permanent disabilities, missed work time, millions of hospitalizations, and thousands of deaths. Before the COVID-19 pandemic, roughly 50,000 adults died from vaccine-preventable diseases in the United States (CDC, n.d.-a). Vaccines work synergistically with the body's defense system to protect against certain bacteria, viruses, and diseases. Some examples include immunizations for HBV, which lower the risk of liver cancer; HPV, which lower the risk of cervical cancer; and influenza, which lower the risk of heart attacks and other influenza-related complications (NCIRD, n.d.-d). Unvaccinated individuals are vulnerable to illnesses such as shingles, pneumococcal disease, influenza, HPV, and HBV. Both HPV and HBV are leading causes of cancer. Furthermore, unvaccinated persons can spread disease to vulnerable children and older adults. Adults 65 years and older carry amplified risks, such as (a) six times greater risk for hospitalization from pneumococcal

pneumonia; (b) higher risk of complications; (c) six times greater risk of dying from influenza and related complications; and (d) in the United States, one-third of older adults will develop shingles in their lifetime (CDC, n.d.-a). Resources for adult and older adult vaccine schedules can be found in Table 5.3.

Screening

APPs are obligated to monitor available cancer screening and chronic disease guidelines for the patients they serve. Screening for specific health diseases can be found in Table 5.2.

Cancer. According to estimations by the NCI (n.d.-b), approximately 1,918,030 new cancer diagnoses will occur in 2022 in the United States, and 31.9% of these will die from the disease. The most common types of cancer include breast, prostate, lung, colorectal, melanoma, bladder, non-Hodgkin lymphoma, kidney/renal pelvis, uterine, and pancreatic. Roughly 39.9% of people will develop cancer during their lifetime, with men at higher incidence rates than women (NCI, n.d.-b). The USPSTF (2016a) recommends biennial breast cancer screening in women 50 to 74 years old. However, the American Cancer Society (n.d.) recommends that women who are 40 to 44 years old should have the option to start annual breast cancer screening with a mammogram if they choose to, and women who are 45 to 54 years old should get a mammogram every year.

Abdominal Aortic Aneurysm. Abdominal aortic aneurysm (AAA) screening via ultrasound is a USPSTF Grade B recommendation for men 65 to 75 years old who have ever smoked (USPSTF, 2019b). APPs may selectively offer screening to males who have never smoked. For women, the current evidence is insufficient for AAA screening in women 65 to 75 years old who have ever smoked or have a family history of AAA. The USPSTF does not recommend screening in women who have never smoked and who have no family history of AAA (USPSTF, 2019b).

Occupational Health Concerns. APPs may also screen for occupational health hazards as part of the wellness exam. The most frequent occupational health concerns are chronic respiratory diseases, musculoskeletal ailments, and hearing loss secondary to noise exposure (WHO, 2017). Millions of workers are vulnerable to loud noises and chemicals that can cause hearing problems (National Institute for Occupational Safety and Health, n.d.). Lack of sleep can contribute to errors at work and motor vehicle crashes (NCCDPHP, n.d.-c). Some employers may create an environment of health in the workplace as an added layer of care. The CDC characterizes workplace health programs as coordinated and comprehensive strategies that encompass programs, policies, benefits, environmental supports, and connections to the surrounding resources that provide employees with health and safety access (Linnan et al., 2019; NCCDPHP, n.d.-f).

Older Adults. Today's individuals are living longer compared with prior generations. According to the U.S. Census Bureau, prior to COVID-19, statistics predicted that approximately 20% of the population would be 65 years or older by 2050 (Reuben & Leonard, 2022) and approximately 25% of the U.S. population will be age 65 or older by 2060 (Mather et al., 2015). Additionally, older persons will be progressively diverse regarding sociodemographic and health status considerations. APPs will need to approach geriatrics comprehensively, incorporating all domains of health and looking beyond older adult age to predict prognosis, morbidity, and mortality (Reuben & Leonard, 2022). Reducing health problems and improving quality of life are the cornerstones for older adults in *Healthy People 2030* (ODPHP, n.d.-c).

Health Promotion Research Study

Workplace Health in America

Background: More than 60% of U.S. adults are employed and spend a good portion of their time at work. Consequently, the workplace plays an important role in promoting health and safety. The 2017 Workplace Health in America Survey was conducted to provide documentation of the quality and effectiveness of workplace health promotion programs.

Methodology: A survey was conducted across a cross-sectional, nationally representative sample of 2,843 U.S. workplaces.

Findings: The results indicate that workplace health promotion programs have increased but that only 46.1% of the final sample supported this type of program. Smaller workplaces were more likely to lack programs and adequate support. The percentage of commeasurable workplaces with comprehensive programs (as defined by *Healthy People 2010* standards) increased from 6.9% to 17.1% from 2004 to 2017.

Implications for Advanced Practice: Although workplace health promotion programs have increased, their existence remains low. Occupational safety and help, as well as workplace health promotion programs, may help with smaller workplaces that have continual deficiencies.

Reference: Data from Linnan, L. A., Cluff, L., Lang, J. E., Penne, M., & Leff, M. S. (2019, April 22). Results of the Workplace Health in America Survey. *American Journal of Health Promotion*, *33*(5), 652–665. https://doi.org/10.1177/0890117119842047

Supplemental Resource: Office of Disease Prevention and Health Promotion. (n.d.). *Increase the proportion of worksites that offer an employee health promotion program.* Retrieved May 1, 2023, from https://health.gov/healthypeople/objectives-and-data/browse-objectives/workplace /increase-proportion-worksites-offer-employee-health-promotion-program-ecbp-d03

Reuben and Leonard (2022) advise that APPs prioritize six key areas for screening the older adult population, including hearing, vision, polypharmacy, mobility, cognition, and depression. The authors also recommend assessments regarding social, functional, frailty, economics, psychosocial, and environmental concerns that intersect with the key areas. Advance directives and goals of care should also be included in the scope of older adult care.

Fall Risk. Approximately one in three older adults falls every year. Falls are a leading cause of injury and death in the older adult population (CDC, n.d.-b). In addition to fall risk assessment, it is important to assess physical activity levels, including balance training, aerobic, and muscle-strengthening exercises (Piercy et al., 2018).

Functional Status. Reuben and Leonard (2022) endorse that the older adult's functional status may reveal signs of disease onset, deconditioning, or the need for other support. Assessing functional status helps APPs to identify goals for medical care, monitor the progression of chronic disabilities, and manage acute illnesses. Frequently used indicators of function include three levels of activities of daily living:

1. Activities of daily living (ADLs), such as bathing, dressing, or toileting
2. Instrumental activities of daily living (IADLs), such as shopping, preparing meals, driving, or taking medications
3. Advanced activities of daily living (AADLs), such as recreational or travel activities.

Mental Status. Assessing brain function is essential for cognition ability or impairment and is a part of the Medicare Annual Wellness Visit for older adults. Mendez (2022) describes three levels of screening:

1. Short instruments (≤30 minutes), such as mental status scales that assess memory and other cognitive domains. They include structured administration, scoring, and predetermined cutoff scores.

2. Extended mental status examinations (30–60 minutes to perform) include more extensive observations and assessments. This exam helps determine which brain areas may be affected and provides signals for underlying neuropathology disease.
3. Formal neuropsychological testing involves the most detailed assessments with standardized values that may capture a wide range of demographic considerations. This type may last several hours and can be administered over multiple visits.

Lifestyle Counseling

The CDC lists the leading causes of death and disability in the United States as heart disease, cancer, and T2DM (NCHS, n.d.). One in three deaths each year is from cardiovascular diseases, such as heart disease or stroke. These noncommunicable diseases result from risky behaviors such as poor diet, lack of physical exercise, and use of tobacco and alcohol and thus are largely preventable. APPs can help mitigate and ameliorate these risks by encouraging smokers to quit, moderating or eliminating alcohol, encouraging physical activity, educating patients about best nutrition and preventing weight gain, and promoting healthy sleep.

Diet. Eating a healthy diet can help counteract weight gain, heart disease, stroke, T2DM, and some types of cancer. However, only 10% of U.S. adults eat sufficient amounts of fruits and vegetables, and 90% consume over the recommended amount of sodium per day (NCCDPHP, n.d.-c). Fiolet et al. (2018) looked at data from 2009 through 2017 in a population-based cohort study and found that a 10% increase in ultra-processed foods in a person's diet correlated with a 12% increased risk for any type of cancer and an 11% increased risk for breast cancer. Zheng and colleagues (2019) designed two prospective cohort studies to examine the association between red meat consumption and mortality. The studies included recurrent assessments of diet and lifestyle factors in 81,469 male and female participants. The findings concluded that eating red meat, especially processed meat, was associated with a higher risk of death for both men and women. Additionally, it was found that substituting red or processed meat with healthy proteins, whole grains, or vegetables yielded health benefits.

Physical Activity. Only 50% of U.S. adults get enough physical exercise (NCCDPHP, n.d.-c). Adults should complete one of the following every week: 150 to 300 minutes of moderate-intensity exercise, 75 to 150 minutes of vigorous-intensity aerobic exercise, or an equivalent combination of moderate- and vigorous-intensity aerobic activity. Additionally, adults should complete at least two days of muscle-strengthening exercises every week. Those with chronic conditions or disabilities should follow the recommended guidelines for adults and do aerobic and muscle-strengthening activities to the best of their ability (Piercy et al., 2018).

Tobacco and Alcohol Use. In the United States, tobacco use is the highest cause of avoidable disease, disability, and death. Roughly 34 million U.S. adults smoke cigarettes, and 58 million nonsmokers are exposed to secondhand smoke each year (NCCDPHP, n.d.-c). Smoking cessation strategies should include positive and supportive communication grounded in evidence-informed therapies to yield efficacious outcomes (Jameson et al., 2018). For adults who drink alcohol, maximum daily consumption should be two drinks for men and one drink for nonpregnant women (USDA & HHS, 2020).

Sleep. One-third of adults report getting less than the recommended seven hours of sleep each night. Lack of sleep is associated with many chronic diseases such as heart disease, T2DM, obesity, and depression (NCCDPHP, n.d.-c).

Obesity. Approximately 74% of U.S. adults are overweight or obese, with the highest rates in those who are 40 to 59 years old (43%), followed by adults who are 60 years and older (41%) (NCCDPHP, n.d.-a; NCHS, 2020b; USDA & HHS, 2020). Some cancers, such as endometrial, breast, colon, kidney, gallbladder, and liver, are related to obesity (NCCDPHP, n.d.-a). In addition to cancer, diabetes, and cardiovascular diseases, there are a plethora of health consequences for patients who are overweight or obese, such as gallbladder disease, osteoarthritis, sleep apnea, body pain, and lower quality of life. Provider counseling can significantly affect weight loss in overweight patients (Davis et al., 2019).

Chemoprevention

The USPSTF (2021a) and others are actively seeking clarification about the benefits or harms of prescribing vitamin, mineral, and multivitamin supplements for patients to prevent heart disease and cancer. Statin medications are often prescribed to prevent hypercholesteremia (Fletcher, 2022). Salami et al. (2017) reported that the use of statins among adults 40 years and older grew from 17.9% in 2002–2003 to 27.8% in 2012–2013. Currently, statins persist as a cornerstone in preventing and treating atherosclerotic cardiovascular disease.

Summary

Each stage of life signifies varied healthcare needs. APPs are instrumental in helping patients prevent and manage their health needs and set individualized goals. Clinical preventive efforts that include immunizations, screenings, lifestyle counseling, and chemoprevention have yielded a prodigious decline in the consequences of common debilitating illnesses.

Many chronic diseases, such as obesity, are preventable. Obesity is a profound problem in

---

Health Promotion Activity: Preventive Care for Young Adult

P.T. is a 25-year-old obese bisexual male who presents to a primary care office as a new patient to establish care. He has not seen a provider since he began college seven years ago and moved to the area. He is unclear about his immunization record. He is having difficulty getting his old records and states, "I am working on it." He admits that he has been stressed due to working the night shift and is looking for a new job. He studied computer science in college but is having trouble finding work in his field. Social history includes smoking 10 to 12 cigarettes a day and drinking a few beers on the weekend with friends.

- What are the priority concerns for this visit?
- Using Fletcher's (2022) framework for clinical preventive care (immunizations, screenings, lifestyle changes and behavioral counseling, chemoprevention), what health promotion needs might you anticipate P.T. needing?
- What A-SMART lifestyle behaviors will you address as part of the lifestyle counseling provided during this visit?
- What evidence-based resources support your plan of care?
- When will you bring him back for a follow-up appointment?
- What are the patient goals for the next visit?

Data from Fletcher, G. S. (2022). *Evidence-based approach to prevention*. UpToDate. https://www.uptodate.com/contents/evidence-based-approach-to-prevention

the United States for children and adults with a propensity for serious lifelong health issues. APPs can help overweight or obese patients across the life span to recalibrate a healthy diet and exercise at any age. All persons from one year through adulthood should follow a healthful diet to meet their nutritional needs, maintain a healthy body weight, and reduce the risk of chronic diseases (USDA & HSS, 2020).

APPs and other primary care providers should teach patients about their modifiable risk factors and encourage lifestyle choices that minimize those risks. Empowering patients to adopt A-SMART lifestyle behaviors, receive preventive services such as vaccines, and leverage risks with screenings contributes to ways APPs can help patients cultivate a healthy lifestyle.

Acronyms

AAA: abdominal aortic aneurysm

AAP: American Academy of Pediatrics

ACE: adverse childhood experience

ACOG: American College of Obstetricians and Gynecologists

APA: American Psychiatric Association

APP: advanced practice provider

ASCVD: atherosclerotic cardiovascular disease

A-SMART: adopt healthy eating, stress less, move often, avoid alcohol, rest more, treat tobacco use

BMI: body mass index

CDC: Centers for Disease Control and Prevention

COVID-19: coronavirus disease 2019

DHQP: CDC Division of Healthcare Quality Promotion

DSTDP: CDC Division of STD Prevention

DVD: CDC Division of Viral Diseases

HBV: hepatitis B virus

HCV: hepatitis C virus

HHS: U.S. Department of Health and Human Services

HIV: human immunodeficiency virus
HPV: human papilloma virus
hrHPV: high-risk HPV
MMR: measles, mumps, and rubella
MVA: motor vehicle accident
NCBDDD: National Center on Birth Defects and Developmental Disabilities
NCCDPHP: National Center for Chronic Disease Prevention and Health Promotion
NCHS: National Center for Health Statistics
NCI: National Cancer Institute
NCIRD: National Center for Immunization and Respiratory Diseases
NIH: National Institutes of Health

ODPHP: U.S. Department of Health and Human Services, Office of Disease Prevention and Health Promotion
PHQ: Patient Health Questionnaire
RPR: rapid plasma reagin test
SIDS: sudden infant death syndrome
STD: sexually transmitted disease
T2DM: type 2 diabetes
Tdap: tetanus, diphtheria, and pertussis
USDA: U.S. Department of Agriculture
USPSTF: U.S. Preventive Services Task Force
UTI: urinary tract infection
VDRL: venereal disease research laboratory test
WHO: World Health Organization

References

American Academy of Pediatrics. (n.d.-a). *AAP schedule of well-child care visits.* Retrieved October 1, 2022, from https://healthychildren.org/English/family-life/health-management/Pages/Well-Child-Care-A-Check-Up-for-Success.aspx

American Academy of Pediatrics. (n.d.-b). *Coming out: Information for parents of LGBTQ teens.* Retrieved October 1, 2022, from https://healthychildren.org/English/ages-stages/teen/dating-sex/Pages/Four-Stages-of-Coming-Out.aspx

American Academy of Pediatrics. (n.d.-c). *Where we stand: Vitamin supplements for children.* Retrieved October 1, 2022, from https://www.healthychildren.org/English/healthy-living/nutrition/Pages/Where-We-Stand-Vitamins.aspx

American Cancer Society. (n.d.). *American Cancer Society recommendations for the early detection of breast cancer.* Retrieved October 1, 2022, from https://www.cancer.org/cancer/breast-cancer/screening-tests-and-early-detection/american-cancer-society-recommendations-for-the-early-detection-of-breast-cancer.html

American College of Obstetricians and Gynecologists. (n.d.-a). *FAQs: Diabetes and women.* Retrieved October 1, 2022, from https://www.acog.org/womens-health/faqs/diabetes-and-women

American College of Obstetricians and Gynecologists. (n.d.-b). *FAQs: Exercise during pregnancy.* Retrieved October 1, 2022, from https://www.acog.org/womens-health/faqs/exercise-during-pregnancy

American College of Obstetricians and Gynecologists. (n.d.-c). *FAQs: Nutrition during pregnancy.* Retrieved October 1, 2022, from https://www.acog.org/womens-health/faqs/nutrition-during-pregnancy

American College of Obstetricians and Gynecologist. (n.d.-d). *Infographic: Breastfeeding benefits.* Retrieved October 1, 2022, from https://www.acog.org/womens-health/infographics/breastfeeding-benefits

American College of Obstetricians and Gynecologists. (2017). *Guidelines for perinatal care* (8th ed.). https://www.acog.org/clinical-information/physician-faqs/-/media/3a22e153b67446a6b31fb051e469187c.ashx

American Psychiatric Association. (n.d.-a). *What are eating disorders?* Retrieved May 20, 2022, from https://www.psychiatry.org/patients-families/eating-disorders/what-are-eating-disorders

American Psychiatric Association. (n.d.-b). *What is gender dysphoria?* Retrieved June 19, 2022, from https://psychiatry.org/patients-families/gender-dysphoria/what-is-gender-dysphoria

Andrasfay, T., & Goldman, N. (2021). Reductions in 2020 US life expectancy due to COVID-19 and the disproportionate impact on the Black and Latino populations. *Proceedings of the National Academy of Sciences of the United States of America, 118*(5), e2014746118. https://doi.org/10.1073/pnas.2014746118

Arias, E., Tejada-Vera, B., Ahmad, F., & Kochanek, K. D. (2021, July). Provisional life expectancy estimates for 2020. *NVSS Vital Statistics Rapid Release, Report No. 015.* https://doi.org/10.15620/cdc:107201

Arnett, D. K., Blumenthal, R. S., Albert, M. A., Buroker, A. B., Goldberger, Z. D., Hahn, E. J., Himmelfarb, C. D., Khera, A., Lloyd-Jones, D., McEvoy, J. W., Michos, E. D., Miedema, M. D., Muñoz, D., Smith, S. C., Jr., Virani, S. S., Williams, K. A., Sr., Yeboah, J., & Ziaeian, B. (2019). 2019 ACC/AHA guideline on the primary prevention of cardiovascular disease. *Circulation, 140*(11), e596–e646. https://doi.org/10.1161/cir.0000000000000678

Bahreynian, M., Qorbani, M., Khaniabadi, B. M., Motlagh, M. E., Safari, O., Asayesh, H., & Kelishadi, R. (2017).

Association between obesity and parental weight status in children and adolescents. *Journal of Clinical Research in Pediatric Endocrinology, 9*(2), 111–117. https://doi.org/10.4274/jcrpe.3790

Centers for Disease Control and Prevention. (n.d.-a). *10 Reasons to get vaccinated.* National Foundation for Infectious Diseases. Retrieved May 20, 2022, from https://www.nfid.org/immunization/10-reasons-to-get-vaccinated

Centers for Disease Control and Prevention. (n.d.-b). *Facts about falls.* Retrieved May 20, 2022, from https://www.cdc.gov/falls/facts.html

Centers for Disease Control and Prevention. (n.d.-c). *Newborn screening portal.* Retrieved October 1, 2022, from https://www.cdc.gov/newbornscreening/index.html

Centers for Disease Control and Prevention. (2021). *Sexually transmitted diseases (STDs).* https://www.cdc.gov/std/default.htm

Davis, J. P. E., Henry, Z. H., Argo, C. K., & Northup, P. G. (2019). Relationship of physician counseling to weight loss among patients with nonalcoholic fatty liver disease: An observational cohort study using National Health and Education Survey data. *Clinical Liver Disease, 14*(4), 156–160. https://doi.org/ 10.1002/cld.832

Debiec, K. E., Paul, K. J., Mitchell, C. M., & Hitti, J. E. (2010). Inadequate prenatal care and risk of preterm delivery among adolescents: A retrospective study over 10 years. *American Journal of Obstetrics & Gynecology, 203*(122), e1–e6. https://doi.org/10.1016/j.ajog.2010.03.001

DeFranco, E. A., Ehrlich, S., & Muglia, L. J. (2014). Influence of interpregnancy interval on birth timing. *BJOG, 121*(13), 1633–1640. https://doi.org/10.1111/1471-0528.12891

Deloitte Access Economics. (2020, June). *The social and economic cost of eating disorders in the United States of America: A report for the Strategic Training Initiative for the Prevention of Eating Disorders and the Academy for Eating Disorders.* Harvard School of Public Health. https://cdn1.sph.harvard.edu/wp-content/uploads/sites/1267/2020/07/Social-Economic-Cost-of-Eating-Disorders-in-US.pdf

Division of Healthcare Quality Promotion. (n.d.). *Vaccines during pregnancy FAQs.* Centers for Disease Control and Prevention, National Center for Emerging and Zoonotic Infectious Diseases. Retrieved May 20, 2022, from https://www.cdc.gov/vaccinesafety/concerns/vaccines-during-pregnancy.html

Division of STD Prevention. (n.d.-a). *Sexually transmitted diseases (STDs).* Centers for Disease Control and Prevention, National Center for HIV, Viral Hepatitis, STD, and TB Prevention. Retrieved May 20, 2022, from https://www.cdc.gov/std/default.htm

Division of STD Prevention. (n.d.-b). *Which STD tests should I get?* Centers for Disease Control and Prevention, National Center for HIV, Viral Hepatitis, STD, and TB Prevention. Retrieved May 20, 2022, from https://www.cdc.gov/std/prevention/screeningreccs.htm

Division of Violence Prevention. (n.d.). *Preventing adverse childhood experiences.* Centers for Disease Control and Prevention, National Center for Injury Prevention and Control. Retrieved May 20, 2022, from https://www.cdc.gov/violenceprevention/aces/fastfact.html

Division of Viral Diseases. (2022a). *COVID-19 vaccines for people who would like to have a baby.* Centers for Disease Control and Prevention, National Center for Immunization and Respiratory Diseases. https://www.cdc.gov/coronavirus/2019-ncov/vaccines/planning-for-pregnancy.html

Division of Viral Diseases. (2022b). *Stay up to date with your COVID-19 vaccines.* Centers for Disease Control and Prevention, National Center for Immunization and Respiratory Diseases. https://www.cdc.gov/coronavirus/2019-ncov/vaccines/stay-up-to-date.html

Duryea, T. K. (2022). *Dietary recommendation for toddlers, preschool, and school-age children.* UpToDate. https://www.uptodate.com/contents/dietary-recommendations-for-toddlers-preschool-and-school-age-children

Fiolet, T., Srour, B., Sellem, L., Kesse-Guyot, E., Allès, B., Méjean, C., Deschasaux, M., Fassier, P., Latino-Martel, P., Beslay, M., Hercberg, S., Lavalette, C., Monteiro, C. A., Julia, C., & Touvier, M. (2018). Consumption of ultra-processed foods and cancer risk: Results from NutriNet-Santé prospective cohort. *British Medical Journal, 360*(K322). http://doi.org/10.1136/bmj.k322

Fletcher, G. S. (2022). *Evidence-based approach to prevention.* UpToDate. https://www.uptodate.com/contents/evidence-based-approach-to-prevention

Fowler, T., Garr, D., Mager, N. D. P., & Stanley, J. (2020). Enhancing primary care and preventive services through interprofessional practice and education. *Israel Journal of Health Policy Research, 9*(12). https://doi.org/10.1186/s13584-020-00371-8

Hagan, J. F., Shaw, J. S., & Duncan, P. M. (Eds.). (2017). *Bright futures: Guidelines for health supervision of infants, children, and adolescents* (4th ed.). American Academy of Pediatrics.

Hales, C. M., Carroll, M. D., Fryar, C. D., & Ogden, C. L. (2017). Prevalence of obesity among adults and youth: United States, 2015–2016. *NCHS Data Brief, No. 288.* U.S. Department of Health and Human Services, Centers for Disease Control and Prevention, National Center for Health Statistics. https://www.cdc.gov/nchs/data/databriefs/db288.pdf

Hernández-Ledesma, B., & Hsieh, C. C. (2017). Chemopreventive role of food-derived proteins and peptides: A review. *Critical Reviews in Food Science and Nutrition, 57*(11), 2358–2376. https://doi.org/10.1080/10408398.2015.1057632

Hornberger, L. L., Lane, M. A., & Committee on Adolescence. (2021). Identification and management of eating disorders in children and adolescents. *Pediatrics, 147*(1), e2020040279. https://doi.org/10.1542/peds.2020-040279

Jameson, J. L., Fauci, A. S., Kasper, D. L., Hauser, S. L., Longo, D. L., & Losclzo, J. (2018). *Harrison's principles of internal medicine* (20th ed.). McGraw-Hill.

Kerr, S. M., Parker, S. E., Mitchell, A. A., Tinker, S. C., & Werler, M. M. (2017). Periconceptional maternal fever, folic acid intake, and the risk for neural tube defects. *Annals of Epidemiology, 27*(12), 777–782. https://doi.org/10.1016/j.annepidem.2017.10.010

Klein, D. A., Paradise, S. L., & Goodwin, E. T. (2018, December 1). Caring for transgender and gender-diverse persons: What clinicians should know. *American Family Physician, 98*(11), 645–653.

Lee, K. C., Ngo-Metzger, Q., Wolff, T., Chowdhury, J., Lefevre, M. L., & Meyers, D. S. (2016). Sexually transmitted infections: Recommendations from the U.S. Preventive Services Task Force. *American Family Physician, 94*(11), 907–915.

Linnan, L. A., Cluff, L., Lang, J. E., Penne, M., & Leff, M. S. (2019, April 22). Results of the Workplace Health in America Survey. *American Journal of Health Promotion, 33*(5). https://doi.org/10.1177/0890117119842047

Mather, M., Jacobsen, L. A., & Pollard, K. M. (2015). Aging in the United States. *Population Reference Bureau Population Bulletin, 70*(2). https://www.prb.org/wp-content/uploads/2016/01/aging-us-population-bulletin-1.pdf

Maurer, D. M., Raymond, T. J., & Davis, B. N. (2018, October 15). Depression: Screening and diagnosis. *American Family Physician, 98*(8), 508–515.

Mendez, M. F. (2022). *Mental status scales to evaluate cognition.* UpToDate. https://www.uptodate.com/contents/mental-status-scales-to-evaluate-cognition

Merriam-Webster. (n.d.-a). Chemoprophylaxis. In *Merriam-Webster.com dictionary.* https://www.merriam-webster.com/dictionary/chemoprophylaxis

Merriam-Webster. (n.d.-b). LGBTQIA. In *Merriam-Webster.com dictionary.* Retrieved March 6, 2022, from https://www.merriam-webster.com/dictionary/LGBTQIA

Merrick, M. T., Ford, D. C., Ports, K. A., & Guinn, A. S. (2018). Prevalence of adverse childhood experiences from the 2011–2014 Behavioral Risk Factor Surveillance System in 23 states. *JAMA Pediatrics, 172*(11), 10381044. https://doi.org/10.1001/jamapediatrics.2018.2537

Nasreddine, Z. S., Phillips, N. A., Bédirian, V., Charbonneau, S., Whitehead, V., Collin, I., Cummings, J. L., & Chertkow, H. (2005). The Montreal Cognitive Assessment, MoCA: A brief screening tool for mild cognitive impairment. *Journal of the American Geriatrics Society, 53*(4), 695–699. https://doi.org/10.1111/j.1532-5415.2005.53221.x

National Cancer Institute. (n.d.-a). *NCI's dictionary of cancer terms.* U.S. Department of Health and Human Services, National Institutes of Health. Retrieved May 20, 2022, from https://www.cancer.gov/publications/dictionaries/cancer-terms/def/chemoprevention

National Cancer Institute. (n.d.-b). *SEER cancer stat facts: Cancer of any site.* Retrieved June 20, 2022, from https://seer.cancer.gov/statfacts/html/all.html

National Center on Birth Defects and Developmental Disabilities. (n.d.). *Commit to healthy choices to help prevent birth defects.* Centers for Disease Control and Prevention. Retrieved May 20, 2022, from https://www.cdc.gov/ncbddd/birthdefects/prevention.html

National Center for Chronic Disease Prevention and Health Promotion. (n.d.-a). *About adult BMI.* Centers for Disease Control and Prevention, Division of Nutrition, Physical Activity, and Obesity. Retrieved May 20, 2022, from https://www.cdc.gov/healthyweight/assessing/bmi/adult_bmi/index.html#Children

National Center for Chronic Disease Prevention and Health Promotion. (n.d.-b). *Childhood obesity facts: Prevalence of childhood obesity in the United States.* Centers for Disease Control and Prevention, Division of Nutrition, Physical Activity, and Obesity. Retrieved May 20, 2022, from https://www.cdc.gov/obesity/data/childhood.html

National Center for Chronic Disease Prevention and Health Promotion. (n.d.-c). *Promoting health for adults.* Centers for Disease Control and Prevention. Retrieved May 20, 2022, from https://www.cdc.gov/chronicdisease/resources/publications/factsheets/promoting-health-for-adults.htm

National Center for Chronic Disease Prevention and Health Promotion. (n.d.-d). *Promoting health for children and adolescents.* Centers for Disease Control and Prevention. Retrieved May 20, 2022, from https://www.cdc.gov/chronicdisease/resources/publications/factsheets/children-health.htm

National Center for Chronic Disease Prevention and Health Promotion. (n.d.-e). *Promoting health for infants.* Centers for Disease Control and Prevention. Retrieved May 20, 2022, from https://www.cdc.gov/chronicdisease/resources/publications/factsheets/infant-health.htm

National Center for Chronic Disease Prevention and Health Promotion. (n.d.-f). *Workplace health model.* Centers for Disease Control and Prevention, Division of Population Health. Retrieved May 20, 2022, from https://www.cdc.gov/workplacehealthpromotion/model/index.html

National Center for Health Statistics. (n.d.). *Leading causes of death.* Centers for Disease Control and Prevention. Retrieved May 20, 2022, from https://www.cdc.gov/nchs/fastats/leading-causes-of-death.htm

National Center for Health Statistics. (2017). *Prevalence of obesity among adults and youth: United States, 2015–2016, NCHS Data Brief No. 288.* Centers for Disease Control and Prevention. https://www.cdc.gov/nchs/products/databriefs/db288.htm

National Center for Health Statistics. (2018). *Health, United States, 2018.* Centers for Disease Control and Prevention. https://www.cdc.gov/nchs/data/hus/hus18.pdf

National Center for Health Statistics. (2020a). *Percentage of having a doctor visit for any reason in the past 12 months for adults aged 18 and over, United States, 2019–2020.* National Health Interview Survey. https://wwwn.cdc.gov/NHISDataQueryTool/SHS_adult/index.html

National Center for Health Statistics. (2020b). *Prevalence of obesity and severe obesity among adults: United States 2017–2018, NCHS Data Brief No. 360.* Centers for Disease Control and Prevention. https://www.cdc.gov/nchs/products/databriefs/db360.htm

National Center for Health Statistics. (2021). *Characteristics of office-based physician visits, 2018, NCHS Data Brief No. 408.* Centers for Disease Control and Prevention. https://www.cdc.gov/nchs/products/databriefs/db408.htm

National Center for Immunization and Respiratory Diseases. (n.d.-a). *Immunization schedules.* Centers for Disease Control and Prevention. Retrieved May 20, 2022, from https://www.cdc.gov/vaccines/schedules/index.html

National Center for Immunization and Respiratory Diseases. (n.d.-b). *People at higher risk of flu complications.* Centers for Disease Control and Prevention. Retrieved May 20, 2022, from https://www.cdc.gov/flu/highrisk/index.htm

National Center for Immunization and Respiratory Diseases. (n.d.-c). *Who needs a flu vaccine?* Centers for Disease Control and Prevention. Retrieved May 20, 2022, from https://www.cdc.gov/flu/prevent/vaccinations.htm

National Center for Immunization and Respiratory Diseases. (n.d.-d). *Reasons for adults to be vaccinated.* Retrieved May 20, 2022, fromhttps://www.cdc.gov/vaccines/adults/reasons-to-vaccinate.html

National Center for Immunization and Respiratory Diseases. (2022a). *Adult immunization schedule: Recommendations for ages 19 years or older, United States, 2022.* Centers for Disease Control and Prevention. https://www.cdc.gov/vaccines/schedules/hcp/imz/adult.html

National Center for Immunization and Respiratory Diseases. (2022b). *Child and adolescent immunization schedule: Recommendations for ages 18 years or younger, United States, 2022.* Centers for Disease Control and Prevention. https://www.cdc.gov/vaccines/schedules/hcp/imz/child-adolescent.html

National Child Traumatic Stress Network. (2019). *What is child trauma?* https://www.nctsn.org/what-is-child-trauma

National Institute for Occupational Safety and Health. (n.d.). *Noise and occupational hearing loss.* Centers for Disease Control and Prevention. Retrieved June 22, 2022, from https://www.cdc.gov/niosh/topics/noise/default.html

National Institutes of Health. (n.d.). *What is prenatal care and why is it important?* U. S. Department of Health and Human Services. Retrieved May 20, 2022, from https://www.nichd.nih.gov/health/topics/pregnancy/conditioninfo/prenatal-care

National Safety Council. (n.d.). *Community safety.* Retrieved May 20, 2022, from https://www.nsc.org/community-safety/safety-topics/child-safety/child-safety-home

Nationwide Children's Hospital. (n.d.). *Sleep in adolescents.* Retrieved May 20, 2022, from https://www.nationwidechildrens.org/specialties/sleep-disorder-center/sleep-in-adolescents

Office of Dietary Supplements. (2021). *Folate: Fact sheet for health professionals.* National Institutes of Health. https://ods.od.nih.gov/factsheets/Folate-HealthProfessional/

Office of Disease Prevention and Health Promotion. (n.d.-a). Healthy People 2030 framework. *Healthy People 2030.* U.S. Department of Health and Human Services. Retrieved May 1, 2023, from https://health.gov/healthypeople/about/healthy-people-2030-framework

Office of Disease Prevention and Health Promotion. (n.d.-b). *Increase the proportion of worksites that offer an employee health promotion program.* Retrieved May 1, 2023, from https://health.gov/healthypeople/objectives-and-data/browse-objectives/workplace/increase-proportion-worksites-offer-employee-health-promotion-program-ecbp-d03

Office of Disease Prevention and Health Promotion. (n.d.-c). LGBT. *Healthy People 2030.* U.S. Department of Health and Human Services. Retrieved May 1, 2023, from https://health.gov/healthypeople/objectives-and-data/browse-objectives/lgbt

Office of Disease Prevention and Health Promotion. (n.d.-d). Older adults. *Healthy People 2030.* U.S. Department of Health and Human Services. Retrieved May 1, 2023, from https://health.gov/healthypeople/objectives-and-data/browse-objectives/older-adults

Office of Disease Prevention and Health Promotion. (n.d.-e). Overweight and obesity. *Healthy People 2030.* U.S. Department of Health and Human Services. Retrieved May 1, 2023, from https://health.gov/healthypeople/objectives-and-data/browse-objectives/overweight-and-obesity

Office of Population Affairs. (n.d.). *Recommended clinical preventive services for adolescents.* U.S. Department of Health and Human Services, Office of the Assistant Secretary for Health. Retrieved June 19, 2022, from https://opa.hhs.gov/adolescent-health/physical-health-developing-adolescents/clinical-preventive-services/recommended

Paladine, H. L., Ekanadham, H., & Diaz, D. C. (2021, February 15). Health maintenance for women of reproductive age. *American Family Physician, 103*(4), 209–217. https://www.aafp.org/afp/2021/0215/p209.html

Pfaller, B., Siu, S. C., D'Souza, R., Wichert-Schmitt, B., Nair, G. K., Haberer, K., Maxwell, C., & Silversides, C. K. (2021, March). Impact of obesity on outcomes of pregnancy in women with heart disease. *Journal of the American College of Cardiology, 77*(10), 1317–1326. https://www.jacc.org/doi/pdf/10.1016/j.jacc.2021.01.010

Piercy, K. L., Troiano, R. P., Ballard, R. M., Carlson, S. A., Fulton, J. E., Galuska, D. A., George, S. M., & Olson, R. D. (2018). The physical activity guidelines for Americans. *Journal of the American Medical Association, 320*(19), 2020–2028. https://doi.org/10.1001/jama.2018.14854

Reilly, J. J., Armstrong, J., Dorosty, A. R., Emmett, P. M., Ness, A., Rogers, I., Steer, C., Sherriff, A., & Avon Longitudinal Study of Parents and Children Study Team. (2005). Early life risk factors for obesity in childhood: Cohort study. *British Medical Journal, 330*(7504), 1357. https://doi.org/10.1136/bmj.38470.670903.E0

Reuben, D. B., & Leonard, S. D. (2022). *Office-based assessment of the older adult*. UpToDate. https://www.uptodate.com/contents/office-based-assessment-of-the-older-adult

Salami, J. A., Warraich, H., Valero-Elizondo, J., Spatz, E. S., Desai, N. R., Rana, J. S., Virani, S. S., Blankstein, R., Khera, A., Blaha, M. J., Blumenthal, R. S., Lloyd-Jones, D., & Nasir, K. (2017). National trends in statin use and expenditures in the US adult population from 2002 to 2013: Insights from the Medical Expenditure Panel Survey. *Journal of the American Medical Association Cardiology, 2*(1), 56–65. https://doi.org/10.1001/jamacardio.2016.4700

Scholl, T. O., & Johnson W. G. (2000). Folic acid: Influence on the outcome of pregnancy. *American Journal of Clinical Nutrition, 71*(5), 1295S–1303S. https://doi.org/10.1093/ajcn/71.5.1295s

Sonneville, K. R., & Lipson, S. K. (2018, June). Disparities in eating disorder diagnosis and treatment according to weight status, race/ethnicity, socioeconomic background, and sex among college students. *International Journal of Eating Disorders, 51*(6), 518–526. https://doi.org/10.1002/eat.22846

Styne, D. M., Arslanian, S. A., Connor, E. L., Farooqi, I. S., Murad, M. H., Silverstein, J. H., & Yanovski, J. A. (2017, January). Pediatric obesity-assessment, treatment, and prevention: An Endocrine Society clinical practice guideline. *Journal of Clinical Endocrinology and Metabolism, 102*(3), 709–757. https://doi.org/10.1210/jc.2016-2573

Szweda, H., & Jóźwik, M. (2016). Urinary tract infections during pregnancy: An updated overview. *Developmental Period Medicine, 20*(4), 263–272.

U.S. Department of Agriculture and U.S. Department of Health and Human Services. (2020). *Dietary Guidelines for Americans, 2020-2025* (9th ed.). https://www.dietaryguidelines.gov/sites/default/files/2020-12/Dietary_Guidelines_for_Americans_2020-2025.pdf

U.S. Preventive Services Task Force. (n.d.-a). *About the USPSTF*. Retrieved October 1, 2022, from https://www.uspreventiveservicestaskforce.org/uspstf/about-uspstf

U.S. Preventive Services Task Force. (n.d.-b). *A & B recommendations*. Retrieved June 25, 2022, from https://www.uspreventiveservicestaskforce.org/uspstf/recommendation-topics/uspstf-and-b-recommendations

U.S. Preventive Services Task Force. (n.d.-c). *Final recommendation statement: Aspirin use to prevent preeclampsia and related morbidity and mortality: Preventive medication*. Retrieved October 1, 2022, from https://www.uspreventiveservicestaskforce.org/uspstf/recommendation/low-dose-aspirin-use-for-the-prevention-of-morbidity-and-mortality-from-preeclampsia-preventive-medication

U.S. Preventive Services Task Force. (2015). *Final recommendation statement: Iron deficiency anemia in pregnant women: Screening and supplementation*. https://www.uspreventiveservicestaskforce.org/uspstf/recommendation/iron-deficiency-anemia-in-pregnant-women-screening-and-supplementation#fullrecommendationstart

U.S. Preventive Services Task Force. (2016a). *Final recommendation statement: Breast cancer screening*. https://www.uspreventiveservicestaskforce.org/uspstf/recommendation/breast-cancer-screening

U.S. Preventive Services Task Force. (2016b). *Final recommendation statement: Breastfeeding: Primary care interventions*. https://www.uspreventiveservicestaskforce.org/uspstf/recommendation/breastfeeding-primary-care-interventions

U.S. Preventive Services Task Force. (2016c). *Final recommendation statement: Screening for depression in adults*. https://www.uspreventiveservicestaskforce.org/uspstf/recommendation/depression-in-adults-screening

U.S. Preventive Services Task Force. (2016d). *Final recommendation statement: Depression in children and adolescents: Screening*. https://www.uspreventiveservicestaskforce.org/uspstf/recommendation/depression-in-children-and-adolescents-screening

U.S. Preventive Services Task Force. (2017a). *Final recommendation statement: Folic acid for the prevention of neural tube defects: Preventive medication*. https://www.uspreventiveservicestaskforce.org/uspstf/recommendation/folic-acid-for-the-prevention-of-neural-tube-defects-preventive-medication

U.S. Preventive Services Task Force. (2017b). *Final recommendation statement: Obesity in children and adolescents: Screening*. https://www.uspreventiveservicestaskforce.org/uspstf/recommendation/obesity-in-children-and-adolescents-screening

U.S. Preventive Services Task Force. (2017c). *Final recommendation statement: Vision in children ages 6 months to 5 years: Screening*. https://www.uspreventiveservicestaskforce.org/uspstf/recommendation/vision-in-children-ages-6-months-to-5-years-screening

U.S. Preventive Services Task Force. (2018). *Final recommendation statement: Syphilis infection in pregnant women: Screening.* https://www.upreventiveservicestaskforce.org/uspstf/recommendation/syphilis-infection-in-pregnancy-screening

U.S. Preventive Services Task Force. (2019a). *Final recommendation statement: Asymptomatic bacteriuria in adults: Screening.* https://www.upreventiveservicestaskforce.org/uspstf/recommendation/asymptomatic-bacteriuria-in-adults-screening

U.S. Preventive Services Task Force. (2019b). *Final recommendation statement: Abdominal aortic aneurysm: Screening.* https://www.upreventiveservicestaskforce.org/uspstf/recommendation/abdominal-aortic-aneurysm-screening

U.S. Preventive Services Task Force. (2019c). Interventions to prevent perinatal depression: Recommendation statement. *American Family Physician, 100*(6).

U.S. Preventive Services Task Force. (2020). *Final recommendation statement: Tobacco use in children and adolescents: Primary care interventions.* https://www.upreventiveservicestaskforce.org/uspstf/recommendation/tobacco-and-nicotine-use-prevention-in-children-and-adolescents-primary-care-interventions

U.S. Preventive Services Task Force. (2021a). *Draft recommendation statement: Vitamin, mineral, and multivitamin supplementation to prevent cardiovascular disease and cancer.* https://www.upreventiveservicestaskforce.org/uspstf/draft-recommendation/vitamin-supplementation-to-prevent-cvd-and-cancer-preventive-medication

U.S. Preventive Services Task Force. (2021b). *Final recommendation statement: Gestational diabetes: Screening.* https://www.upreventiveservicestaskforce.org/uspstf/recommendation/gestational-diabetes-screening

U.S. Preventive Services Task Force. (2021c). *Final recommendation statement: Prevention of dental caries in children younger than 5 years: Screening and interventions.* https://www.upreventiveservicestaskforce.org/uspstf/recommendation/prevention-of-dental-caries-in-children-younger-than-age-5-years-screening-and-interventions1

U.S. Preventive Services Task Force. (2021d). *Final recommendation statement: Tobacco smoking cessation in adults, including pregnant persons: Interventions.* https://www.upreventiveservicestaskforce.org/uspstf/recommendation/tobacco-use-in-adults-and-pregnant-women-counseling-and-interventions

Whitaker, K. L., Jarvis, M. J., Beeken, R. J., Boniface, D., & Wardle, J. (2010). Comparing maternal and paternal intergenerational transmission of obesity risk in a large population-based sample. *American Journal of Clinical Nutrition, 91*(6), 1560–1567. https://doi.org/10.3945/ajcn.2009.28838

Woolf, S. H., Jonas, S., & Kaplan-Liss, E. (2008). *Health promotion and disease prevention in clinical practice.* Lippincott Williams & Wilkins.

World Health Organization. (n.d.). *Coronavirus disease (COVID-19).* Retrieved October 1, 2022, from https://www.who.int/health-topics/coronavirus

World Health Organization. (2017, November 30). *Protecting workers' health.* https://www.who.int/news-room/fact-sheets/detail/protecting-workers'-health

World Health Organization. (2021). *Noncommunicable diseases.* https://www.who.int/en/news-room/fact-sheets/detail/noncommunicable-diseases

Yuan, M., Cross, S. J., Loughlin, S. E., & Leslie, F. M. (2015). Nicotine and the adolescent brain. *Journal of Physiology, 593*(16), 3397–3412. https://doi.org/10.1113/JP270492

Zheng, Y., Li, Y., Satija, A., Pan, A., Sotos-Prieto, M., Rimm, E., Willett, W. C., & Hu, F. B. (2019, June 12). Association of changes in red meat consumption with total and cause specific mortality among U.S. women and men: Two prospective cohort studies. *British Medical Journal, 365,* 2110. https://doi.org/10.1136/bmj.l2110

CHAPTER 6

Person-Centered Strategies for Promoting Healthy Lifestyles

Darlene Trandel, PhD, CNS, FNP, NBC-HWC, ICF
Lilly Tryon, DNP, FNP-BC, DipACLM, NBC-HWC

There are risks and costs to action. But they are far less than the long-range risks of comfortable inaction.

John F. Kennedy

OBJECTIVES

This chapter will enable the reader to:

1. Define a person-centered care approach to health promotion.
2. Apply person-centered strategies when promoting healthy lifestyles.
3. Utilize a partnership model of care approach to empower patients in self-care and self-management activities.
4. Integrate motivational interviewing concepts when communicating with patients about lifestyle change or self-care management of their disease or health condition.

Overview

Chronic disease management and care in the United States is a costly endeavor. Over $4.1 trillion was spent in 2020 (Centers for Medicare and Medicaid Services, 2022). This is an unsustainable amount that could bankrupt the country if the system of care doesn't change. Moreover, 90% of the annual health-care expenditures are for people with chronic diseases that require long-term treatment and management (National Center for Chronic Disease Prevention and Health Promotion [NCCDPHP], n.d.-b). These chronic diseases

© Kathleen Gail/Shutterstock; © StoryTime Studio/Shutterstock; © kali9/Getty Images

are predominantly a result of unhealthy lifestyle habits, such as tobacco use, poor nutrition, physical inactivity, and excessive alcohol use (NCCDPHP, n.d.-a).

It is well established that much of the burden of chronic disease could be prevented if individuals adopted healthy lifestyles (NCCDPHP, n.d.-c). Several large, long-term epidemiological studies, such as Adventist Health Studies, the Framingham Heart Study, and the Nurses' Health Study, have found connections between daily lifestyle habits and chronic disease (Rippe, 2019). Although these findings have been integrated into evidence-based clinical guidelines, little progress has been made in improving patient habits and actions (Rippe, 2018). Despite the recommendations and education provided to patients by advanced practice providers (APPs) about lifestyle change, many patients continue their unhealthy habits. Clearly, APPs need a more effective approach to promote healthier lifestyles in their patients.

Over the past decade, patient- or person-centered care (PCC) has changed healthcare delivery so that patients are no longer passive recipients of healthcare services but rather are at the center of their healthcare decisions. A PCC approach "consciously adopts the perspectives of individuals, families and communities, respects and responds to their needs, values and preferences and sees them as participants in their own healthcare rather than just beneficiaries" (Giusti et al., 2020, p. 2). Likewise, a PCC approach to health promotion sees the patient as a self-care manager in preventing chronic disease. The role of the provider in person-centered health promotion is that of a knowledgeable health advisor skilled in empowering patients to adopt the lifestyle behaviors needed for decreased disease risk and improved health outcomes. This chapter provides an overview of some foundational concepts for understanding health behavior change. It also offers evidence-informed strategies for promoting healthy lifestyles and assisting patients in developing the knowledge, skills, and confidence they need to make and sustain positive lifestyle changes.

Foundational Frameworks for Health Behavior Change

Many theoretical frameworks and models have been conceptualized to understand behavior change better. This chapter will review whole-person care, self-determination theory, the information-motivation-strategy (IMS) model, and the transtheoretical model. These frameworks provide insights for APPs as they identify patients' needs and design person-centered strategies for promoting health.

Whole-Person Care

An old maxim states that it is much more important to know what sort of person has a disease than what sort of disease a person has. The concept of whole-person care is premised on the understanding that the best way to promote healthy lifestyles and treat patients with chronic disease is to consider the many biological, behavioral, social, environmental, and cultural factors that commonly affect well-being and contribute to health outcomes. Instead of viewing the patient through a reductionistic lens of physiology, disease, and treatment, a whole-person care orientation weighs medical and nonmedical contributors in health care and self-care support (National Center for Complementary and Integrative Health [NCCIH], 2021) (see **Figure 6.1**). For instance, most chronic conditions increase the risk of depression; social connections can affect morbidity and mortality; environmental conditions affect health behavior and outcomes; cultural beliefs, attitudes, and behaviors affect disease risks and treatment adherence; and racial and sexual disparities affect access to health care as well as treatment and outcomes. Social determinants of health can contribute to and exacerbate disease as well as limit access to health care.

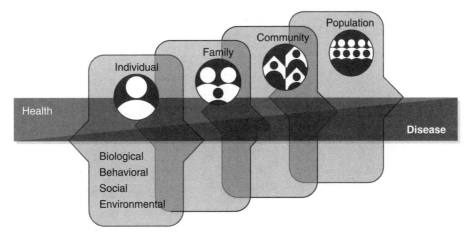

Figure 6.1 Whole-person care.

National Center for Complementary and Integrative Health. (2021). *Whole person health: What you need to know.* U.S. Department of Health and Human Services, National Institutes of Health. https://www.nccih.nih.gov/health/whole-person-health-what-you-need-to-know

A whole-person integrative approach to primary care improves the patient experience and clinical outcomes and reduces cost (Jonas & Rosenbaum, 2021). For example, the Veterans Health Administration piloted a model of care called Whole Health to reduce opioid addiction and improve chronic pain management. Veterans who received this care approach reported engaging in healthier behaviors, being more involved in healthcare decisions, improved pain management, and decreased opioid use than veterans who received the usual care (Bokhour et al., 2020).

Whole-Person Care Strategies

Instead of focusing on treating a patient's condition or disease, the APP who understands the concept of whole-person health will focus on restoring health, promoting resilience, and preventing disease across the life span (NCCIH, 2021). Consequently, many factors will be considered when promoting and supporting healthier lifestyles, including a patient's values, personality, literacy, interests, schedule, resources, living/work conditions, and support system. Furthermore, lifestyle change interventions will be tailored to each patient.

Self-Determination Theory

One of the foundational theories for understanding human motivation is the self-determination theory (SDT), developed by psychologists Deci and Ryan (1985). At the time, the dominant belief was that the best way to get people to change their behavior was by using rewards. Deci and Ryan proposed a different perspective, that of self-determination. *Self-determination* is a person's ability to reach their highest level of motivation, engagement, and performance. This autonomous motivation and resulting behaviors originate from self and are consistent with intrinsic goals or outcomes rather than external control or pressure from other forces. The SDT maintains that people have three basic psychological needs that must be met to experience self-determination: (a) *competence*, the need to feel effective at carrying out a specific behavior within their environment; (b) *autonomy*, the need to feel in control of one's own behavior and the course of their life; and (c) *relatedness*, the need for close connections with others (see **Figure 6.2**). To the extent that a patient's environment nurtures and meets these basic needs, autonomous motivation (or self-determination) can occur.

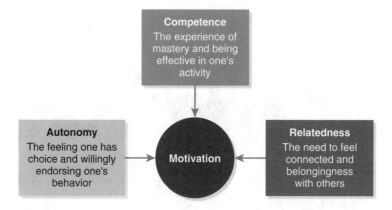

Figure 6.2 Self-determination theory.

Reproduced with permission from Ryan, R., & Deci, R. (n.d.). Self-determination theory. Behavior Institute. https://www.besci.org/models
/self-determination-theory

SDT-Informed Strategies

The APP who understands the SDT will use person-centered strategies that support the patient's needs for competence, autonomy, and relatedness (Patrick & Williams, 2012). For example, competence support strategies might include affirming the patient's strengths and change efforts, helping the patient develop a realistic plan for change, problem-solving, and identifying resources needed. Autonomy support strategies might include eliciting the patient's perspectives before making a recommendation, giving rationale for recommended interventions, and providing a menu of evidence-informed options for change. Support for relatedness might include expressing empathy for the patient's concerns and providing unconditional positive regard for the patient.

Information-Motivation-Strategy Model

Healthcare providers often express frustration at patient noncompliance with recommendations for lifestyle modification. A perspective shift from *compliance* to *adherence* can be helpful. Compliance implies a one-way relationship in which the provider prescribes a treatment plan and the patient is expected to comply. Adherence, on the other hand, is defined as "the extent to which health behavior reflects a health plan constructed and agreed to by the patient as a partner with the clinician in healthcare decision making" (Gould & Mitty, 2010, p. 290). This perspective, combined with an understanding of the SDT, encourages the APP to use strategies that foster patient–provider collaboration rather than relying on prescribing behavior change.

Martin and colleagues (2010) developed the information-motivation-strategy (IMS) model to promote health behavior change and patient adherence to treatment management. This model maintains that before a person can change, they must (1) *know* what change is necessary (information), (2) *desire* the change (motivation), and (3) have the tools to achieve and maintain the change (the *how*, or self-efficacy). A simple way of looking at the components of this model is "I know," "I want," and "I can"; therefore, "I act" (see **Figure 6.3**).

IMS-Related Strategies

The IMS model offers three reasons for patient nonadherence. This framework is also

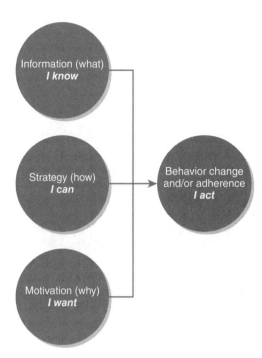

Figure 6.3 Information-motivation-strategy model.

Data from Martin, L. R., Haskard-Zolnierek, K. B., & DiMatteo, M. R. (2010). *Health behavior change and treatment adherence: Evidence-based guidelines for improving healthcare.* Oxford University Press.

helpful for identifying related person-centered strategies that match the patient's reasons for nonadherence (see **Figure 6.4**). Although APPs honor the adage "knowledge is power" when providing patient education, inspiration and implementation are also necessary for successful lifestyle change. Using this model builds trust and encourages patients to participate in decision-making and be partners in their health care, thus improving patient adherence and supporting autonomy.

Transtheoretical Model

A widely used model in health behavior change research is the transtheoretical model (TTM), also known as the stages of change model (Prochaska et al., 1992). The premise of the TTM is that change is a continuum, not a discrete event. Prochaska and colleagues noted that individuals cycle and recycle through five stages several times before successfully adopting healthy behaviors or stopping unhealthy behaviors (see **Table 6.1**). Guided by the TTM, the APP can assess readiness for change by noticing the patients' language when discussing a particular behavior (e.g., "I'd like to, but . . ." or "I am going to start next week.").

Stage-Matched Strategies

Fewer than 20% of at-risk individuals are prepared to act on a problem behavior at any given time (Prochaska et al., 1994). Ironically, more than 90% of behavior change programs are geared toward individuals in the action stage. Understanding the patients' stage and readiness to change helps the APP choose the appropriate approaches and specific intervention strategies for each patient to move to the next stage of change. In addition, patients may be in a different stage of change for each behavioral change. For instance, they may be in contemplation for considering an exercise program but may be in preparation for engaging in a healthy meal plan.

The goal for patients in precontemplation is to build awareness of the need for change and get them thinking about the possibility of changing their behavior. Patients in contemplation need to resolve their ambivalence to change by increasing the pros for change and decreasing the cons. Once they reach the preparation stage, patients have made a commitment to change. Therefore, the APP can help them develop a realistic plan. Patients in the action stage need to revise their plan as they identify what works and what doesn't. They are also at high risk for relapse, so the APP can help them explore solutions for getting around obstacles and plan for high-risk situations. Patients in maintenance will need ongoing support for sustaining change and assistance if they relapse.

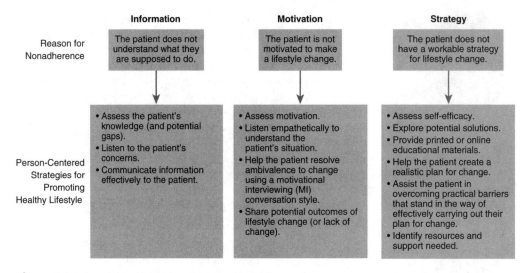

Figure 6.4 Information-Motivation-Strategy Model Categories

Data from DiMatteo, M. R., Haskard-Zolnierek, K. B., & Martin, L. R. (2012). Improving patient adherence: A three-factor model to guide practice. *Health Psychology Review*, 6(1), 74–91. https://doi.org/10.1080 /17437199.2010.537592

Table 6.1 Transtheoretical Model

Stage of Change	Characteristics	Examples of Person-Centered Strategies
Precontemplation ("I won't" or "I can't")	Patients may not be aware of or acknowledge a problem behavior. Therefore, there is no intention to change.	▪ Build a therapeutic relationship with patients. Remain nonjudgmental. ▪ Personalize information on risks and benefits of change. ▪ Help patients explore how their current behavior affects others. ▪ Share success stories.
Contemplation ("I might" or "I'd like to, but . . .")	The problem is recognized, but patients are not ready or sure they want to commit to change. They begin to think about change but are ambivalent as they weigh the pros and cons of changing or maintaining the status quo.	▪ Explore patients' reasons for change. ▪ Assist patients in weighing the pros and cons. ▪ Identify barriers and misconceptions. ▪ Help patients explore their options and address concerns.
Preparation ("I will")	Patients intend to take action and are preparing to change soon (within one month).	▪ Develop a plan for change with realistic goals and a timeline.

Stage of Change	Characteristics	Examples of Person-Centered Strategies
Action ("I am")	Patients initiate a change and commit considerable time and energy to modify their behavior.	■ Provide positive reinforcement. ■ Identify support system, tracking methods, accountability, and rewards. ■ Plan for high-risk situations. ■ Identify barriers and assist with problem-solving.
Maintenance ("I still am")	Patients have been doing the changed behavior for more than six months, have noted the gains from the change, and work to prevent relapse.	■ Provide positive reinforcement. ■ Provide ongoing support. ■ Address slips and relapses.

A Partnership Model of Care Approach to Health Promotion

Effective person-centered health promotion requires a partnership model for patient care that considers the patients' whole-person health, self-determination, reasons for nonadherence, and readiness to change. This partnership approach avoids promoting resistance to lifestyle modification interventions. Rather than advising or prescribing, the APP forms a cooperative working relationship with patients, encouraging them to participate in shared decision-making and exploring strategies for improved health outcomes (Emmons & Rollnick, 2001). The partnership approach also encompasses collaboration with other professionals and access to community resources that further empower patients in self-care and self-management activities (see **Figure 6.5**).

The partnership model of care (PMC) approach to health promotion represents a paradigm shift in how providers interact and communicate with patients. Specifically, the APP partners with patients around a holistic agenda for preventing and managing chronic disease. The relationship shifts from a hierarchal perspective to a cooperative working relationship in which each partner has much to offer toward health achievement. While the APP is the expert on health promotion and evidence-informed strategies for disease prevention, patients are recognized as experts on their own lives (Bodenheimer et al., 2002; Wiggins, 2008). Accordingly, the patient–provider partnership in this model involves the APP and patient sharing their unique expertise and making healthcare decisions together (Wiggins, 2008). For example, instead of merely advising lifestyle modification, the APP helps patients to explore how their lifestyle choices positively and negatively affect their life and why they might consider a change. Patients are guided to make informed choices for health behavior change, set health goals, and design a realistic plan that fits their unique situation. The traditional perception of "we know better" is replaced by "no decision about you, without you" (Wiggins, 2008, p. 4).

In the traditional model, the patients' role is passive, listening to the providers' directives and knowing their progress will be evaluated at the next visit. With a whole-person orientation in the PMC, the spotlight is on patients as self-care managers of their risk factors and health conditions. The APP recognizes that

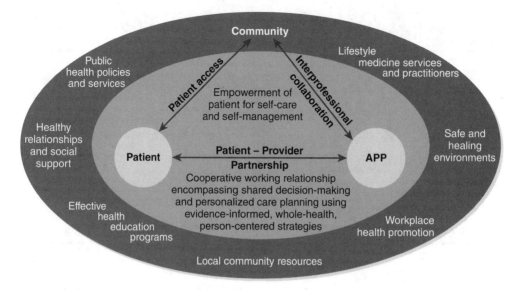

Figure 6.5 A partnership model of care approach to health promotion.

Data from Harrison, S. R., & Jordan, A. M. (2022). Chronic disease care integration into primary care services in sub-Saharan Africa: A "best fit" framework synthesis and new conceptual model. *Family Medicine and Community Health, 10*(3), e001703. https://doi.org/10.1136/fmch-2022-001703

most patient care is self-care delivered outside the healthcare setting by patients in their own homes. Patients control important self-management decisions such as choosing what to eat, taking prescribed medications, managing stress, and watching for complications. Bodenheimer et al. (2002) note that it isn't an issue of whether patients self-manage but how well they self-manage their health conditions. Therefore, the APP assesses knowledge, motivation, and self-efficacy before co-creating a personalized plan for change. Evidence-informed, whole-health, person-centered strategies are relevant to patients' goals for health and well-being.

Effective interventions for behavior change must include behavioral counseling to engage patients in self-management practices that support their efforts to change and maintain healthy behaviors (U.S. Preventive Services Task Force, 2013). However, providing education to those who are not ready or even thinking about change is a mismatch of interventions. That is why just providing patient

education, while important, is not sufficient to empower patients to effectively self-manage their health. The education model is built on the belief that the more information patients have, the better their self-management and outcomes. In contrast, the PMC targets patients' perspective in defining their problem, evoking internal motivation, setting health goals, exploring solutions based on their experiences and strengths, and increasing their self-efficacy to achieve their goals. In this model, the APP becomes a behavior change agent.

In the PMC approach to health promotion, the APP will consider the expertise and skill of other health professionals who can support patients in lifestyle modification (e.g., dietitians, physical therapists, and health coaches). In addition to interprofessional collaboration and care coordination, the APP will assess patients' access to community resources that can further empower them in self-management, such as health education programs, workplace health promotion, and public health policies

---

Health Promotion Research Study

Self-Development Theory and Motivational Interviewing for Type 2 Diabetes Mellitus

Background: Obesity, prediabetes, and type 2 diabetes mellitus (T2DM) have become a global epidemic. The modifiable risk factors for these diseases are behaviorally based, making lifestyle modification the primary goal for prevention and treatment. Thus, the current challenge is to develop lifestyle modification interventions that produce long-term behavior change.

Methodology: A systematic review of SDT-based and MI interventions for obesity, prediabetes, and T2DM was conducted with a specific focus on their quality and effectiveness.

Results: The review included 54 publications and 42 independent samples using SDT and MI interventions. Interventions to treat overweight and obesity ($n = 15$), prediabetes ($n = 4$), and T2DM ($n = 23$) were summarized and evaluated using the Quality Rating Scale. While the results of these studies were mixed, most of the interventions resulted in health benefits. The overweight and obese intervention groups showed improved weight loss, physical activity, and nutrition compared to control groups in 12 of the 15 samples. All four prediabetes studies led to positive outcomes, including weight loss, reduced risk of T2DM, and return to normal glucose tolerance. The T2DM intervention groups showed improved glucose control, weight loss, and fat consumption compared to control groups in 10 of the 23 samples.

Implications for Advanced Practice: APPs may find that their patients achieve better health outcomes when they integrate SDT and MI constructs into interventions for preventing and treating T2DM and other lifestyle-related chronic diseases.

Reference: Phillips, A. S., & Guarnaccia, C. A. (2020). Self-determination theory and motivational interviewing interventions for type 2 diabetes prevention and treatment: A systematic review. *Journal of Health Psychology, 25*(1), 44–66. https://doi.org/10.1177/1359105317737606

---

and services. The patients' environment and relationships will also be explored when identifying barriers to lifestyle modification and discovering individualized strategies to adhere to healthy living habits.

Communicating with Patients About Lifestyle Change

J.T., a 42-year-old recently divorced middle-school teacher, presents to her APP with a primary complaint of urinary frequency. Her blood pressure is 148/89 mmHg, and she has a body mass index of 36 kg per m². A dipstick urinalysis in the office shows 2+ sugar, and finger-stick blood glucose is 240 mg/dL.

As the APP indicates her suspicion about diabetes and plans for additional blood tests, J.T. remembers the complications her mother had experienced with T2DM. She expresses concern that as a single working mother with two teenage children, she doesn't have the time to exercise or cook. A typical breakfast consists of a pastry and coffee; she skips lunch to grade or prepare lesson plans; dinner is often picked up at a fast-food restaurant while taking her children to music lessons and soccer games. She laughingly admits that she is fueled by Coke. The APP, busy adding lab orders and a follow-up plan to the electronic health record, doesn't acknowledge J.T.'s concerns. Instead, she advises J.T. that weight loss is critical for improving her health outcomes and preventing diabetic complications in the future. She recommends that J.T. eat a low-fat, high-fiber diet and exercise 150 minutes weekly. The APP notices that J.T.'s attention is distracted by notifications on her mobile phone and wonders how compliant the patient will be with the plan of care.

It is easy to conclude that J.T. lacks motivation or that she doesn't truly understand the effects of her current lifestyle on her health. These conclusions may lead the APP to adopt an authoritative communication style and warn J.T. of the risks to her health, provide patient education, and recommend lifestyle changes. In subsequent visits, when J.T.'s behavior hasn't changed and her health has worsened, it would be easy to label her as un-motivated or noncompliant and stop recommending lifestyle changes altogether.

While it is good practice for APPs to recommend lifestyle changes to their patients, a directing style is often used instead of a person-centered approach. As the APP attempts to address and fix what seems wrong, recommendations are prefaced with phrases such as "You really need to . . ." "It would be so much better for you if . . ." "Have you tried . . . ?" and "You should . . ." Miller and Rollnick (2013) refer to this style of helping people to change as the *righting reflex*. Unfortunately, this approach doesn't work when it comes to behavior change. Over half of patients fail to recall recommendations received during a healthcare visit due to ineffective communication with their healthcare providers (Laws et al., 2018). To make matters worse, APPs can inadvertently increase patients' resistance to behavior change because their directing style naturally brings out patients' arguments against change (Miller & Rose, 2009). The truth is, "people do not resist change; they resist being changed" (Senge, 2010, p. 144).

Ambivalence

One would think that threats of blindness, amputations, and kidney failure from diabetes complications would be enough to motivate weight loss or that a heart attack would awaken the urge to quit smoking and eat a healthy diet. However, these situations often do not lead to lasting change. APPs who regularly engage in conversations about lifestyle change often ask themselves, "How can I help my patients make and maintain self-defined changes?" Sometimes they may think that patients lack information, are lazy, have an oppositional personality, are in denial, or are resistant. But this is not usually the case. The reason change is difficult is because of ambivalence.

Ambivalence is simultaneously wanting and not wanting something. It is one's argument both for and against change. People think about reasons to change, then think of reasons not to change, then stop thinking about it. Ambivalence can be uncomfortable, cause anxiety, lead to procrastination, and often make patients stuck in their decision-making about change. When faced with a patient ambivalent about lifestyle change, healthcare professionals may be tempted to push them toward a healthier behavior (the righting reflex). However, this approach can be counterproductive.

Miller and Rollnick (2013) found that ambivalence is a normal part of the change process and noted better outcomes when healthcare professionals altered how they communicated with patients to engage them as active partners in their own health behavior change. Their finding aligns with the self-perception theory (Bem, 1972), which states that when people are unsure about their feelings and motivations, they will use their own behavior to infer what they feel. In other words, they believe what they hear themselves say. For example, if patients hear themselves talk about the disadvantages of the status quo (not changing), all the good reasons for changing, and their optimism for making that change, they are more likely to be motivated for change and move toward an intention to commit to change. As French philosopher Blaise Pascal noted in the 1600s, "people are generally better persuaded by the reasons which they have themselves discovered than by those which have come into the mind of others" (Pascal, 1958, p. 4).

Motivational Interviewing

For the PMC approach to health promotion to be effective, APPs need a different conversation style when communicating with patients about lifestyle modification. *Motivational interviewing* (MI) is a communication approach defined as a "collaborative conversation style for strengthening a person's own motivation and commitment to change" (Miller & Rollnick, 2013, p. 12). The increased motivation for change is accomplished within an atmosphere of acceptance and compassion, without pressure or coercion to change. This guiding style of communication supports the PMC approach to health promotion by helping patients understand their reasons for and against change and allowing for more informed and intrinsically invested decisions around these concerns.

Simply put, MI is an effective way of conversing with people about change, specifically their *own* reasons for change. MI increases patients' intrinsic motivation for change by capitalizing on the idea that if people can talk themselves out of change, they can also talk themselves into change. Therefore, primary aim of MI is to elicit from patients their own *change talk* (positive statements about change) and their own reasons and arguments for change. The act of speech, of verbally defending change in the absence of coercion, causes patients to change in attitude and behavior. The more patients hear their own arguments for change based on their values and interests, the more committed they become to that change. This MI-informed conversation sharply contrasts the traditional approach that healthcare professionals often use when conversing with patients (see **Table 6.2**).

MI recognizes that every person faced with recommendations for lifestyle change will

Table 6.2 Distinctions Between Traditional and MI-Informed Approaches to Lifestyle Change

Traditional Approach	MI-Informed Approach
Focused on fixing the problem	Focused on the patient's concerns and perspective
Unequal relationship, with power residing with the provider	Collaborative equal partnership
Assumes the patient is motivated	Matches intervention to the patient's readiness
Advises, persuades, warns	Emphasizes personal choice and autonomy
Prescribes goals	Collaborates with the patient for setting goals
Interprets ambivalence as the patient is in denial	Recognizes ambivalence as a normal part of the change process
Resistance met with pushback and correcting	Resistance acknowledged and influenced by provider behavior

experience ambivalence. The goal of MI is to resolve this ambivalence and increase internal motivation by (1) having patients talk about why they want to change, (2) having patients talk about their discontent with their current situation, and (3) having patients develop strategies to overcome barriers to change. Following are some questions to help patients voice their reasons for change:

- "Why would you want to change?"
- "What are the three best reasons for you to change?"
- "What makes it important for you to make this change?"
- "If you considered changing, how might you be successful in making this change?"

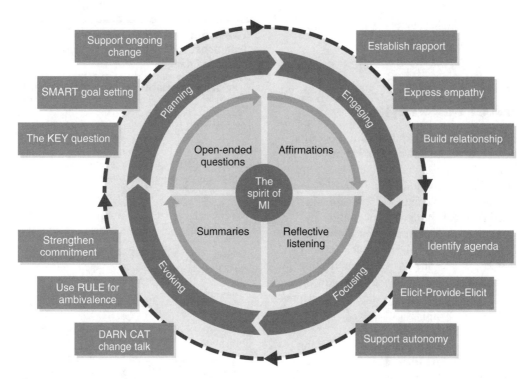

Figure 6.6 The MI communication approach.

These questions help patients feel engaged (interested, cooperative), empowered (hopeful, optimistic, confident), open (accepted, comfortable, safe, respected), and understood (connected, heard, listened to).

MI theory was first published in 1983, and changes in the approach continue with the last updated book edition released in 2013. The first focus of MI was on addiction, and later the focus was expanded to people in change. MI continues to be a living approach with its expansion based on research, including clinical trials, efficacy reviews, and meta-analyses. The effectiveness of an MI approach has been noted in cardiovascular rehabilitation, diabetes management, dietary change, hypertension, illicit drug use, infection risk reduction, management of chronic mental disorders, problem drinking, problem gambling, smoking, and concomitant mental and substance use disorders (Miller & Rose, 2009). Currently, it's one of the most

well-known behavior approaches to helping patients change their behavior to improve healthcare outcomes, particularly in chronic care.

This chapter introduces the APP to selected components of MI, including the Spirit of MI and the MI Processes. Basic MI communication methods to use when talking with patients about lifestyle change and examples of each are reviewed, although advanced training in MI is recommended for APPs to become competent MI practitioners. **Figure 6.6** provides an overview of the MI communication approach.

The Spirit of MI

An empathic, person-centered approach is the heart and foundation of MI. It is through the positive regard and respectful understanding of patients' experiences and the belief that they have the motivation and solutions within to take charge of their health that the

Table 6.3 The Spirit of MI Contrasted with an Authoritative Communication Style

Element	Spirit of MI	Authoritative Communication Style
Partnership (collaboration between the practitioner and the patient)	▪ Recognizes patients' expertise about themselves. There is a collaboration of expertise (e.g., "You have what you need, and together we will find it."). ▪ Facilitates shared decision-making	▪ Based on the deficit model. Implies, "I have what you need, and I will give it to you." ▪ Attempts to persuade change ▪ Confrontation can occur
Acceptance (respecting the autonomy of the patient)	▪ Considers the absolute worth of each patient. Affirms patients' strengths and efforts. ▪ Believes that there is no right way to change and that the solutions for how to make the change may reside in patients ▪ Takes a nonjudgmental stance about patients' readiness to change and respects their choices ▪ Shows empathy (e.g., "You are frustrated by trying to lose weight," or "You are discouraged in finding time to fit in your gym workouts.").	▪ Uses authority to instruct patients to make changes ▪ Labels low readiness to change as noncompliance
Compassion	▪ Actively promotes patients' welfare and gives priority to their needs ▪ Seeks to understand patients' experiences, values, and motivation (e.g., "I want to understand your experience.").	▪ Disregards or shows indifference to patients' experience, values, motivation, and needs
Evocation (evoking or drawing out patients' ideas about change)	▪ Believes that change is fundamentally self-change and that people make their own decisions about what they will and will not do ▪ Recognizes that motivation for change is present in patients and activated by the provider eliciting change talk ▪ Connects lifestyle change to the things patients care about	▪ Gives unsolicited education or imposes ideas, presuming that patients lack the insight, knowledge, or skills for lifestyle change

Data from Miller, W. R., & Rollnick, S. (2013). *Motivational interviewing: Helping people change* (3rd ed.). Guilford Press.

principles and strategies of MI are successful. The Spirit of MI is the overarching "way of being" with patients that communicates partnership, acceptance, compassion, and evocation (Miller & Rollnick, 2013) (see **Table 6.3**). These elements establish a safe, exploratory atmosphere for patients to verbalize their ambivalence and explore the possibility of behavior change.

As previously noted, change requires a *partnership* of expertise. The APP works collaboratively with patients to identify their problems and health goals and a realistic plan for change. This partnership approach builds trust between patients and the APP, as the APP guides rather than tells and recognizes patients as competent to make decisions about their lifestyle habits and be accountable for them. A second element in the Spirit of MI is *acceptance*, in which the APP respects patients' autonomy and readiness to change. Empathy toward patients increases as the APP seeks to understand the reasons behind their behaviors. The APP demonstrates *compassion* when actively promoting patients' welfare and giving priority to their needs rather than operating from a place of self-interest. The fourth element in the Spirit of MI, *evocation*, recognizes that patients already have much of the motivation, wisdom, and resources needed for behavior change. The provider's role is to *evoke* or draw it out.

MI Methods

MI not only defines the overarching spirit for communicating with patients about lifestyle change but also offers basic communication methods to guide them. These include open-ended questions, affirmations, reflections, and summaries—referred to by the acronym OARS (Miller & Rollnick, 2013).

Open-Ended Questions

While time and schedules are often tight for the APP, taking a few extra moments to ask open-ended questions enables collaboration and yields more accurate information. *Closed-ended questions*, which require a yes; no; or simple, direct response are often utilized in health care to get to the bottom of things in a time-efficient manner. An example is, "Have you been taking your medicine regularly?" Closed-ended questions are appropriate when a quick, definitive answer is needed. However, due to the simplicity and limitation of the responses elicited by closed-ended questions, they may not offer patients choices that accurately reflect their situation. In addition, closed-ended questions can convey a lack of understanding and interest on the APP's part, present a conversational dead end, and negatively influence the relationship and patient outcome.

While APPs need to collect information to assess, diagnose, treat, and document, using more open-ended questions elicits more facts about the issue and leads to a fuller picture of what is happening with patients. *Open-ended questions* often begin with the words "what" and "how," allowing patients to provide extra

detail and information such as feelings, attitudes, and understanding of their situation (Moore et al., 2016). For example, questions such as "What concerns you most about your diabetes?" "Tell me about your sleep routine," and "I am interested in hearing more about what a typical dinner looks like" would yield more accurate information and actionable insight for the APP.

Affirmations

Affirmations are at the core of the values that support MI because they validate patients' capability to make change. An *affirmation* acknowledges patients' attributes and steps taken in the direction of change. Rather than providing general praise (e.g., "Good job on losing weight this month") or a compliment (e.g., "You look great!"), the APP can call attention to something patients have done, recognize an underlying strength or value, or describe the effect of patients' actions. Following are some examples:

- "You were committed to fitting in exercise this week and made it to all your workouts."
- "You've shown a lot of persistence in keeping your pantry stocked with healthy choices so you can make and carry nutritious lunches to work."
- "Your willingness to cook healthy dinners helped lower your blood sugars."

Self-affirmations can also be evoked by asking patients questions such as "What enabled your success staying sober when everyone around you was drinking?" Affirmations have the effect of strengthening patients' self-efficacy and capacity for change. Additionally, they can support the patient–provider relationship while fostering engagement and reducing defensiveness.

Reflective Listening

In the MI communication style, there is a strong emphasis on the intentional use of reflective listening for enhancing rapport, expressing empathy, and evoking change talk. *Reflective listening* involves listening to truly understand the meaning of what patients say rather than filtering their words through the APP's assumptions, experience, stereotyping, or prejudices. Reflections not only convey to patients that the APP is listening but also help both the APP and the patients better understand the content, feeling, and meaning of messages. Patients hear what they just said from the APP's perspective, which can provide the opportunity to correct any misunderstanding that might have occurred in the exchanged communication. Effective reflections also help patients think more deeply about their situation and encourage them to continue their exploration of problems, motivations, and feelings.

An extension of active listening skills, reflective listening requires that the APP be present and free from external distractions (e.g., computers, texts, noise) and internal distractions (e.g., their own thoughts or feelings) and not interrupt patients as they disclose their concerns and experiences. Additionally, active listening necessitates that the APP becomes comfortable with moments of silence to allow patients to process what was just said instead of filling the space with questions or other logistics. Also important is that the APP give full attention to multiple dimensions: the content of the words, body language, qualities of the voice (e.g., tone, energy), and meaning behind the words (e.g., needs, emotions, ambivalence) (Moore et al., 2016). The simplest reflection paraphrases the significant part of what the APP understood from the content of the patients' messages. More complex reflections go beyond the surface as the APP makes an educated guess about the patients' meaning. Empathetic reflections acknowledge patients' emotion and experience behind the words. Giving empathy is widely recognized as a predictor of behavior change (Yu et al., 2022). **Table 6.4** offers descriptions and examples of several types of reflections. The MI rule of thumb is to use two or three reflections for every open-ended question during a patient conversation.

Summaries

Finally, MI suggests using *summaries*, which are statements linking, highlighting, and reinforcing selected important points that have been discussed. An example of a summary statement is, "Let me stop and sum up what we've just talked about. You're not sure you want to be here today, and you only came because your spouse insisted. At the same time, you have had some nagging thoughts about how much you've been smoking, how it might affect your ability to keep up with your kids on the basketball court, and your chronic cough. Did I miss anything? I'm curious what you make of all those things." Summaries communicate interest and understanding of the patient's perspective. They can be helpful in highlighting both sides of a patient's ambivalence about change or when transitioning to the question of the patient's next step in moving toward their health goal.

Complex Methods

In addition to the basic methods of OARS, MI utilizes complex methods such as reframing and reviewing past successes. *Reframing* helps the patient consider a different (and more positive) perspective of a negative experience. For example, a failed attempt at behavior change can be reframed as a learning experience: "Although you weren't able to stop your smoking habit completely, you did successfully stop for the first several days in the many times you tried to quit." *Reviewing past successes* at changing can help increase a patient's self-efficacy.

MI Processes

MI helps to guide patients through the stages of change by using four processes: engaging, focusing, evoking, and planning (Miller & Rollnick, 2013). Although these processes have a natural sequence of emergence within

Table 6.4 Types of Reflections

Reflection	Description	Example
Simple	Stays close to the meaning of the message by paraphrasing without sounding like parroting	Patient: "I don't want to quit smoking." APP: "You don't want to give up your cigarettes."
Rephrasing	Substitutes synonyms	Patient: "I hear what you are saying about my drinking, but I don't think it's a big issue." APP: "So at this moment, you are not too concerned about your drinking."
Complex	More effective than simple reflection, as the APP provides a statement back to the patient that goes beyond the words spoken and attempts to get at the meaning, significance, or feeling implied by the patient Sometimes APPs worry that the reflection may be overreaching. However, if they miss the point, the patient will usually provide a more accurate interpretation.	Patient: "I just don't want to take pills. I want to handle this on my own." APP: "You don't want to depend on a drug. It seems like you should be able to do this yourself without help."
Double-sided	Reflects both sides of the ambivalence the patient experiences, especially after they share the pros and cons of change It is more effective to reflect the cons of changing first and then reflect the pros of changing in the hope that the patient's next comment will go in the direction of what was last reflected. A good way to start a double-sided reflection is "On the one hand, (cons/negative side of change), and on the other hand (pros/positive side of change).	APP: "On the one hand, you are not happy about having to make changes to the way you eat, and on the other hand, you are concerned about your elevated blood sugar and weight."
Empathy	An empathy reflection recognizes the feeling, emotion, or need that is unspoken but conveyed by the patient's tone or body language. It requires deep listening and going beyond what is said.	Patient: "My wife decided not to come today. After all these years of my helping her go through her surgeries and treatment, and now she doesn't want to help me with my health issues!" APP: "Her choosing not to attend today's visit was a big disappointment for you."

a patient encounter, they can overlap and may not follow a linear progression.

Engaging

The *engaging* process involves establishing rapport and building a positive, trusting relationship with patients. Engaging is critical at the beginning of the patient–provider relationship and at each patient visit. The goal is to build a cooperative working relationship and create a safe atmosphere in which patients feel comfortable discussing lifestyle change. Important in this process is the ability of the APP to accept patients where they are; respond with a nonjudgmental attitude; and validate patients' issues, views, or choices in both their verbal and their nonverbal behavior. Key skills to use in the engaging process include actively listening to patients, expressing empathy, and striving to understand their perspective. General first questions might include "What brings you here today?" or "What's been happening since we last met?" It is essential to resist the righting reflex so as not to provoke resistance or defensiveness in patients.

Focusing

With the engaging foundation in place, the *focusing* process identifies a clear direction and agenda for the patient visit. This focus may not be clear from the outset. Some patients come in with issues they are ready to work on while others lack insight regarding direction. Focusing is about helping patients determine what is truly important to them in the visit and using that information to set the tone and agenda for the care. Allowing patients to identify the focus empowers them to be more actively engaged and invested in the topic. The APP might ask, "What would you like to talk about today? What are you most concerned about?" Sometimes patients may need a list of options: "We could talk about monitoring your blood sugar, eating a healthy diet, exercising, or taking your medication. Or perhaps there is something else?"

After patients' concerns are addressed, the door might be open to the APP's agenda. By eliciting what is important to patients using open-ended questions, reflections, clinical judgment, and a balance of the patients' and APP's expertise, shared goals for a visit can be negotiated. The structure and agenda of the visit can be collaborated, keeping in mind the patients' most pressing needs, the most clinically compelling issue, and the visit time boundaries.

Elicit-Provide-Elicit. While the MI communication style is person centered, there are times when it is appropriate and desirable to provide information or contribute ideas to patients. Providing information can be vital in finding a clear focus. The need for information or strategies can also arise during evoking and is a central task to planning. MI considers this exchange a respectful, thoughtful, and reciprocal flow of information and ideas that champions patients' needs and autonomy. The method of providing information in MI is called *Elicit-Provide-Elicit* (see **Table 6.5**). It's easy to overestimate how much information patients need. Therefore, the APP should first inquire about patients' prior knowledge to prevent wasting time giving information they already have. It is also important to query patients' interest in the information, mindful that their desires and needs might differ from initially thought. After filling patients' information gap, always turn the conversation back to them to determine their response to the information shared.

Patients may feel stuck or be unable to think of any solutions and ask the APP for advice. At these times, it may be helpful for the APP to offer ideas but to do so in a manner consistent with the Spirit of MI. Rather than make a single suggestion that may make patients feel compelled to accept, it is more effective to provide several options for them to consider and evaluate whether they would work in their situation. When the information is related to changing behavior, it is also helpful to honor patients' autonomy by including

Table 6.5 Steps to Elicit-Provide-Elicit

Step	Examples
1. Prioritize by focusing on what patients most want or need to know.	"What do you know about relaxation methods?" "I wonder if there is anything that you might like to know about that strategy?" "What have you been wondering about that I might be able to clarify for you?"
2. Use autonomy-supportive language versus talking down authoritatively, giving information without permission, or telling patients what they must do.	"If it's all right with you, we could discuss changes you could make to your stress management practices. May I tell you about a way of deep breathing that might be helpful for you?" "Would it be OK if I share some information about the kinds of foods that support heart health?" "It sounds like you're doing well with your diet. Can I ask you about your physical activity?"
3. Present information clearly, in a level of language patients can understand. Give information in small doses without overloading patients with more than they need.	"There are four keys to this way of eating: (1) several daily servings of vegetables and fruits; (2) whole grains instead of refined; (3) less red meat and more legumes; (4) and nuts for snacks instead of sugary foods."
4. Inquire about patients' understanding, interpretation, questions, or response to the information shared.	"What resonated most with you from the information I shared about ways to manage stress?" "What are your thoughts about this way of eating?" "Sometimes people find it easier to change one part of their diet at a time. Is there one aspect I mentioned that you feel ready to work on?" "What questions or concerns do you have about becoming more physically active?"

statements that offer empathy and not pressuring patients to change. For example, "Making changes to your longtime lifestyle is hard. From what you are saying, together with your health data, the best thing you might do for your diabetes right now is to consider quitting smoking. I cannot make you quit. Only you can make that choice, and that decision is totally up to you. I know these decisions can sometimes be difficult to make."

Evoking

Miller and Rollnick (2013) define *evoking* as the process that involves eliciting the individuals' own motivation for a particular change. Evoking is an emergent, co-creative process sensitive to in-the-moment interactions through which the patients' potential for change is released. In other words, the motivation for change emerges as the conversation unfolds. During the evoking process, the APP elicits the patients' own reasons for change and thus strengthens their motivation in the direction of the change goal. This evoking is accomplished by listening to the language of change and selectively focusing on and emphasizing patients' statements that favor change.

Language of Change. APPs trained to diagnose and treat often fail to hear the language of change in their patients. In the MI style of communication, however, APPs seek to understand patients' views on their health status, self-management efforts, challenges, and priorities while listening for their change talk. As mentioned previously, ambivalence is a normal part of the change process in which a person has simultaneous conflicting motivations about change. This internal struggle of ambivalence can be a long-lasting and tiring debate, leaving patients to feel stuck, stop thinking about change, or resolve to stay in the status quo.

Recognizing and eliciting change talk is a critical skill for helping patients with lifestyle change (Matthews et al., 2022). MI categorizes change talk as (a) early change talk, when the patient is beginning to consider a behavior change, and (b) later change talk, when the patient begins to move into action to make a change (Miller & Rollnick, 2013). In early change talk, patients will talk about their desire, ability, reasons, and needs (DARN) to change their behavior. In later change talk, patients make statements about commitment, activation, or taking steps (CAT) toward change (see **Table 6.6**). Sustain talk, or arguments favoring the status quo, have a similar pattern.

It is normal to hear change talk and sustain talk intertwined; that's the nature of ambivalence. For example, a patient might state, "I know smoking is bad for me and wish I could quit. Then maybe I could join my kids when they play football and run around the field without getting out of breath. But it's hard to quit because my job is so stressful and smoking is my only relaxation." Early in

Table 6.6 Recognizing the Language of Change

Language of Change	Change Talk	Sustain Talk
Early		
Desire (wanting)	"I want to lose weight."	"I want to eat whatever I want."
Ability (perceived ability to achieve)	"I could lose weight by skipping suppers."	"I've tried, but I can't keep the weight off."
Reasons (specific rationalization)	"Losing weight would help me control my diabetes."	"I don't have time to prepare my meals."
Need (importance or urgency)	"I have to lose weight to prevent diabetic complications."	"I just have to accept that my genes keep me from losing weight."
Later		
Commitment (making a promise or guarantee)	"I will lose weight."	"I'm not trying anymore diets. They never work."
Activation (indicates movement toward action)	"I'm ready to lose weight."	"I'm not willing to give up junk foods or sweets."
Taking steps (something in the direction of change has already been done)	"I've cooked oatmeal for my breakfast three days this week."	"I threw away the diet plan that you gave me."

ambivalence, the drawbacks of change generally outnumber the benefits. As patients move closer to change, the pros and cons can equalize. Ambivalence resolves when the balance tips in favor of the benefits and the pros of changing begin to outweigh the cons. Increases in change talk (relative to sustain talk) are associated with subsequent change. Therefore, paying close attention to patients' language of change is imperative. When the APP hears both change talk and sustain talk, they can intentionally reflect the change talk stated by patients: "It's important for you to be able to play with your kids." This reflection of change talk can evoke more change talk and influence the direction of change. Hence, change talk begets more change talk, and sustain talk evokes more sustain talk.

APPs must keep in mind that patients who are ambivalent about change have a natural tendency to present arguments from the opposing side of their ambivalence when they hear or speak sustain talk. Consequently, if the APP states the reasons for initiating change, patients will likely argue the reasons for not changing, thus literally talking themselves out of change. This is one explanation for why education can sometimes have a paradoxical effect on motivation and reduce, rather than increase, patients' desire to change. People also tend to believe what they hear themselves say over what others tell them. Consequently, the patients, not the APP, need to verbalize the change talk. The role of the APP is to make reflections or ask open-ended questions that help patients talk themselves into change by continuing to voice arguments in favor of change.

Evoking Change Talk. MI uses open-ended questions to evoke four types of change talk: (1) the disadvantages of the status quo (staying the same or not changing), (2) the advantages of changing, (3) patients' optimism for changing, and (4) patients' intention to change. **Table 6.7** provides examples of open-ended questions in each of these categories.

Table 6.7 Questions for Evoking Change Talk

Change Talk	Examples of Open-Ended Questions
Disadvantages of the status quo	"What worries you about (your current behavior)?" "What makes you think you need to do something about (your current behavior)?" "What difficulties or hassles have you had relative to (your current behavior)?" "Is there anything about (your current behavior) you might see as a reason for concern?" "Is there anything about (your current behavior) that other people might see as a reason for concern?" "In what ways does (your current behavior) concern you?" "How has (your current behavior) stopped you from doing what you want in life?" "What do you think will happen if you don't change anything?"
Advantages of changing	"How would you like for things to be different?" "What would be the good things about changing?" "What would you like your life to be like five years from now?" "If you woke up tomorrow and this problem was gone, how would things be different?" "The fact that you're interested in talking to me says that you're at least considering doing something different. What are the main reasons you see for making a change?" "What would be the main advantages of making this change?"

Change Talk	Examples of Open-Ended Questions
Optimism for changing	"What makes you think that if you did decide to change, you could do it?" "What encourages you that you can change if you want to?" "What do you think would work for you if you decided to change?" "When else have you made a significant change like this? How did you do it?" "How confident are you that you can make this change?" "What personal strengths do you have that will help you succeed?" "Who could offer you helpful support in making this change?"
Intention to change	"What are you thinking about changing your current behavior?" "I can see that you're feeling stuck at the moment. What will need to change?" "What do you think you might do?" "How important is this to you? How much do you want to do this?" "What would you be willing to try?" "Of the options we've discussed, which one sounds like it fits you the best?" "Never mind the 'how' for right now. What do you want to happen?" "What do you intend to do?"

Data from Miller, W. R., & Rollnick, S. (2013). *Motivational interviewing: Helping people change* (3rd ed.). Guilford Press.

Using OARS to Evoke Motivation. The basic MI methods of open-ended questions, affirmations, reflections, and summaries can evoke more change talk and increase motivation to change (see **Table 6.8**). Other ways to increase change talk include the following:

- Inquiring about the extremes: "What concerns you most in the long run about___?" "If you stopped smoking today, how would your life be better?"
- Looking backward: "How were things before you were smoking?"
- Looking forward: "How would you like your life to be a year from now?" "How might things be if you don't change your lifestyle?"
- Elaborating: "Can you give me examples?"
- Exploring values and asking about any discrepancy between patients' stated values and their behaviors: "How is it you don't smoke in front of your children?" "How would not smoking honor your values?"

Using RULE to Resolve Ambivalence. Rollnick et al. (2008) developed four guiding principles, easily remembered by the mnemonic RULE, to simplify the implementation of MI in healthcare settings. The *R* in RULE stands for *resist the righting reflex*. MI requires that the APP suppress the tendency to tell, direct, or advise patients and instead explore their motivation for change. The patients, not the APP, should be voicing arguments for change. If the APP argues for change, they take all the best lines, leaving patients to resist and argue against change. The second principle, *understand patients' motivations*, is a good reminder that patients' reasons for change, not the APP's, are more important. The APP should seek to understand patients' motivation, values, needs, abilities, and potential barriers. *Listen with empathy* involves having a compassionate interest in patients and their welfare. This principle is demonstrated by naming the feeling or need that the APP hears expressed by patients but is unspoken. Finally, *empower patients* involves helping them draw on their knowledge about their lives and explore their ideas to accomplish lifestyle changes to improve health. While the RULE principles are appropriate during any part of an MI-guided

Table 6.8 Using OARS as a Strategy for Evoking Change Talk

Strategy	Example
Open-ended questions: Ask questions to evoke change talk from patients.	
Desire: Ask what patients want, wish, and like around their desire for change.	"How would you like for things to change?"
Ability: Ask what patients could do or are able to do.	"What ideas do you have for how you could change?"
Reasons: Ask questions about specific reasons.	"What is the downside of how things are now?"
Need: Ask what makes this change urgent or important.	"What is the need for you to change at this moment?"
Affirmations: Recognize and value what patients say about change. Comment positively in response.	Patient: "I've got to do something about my weight!" APP: "Your health is important to you."
Reflections: Strengthen change talk by reflecting it to patients when you hear it. (Note that if you reflect sustain talk, you will encourage patients to talk more about the reasons for not changing.)	Patient: "I could do better at losing weight if I really tried, but I love to eat desserts and ice cream!" APP: "You love eating sweet things and know you could lose weight if you tried harder to reduce the number of treats you consume."
Summaries: Reflect a summary of the change talk heard so far, and then ask if there are any other reasons for the change.	"So far, you have shared that managing your blood sugar levels is important because you don't want to experience the diabetic complications your mother had. You were able to drop your HgA1c last year by eating a low-fat plant-based diet, and you think that is something you can do again. And you want to model a healthier lifestyle for your son. Is there anything else?"

conversation, they are beneficial during the evoking process, when helping patients to resolve ambivalence.

Responding to Resistance. MI distinguishes between two types of resistance, sustain talk and discord (Miller & Rollnick, 2013). *Sustain talk* is a natural response to change and represents the other side of patients' ambivalence about changing the target

behavior. In *discord*, the focus is on the relationship or rapport, not the behavior, between patients and providers. Discord often occurs as a response to something the providers do or how they communicate that causes resistance or defensiveness. Both sustain talk and discord predict poor outcomes. Therefore, the goal is for the APP to recognize them and respond appropriately to diffuse resistance. **Table 6.9** compares these two types of resistance and suggests actions the APP can take in response.

Strengthening Commitment to Change.

Patients' commitment to change is influenced by motivation and confidence (Miller & Rollnick, 2013). *Motivation*, or importance, is based on factors such as how significant the change is to patients. *Confidence*, or self-efficacy, is the patients' belief that change is possible and within their ability to make happen. **Figure 6.7** shows the relationship between motivation and confidence. The y-axis shows how important the change is to patients. The x-axis displays the level of patients' confidence in their ability to change. Patients can fall into one of four quadrants:

- *Bottom left*, low importance and low confidence. Change is neither important nor perceived as possible by patients.
- *Top left*, high importance and low confidence. Patients are motivated to change but lack confidence in their ability to change.

Table 6.9 Recognizing and Responding to Resistance

Characteristic	Sustain Talk	Discord
Description	Patients' statements about their desire to maintain the status quo around the target behavior, reasons not to change, and concerns about change. Note: Patients' statements include the target behavior.	Patients' statements about the intervention process or relationship to the provider in response to feeling pressured or challenged to do something about which they are ambivalent.
Example	"I don't know what I'd do without my cigarettes. They are a great stress reliever for me."	"You don't understand what I'm going through."
Contributing factors	Sustain talk is expected in any conversation about change, especially when patients are ambivalent. Patients ambivalent about change have a natural tendency to present arguments from the opposing side of their ambivalence.	The provider exhibits the righting reflex by assuming an expert role, arguing for change, disagreeing about what to change (e.g., the patient comes to talk about arthritis and the provider pushes smoking cessation), claiming to know what is best for patients, criticizing, blaming, shaming, labeling, or being in a hurry.
Signals	Patients push against change by bringing up reasons to maintain the status quo or expressing concerns about changing.	Patients push back by arguing, interrupting, blaming, or ignoring. There is no longer a feeling of collaboration but a deterioration of the patient–provider alliance.
Effect	The concern of sustain talk is that the more patients argue on behalf of the status quo, the more likely they will talk themselves out of any change.	Discord signals a breakdown in the relationship and is inversely related to subsequent change.

(continues)

Table 6.9 Recognizing and Responding to Resistance *(continued)*

Characteristic	Sustain Talk	Discord
Provider response to diffuse resistance	Do not argue for change. It only pushes patients to the other side of ambivalence (status quo). Use reflections without adding anything that would elicit more sustain talk. Reflecting sustain talk lets patients know they are heard. After the reflection, ask an open-ended question to keep patients engaged in exploring the possibility of change and increasing more change talk. Patient: "I don't have any desire to stop smoking, and the one time I tried it, it only lasted a day or two. It was not fun." Provider: "It's a combination of not wanting to change and not being certain about whether you can stop. What would increase your confidence?" Emphasize autonomy. Patient: "It's too much trouble to think about quitting smoking when I have other stresses to deal with." Provider: "It's more effort than you want to make right now. Certainly, only you can decide to change. If you did decide to quit later, what would make you want to?"	Pause and assess how provider behavior influenced discord. Use reflections: "It's difficult for you to see how you can cut down your cigarettes." Empathize: "You feel angry that your spouse made you come today to talk about quitting smoking." Apologize if needed: "I apologize for pushing you to reduce your cigarette consumption when you are not ready to take that step." Emphasize choice and control: "It is really up to you whether to make this change." Shift the focus away from the stumbling block: "I'm not interested in placing blame. What matters most is how you would like your health to improve and your ideas for getting there."

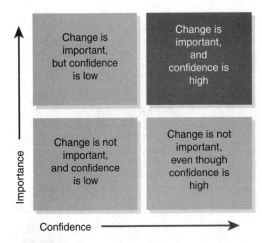

Figure 6.7 Relationship between importance and confidence.

- *Bottom right*, low importance and high confidence. Patients believe that change is possible but don't consider it important.
- *Top right*, high importance and high confidence. Patients are primed for change.

Each quadrant represents a different readiness for change and needs a different approach from the APP.

Assessing Importance and Confidence.
The Readiness Ruler is a useful MI tool for assessing motivation and self-efficacy and guiding conversations about behavior change (Miller & Rollnick, 2013). This imaginary ruler has two sides, each with a question and a 0 to 10 scale to help patients evaluate the

importance of the change and their confidence about making a change.

The *motivation* side of the Readiness Ruler is designed to help patients express their desire, ability, reasons, and need for change. The APP can ask, "On a scale of 0 to 10, with 1 being not at all important and 10 being extremely important, how important is it for you to change (behavior)?" After patients rate the importance of the change, the APP can ask, "What makes you choose that number rather than a lower number?" Asking why patients don't choose a *lower* number evokes change talk from them as they share their reasons for why the change is important to them. It is critical to note that if the APP were to ask why patients chose that number and not a *higher* number, they might respond defensively.

The *confidence* side of the Readiness Ruler is designed to help patients express their feelings or beliefs about their abilities to change. In a similar fashion to the motivation side, the APP asks patients to choose a number from 0 to 10 that best reflects how confident they are in their ability to change the behavior. Then the APP asks about the patients' response. For example, the APP may ask a patient, "On a scale of 0 to 10, with 1 being not at all confident that you can substitute a bowl of fruit for ice cream during the weekdays this week, and 10 being absolutely confident that you can do this, how confident are you that you can achieve this goal?" If patients rate their confidence at an 8/10, the APP can respond, "Why 8 and not 7?" Patients may reply, "Because I already bought some fresh berries that are my favorite at my last shopping trip. And I lost a few pounds last winter just by focusing on healthier options for my sweet tooth!" When asked why patients chose a particular number and not a lower one, they will respond with statements about their ability to change, previous successes, or small steps that they are already taking.

Raising Importance by Developing Discrepancy. A *discrepancy* becomes apparent when patients' current behavior or action is inconsistent with a core belief or value (i.e., what is important to them). This discrepancy can heighten patients' internal conflict and enhance motivation to change (Miller & Rollnick, 2013). To develop discrepancy and strengthen the commitment to change, the APP can help patients explore their goals, values, and hopes for the future. Once identified, the APP can ask questions to guide patients to elaborate further: "How important are these goals to you?" "How do you demonstrate these values in your daily life?" "How does your current situation connect with your hopes for the future?" "How does (current unhealthy behavior or target healthy behavior) fit in with your most important values? How does the current behavior help you honor your values (or conflict with them)?" The APP usually won't need to point out the inconsistencies since these will become apparent to patients. However, listening for discrepancies and then briefly summarizing and reflecting them to patients can be useful: "On the one hand, taking your medication supports your goal of lowering your blood pressure and your value of good health. On the other hand, smoking raises your blood pressure and interferes with your goal." It is essential to honor patients' autonomy when discussing discrepancies. Ultimately, it is the patients' decision what, if anything, to change.

Raising Confidence by Increasing Self-Efficacy. *Self-efficacy* refers to individuals' confidence in managing their health or changing health habits (Bandura, 1986). A lack of confidence may keep patients from engaging in self-management or behavior change. Self-efficacy is affected by what people believe and how they feel about what they can do (personal factors), their support networks and role models (external environment factors), and their own experience and accomplishments (behavioral factors). Patients with higher self-efficacy will exert more effort, avoid focusing on doubts, and have an "I can do it" attitude toward challenges. In contrast, those with low self-efficacy will avoid challenges and have lower hopes and decreased performance. APPs can help increase self-efficacy by using the following strategies (Moore et al., 2016):

- Use Elicit-Provide-Elicit to identify and fill any knowledge gaps.
- Apply personal strengths: "What would your friends say are your top three strengths? Which of these strengths might be useful to you in making this change? How might you use that strength in this situation?"
- Review past successes: "What changes have you made successfully in the past? What contributed to your success? How might those insights be helpful when making this change?"
- Identify barriers and strategies to overcome them: "What barriers are in the way? Would it be helpful to brainstorm solutions together?"
- Identify realistic role models for social support: "Whom do you know who has made the change you are considering?"
- Reframe previous failed attempts at changing as learning opportunities: "What did you learn from that experience?"
- Hypothetical thinking: "Suppose that this one big obstacle wasn't there. How might you make the change? How could you go about it in order to succeed?" This approach explores strategies for overcoming barriers and sends patients the message that they have the wisdom, insight, and creativity needed to find the way around the obstacle.

Planning

The essence of the planning process in MI is to move from discussing the importance of the change to developing a specific change plan that individuals are willing to implement (Miller & Rollnick, 2013). Planning involves applying the Spirit of MI to goal-setting techniques, thus evoking from patients what they plan to do (rather than giving them an action plan to implement). When guided to select

their own goal or action step, patients will likely come up with something they believe to be achievable and appropriate for their lives. This approach supports patients' autonomy and gives them confidence in setting future health goals independently.

The Key Question. Ambivalence may still occur in the planning process, but it doesn't necessarily indicate a lack of commitment to change. The balance between the pros and the cons of changing has just tipped toward the pro side enough for patients to start moving forward. When transitioning to the planning process, the APP first needs to assess the patients' readiness to move from discussing the why of change to how. This assessment is a judgment call, but there are signs that signal readiness for planning, such as increased frequency and strength of change talk, diminished sustain talk, envisioning what it would be like to make a change, questions about change (e.g., "How do other people manage their blood sugar?"), and experimentation with new behavior (Miller & Rollnick, 2013). The APP might test the waters by asking a key question such as "I'm curious whether you would like to consider how you might go about making this change?" "Would it make sense to think about how you might change, or is that getting ahead of things?" "What do you think you might do?" or "After all we've discussed, what's your next step?" How patients respond to this key question will determine whether the APP should move forward in guiding the discussion toward developing a change plan. If the APP gets ahead of the patients' readiness, the result can be reluctance, increased sustain talk, and discord.

Supporting Patient Autonomy. Providers often feel tempted to give suggestions for how to make the change. It is also common for patients to ask for solutions. While the APP may have many solutions to help patients move forward, the goal in MI is to support their autonomy in developing their own action plan. The APP can remind patients of their autonomy by responding, "You are the expert on your life and what will work for you. But if it would be helpful to your planning, I can share what the evidence shows and some ideas that have worked for others."

SMART Goal Setting. People often think about lifestyle change by considering the outcomes they want to achieve: "I want to lose weight" or "I want my blood sugars under control." When patients are ready to make a plan for change, the APP should help them to explore the behaviors and habits that will lead to their desired outcome and assist them in setting goals using the SMART criteria: specific, measurable, attainable, relevant, and time-bound (see **Figure 6.8**). SMART goals are target behaviors that can be achieved in a one- to three-month time frame and that will move patients toward the larger outcome they would like to achieve. For example, patients who want to control their blood sugars may set a SMART goal such as "By my next appointment, I will be walking 30 minutes after dinner five days per week."

SMART goals assist patients with being *specific* about the actions they will take to achieve their desired health outcome. Being specific about how and when is crucial because it helps patients pin down the details needed to accomplish the goal. SMART goals delineate a means to *measure* progress. The APP should also guide patients in choosing a realistic and *attainable* goal. Setting too large of a goal can de-motivate patients while smaller, incremental goals build confidence and momentum because they are more easily achieved. SMART goals are patient defined and always *relevant* to patients' values. They also are *time-bound*, providing a designated time for inserting the new behavior into the patients' schedule and a deadline for goal achievement.

It is often easier for patients to agree to take a small step in the direction of change than to commit to the ultimate change goal itself. Therefore, the APP should guide patients to take the bigger vision for health (their desired outcome) and break it down into SMART goals and even smaller action steps that build confidence and momentum toward success. For example, the patient who sets a goal to

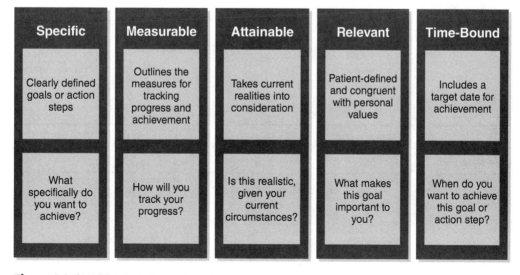

Figure 6.8 SMART criteria for goals and action steps.

walk 30 minutes after dinner five days per week may begin by taking 10-minute walks after dinner on the weekends. The objective is to help patients scale the goal down to an action that is easy to start immediately. It is also important to help patients address potential barriers and consider what is needed to support success in reaching the goal.

Strengthening Commitment. Once the change plan has been defined, the APP should assess whether patients are ready to implement it. A summary reflection of the broader goal, change talk (as a reminder of the patients' desire, ability, reasons, and need for change), and change plan can help pull all the pieces together. The APP can then ask one of the following questions to focus on commitment:

- Evoking activation: "Are you willing to give that a try?" "What steps are you willing to take this week?" "What part of this plan do you think you are ready to do?"
- Asking for commitment: "Is that what you're going to do?" "How ready are you to do this?" "What might help you reinforce your commitment to this plan?"
- Getting more specific: "How would you get ready?"
- Setting a date: "When would you start?"
- Preparing: "What would be the first step?"
- Troubleshooting: "What could get in the way?" "Knowing yourself as well as you do, how could you handle that?"

Supporting Ongoing Change. People generally are accountable only to themselves when it comes to health and well-being, which often isn't enough for change to happen. Patient accountability can be established at subsequent visits when the APP checks on patients' experience with their goals. Questions about progress should be asked in a nonjudgmental way such as "Catch me up on the action steps you set at our last visit." "Tell me about your experience implementing your change plan last month." "What new learning and insight did you gain from the successes and challenges you experienced?" or "How have the actions you've taken so far been helpful?"

Often unexpected aspects of implementing change can pose new problems that weren't anticipated. This discussion allows the APP to catch setbacks early and normalize them. By reframing patients' failure as partial progress or a learning opportunity, the APP can affirm their efforts, evoke their wisdom and solutions for the next step, and support their ownership of the change process. Some changes require sustained attention and effort over time, thus necessitating ongoing support. The APP can revisit the process and tweak plans or regroup where needed.

MI in Practice

In summary, the APP can use MI to strengthen patients' motivation and commitment to

---

Health Promotion Case Study Use of Person-Centered Strategies with an Obese Female

Case description: J.T., a 42-year-old female, presents to her APP with a primary complaint of urinary frequency.

- Past medical history: Denies. Admits to occasional heartburn.
- Family history: Mother with insulin dependent T2DM, chronic kidney disease, and left below-knee amputation. Father deceased in a motor vehicle accident.
- Medications: Prilosec OTC PRN heartburn; Benadryl OTC PRN sleep.

- Allergies: NKDA.
- Social history: Recently divorced. Works as a middle-school teacher. Lives with her two teenage children, aged 13 and 15.
- Vital signs: BP 148/89 mmHg right arm, heart rate 84 bpm, respiratory rate 20/min, temperature 98.4°F, BMI 36 kg per m^2.
- Physical exam: Obese female who appears distracted by her mobile phone. A dipstick urinalysis in the office shows 2+ sugar, and finger-stick blood glucose is 240 mg/dL. The rest of the exam is unremarkable.

Lifestyle Vital Signs

- Adopt healthy eating: J.T. makes the following statement when asked about her typical eating pattern. *I always make sure the kids eat breakfast, and I pack them a lunch every day. But I don't have time to sit down to eat, so my breakfast is usually coffee and a granola bar in the car. I usually skip lunch to grade or prepare lesson plans. Dinner is picked up at a drive-through to eat while taking the kids to their music lessons and soccer games. I try to choose salads when I can, but my options are limited. I guess you could say that I'm fueled by Coke.*
- Stress less: Not assessed.
- Move often: Has membership to a fitness center through work benefit but doesn't use it. J.T. makes the following comment in response to the APP's inquiry about physical activity: *I know exercise is important for losing weight. Sometimes I join a friend for a walk on Saturday, and I feel much better afterward. Plus, I get to sleep easier. But I can't fit one more thing into my day. Mornings are rushed getting everyone out the door on time, and evenings are busy with the kids' extracurricular activities. I usually have grading or lesson plans to finish before I can go to bed. I'm just pulled in a million different directions.*
- Avoid alcohol: Drinks wine 3–4x/week to unwind in the evening after the kids are in bed. Denies recreational drug use.
- Rest more: Occasional insomnia. Wakens unrefreshed when the alarm rings at 5:00 a.m.
- Treat tobacco use: Denies recent smoking. Ten pack-year history, quit when pregnant with first child.

Critical Thinking Questions

- What stage of change do you think J.T. is in for healthy eating and for moving/activity, and why?
- MI emphasizes eliciting the patient's reasons for change rather than advising them why they should change their lifestyle. In J.T.'s comments about physical activity, which statements represent change talk? Which statements best represent sustain talk? Give an example of a reflection and an open-ended inquiry that you could use in this conversation to elicit more change talk.
- What strengths do you observe in J.T.? Form two affirmations based on those strengths that the APP could use in the conversation with the patient.
- In J.T.'s comments about diet, what inconsistencies do you notice between her values and her actions? Provide an example of how you might develop this discrepancy and strengthen her commitment to change.
- Read the following advice. What are the concerns with this advice? How can you improve it using the Elicit-Provide-Elicit technique? *You need to lose weight; eat a low-fat, high-fiber diet; and exercise daily to control your blood sugars. If you don't, you are at risk for the same diabetic complications your mother has experienced. Your weight also puts you at risk for heart disease and other health problems. The bottom line is you need to start putting yourself first.*

change by exploring and resolving ambivalence and helping the patient to do the following:

- Recognize the disadvantages of the status quo: "What concerns you about your current situation?"
- Recognize the advantages of change: "What would be the benefits of (new behavior) for you?"
- Expressing optimism about change: "What kind of support would be helpful in making this change?"
- Expressing intention to change: "How important is it for you to . . . ?"

Implementing MI When Time Is Short

Time constraints can be a barrier to promoting healthy lifestyles and assisting patients in developing a plan for lifestyle change. However, even in brief patient encounters, the APP can express the Spirit of MI and implement the following MI-inspired person-centered strategies in the discussion.

- Connect: Even when time is short, it is essential to establish rapport with eye contact, a handshake, the use of their name, and a warm welcome (e.g., "It's lovely to see you, (name). I appreciate your visit today.").
- Explore: "What is important to you to take away from our visit today? How can I most help you?"
- Assess, diagnose, and discuss the treatment plan.
- Collaborate: "Was my explanation understandable? What else do you want to know? How else can I help?" (Use Elicit-Provide-Elicit as needed.)
- Plan: "What's one small goal that feels achievable as it relates to this topic? What are your best next steps? What would strengthen your motivation (or your confidence)? What might come up as you attempt to make that change? What support do you need? How would you like to set up accountability?"

> **Health Promotion Case Study**
> **Reflect on the Spirit of MI in Practice**
>
> Think about your previous experiences with patients in the context of your new understanding of MI. Give an example of when you demonstrated the Spirit of MI. When did you use the righting reflex? What were the outcomes of these experiences?

- Appreciate: "Thank you for your commitment to your health. I am glad we had this time together today, and I look forward to hearing about your change journey at our next visit."

Summary

It is recognized that directing patients what to do or only offering information is not sufficient for behavior change (Miller & Rollnick, 2013). Before making recommendations or providing health information, it is imperative to build rapport and develop a partnership of care (Wiggins, 2008). APPs utilizing a partnership approach avoid provoking resistance to behavior change by emphasizing the patients' role and supporting their autonomy in the change process, engaging them in shared decision-making, and empowering them in improved self-care and self-management. The partnership model of care approach to health promotion conceptualizes this partnership of informed, activated patients and integrates several foundational frameworks and strategies for health behavior change. Supported by the guiding communication style of motivational interviewing, APPs will evoke patients' motivation, support them in increasing their self-efficacy, and empower them to adopt the lifestyle behaviors needed to achieve their goals for their health and well-being. See **Table 6.10** for additional resources to promote person-centered care.

TABLE 6.10	Evidence-Based Resources for Person-Centered Health Promotion

Resource	URL
Center for Self-Determination Theory	https://selfdeterminationtheory.org
Guilford Press (a large publisher of MI books related to health care, psychology, education, etc.)	https://www.guilford.com/search/motivational+interviewing
Motivational Interviewing Network of Trainers (MINT)	https://motivationalinterviewing.org
National Board for Health and Wellness Coaching	https://nbhwc.org
ProChange (TTM)	https://prochange.com
Wellcoaches Center for Coaching Excellence	https://www.wellcoachesschool.com

Acronyms

APP: advanced practice provider

DARN CAT: desire, ability, reasons, needs, commitment, activation, taking steps

IMS: information-motivation-strategy model

MI: motivational interviewing

NCCDPHP: National Center for Chronic Disease Prevention and Health Promotion

OARS: open-ended questions, affirmations, reflections, summaries

PCC: patient- or person-centered care

PMC: partnership model of care

RULE: resist the righting reflex, understand patients' motivations, listen with empathy, empower patients

SDT: self-determination theory

SMART: specific, measurable, attainable, relevant, time-bound

T2DM: type 2 diabetes mellitus

TTM: transtheoretical model

References

Bandura, A. (1986). *Social foundations of thought and action: A social cognitive theory*. Prentice Hall.

Bem, D. J. (1972). Self-perception theory. *Advances in Experimental Social Psychology, 6*, 1–62. https://doi.org/10.1016/S0065-2601(08)60024-6

Bodenheimer, T., Lorig, K., Holman, H., & Grumbach, K. (2002). Patient self-management of chronic disease in primary care. *JAMA, 288*(19), 2469–2475. https://doi.org/10.1001/jama.288.19.2469

Bokhour, B., Hyde, J., Zeliadt, S., & Mohr, H. (2020). *Whole Health System of Care evaluation—A progress report on outcomes of the WHS pilot at 18 flagship sites*. Veterans Health Administration, Center for Evaluating Patient-Centered Care in VA (EPCC-VA).

https://www.va.gov/WHOLEHEALTH/professional-resources/clinician-tools/Evidence-Based-Research.asp

Centers for Medicare and Medicaid Services. (2022). *NHE fact sheet*. https://www.cms.gov/Research-Statistics-Data-and-Systems/Statistics-Trends-and-Reports/NationalHealthExpendData/NHE-Fact-Sheet

Deci, E. L., & Ryan, R. M. (1985). *Intrinsic motivation and self-determination in human behavior*. Plenum Press.

DiMatteo, M. R., Haskard-Zolnierek, K. B., & Martin, L. R. (2012) Improving patient adherence: a three-factor model to guide practice. *Health Psychology Review, 6*(1), 74–91. https://doi.org/10.1080/17437199.2010.537592

Emmons, K. M., & Rollnick, S. (2001). Motivational interviewing in health care settings. Opportunities and limitations. *American Journal of Preventive Medicine, 20*(1), 68–74. https://doi.org/10.1016/S0749-3797(00)00254-3

Giusti, A., Nkhoma, K., Petrus, R., Petersen, I., Gwyther, L., Farrant, L., Venkatapuram, S., & Harding, R. (2020). The empirical evidence underpinning the concept and practice of person-centred care for serious illness: A systematic review. *BMJ Global Health, 5*(12), e003330. https://doi.org/10.1136/bmjgh-2020-003330

Gould, E., & Mitty, E. (2010). Medication adherence is a partnership, medication compliance is not. *Geriatric Nursing, 31*(4), 290–298. https://doi.org/10.1016/j.gerinurse.2010.05.004

Günter, A. V., Endrejat, P. C., & Kauffled, S. (2019). Guiding change: Using motivational interviewing within organizations. *Gruppe. Interaktion. Organisation.* https://doi.org/10.1007/s11612-019-00459-z

Harrison, S. R., & Jordan, A. M. (2022). Chronic disease care integration into primary care services in sub-Saharan Africa: A 'best fit' framework synthesis and new conceptual model. *Family Medicine and Community Health, 10*(3), e001703. https://doi.org/10.1136/fmch-2022-001703

Jonas, W. B., & Rosenbaum, E. (2021). The case for whole-person integrative care. *Medicina, 57*(7), 677. https://doi.org/10.3390/medicina57070677

Laws, M. B., Lee, Y., Taubin, T., Rogers, W. H., & Wilson, I. B. (2018). Factors associated with patient recall of key information in ambulatory specialty care visits: Results of an innovative methodology. *PLoS ONE, 13*(2). https://doi.org/10.1371/journal.pone.0191940

Martin, L. R., Haskard-Zolnierek, K. B., & DiMatteo, M. R. (2010). *Health behavior change and treatment adherence: Evidence-based guidelines for improving healthcare.* Oxford University Press.

Matthews, J. A., Moore, M., & Collings, C. (2022). A coach approach to facilitating behavior change. *Journal of Family Practice, 71*(Suppl 1 Lifestyle), eS93–eS99. https://doi.org/10.12788/jfp.0246

Miller, W. R., & Rollnick, S. (2013). *Motivational interviewing: Helping people change* (3rd ed.). Guilford Press.

Miller, W. R., & Rose, G. S. (2009). Toward a theory of motivational interviewing. *American Psychologist, 64*(6), 527–537. https://doi.org/10.1037/a0016830

Moore, M., Jackson, E., & Tschannen-Moran, B. (2016). *Coaching psychology manual* (2nd ed.). Wolters Kluwer.

National Center for Chronic Disease Prevention and Health Promotion. (n.d.-a). *About chronic diseases.* Centers for Disease Control and Prevention. Retrieved September 26, 2022, from https://www.cdc.gov/chronicdisease/about/index.htm#risks

National Center for Chronic Disease Prevention and Health Promotion. (n.d.-b). *Health and economic costs of chronic diseases.* Centers for Disease Control and Prevention. Retrieved September 26, 2022, from https://www.cdc.gov/chronicdisease/about/costs/index.htm

National Center for Chronic Disease Prevention and Health Promotion. (n.d.-c). *How you can prevent chronic diseases.* Centers for Disease Control and Prevention. Retrieved September 26, 2022, from https://www.cdc.gov/chronicdisease/about/prevent/index.htm

National Center for Complementary and Integrative Health. (2021). *Whole person health: What you need to know.* U.S. Department of Health and Human Services, National Institutes of Health. https://www.nccih.nih.gov/health/whole-person-health-what-you-need-to-know

Pascal, B. (1958). *Pascal's pensées.* E. P. Dutton. (Original work published 1623–1662)

Patrick, H., & Williams, G. C. (2012). Self-determination theory: Its application to health behavior and complementarity with motivational interviewing. *International Journal of Behavioral Nutrition and Physical Activity, 9*(18). https://doi.org/10.1186/1479-5868-9-18

Phillips, A. S., & Guarnaccia, C. A. (2020). Self-determination theory and motivational interviewing interventions for type 2 diabetes prevention and treatment: A systematic review. *Journal of Health Psychology, 25*(1), 44–66. https://doi.org/10.1177/1359105317737606

Prochaska, J. O., Diclemente, C. C., & Norcross, J. C. (1992). In search of how people change. *American Psychologist, 47*(9), 1102–1114. https://doi.org/10.1037/0003-066X.47.9.1102

Prochaska, J. O., Norcross, J. C., & Diclemente, C. C. (1994). *Changing for good: A revolutionary six-stage program for overcoming bad habits and moving your life positively forward.* William Morrow.

Rippe, J. M. (2018). Lifestyle medicine: The health promoting power of daily habits and practices. *American Journal of Lifestyle Medicine, 12*(6), 499–512. https://doi.org/10.1177/1559827618785554

Rippe, J. M. (2019). *Lifestyle medicine* (3rd ed). CRC Press.

Rollnick, S., Miller, W. R., & Butler, C. C. (2008). *Motivational interviewing in health care: Helping patients change behavior.* Guilford Press.

Senge, P. M. (2010). *The fifth discipline: The art and practice of the learning organization.* Crown.

U.S. Preventive Services Task Force. (2013). *Behavioral counseling interventions: An evidence-based approach.* https://www.uspreventiveservicestaskforce.org/uspstf/about-uspstf/methods-and-processes/behavioral-counseling-interventions-evidence-based-approach#rationale

Wiggins, M. S. (2008). The partnership care delivery model: An examination of the core concept and the need for a new model of care. *Journal of Nursing Management, 16*, 629–638. https://doi.org/10.1111/j.1365-2834.2008.00900.x

Yu, C. C., Tan, L., Le, M. K., Tang, B., Liaw, S. Y., Tierney, T., Ho, Y. Y., Lim, B., Lim, D., Ng, R., Chia, S. C., & Low, J. A. (2022). The development of empathy in the healthcare setting: A qualitative approach. *BMC Medical Education, 22*(1), 245. https://doi.org/10.1186/s12909-022-03312-y

© Kathleen Gail/Shutterstock; © StoryTime Studio/Shutterstock; © kali9/Getty Images

CHAPTER 7

The Use of Technology in Health Promotion

Katherine Chike-Harris, DNP, APRN, CPNP-PC, FNP-BC, CNE
Kelli Garber, DNP, APRN, PPCNP-BC
Mollie Dwivedi, MS, PA-C, DipACLM
Michelle Nichols, PhD, RN

Telehealth exceeds our expectations when we leverage it to focus on the care needs of an individual, as opposed to extending a clinic-based health ecosystem. To this end, there is huge potential to enhance wellness by engaging patients intelligently at the right moment in time. This can be passive health literacy support, having a wide-open door when the individual is ready to reach out, and in the prescribing of digital interventions that conform to the daily life and environment of the patient in need.

Jimmy McElligott, MD, MSCR, Executive Medical Director
Center for Telehealth at the Medical University of South Carolina

OBJECTIVES

This chapter will enable the reader to:

1. Define telemedicine.
2. Differentiate between telemedicine and telehealth.
3. Identify the benefits and barriers of telehealth.
4. Evaluate the usefulness of telehealth technology in health promotion and lifestyle management.
5. Examine the use of mobile health for the management of chronic diseases.
6. Discuss how electronic medical records can be harnessed to increase lifestyle management by both advanced practice providers and patients.

Overview

This chapter aims to provide the advanced practice provider (APP) with a high-level overview of the various technological modalities used in health promotion for the lifestyle management and prevention of chronic disease. Key terms are defined, and examples are provided to give the reader a general understanding of how they can be used for lifestyle management as well as their benefits and barriers.

Technology in Health Care

Information technology has evolved to be an integral part of health care. The healthcare landscape has changed dramatically over the past several decades, from the digitalization of health records to the ability to collect, process, and use large amounts of data for analytics (Tuman, 2019). Telehealth is becoming an accepted and widely used healthcare delivery modality within the United States and globally (Centers for Disease Control and Prevention [CDC], 2020). Telehealth is defined as follows:

> The delivery of health care services, where patients and providers are separated by distance. Telehealth uses technology for the exchange of information for the diagnosis and treatment of disease and injuries, research and evaluation, and for the continuing education of health professionals. Telehealth can contribute to achieving universal health coverage by improving access for patients to quality, cost-effective, health services wherever they may be. It is particularly valuable for those in remote areas, vulnerable groups, and ageing populations. (World Health Organization, 2020, line 4)

Telemedicine is often used interchangeably with telehealth but has subtle differences (see **Figure 7.1**). Telemedicine focuses on patients' health-related care (i.e., clinical services) and is a subcategory of telehealth. Telehealth includes clinical services and the education of providers, staff, and patients; health-focused

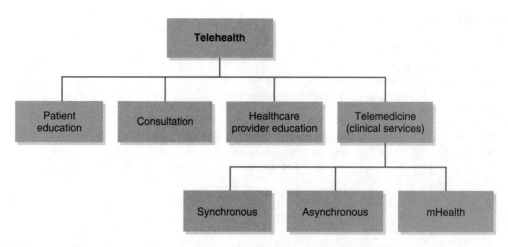

Figure 7.1 Diagram illustrating the differences between telehealth and telemedicine.

meetings; mobile health (mHealth); distance health administration; and implementation of public health interventions (Bates et al., 2020; Rutledge et al., 2017). This chapter does not distinguish between telehealth and telemedicine; instead, it uses the broad term *telehealth* throughout.

Telemedicine consists of mobile health (mHealth), remote patient monitoring (RPM), and both synchronous and asynchronous service modalities (Bates et al., 2020; Rutledge et al., 2017). The use of mHealth technology improves patient health outcomes and involves using healthcare applications (apps), wearable devices, and social media (Sim, 2019). This technology can be used with mobile phones, tablets, personal computers, and other devices and plays a vital role in managing chronic diseases, such as hypertension (Thangada et al., 2018). RPM is similar to mHealth and uses sensors with Wi-Fi or internet capabilities to transmit biometric data (e.g., heart rate, blood pressure [BP], weight, or glucose measurements). This is also known as patient-generated health data (PGHD); it is sent in real time to a monitoring facility or provider's office to detect and prevent a medical emergency or hospital readmission (Sim, 2019).

Asynchronous telehealth, often referred to as store and forward, is where patient information (e.g., history information, radiographs, lab results, pathology reports, and images) is collected and stored, then transmitted to a healthcare provider for review (Bates et al., 2020; Rutledge et al., 2017). This offers APPs and patients the ability to interact independently of one another since questions or data transmittal, with or without images or videos, can be uploaded into a secure platform and viewed by the APP or support staff for response at a later time. In contrast, synchronous telehealth involves real-time communication between two participants using audiovisual equipment and a secure videoconferencing platform (Bates et al., 2020; Rutledge et al., 2017). This communication can be between providers (e.g., primary care providers and specialists) or patients and providers. Synchronous telehealth visits may include clinical assessment using telehealth equipment (e.g., carts, kiosks, and mobile kits) and associated peripheral attachments (e.g., electronic stethoscopes, lenses, and otoscopes).

As healthcare technology and telehealth have advanced, artificial intelligence (AI) has evolved. The term *AI* was coined in 1956 by John McCarthy (a computer and cognitive scientist); it relates to a machine's ability to imitate human intelligence (Mintz & Brodie, 2019). AI can absorb and analyze a large amount of data (i.e., big data) to recognize and predict patterns, emulating human thought processes (Chaikijurajai et al., 2020). This technology is already well established within daily activities, such as smartphone apps that assist in internet searches, turning lights and appliances on and off, and solving mathematical problems with a simple voice command (e.g., Siri, Alexa, and Bixby). Though AI is not considered a telehealth modality, it is essential to mention since AI is becoming increasingly more integrated into medicine. Its most significant application may be in assisting radiologists with identification and diagnoses, but it is also used in gastroenterology, oncology, cardiology, ophthalmology, and surgery. In combination with AI, mHealth is currently being evaluated for the management of chronic diseases. Stein and Brooks (2017) tested the use of a text-based coaching service integrated with conversational AI to promote healthcare behaviors to prevent diabetes. The study results showed that lifestyle modification coaching via an AI coaching app was comparable to in-person visits regarding increased healthy meal choices and satisfaction scores. The future application of AI for the predisposition and diagnosis of hypertension is also promising by utilizing mHealth and RPM data to develop algorithms to predict which individuals are at high risk for cardiovascular disease (Chaikijurajai et al., 2020).

Integrating telehealth into the management of chronic diseases through patient interactions regarding lifestyle modification shows great potential (Hanlon et al., 2017). Traditional methods of addressing lifestyle changes for chronic illnesses are plagued with low patient adherence and high no-show visit rates (VSee, 2017). Telehealth can help APPs overcome barriers and increase referrals to dieticians, lifestyle coaches, and mental health providers to facilitate permanent lifestyle changes and increase patient success (VSee, 2017). According to a special report from Press Ganey, overall patient satisfaction with telehealth is high. Most patients were likely to recommend a video telehealth visit, supporting acceptance of the modality and confirming that it meets patient needs (Press Ganey, 2020). The use of telehealth can enhance the role of lifestyle medicine in chronic disease prevention and management through technologies and is the focus of this chapter.

Benefits of Telehealth in Health Promotion

Telehealth is a way of implementing care that is efficient, effective, convenient, person centered, and accessible; for these reasons, telehealth is well suited for the delivery of lifestyle medicine. Regardless of whether care is provided in person or virtually, the standard of care for any condition remains the same (Olson et al., 2018). Therefore, telehealth is not considered a new or different type of care but offers a mechanism to deliver health care regardless of distance or patient location (Committee on Pediatric Workforce, 2015). For many clinical domains, including mental health, cardiology, and type 1 diabetes mellitus management, telehealth has proven to be equivalent or better than in-person care (Shigekawa et al., 2018; Wood et al., 2016). Specialty care, such as that for type 1 diabetes mellitus, delivered via telehealth is safe and effective while contributing to high appointment adherence rates, healthcare cost savings, and high patient satisfaction (Xu et al., 2018).

Telehealth provides many benefits, particularly for those living in rural or underresourced areas (see **Table 7.1**). Approximately one in five Americans lives in a rural community (U.S. Census Bureau, 2017). It is well documented that those living in rural areas experience increased health disparities and poor access to health care (Warshaw, 2017). Challenges include few local providers, transportation, higher poverty levels, and large distances between where patients reside and providers practice, all of which contribute to barriers to health care (Warshaw, 2017). Access to specialty care in rural areas is of particular concern because specialists are more likely to be in urban locales, particularly those with a medical school (Naylor et al., 2019). Patients with chronic conditions often rely on specialized care and can benefit from lifestyle-focused services. Telehealth provides a way to overcome these barriers, increase access to care, and improve patient outcomes (Rural Health Information Hub, 2019). Telehealth also extends the care continuum, allowing

Telehealth Benefits in Practice

Where telehealth seems most beneficial in my practice is meeting patients where they are—literally. Telehealth allows our patients to join our lifestyle and chronic disease prevention programs while engaging fully in their lives at work, school, home and in our communities without the need to travel to a clinic or hospital to receive services. With lifestyle change programs such as these, it's essential that people are engaged in their treatment, and telehealth allows them to do this more efficiently.

Sarah Hales, PhD, LISW-CP, CSOWM
Assistant Professor
Department of Psychiatry & Behavioral Sciences
Medical University of South Carolina

Table 7.1 Telehealth Benefits and Limitations

Benefits of Telehealth	Telehealth Limitations
Increased contact with a provider or nurse Frequent reinforcement of lifestyle changes Increased self-monitoring Improved compliance with lifestyle modifications Improved health outcomes Reduced no-show rates Reduced hospitalizations and length of stay	Digital divide (limited access to broadband or technology to conduct telehealth visits) Digital literacy Accessibility Visit types limited by exam requirements or necessary testing Cost of equipment and reimbursement limitations for providers Technophobia

care to be provided to patients in multiple locations, including homes, clinics, hospitals, rehabilitation centers, and nursing homes.

In addition to increasing access to care, telehealth may improve the care system's efficiency. The evolution of the eConsult, also known as eReferral, refers to an asynchronous electronic consultation between primary care providers and specialists (Center for Connected Health Policy, n.d.), which contributes to the system's efficiency. eConsults reduce the number of inappropriate in-person referrals, allowing for increased availability of specialty appointments for those who truly need to be seen in person and reduced wait times (Chen et al., 2013). Additional benefits of eConsults include increased care coordination, improved previsit workups, decreased low-value specialty visits, reduced missed appointments, improved bidirectional communication between specialists and primary care providers, reduced missed workdays, and decreased travel time for patients (Center for Connected Health Policy, n.d.). Telehealth may also reduce redundant diagnostic studies by allowing efficient and timely sharing of study results between providers (Marcin et al., 2015). The strong relationship between lifestyle and chronic disease necessitates clear and timely communication between primary care and specialty providers. These services facilitate the often complex care coordination challenges of chronic disease management.

Initiatives such as Project ECHO (Extension for Community Healthcare Outcomes) also contribute to improved efficiency of the care system by enhancing the care provided by rural clinicians through telementoring, which is mentoring done through electronic communications, by specialists (University of New Mexico School of Medicine, 2020). Telementoring enables the education of rural providers in the management of chronic diseases, such as diabetes, obesity, and hypertension, through the sharing and discussion of complex cases, which can mitigate the barriers related to the insufficient number of specialists within rural and underresourced communities (Lewiecki & Rochelle, 2019). Enhancing the care patients receive from their local provider allows patients to remain in their local community and may contribute to the same benefits as those noted for eConsults.

Telehealth benefits APP practice through improved clinical workflows, increased practice efficiency, increased revenue from a reduction in overall practice overhead costs, reduction in patient no-show rates, and increased provider productivity (Ortholive, 2018). It also provides a reduction in healthcare costs through reduced hospital admissions and readmissions (Becker's Health IT, 2014; O'Connor et al., 2016); decreased lengths of stay for both physical and mental health issues (Department of Veterans Affairs, 2020); and a reduction in emergency department visits, particularly for those with chronic diseases (Bashshur et al., 2014).

With 60% of the U.S. population suffering from a chronic disease (CDC, 2021), chronic disease management is a significant concern for patients and healthcare providers. Telehealth can reduce the cost of care through modalities such as RPM (Bashshur et al., 2014; InTouch Health, 2020). Patients may participate in their care through this modality, receive continuous monitoring by their healthcare providers, and benefit from early symptom identification regarding potential illness exacerbation with a prompt intervention (Bashshur et al., 2014). In addition, necessary lifestyle changes, such as medication adherence, diet, smoking cessation, and increased exercise, may be monitored more closely by a care team member, allowing for more timely intervention should a patient not be adhering to the recommended care plan (InTouch Health, 2020).

Limitations of Telehealth

In addition to its many benefits, telehealth has some limitations (see Table 7.1). Economic, educational, and social inequities contribute to the digital divide, creating gaps between those who have access to technology and digital services and those who do not (Vassilakopoulou & Hustad, 2021). Many members of society are considered underresourced and may not have internet access, such as those residing in rural communities, the poor, or the elderly, which prohibits their use of telehealth (Kaufman et al., 2006). The Federal Communications Commission (2018) estimated that one-quarter of rural Americans and one-third of those living on tribal lands did not have access to broadband while less than 2% of those living in urban areas lacked access. Between 2016 and 2021, only a 9% increase in home broadband adoption was noted, resulting in 72% of rural Americans reporting a broadband internet connection at home (Vogels,

2021). Moreover, according to a 2019 Pew Research Center survey, among adults who live in households earning less than $30,000 per year, 29% do not own a smartphone, 44% do not have broadband access, and 46% do not own a computer (Anderson & Kumar, 2019). This translates to a major barrier to telehealth usage for these populations. While programs are implemented to combat the digital divide by expanding broadband access, many patients still lack electronic connectivity or digital literacy, leading to digital exclusion (Castilla et al., 2018). Also, an emotional fear of interacting with computers, known as technophobia, may lead to computer avoidance, a phenomenon more prevalent among the elderly and those who did not grow up with technology (Nimrod, 2018; Van Houwelingen et al., 2018).

Telehealth is a method of care delivery rather than a different type of health care and is not intended to replace all in-person visits. Depending on the modality implemented, there may be limitations to the care provided, requiring some telehealth visits to be rescheduled as in-person visits. Emergencies, procedures, and vaccinations are among the reasons some visits may not be completed solely through telehealth. Obtaining a thorough history and ensuring that enough of a physical exam can establish an appropriate diagnosis is the responsibility of the provider conducting the telehealth encounter (Joshi & Hollander, 2017). APPs must be creative in conducting exams when telehealth peripheral devices are not available. Using household items and guiding patients through self-exams may be necessary, depending on the nature of the visit.

The American Heart Association emphasized another barrier for telehealth: digital health literacy (Magnani et al., 2018). Digital health literacy, or eHealth literacy, is "the ability to seek, find, understand, and appraise health information from electronic sources and apply the knowledge gained to addressing or solving a health problem" (Ortiz, 2017, p. 8).

With the increasing number of patients using the internet and social media, APPs provide an important role in educating patients about reliable and trustworthy online health information and digital tools. To ensure that the patient is engaged and understands the plan of care, Conard (2019) recommends three steps in his health literacy instructional model:

1. Evaluate and address the emotional state of the patient.
2. Engage and build commitment through the use of motivational interviewing.
3. Provide the education using language and terms that the patients are familiar with and then slowly build their vocabulary and knowledge through the use of a digital library system that can be integrated into a mobile app.

Financial barriers to telehealth may also limit its utility for APPs. Technology costs may be prohibitive, necessitating a diversity of funding, including grants and governmental support. Reimbursement for telehealth services has long been cited as a barrier to telehealth adoption (Weinstein et al., 2014). However, coverage for communication technology-based services or "virtual check-ins" and specific codes for remote physiological management were introduced in the 2019 Physician Fee Schedule (Center for Connected Health Policy, 2020; Wecklund, 2018). During the novel coronavirus 2019 (COVID-19) pandemic, the Centers for Medicare and Medicaid Services reduced coverage restrictions for Medicare fee-for-service recipients and allowed expanded coverage for Medicare Advantage plan members (Weigel et al., 2020). State Medicaid programs and commercial insurers also expanded coverage for telehealth services (Weigel et al., 2020). The Coronavirus Aid, Relief, and Economic Security (CARES) Act was passed and provided over $2 trillion in economic relief. This funding enabled healthcare providers to increase access to care using telehealth through the COVID-19 Telehealth Program (EMS GrantsHelp Team, 2020).

Health Promotion Research Study

Use of Mobile Technology in Managing Disease

Background: Mobile technology shows promise for day-to-day chronic disease management in resource-limited areas. The primary objective of the Phone-based Intervention under Nurse Guidance after Stroke (PINGS) study was to assess feasibility and pilot test a multilevel, theoretically designed, mHealth technology-enabled approach for BP control and lifestyle modification among stroke survivors through a nurse-guided intervention.

Methodology: The study design was structured as a two-arm, cluster randomized controlled trial with randomization occurring at the provider level within a tertiary referral hospital in Kumasi, Ghana. Cluster randomization included assignment allocation of two physicians to the intervention arm and two to the control, with data collected at the participant level. Stroke survivors with uncontrolled hypertension within the first month poststroke were enrolled (n = 60) following informed consent and randomized to either the intervention or the control group with 15 participants per physician.

Intervention group participants (n = 30) underwent a three-month pilot intervention and received a Bluetooth-enabled BP machine, a medication pillbox, and a smartphone to enable transmission of BP data and communication with the study team. Intervention participants received nurse support via training on BP self-assessment techniques. Daily BP readings and medication adherence data obtained from the digital pillbox were transmitted to a secure server. Targeted short message service (SMS) messages based on the data received were sent via mobile devices to encourage BP and medication adherence along with lifestyle recommendations and motivational encouragement. Study nurses also provided ongoing telephone support and more frequent access to care.

Control group participants ($n = 30$) used their mobile phones. They received healthy lifestyle SMS messages to control for attention exposure. However, control participants did not receive medication reminder messages or have access to at-home BP monitoring and received standard of care treatment for hypertension.

Results: Overall, the PINGS intervention was associated with increased odds of achieving BP control compared with the control group based on systolic BP <140 mmHg at nine months. The majority of intervention participants (73%) achieved this goal, compared with only 43% of control group participants. Additionally, there was an overwhelmingly positive response from patients, caregivers, and clinical team members regarding the use of mobile technology to address BP control, medication adherence, and lifestyle modification among poststroke survivors in Sub-Saharan Africa.

Implications for Advanced Practice: While sufficient developmental infrastructure is needed in designing an mHealth intervention, once established, it can serve as a low-cost mechanism to provide high-quality care. Furthermore, mHealth may mitigate both the burden of disease and the ever-increasing costs associated with care delivery.

References: Nichols, M., Sarfo, F. S., Singh, A., Qanungo, S., Treiber, F., Ovbiagele, B., Saulson, R., Patel, S., & Jenkins, C. (2017). Assessing mobile health capacity and task shifting strategies to improve hypertension among Ghanaian stroke survivors. *American Journal of Medical Sciences*, *354*(6), 573–580. https://doi.org/10.1016/j.amjms.2017.08.005

Nichols, M., Singh, A., Sarfo, F. S., Treiber, F., Tagge, R., Jenkins, C., & Ovbiagele, B. (2019). Post-intervention qualitative assessment of mobile health technology to manage hypertension among Ghanaian stroke survivors. *Journal of the Neurological Sciences*, *406*, 116462. https://doi.org/10.1016/j.jns.2019.116462

Sarfo, F. S., Treiber, F., Gebregziabher, M., Adamu, S., Nichols, M., Singh, A., Obese, V., Sarfo-Kantanka, O., Sakyi, A., Adu-Darko, N., Tagge, R., Agyei-Frimpong, M., Kwarteng, N., Badu, E., Mensah, N., Ampofo, M., Jenkins, C., Ovbiagele, B., & PINGS Team. (2019). Phone-based intervention for blood pressure control among Ghanaian stroke survivors: A pilot randomized controlled trial. *International Journal of Stroke*, *14*(6), 630–638. https://doi.org/10.1177/17474493018816423

Sarfo, F. S., Treiber, F., Jenkins, C., Patel, S., Gebregziabher, M., Singh, A., Sarfo-Kantanka, O., Saulson, R., Appiah, L., Oparebea, E., & Ovbiagele, B. (2016). Phone-based Intervention under Nurse Guidance after Stroke (PINGS): Study protocol for a randomized controlled trial. *Trials*, *17*(436). https://doi.org/10.1186/s13063-016-1557-0

Synchronous Telehealth in Health Promotion

Synchronous telehealth encounters are similar to in-person visits, though they are conducted remotely using videoconferencing. Workflows (see **Figure 7.2**) follow typical office visit procedures with the addition of a team member confirming the patient has the necessary technology and digital literacy to participate in the encounter. Before the appointment, a front office staff member contacts the patient to complete required paperwork, such as consent, and collect a copay if indicated. The office staff member works with the patient to establish access to the live, two-way video visit

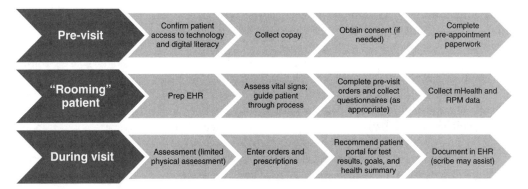

Figure 7.2 Example of a workflow process for synchronous telehealth.

platform and ensure the patient is prepared for the visit. The office staff member can then instruct patients to check their vital signs and complete any previsit orders in preparation for the appointment. If available, a medical assistant can then "room" the patient by preparing the electronic health record (EHR), collecting vital signs (including lifestyle vital signs), asking review of systems questions, addressing concerns for the visit, collecting pertinent assessments or questionnaires, and collecting patient mHealth and RPM data. Patients can alternatively share their PGHD through a patient portal or verbal discussion. A scribe may assist APPs with documentation, orders, and prescriptions during a virtual appointment. The provider visit proceeds similarly to in-office visits, except for the physical exam, which is limited to inspection and observation. APPs may conclude the visit by recommending the patient portal to view results, trends, goals, and plans.

Use of mHealth and RPM Tools in Health Promotion

Mobile applications, or apps, are software programs that run on smartphones or other mobile devices (U.S. Food and Drug Administration [FDA], 2019). Health apps are mobile programs that provide health-related services on smartphones, tablets, and other communication devices (Rouse, 2011). Other mHealth technologies available include point-of-care testing, medical-grade imaging, cardiac electrical impulses, and automated clinical decision-support tools for the patient (Steinhubl et al., 2015). Instead of providing the APP with feedback, mHealth apps are typically for the patients' use, with no provider-to-patient interaction. There were 350,000 health apps available in 2021, with 47% focused on managing specific diseases, including mental health, diabetes, and cardiovascular disease (Kent, 2021). In some cases, health apps meet a medical device definition and are referred to as mobile medical apps (MMAs). Health apps and MMAs may assist with managing patients' health and wellness, promote a healthy lifestyle, and access information as needed or provide healthcare guidance for consumers or clinicians (FDA, 2019).

There are several ways that mHealth can assist patients in managing their chronic disease, such as reminding them to take medications or to exercise and by providing feedback regarding their health data (e.g., BP or glucose measurement trends) (Thangada et al., 2018). This technology puts patients in charge of their health and allows them to set goals to monitor or improve their chronic conditions. For example, real-time remote monitoring of blood glucose increased patient education and lifestyle interventions to improve glycemic control of patients with type 2 diabetes mellitus (T2DM) (Hanlon et al., 2017). Glucose monitoring by certified diabetes health educators combined with remote lifestyle coaching has demonstrated significant improvements in blood glucose control among patients with T2DM (Bollyky et al., 2018).

RPM has multiple utilities with various other chronic diseases, such as management of asthma through the use of a *smart* inhaler, which tracks the time, frequency, and location of inhaler use; digital cognitive behavior therapies to assist patients with lifestyle modification or management of insomnia; and reminder or behavior management programs to increase control of BP in patients with hypertension (Sim, 2019). In addition to chronic disease management, mHealth technology appears to increase patient participation in healthful behaviors. Engaging patients in physical activity interventions that utilize technology, such as wearables, may significantly increase weekly minutes of physical activity when supported by the clinical team for setup, goal setting, and individualized coaching (Cadmus-Bertram et al., 2019). The information provided by these devices can be used as educational tools to increase patient self-management and positively affect healthcare outcomes.

Remote Health Monitoring in Practice

Remote monitoring gives providers the opportunity to think beyond the traditional approach to managing chronic diseases with a 15-minute office visit every three months and ask themselves, "Could I better manage this disease process by asking my patient one question every day?"

Kathryn King, MD, MHS
Associate Executive Medical Director
Center for Telehealth
Medical University of South Carolina

Lentferink et al. (2017) conducted a scoping review of lifestyle interventions utilizing self-tracking and persuasive eCoaching. In this process, technology is used during coaching to motivate and stimulate behavior change. This review outlined lifestyle intervention characteristics that positively influence health outcomes and usability. Components of eCoaching interventions that appear to affect both outcomes and usability positively were short-term goal setting to reach long-term goals, personalization of goals, delivery of praise, reminders to input self-tracking data, use of devices that are validity tested, integration of self-tracking and persuasive eCoaching, and face-to-face instruction during implementation. Participants indicated mobile phones as the preferred intervention platform and desired access to a healthcare professional for the intervention. APPs integrating a lifestyle approach can browse apps with these characteristics in mind to identify potentially effective apps for patients to use in the active phase of behavior change (Lentferink et al., 2017).

A growing number of apps are available to facilitate dietary change. A systematic review and meta-analysis conducted by Teasdale et al. (2018) found that remotely delivered interventions (digital and nondigital) that use self-monitoring and tailored feedback had a significant but small, positive effect on dietary change. These results are consistent with a systematic review and meta-analysis of app-based mobile interventions that found significant improvements in nutrition behaviors and nutrition-related health outcomes among adults and adolescents (Villinger et al., 2019). A wide variety of study methodologies and participant populations were analyzed in this review. Roughly half of the interventions evaluated used commercial apps. A majority of interventions used additional strategies such as in-person contact and digital messaging, whereas 18 of the 41 studies were stand-alone app-based interventions. This analysis found comparable results whether or not additional strategies were utilized. Although the effect size is likely small and may not produce long-term results without further intervention, these results give more support for apps as a tool for nutrition lifestyle intervention.

Apps for mental and emotional well-being are also widely available on mobile devices. However, an analysis by Lau et al. (2020) found that only 2% of apps marketed for psychological wellness and stress management had supporting research. Most of these apps had only one publication. Mindfulness meditation was the most common therapeutic component among these evidence-informed apps. Although the number of studies on the benefits of app-based mindfulness meditation is limited, the mental health effects appear to be positive. A randomized wait-list control trial of 238 office-based, healthy employees found that the use of a commercial mindfulness meditation app resulted in significant improvements in well-being, psychological distress, job strain, and perceptions of workplace social support after eight weeks when compared to the control group (Bostock et al., 2019). The improvements in well-being and job strain continued to be evident at 16 weeks. Participants who completed more meditation sessions showed greater improvements than those who completed fewer, suggesting a dose-response relationship. However, improvements in stress, resilience, and satisfaction with life were observed even after just 10 days of using a commercial mindfulness meditation app, which suggests benefits from short-term engagement (Champion et al., 2018). These positive effects are supported by a meta-analysis of 34 randomized controlled trials conducted by Gál et al. (2021), who found that mindfulness meditation apps significantly affected perceived stress, symptoms of anxiety and depression, life satisfaction, quality of life, burnout, psychological well-being, and positive and negative emotions. Mindfulness meditation apps appear to be a promising adjunctive tool for improving mental health in patients with and without clinical diagnoses. Given the availability of these apps to the public, APPs should be familiar with the current evidence base for these apps and feel comfortable recommending specific apps to interested patients. However, it is important to note that many evidence-informed apps require a fee to access additional meditations, contributing to health inequities. Thus, APPs should familiarize themselves with free evidence-informed content and comparable alternatives on streaming services, such as YouTube.

As the use of health apps increases, many users are not aware of potential quality limitations and security risks (see **Table 7.2**). The FDA oversees medical device safety and effectiveness, including MMAs, and typically focuses on those that present a greater risk to

Table 7.2 Key App Considerations

Quality	Security
Not regulated unless it meets the definition of a medical device May interfere with a medical device Content quality depends on the app developer: ■ Evidence informed? ■ Current? ■ Frequency of content review and updates? No established criteria to evaluate app quality Little tracking or documentation of app problems and clinical problems associated with app use	Data sharing with third parties May not guard sensitive data May not have or enforce privacy policies Data fall outside HIPAA regulations, putting patients at risk

patients if they do not function properly and those that may cause interference with traditional medical devices (FDA, 2019). However, the FDA does not regulate apps that do not meet the definition of medical devices established in the Federal Food, Drug, and Cosmetic (FD&C) Act section 201(h). Additionally, popular wearable activity and health monitors (e.g., Fitbit and smartwatches) are often not considered medical devices because they do not meet established criteria (Widman, 2019).

Studies have suggested that many health apps share user information with third parties and do not guard sensitive data or enforce privacy policies (Cybrary, 2018; Huckvale et al., 2015, 2019; Iwaya et al., 2020). The Health Insurance Portability and Accountability Act (HIPAA) is a federal law that regulates patient data collected by healthcare providers and their business associates about treatment, payment, or healthcare operations (Glenn & Monteith, 2014). The data from most apps are managed by the vendor, not accessible by healthcare clinicians, and fall outside of HIPAA regulations (Glenn & Monteith, 2014). The data, therefore, are not required to be secured (Wu et al., 2017). Consumers are often unaware that data entered into health apps may be shared with the software vendor for analytics and advertising purposes (Glenn & Monteith, 2014; Huckvale et al., 2015). Not all apps list a privacy policy, and for those that do, it is not necessarily an assurance that the consumer's information will not be shared (Blenner et al., 2016).

APPs should use caution when recommending an app to a patient and when using apps to complement patient care. The question remains whether the responsibility for the data entered extends to the provider. A thorough evaluation of an app's security and privacy is warranted before recommending or using it (Federal Trade Commission, 2021). APPs should critically appraise published scientific literature to evaluate the rigor of the development, testing, and evaluation of mHealth intervention apps before recommending them to patients for clinical application. Beyond security and privacy, the quality of the app's content should also be considered. Limited testing, poor awareness of app quality criteria, and low rates of reporting faulty apps or clinical problems associated with app utilization contribute to an implicit trust in apps without rigorous evaluation (Wyatt, 2018). The content of the app should be current and include a mechanism for updating the information.

Health Promotion Case Study Use of Telehealth for Hospital Discharge Follow-Up

Case Description: A 73-year-old female patient was recently discharged from the hospital for heart failure exacerbation and hyperkalemia two days ago. She wonders when she should be seen in the office for hospital discharge follow-up and what she should eat given her new diagnoses of heart failure and hyperkalemia. She has a laptop at home but does not know how to use it.

Past Medical History: T2DM (recently started on insulin), heart failure with preserved ejection fraction, aortic stenosis, stroke, stage 3 chronic kidney disease, hyperkalemia, hypertension, hyperlipidemia, obesity, and rheumatoid arthritis

Critical Thinking Questions

1. What are the benefits of telehealth for this patient?
2. What needs to be accomplished in person for this patient?
3. What can be monitored via telehealth?
4. What telehealth tools would be helpful for managing this patient?

Many organizations worldwide now recognize that health app privacy and security are lacking and have begun efforts to make digital health tools, such as smartphone apps, more secure and private (Huckvale et al., 2019). To date, however, there are no legal requirements for app developers to comply with any guidelines apart from HIPAA regulations.

Using Telehealth to Deliver Patient Education

Telehealth, as a patient education platform, can meet both APP and patient needs by increasing education and engagement through the delivery of education using digital technologies, which do not have the typical barriers of distance, availability, time, and location (Kuwabara et al., 2019). The utilization of telehealth and mHealth applications to enhance patient education and communication has shown great promise and increased patient health outcomes (Kruse et al., 2017). Telehealth has also demonstrated an impact in the self-management of diabetes by improving hemoglobin A1C measures and in BP monitoring, as previously noted, through enhanced communications and reinforcement of education between patient and provider (Greenwood et al., 2017). Telehealth can provide intensive and frequent interactions, education, and patient reinforcement, which may not be feasible for in-person visits. This has been shown to increase the likelihood of successful lifestyle changes in patients with chronic diseases such as hypertension, diabetes mellitus, stroke, cancer, heart disease, obesity, and renal disease (Kelly et al., 2016).

Application of EHR to Health Promotion

Telehealth modalities may be integrated into the EHR. The EHR is defined, in part, as "real-time, patient-centered records that make information available instantly and securely to authorized users" (HealthIT.gov, 2019, line 2). The EHR plays an integral role in healthcare delivery today and thus can act as a tool to enhance patient health promotion.

Documentation in the EHR is a crucial component of patient care. For example, patients who have a documented diagnosis of obesity are more likely to have an obesity management plan (Bardia et al., 2007). This process can be facilitated by using preset templates and lists. Thaker et al. (2016) found that using a standardized EHR template for well-child visits improved the documentation of childhood obesity and the probability of offering counseling for severe early-onset childhood obesity. Although the EHR provides numerous tools that may facilitate clinical care, APPs may feel burdened by documentation requirements and as a result interact with the EHR during patient encounters. A study by Street et al. (2018) suggested that physician engagement with the EHR (specifically, typing) during patient visits negatively affects patient–provider communication. However, physician conversational tactics such as asking about patient concerns and expressing empathy and encouragement improve patient participation. APPs can use the EHR to design workflows that enhance the quality of patient care while maintaining the integrity of patient–provider communication.

The EHR is a clinical tool that can be leveraged to help patients successfully navigate the lifestyle improvement journey (see **Figure 7.3**). Clinicians are typically the primary users of the EHR, but the use of the *patient portal* may enhance person-centered care. The patient portal, defined as "a secure online website that gives patients convenient 24-hour access to personal health information" (HealthIT.gov, 2017, lines 1–2), provides patients with direct access to select information such as vital signs, medications, forms, immunizations, laboratory results, radiology reports, and clinical notes. In addition, many patient portals offer secure patient messaging with the clinical team.

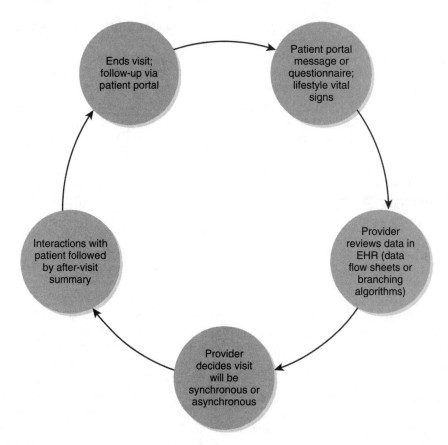

Figure 7.3 Process diagram highlighting examples of EHR tools pertinent to an outpatient lifestyle medicine visit.

Research on patient portal use is limited, but outcomes are conflicting; the studies raise important questions about accessibility and growing health disparities. A systematic review of patient portals conducted by Ammenwerth et al. (2019) did not find clinically significant improvements in patient empowerment or clinical outcomes (such as hemoglobin A1C and BP). Conversely, Han et al. (2019) conducted a systematic review and found that patient portal interventions are effective in some domains. The review identified that portal interventions improve psychological and behavioral outcomes, including health knowledge, self-efficacy, decision-making, medication adherence, and preventive service use (e.g., cancer screening);

portal interventions did not, however, improve patient activation or behavioral goal achievement. The patient portal interventions commonly pursued in these studies were the delivery of tailored educational materials about a patient's condition and tailored alerts for the management of chronic conditions. This review also concluded that evidence was insufficient to link patient portal interventions to improved clinical outcomes such as BP, glucose control, and cholesterol levels. It is important to note that the participants in the analyzed studies were predominantly White, English speaking, and highly educated, limiting these results' generalizability (Han et al., 2019). Lower rates of personal EHR use have been identified in patients without access to the internet or a computer; patients who are elderly or racial minorities; and patients with low socioeconomic status, low health or technical literacy, disabilities, and chronic illness (Showell, 2017). These disparities impede groups of patients who may benefit from this innovative access to care and thus worsen existing health inequities.

Grossman et al. (2019) conducted a systematic review that found that despite the well-described disparities in portal use, few studies have assessed interventions to overcome these disparities. Of the interventions studied, most focused on individual factors (e.g., training), instead of systemic factors, such as internet access and software accessibility standards. Although training and assistance have some evidence for increasing portal use, the authors stated that addressing system-wide inequities may be more effective. Patient portals may potentially enhance the delivery of a lifestyle approach to care; providers and office staff must work with all patients to identify individual barriers to patient portal use and to facilitate access and navigation of the portal so that all patients can equally benefit from this technology.

Telehealth can be integrated into the EHR to provide a seamless visit that is not much different from an in-person office visit except that the patient and provider are located remotely (Jason, 2020). Integrating telehealth into the EHR increases provider efficiency and patient healthcare outcomes since the two systems can communicate using a bidirectional interface instead of the APP needing to switch between two different platforms (Muller, 2020; Vyas, 2017). This integration also decreases the duplication of records and the ordering of multiple or the same diagnostics by allowing all information to be documented in one location, the patient's EHR (Muller, 2020). Another benefit of integrating telehealth into the EHR is that the platform is HIPAA compliant (Al-Maskari, 2020). Even though telehealth's functionality within an EHR system offers both the patient and the APP many benefits, it is essential to realize that functionality is not the same across all EHR systems. It is important to research its flexibility and adaptability before purchasing a system (Al-Maskari, 2020).

Data Monitoring of Behavior Change

The patient–provider alliance offers an opportunity to empower patient self-monitoring, an indispensable component of behavior change (Wadden et al., 2012). The combination of patient self-monitoring and close healthcare provider follow-up appears to produce favorable outcomes. In a randomized controlled trial of 194 patients who utilized EHR-based tracking tools for weight, diet, and physical activity, participants who received personalized EHR-based coaching and real-time progress reporting in addition to the EHR tools were more likely to maintain weight loss after 24 months in comparison to those who used the same EHR tools alone (Conroy et al., 2019). Although patient engagement with technology is growing, the clinical utilization of PGHD is in the early stages and requires further investigation to dismantle health disparities and integrate into clinical workflow effectively (Baig et al., 2017; Demiris et al., 2019).

From the APP's perspective, reviewing patient monitoring data can be expedited through the EHR. Flow sheets built into the EHR allow for visualization of anthropometrics, such as weight and body mass index, over time. In addition, lifestyle vital signs can be completed online at home prior to the appointment or on a tablet upon arrival to the clinic or can be handwritten and scanned into the EHR for provider review. Some EHRs may support customization and direct integration of lifestyle vital signs. Kaiser Permanente, for example, has had EHR exercise vital signs since 2010 (Sallis et al., 2015). These components are visible in the patient portal for transparency and patient self-monitoring. It is beneficial to spend time learning and personalizing the EHR settings to view, trend, and populate data effectively for viewing and documentation purposes.

Documentation in the EHR can conceptually follow the clinical behavior change framework utilized in practice, the 5As (assess, advise, agree, assist, and arrange) (Goldstein et al., 2004). Depending on provider preference, the history of present illness can be problem focused or structured to include the six A-SMART (adopt healthy eating, stress less, move often, avoid alcohol, rest more, treat tobacco use) lifestyle behaviors (Downes et al., 2021).

The *assessment* and plan documented in the EHR include the patient's current medical problems, appropriate guideline-directed medical therapy, risk factors, goals, readiness for change, active lifestyle prescriptions, consulting providers, and maintenance and relapse prevention planning. Some EHR-based problem lists are generated by identifying International Classification of Diseases (ICD) codes. Although this is intuitive for documenting some problems (e.g., hyperlipidemia), some patients may not have a specific ICD problem to code. In this case, the clinician can use an ICD code for *exercise counseling* or *relationship problems*, for example. EHR charting shortcuts (such as Epic SmartTools) provide customizable templates that pull pieces of information (e.g., text, labs, and vital signs) from other parts of the patient's chart. Utilizing and personalizing these shortcuts may improve the organization of patient data. The assessment and plan should be easily accessible in the EHR and updated at each visit.

The patient's goals should be documented in the plan so that the APP understands the patient's motivations. Each documented patient goal should be highly specific and time oriented (e.g., weeks, months, and years). Lifestyle-related problems should include whether readiness for change was assessed and, if so, the corresponding stage in the transtheoretical model of change (Prochaska & Velicer, 1997) noted. The six stages of the transtheoretical model

of change that correspond with a patient's readiness to implement a behavior include precontemplation (no intention to change), contemplation (thinking about making a change), preparation (ready to change within 30 days), action (a recent change in behavior usually within six months), maintenance (ongoing behavior change for at least six months, with plans to sustain the change and prevent relapse), and termination (will not relapse even with challenges). The stages are not linear, but each of the stages must be completed for the behavior change to become an habit.

After *advising* patients on a specific topic, such as the importance of quitting smoking, noting the discussion and the patient response will improve efficiency and maintain focus on the patient's goals. When the patient and the APP collaboratively *agree* on a specific goal, the lifestyle prescription should be documented in the EHR. Documentation for a physical activity plan, for example, may include an exercise prescription and the name of the mHealth app to be used for exercise logging and monitoring. Similarly, for the nutrition prescription, documentation may include a list of app functions utilized (e.g., calorie counting or macronutrient monitoring).

After the encounter, the healthcare team can *assist* patients and caregivers in developing self-monitoring skills that may enhance patient self-efficacy. Clinical team members, such as medical assistants, can instruct patients on PGHD collection techniques and validate patient tools in the clinic. Patients should be instructed to bring their mHealth devices or logs to their follow-up appointment for review.

Care coordination is an essential component of medical care, particularly for patients with multiple chronic conditions. Interprofessional team members work to *arrange* for the implementation of plans created during the visit. The APP enters the specific patient instructions without medical jargon into the EHR for the after-visit summary (AVS). These instructions include the specific details of each lifestyle prescription and other helpful information such as local support groups or websites. It is vital to assess barriers that affect patient use of the AVS, such as vision, literacy, or language. A retrospective cohort study by Mir et al. (2019) found that 15.2% of patients who did not indicate English as their primary language still received an AVS in English. Additionally, 16% of all patients received a non-meaningful AVS because it did not contain information on either the patient's presenting problem (39.2%), the physician intervention (35.6%), or the plan of care (18.4%). Although further study is required to determine the implications these findings have on outcomes, patient–provider communication can be improved by standardizing these practices at checkout.

Substance use is assessed and revisited regularly in primary care practice. Smoking is one element of substance use evaluation well established in the EHR. Government programs created incentives for providers and health systems to document patient smoking status (Centers for Medicare and Medicaid Services, 2014). A content analysis of EHRs that include support for smoking cessation done by Schindler-Ruwisch et al. (2017) found that all studied EHRs provided for the documentation of patient smoking status (*ask* of the 5As) and a majority provided a tool for prescribing medication (*assist*). More than half (57%) provided a function for documenting the patient's willingness to quit (*assess*). These tools function to guide the clinical team through assessment and management of patient tobacco use. Utilizing EHR prompts to involve multiple clinical team members improves APP workload and provides an opportunity for team members to engage in elements of patient care such as advising smoking cessation and assisting in enrollment for external programs.

Ramsey et al. (2019) implemented a point-of-care, EHR-based smoking assessment and cessation model at an outpatient cancer center. The model significantly increased the percentage of cancer patients assessed for tobacco use, referred for cessation counseling, and documented to have medication for smoking cessation. The 5As model can be adapted to any EHR and workflow to increase the reach of smoking cessation treatment. In addition to tobacco, screening for alcohol, marijuana, and other recreational drugs can be completed in the social history or the problem list in the EHR. The frequency of substance use, history of use, current medications, readiness for change, and consultant recommendations are documented in the assessment and plan.

Health Promotion Activity: Telehealth Delivery of Health Promotion

Telehealth visits for health promotion can be enhanced through the use of supplemental resources or activities. Providers can incorporate additional materials and tasks that enhance skills building or lifestyle modification within the standard telehealth visit via screen sharing or opening links to other content. These resources and activities can include, for example, the use of videos, digital workbooks, games, cooking demonstrations, exercise activities, and activities to promote behavioral activation.

Consider yourself as a provider conducting telehealth visits with your patients. What types of things would you want to address regarding health promotion and lifestyle management? What are some approaches you could use to incorporate content into your clinic visits? How could these approaches make learning more engaging and appealing to your patient population?

Identify an existing resource or create your own that could be shared with patients and that supports the clinical recommendations you would provide. How would this resource or approach enhance your practice? In what ways would it need to be tailored to meet the needs of various demographic groups?

TABLE 7.3	Evidence-Based Resources for Health Promotion Technology
Resource	**URL**
American College of Lifestyle Medicine	https://www.lifestylemedicine.org
Center for Connected Health Policy	https://www.cchpca.org
National Consortium of Telehealth Resource Centers	https://www.telehealthresourcecenter.org

Summary

There are many avenues available to utilize technology to address all components of lifestyle medicine, enhance chronic disease management, provide patient education, and improve patient access to care. See **Table 7.3** for additional evidence-based resources for health promotion technology. Telehealth modalities have increased positive health outcomes through synchronous, asynchronous, mHealth, and RPM. EHRs can also improve management through appropriate documentation of patient information (e.g., vital signs, lifestyle vital signs, diagnostic results, and management plans). To fully embrace these technologies, APPs need to become knowledgeable regarding their appropriate use and applications as well as the associated laws, security measures, and limitations of each.

Acronyms

AI: artificial intelligence
APP: advanced practice provider
AVS: after-visit summary
BP: blood pressure
EHR: electronic health record
FDA: U.S. Food and Drug Administration
FD&C: Federal Food, Drug, and Cosmetic Act
HIPAA: Health Insurance Portability and Accountability Act

ICD: International Classification of Diseases
mHealth: mobile health
MMA: mobile medical app
PGHD: patient-generated health data
RPM: remote patient monitoring
T2DM: type 2 diabetes mellitus

References

Al-Maskari, K. (2020, September 2). *Why EHR interoperability is critical for telehealth.* HIT Consultants. https://hitconsultant.net/2020/09/02/why-ehr-interoperability-is-critical-for-telehealth

Ammenwerth, E., Hoerbst, A., Lannig, S., Mueller, G., Siebert, U., & Schnell-Inderst, P. (2019). Effects of adult patient portals on patient empowerment and health-related outcomes: A systematic review. *Studies in Health Technology and Informatics, 21*(264), 1106–1110. https://doi.org/10.3233xSHTI190397

Anderson, M., & Kumar, M. (2019, May 7). *Digital divide persists even as Americans with lower incomes make gains in tech adoption.* https://www.pewresearch.org/fact-tank/2019/05/07/digital-divide-persists-even-as-lower-income-americans-make-gains-in-tech-adoption

Baig, M. M., GholamHosseini, H., Moqeem, A. A., Mirza, F., & Lindén, M. (2017). A systematic review of wearable patient monitoring systems: Current challenges and opportunities for clinical adoption. *Journal of Medical Systems*, *41*(7), 115. https://doi.org//10.1007/s10916-017-0760-1

Bardia, A., Hotan, S. B., Slezak, J. M., & Thompson, W. G. (2007). Diagnosis of obesity by primary care physicians and impact on obesity management. *Mayo Clinic Proceedings*, *82*(8), 927–932. https://doi.org/10.4065/82.8.927

Bashshur, R. L., Shannon, G. W., Smith, B. R., Alverson, D. C., Antoniotti, N., Barsan, W. G., Bashshur, N., Brown, E. M., Coye, M. J., Doarn, C. R., Ferguson, S., Grigsby, J., Krupinski, E. A., Kvedar, J. C., Linkous, J., Merrell, R. C., Nesbitt, T., Poropatich, R., Rheuban, K. S., ... Yellowlees, P. (2014). The empirical foundations of telemedicine interventions for chronic disease management. *Telemedicine and e-Health*, *20*(9), 769–800. https://doi.org/10.1089/tmj.2014.9981

Bates, R. A., Henderson, K., & Rutledge, C. M. (2020). Telehealth basics. In P. A. Schweickert & C. M. Rutledge (Eds.), *Telehealth essentials for advanced practice nursing* (pp. 23–44). Slack.

Becker's Health IT. (2014). *Seven key findings on VA telehealth services outcomes*. Becker's Hospital Review. https://www.beckershospitalreview.com/healthcare-information-technology/7-key-findings-on-va-telehealth-services-outcomes.html

Blenner, S., Kollmer, M., & Rouse, A. (2016). Privacy policies of Android diabetes apps and sharing of health information. *Journal of the American Medical Association*, *315*(10), 1051–1052. https://doi.org/10.1001/jama.2015.19426

Bollyky, J. B., Bravata, D., Yang, J., Williamson, M., & Schneider, J. (2018). Remote lifestyle coaching plus a connected glucose meter with certified diabetes educator support improves glucose and weight loss for people with type 2 diabetes. *Journal of Diabetes Research*, *2018*. https://doi.org/10.1155/2018/3961730

Bostock, S., Crosswell, A. D., Prather, A. A., & Steptoe, A. (2019). Mindfulness on-the-go: Effects of a mindfulness meditation app on work stress and well-being. *Journal of Occupational Health Psychology*, *24*(1), 127–138. https://doi.org/10.1037/ocp0000118

Cadmus-Bertram, L., Tevaarwerk, A. J., Sesto, M. E., Gangnon, R., Van Remortel, B., & Date, P. (2019). Building a physical activity intervention into clinical care for breast and colorectal cancer survivors in Wisconsin: A randomized controlled pilot trial. *Journal of Cancer Survivorship*, *13*, 593–602. https://doi.org/10.1007/s11764-019-00778-6

Castilla, D., Botella, C., Miralles, I., Breton-Lopez, J., Dragomir-Davis, A. M., Zaragoza, I., & Garcia-Palacios, A. (2018). Teaching digital literacy skills to the elderly using a social network with linear navigation: A case study in a rural area. *International Journal of Human-Computer Studies*, *118*, 24–37. https://doi.org/10.1016/j.ijhcs.2018.05.009

Center for Connected Health Policy. (n.d.). *What is eConsult?* Retrieved October 10, 2020, from https://www.cchpca.org/sites/default/files/2018-09/eConsult%20Inforgraph%20Final.pdf

Center for Connected Health Policy. (2020). *Telehealth and Medicare*. https://www.cchpca.org/search?keyword=2019+physician+fee+schedule

Centers for Disease Control and Prevention. (2020, July 8). *Telehealth and telemedicine*. https://www.cdc.gov/phlp/publications/topic/telehealth.html

Centers for Disease Control and Prevention. (2021). *Chronic diseases in America*. https://www.cdc.gov/chronicdisease/resources/infographic/chronic-diseases.htm

Centers for Medicare and Medicaid Services. (2014, May). *Eligible professional meaningful use core measures: Measure 9 of 13*. https://www.cms.gov/Regulations-and-Guidance/Legislation/EHRIncentivePrograms/downloads/9_Record_Smoking_Status.pdf

Chaikijurajai, T., Laffin, L. J., & Tang, W. H. W. (2020). Artificial intelligence and hypertension: Recent advances and future outlook. *American Journal of Hypertension*. Advance online publication. https://doi.org/10.1093/ajh/hpaa102

Champion, L., Economides, M., & Chandler, C. (2018). The efficacy of a brief app-based mindfulness intervention on psychosocial outcomes in healthy adults: A pilot randomised controlled trial. *PLoS ONE*, *13*(12), e0209482. https://doi.org/10.1371/journal.pone.0209482

Chen, A., Murphy, E., Yee, D., & Yee, H. (2013). eReferral: A new model for integrated care. *New England Journal of Medicine*, *368*(26), 2450–2453. https://doi.org/10.1056/NEJMp1215594

Committee on Pediatric Workforce. (2015). The use of telemedicine to address access and physician workforce shortages. *Pediatrics*, *136*(1), 202–209. https://doi.org/10.1542/peds.2015-1253

Conard, S. (2019). Best practices in digital health literacy. *International Journal of Cardiology*, *292*(2019), 277–279. https://doi.org/10.1016/j.ijcard.2019.05.070

Conroy, M. B., McTigue, K. M., Bryce, C. L., Tudorascu, D., Gibbs, B. B., Arnold, J., Comer, D., Hess, R., Huber, K., Simkin-Silverman, L. R., & Fischer, G. S. (2019). Effect of electronic health record–based coaching on weight maintenance. *Annals of Internal Medicine*, *171*(11), 777–784. https://doi.org/10.7326/m18-3337

Cybrary. (2018, May 6). *Is your information on mobile health apps safe?* https://www.cybrary.it/2018/05/information-mobile-health-apps-safe

Demiris, G., Iribarren, S. J., Sward, K., Lee, S., & Yan, R. (2019). Patient generated health data use in clinical practice: A systematic review. *Nursing Outlook*, *67*(4), 311–330. https://doi.org/10.1016/j.outlook.2019.04.005

Department of Veterans Affairs. (2020). *VA telehealth services*. https://www.va.gov/anywheretoanywhere/docs/Telehealth_Services_factsheet.PDF

Downes, L. S., St. Hill, H., & Mays, T. (2021). A-SMART lifestyle behaviors model for health, well-being, and immune system enhancement. *The Nurse Practitioner, 46*(6), 31–39. https://doi.org/10.1097/01.NPR.0000769748.45938.10

EMS GrantsHelp Team. (2020, April 30). *Telehealth funding eligibility under the CARES Act*. EMS1. https://www.ems1.com/telemedicine/articles/telehealth-funding-eligibility-under-the-cares-act-1Dttio NUAN1TCzJ8

Federal Communications Commission. (2018). *Federal Communications Commission report*. https://docs.fcc.gov/public/attachments/FCC-18-181A1.pdf

Federal Trade Commission. (2021). *How to protect your privacy on*. https://www.consumer.ftc.gov/articles/0018-understanding-mobile-apps#privacy

Gál, É., Ştefan, S., & Cristea, I. A. (2021). The efficacy of mindfulness meditation apps in enhancing users' well-being and mental health related outcomes: A meta-analysis of randomized controlled trials. *Journal of Affective Disorders, 279*, 131–142. https://doi.org/10.1016/j.jad.2020.09.134

Glenn, T., & Montieth, S. (2014). Privacy in the digital world: Medical and health data outside of HIPAA protections. *Current Psychiatry Reports, 16*(494). https://doi.org/10.1007/s11920-014-0494-4

Goldstein, M. G., Whitlock, E. P., & Depue, J. (2004). Multiple behavioral risk factor interventions in primary care. *American Journal of Preventive Medicine, 27*(2S), 61–79. https://doi.org/10.1016/j.amepre.2004.04.023

Greenwood, D. A., Gee, P. M., Fatkin, K. J., & Peeple, M. (2017). A systematic review of reviews evaluating technology-enabled diabetes self-management education and support. *Journal of Diabetes Science and Technology, 11*(5), 1015–1027. https://doi.org/10.1177/1932296817713506

Grossman, L. V., Masterson Creber, R. M., Benda, N. C., Wright, D., Vawdrey, D. K., & Ancker, J. S. (2019). Interventions to increase patient portal use in vulnerable populations: A systematic review. *Journal of the American Medical Informatics Association, 26*(8–9), 855–870. https://doi.org/10.1093/jamia/ocz023

Han, H., Gleason, K. T., Sun, C. A., Miller, H. N., Kang, S. J., Chow, S., & Bauer, T. (2019). Using patient portals to improve patient outcomes: Systematic review. *JMIR Human Factors, 6*(4), e15038. https://doi.org/10.2196/15038

Hanlon, P., Daines, L., Campbell, C., McKinstry, B., Weller, D., & Pinnock, H. (2017). Telehealth interventions to support self-management of long-term conditions: A systematic metareview of diabetes, heart failure, asthma, chronic obstructive pulmonary disease, and cancer. *Journal of Medical Internet Research, 19*(5), e172. https://doi.org/10.2196/jmir.6688

HealthIT.gov. (2017, September 29). *What is a patient portal?* https://www.healthit.gov/faq/what-patient-portal

HealthIT.gov. (2019, September 10). *What is an electronic health record (EHR)?* https://www.healthit.gov/faq/what-electronic-health-record-ehr

Huckvale, K., Prieto, J., Tilney, M., Benghozi, P., & Car, J. (2015). Unaddressed privacy risks in accredited health and wellness apps: A cross-sectional systematic assessment. *BMC Medicine, 13*(214). https://doi.org/10.1186/s12916-015-0444-y

Huckvale, K., Torous, J., & Larsen, M. (2019). Assessment of the data sharing and privacy practices of smartphone apps for depression and smoking cessation. *JAMA Network, 2*(4). https://doi.org/10.1001/jamanetworkopen.2019.2542

InTouch Health. (2020). *4 Benefits of telemedicine in chronic disease management: How telemedicine is changing chronic disease management for the better*. https://intouchhealth.com/4-benefits-of-telemedicine-in-chronic-disease-management

Iwaya, L. H., Ahmad, A., & Babar, M. A. (2020). Security and privacy for mHealth and uHealth systems: A systematic mapping study. *IEEEAccess, 8*, 150081–150112. https://doi.org/10.1109/ACCESS.2020.3015962

Jason, C. (2020, June 22). *How EHR telehealth integration evolved patient care during COVID-19*. EHR Intelligence. https://ehrintelligence.com/news/how-ehr-telehealth-integration-evolved-patient-care-during-covid-19

Joshi, A., & Hollander, E. (2017, March 9). *Why the telemedicine physical is better than you think*. http://www.telemedmag.com/telemedicine-physical-better-think

Kaufman, D. R., Pevzner, J., Hilliman, C., Weinstock, R. S., Teresi, J., Shea, S., & Starren, J. (2006). Redesigning a telehealth diabetes management program for a digital divide seniors population. *Home Health Care Management & Practice, 18*(3), 223–234. https://doi.org/10.1177/1084822305281949

Kelly, J. T., Reidlinger, D. P., Hoffmann, T. C., & Campbell, K. L. (2016). Telehealth methods to deliver dietary interventions in adults with chronic disease: A systematic review and meta-analysis. *American Journal of Clinical Nutrition, 104*(6), 1696–1702. https://doi.org/10.3945/ajcn.116.136333

Kent, C. (2021). *Digital health app market booming, finds IQVIA report*. Medical Device Network. https://www.medicaldevice-network.com/news/digital-health-apps

Kruse, C. S., Krowski, N., Rodriguez, B., Tran, L., Vela, J., & Brooks, M. (2017). Telehealth and patient satisfaction: A systematic review and narrative analysis. *British Medical Journal Open, 7*(8), e016424. https://doi.org/10.1136/bmjopen-2017-016242

Kuwabara, A., Su, S., & Krauss, J. (2019). Utilizing digital health technologies for patient education in lifestyle medicine. *American Journal of Lifestyle Medicine*, *14*(2), 137–142. https://doi.org/10.1177/15598276 19892547

Lau, N., O'Daffer, A., Colt, S., Yi-Frazier, J. P., Palermo, T. M., McCauley, E., & Rosenberg, A. R. (2020). Android and iPhone mobile apps for psychosocial wellness and stress management: Systematic search in app stores and literature review. *JMIR MHealth and UHealth*, *8*(5), e17798. https://doi.org/10.2196/17798

Lentferink, A. J., Oldenhuis, H. K. E., de Groot, M., Polstra, L., Velthuijsen, H., & van Gemert-Pijnen, J. E. W. C. (2017). Key components in eHealth interventions combining self-tracking and persuasive eCoaching to promote a healthier lifestyle: A scoping review. *Journal of Medical Internet Research*, *19*(8), 1–19. https://doi.org/10.2196/jmir.7288

Lewiecki, E. M., & Rochelle, R. (2019). Project ECHO: Telehealth to expand capacity to deliver best practice medical care. *Rheumatic Disease Clinics of North America*, *45*(2), 303–314. https://doi.org/10.1016/j .rdc.2019.01.003

Magnani, J. W., Mujahid, M. S., Aronow, H. D., Cené, C. W., Dickson, V. V., Havranek, E., Morgenstern, L. B., Paasche-Orlow, M. K., Pollak, A., & Willey, J. Z. (2018). Health literacy and cardiovascular disease: Fundamental relevance to primary and secondary prevention: A scientific statement from the American Heart Association. *Circulation*, *138*(2), e48–e74. https://doi.org/10.1161/CIR.0000000000000579

Marcin, J. P., Rimsza, M. E., & Moskowitz, W. B. (2015). The use of telemedicine to address access and physician workforce shortages. *Pediatrics*, *136*(1), 201–209. https://doi.org/ 10.1542/peds.2015-1253

Mintz, Y., & Brodie, R. (2019). Introduction to artificial intelligence in medicine. *Minimally Invasive Therapy & Allied Technologies*, *28*(2), 73–81. https://doi.org/10.1080 /13645706.2019.1575882

Mir, T. H., Osayande, A., Kone, K., Bridges, K., & Day, P. (2019). Assessing the quality of the after-visit summary (AVS) in a primary-care clinic. *Journal of the American Board of Family Medicine*, *32*(1), 65–68. https://doi.org/10.3122/jabfm.2019.01.180055

Muller, E. (2020). *Electronic medical records and telemedicine software*. Health Recovery Solutions. https://www .healthrecoverysolutions.com/blog/the-role-of -electronic-medical-records-in-telehealth

Naylor, K., Tootoo, J., Yakusheva, O., Shipman, S., Bynum, J., & Davis, M. (2019). Geographic variation in spatial accessibility of US healthcare providers. *PLoS ONE*, *14*(4), e0215016. https://doi.org/10.1371/journal .pone.0215016

Nichols, M., Sarfo, F. S., Singh, A., Qanungo, S., Treiber, F., Ovbiagele, B., Saulson, R., Patel, S., & Jenkins, C. (2017). Assessing mobile health capacity and task shifting strategies to improve hypertension among Ghanaian stroke survivors. *American Journal of Medical*

Sciences, 354(6), 573–580. https://doi.org/10.1016/j .amjms.2017.08.005

Nichols, M., Singh, A., Sarfo, F. S., Treiber, F., Tagge, R., Jenkins, C., & Ovbiagele, B. (2019). Post-intervention qualitative assessment of mobile health technology to manage hypertension among Ghanaian stroke survivors. *Journal of the Neurological Sciences, 406*, 116462. https://doi.org/10.1016/j.jns.2019.116462

Nimrod, G. (2018). Technophobia among older internet users. *Educational Gerontology, 44*(2–3), 148–162. https://doi.org/10.1080/03601277.2018.1428145

O'Connor, M., Asdornwised, U., Dempsey, M. L., Huffenberger, A., Jost, S., Flynn, D., & Norris, A. (2016). Using telehealth to reduce all-cause 30-day hospital readmissions among heart failure patients receiving skilled home health services. *Applied Clinical Informatics, 7*(2), 238–247. https://doi.org/10.4338 /ACI-2015-11-SOA-0157

Olson, C., McSwain, D., & Curfman, A. (2018). The current pediatric telehealth landscape. *Pediatrics, 141*(3). https://doi.org/10.1542/peds.2017-2334

Ortiz, D. N. (2017, February 27–28). *Digital health literacy*. First Meeting of the WHO GCM/NCD Working Group on Health Literacy for NCDs, Geneva, Switzerland. https://www.who.int/global-coordination-mechanism /working-groups/digital_hl.pdf

Ortholive. (2018, December 13). *Top 10 benefits of telehealth for patients and doctors*. https://www.ortholive .com/blog/top-10-benefits-of-telehealth-for-patients -and-doctors

Press Ganey. (2020, May 19). *The rapid transition to telemedicine: Insights and early trends*. http://images .healthcare.pressganey.com/Web/PressGaneyAssociates Inc/%7B353645d0-ea02-4a11-a012-ba4f0c3debb9% 7D_2020_PG_Telemedicine_Special_Report.pdf

Prochaska, J. O., & Velicer, W. F. (1997). The transtheoretical model of health behavior change. *American Journal of Health Promotion, 12*(1), 38–48. https://doi .org/10.4278/0890-1171-12.1.38

Ramsey, A. R., Chiu, A., Baker, T., Smock, N., Chen, J., Lester, T., Jorenby, D. E., Colditz, G. A., Bierut, L. J., & Chen, L. (2019). Care-paradigm shift promoting smoking cessation treatment among cancer center patients via a low-burden strategy, electronic health record-enabled evidence-based smoking cessation treatment. *Translational Behavioral Medicine, ibz107*. https://doi.org/10.1093/tbm/ibz107

Rouse, M. (2011, March). *Health apps*. TechTarget. https:// searchhealthit.techtarget.com/definition/health -apps#:~:text=Health%20apps%20are%20application %20programs,mHealth)%20programs%20in%20 health%20care

Rural Health Information Hub. (2019, May 21). *Telehealth models for increasing access to specialty care*. https://www.ruralhealthinfo.org/toolkits/telehealth/2 /care-delivery/specialty-care

Rutledge, C. M., Kott, K., Schweickert, P. A., Poston, R., Fowler, C., & Haney, T. S. (2017). Telehealth and eHealth in nurse practitioner training: Current perspectives. *Advances in Medical Education and Practice*, 8, 399–409. https://doi.org/10.2147/AMEP.S116071

Sallis, R., Franklin, B., Joy, L., Ross, R., Sabgir, D., & Stone, J. (2015). Strategies for promoting physical activity in clinical practice. *Progress in Cardiovascular Diseases*, 57(4), 375–386. https://doi.org/10.1016/j.pcad.2014.10.003

Sarfo, F. S., Treiber, F., Gebregziabher, M., Adamu, S., Nichols, M., Singh, A., Obese, V., Sarfo-Kantanka, O., Sakyi, A., Adu-Darko, N., Tagge, R., Agyei-Frimpong, M., Kwarteng, N., Badu, E., Mensah, N., Ampofo, M., Jenkins, C., Ovbiagele, B., & PINGS Team. (2019). Phone-based intervention for blood pressure control among Ghanaian stroke survivors: A pilot randomized controlled trial. *International Journal of Stroke*, 14(6), 630–638. https://doi.org/10.1177/17474493018816423

Sarfo, F. S., Treiber, F., Jenkins, C., Patel, S., Gebregziabher, M., Singh, A., Sarfo-Kantanka, O., Saulson, R., Appiah, L., Oparebea, E., & Ovbiagele, B. (2016). Phone-based Intervention under Nurse Guidance after Stroke (PINGS): Study protocol for a randomized controlled trial. *Trials*, 17(436). https://doi.org/10.1186/s13063-016-1557-0

Schindler-Ruwisch, J. M., Abroms, L. C., Bernstein, S. L., & Heminger, C. L. (2017). A content analysis of electronic health record (EHR) functionality to support tobacco treatment. *Translational Behavioral Medicine*, 7(2), 148–156. http://dx.doi.org/10.1007/s13142-016-0446-0

Shigekawa, E., Fix, M., Corbett, G., Roby, D., & Coffman, J. (2018). The current state of telehealth evidence: A rapid review. *Health Affairs*, 37(12), 1975–1982. https://doi.org/ 10.1377/hlthaff.2018.05132

Showell, C. (2017). Barriers to the use of personal health records by patients: A structured review. *PeerJ*, 5, 1–24. https://doi.org/10.7717/peerj.3268

Sim, I. (2019). Mobile devices and health. *New England Journal of Medicine*, 381, 956–968. https://doi.org/10.1056/NEJMra1806949

Stein, N., & Brooks, K. (2017). A fully automated conversational artificial intelligence for weight loss: Longitudinal observational study among overweight and obese adults. *JMIR Diabetes*, 2(2), e28. https://doi.org/10.2196/diabetes.8590

Steinhubl, S. R., Muse, E. D., & Topol, E. J. (2015). The emerging field of mobile health. *Science Translational Medicine*, 7(283), 1–12. https://doi.org/10.1126/scitranslmed.aaa3487

Street, R. L., Jr., Liu, L., Farber, N. J., Chen, Y., Calvitti, A., Weibel, N., Gabuzda, M. T., Bell, K., Gray, B., Rick, S., Ashfaq, S., & Agha, Z. (2018). Keystrokes, mouse clicks, and gazing at the computer: How physician interaction with the EHR affects patient participation. *Journal of General Internal Medicine*, 33, 423–428. https://doi.org/10.1007/s11606-017-4228-2

Teasdale, N., Elhussein, A., Butcher, F., Piernas, C., Cowburn, G., Hartmann-Boyce, J., Saksena, R., & Scarborough, P. (2018). Systematic review and meta-analysis of remotely delivered interventions using self-monitoring or tailored feedback to change dietary behavior. *American Journal of Clinical Nutrition*, 107(2), 247–256. https://doi.org/10.1093/ajcn/nqx048

Thaker, V. V., Lee, F., & Bottino, C. J. (2016). Impact of an electronic template on documentation of obesity in a primary care clinic. *Clinical Pediatrics*, 55(12). https://doi.org/10.1177/0009922815621331

Thangada, N. D., Garg, N., Pandey, A., & Kumar, N. (2018). The emerging role of mobile-health applications in the management of hypertension. *Current Cardiology Reports*, 20(9), 78. https://doi.org/10.1007/x11886-018-1022-7

Tuman, A. (2019, September 25). *Impact of technological innovations in healthcare*. Health Tech. https://www.healthtechzone.com/topics/healthcare/articles/2019/09/25/443350-impact-technological-innovations-healthcare.htm

University of New Mexico School of Medicine. (2020). *ECHO impact and initiatives: Touching one billion lives by 2025*. https://hsc.unm.edu/echo/echos-impact/

U.S. Census Bureau. (2017, August 9). *One in five Americans live in rural areas*. https://www.census.gov/library/stories/2017/08/rural-america.html#:~:text=Urban%20areas%20make%20up%20only,Census%20Bureau%20%2D%20Opens%20as%20PDF

U.S. Food and Drug Administration. (2019, September 27). *Policy for device software functions and mobile medical applications: Guidance for industry and Food and Drug Administration staff*. https://www.fda.gov/media/80958/download

Van Houwelingen, C., Ettema, R., Antonietti, M., & Kort, H. (2018). Understanding older people's readiness for receiving telehealth: Mixed method study. *Journal of Medical Internet Research*, 20(4). https://doi.org/10.2196/jmir.8407

Vassilakopoulou, P., & Hustad, E. (2021). Bridging digital divides: A literature review and research agenda for information systems research. *Information Systems Frontiers*. Advance online publication. https://doi.org/10.1007/s10796-020-10096-3

Villinger, K., Wahl, D. R., Boeing, H., Schupp, H. T., & Renner, B. (2019). The effectiveness of app-based mobile interventions on nutrition behaviours and nutrition-related health outcomes: A systematic review and meta-analysis. *Obesity Reviews*, 20(10), 1465–1484. https://doi.org/10.1111/obr.12903

Vogels, E. (2021). *Some digital divides persist between rural, urban and suburban America*. Pew Research. https://www.pewresearch.org/fact-tank/2021/08/19/some-digital-divides-persist-between-rural-urban-and-suburban-america

VSee. (2017, January 17). *Why telehealth is the key for lifestyle interventions – Laurence Girard, Fruit Street.* https://vsee.com/blog/health-coach-telehealth-tools

Vyas, S. (2017, October 12). *How telehealth and EHR integration deliver complete, effective care while streamlining provider workflows.* Becker's Hospital Review. https://www.beckershospitalreview.com/healthcare-information-technology/how-telehealth-and-ehr-integration-deliver-complete-effective-care-while-streamlining-provider-workflows.html

Wadden, T. A., Webb, V. L., Moran, C. H., & Bailer, B. A. (2012). Lifestyle modification for obesity. *Circulation, 125*(9), 1157–1170. https://doi.org/10.1161/circulationaha.111.039453

Warshaw, R. (2017, October 31). *Health disparities affect millions in rural US communities.* AACM News. https://www.aamc.org/news-insights/health-disparities-affect-millions-rural-us-communities#:~:text=Rural%20Americans%E2%80%94who%20make%20up,geographic%2C%20and%20health%20workforce%20actors

Wecklund, E. (2018, November 2). *CMS to reimburse providers for remote patient monitoring services.* https://mhealthintelligence.com/news/cms-to-reimburse-providers-for-remote-patient-monitoring-services

Weigel, G., Ramaswamy, A., Sobel, L., Salganicoff, A., Cubanski, J., & Freed, M. (2020, May 11). *Opportunities and barriers for telemedicine in the US during the COVID-19 emergency and beyond.* Kaiser Family Foundation. https://www.kff.org/womens-health-policy/issue-brief/opportunities-and-barriers-for-telemedicine-in-the-u-s-during-the-covid-19-emergency-and-beyond

Weinstein, R., Lopez, A., Joseph, B., Erps, K., Holcomb, M., Barker, G., & Krupinski, E. (2014). Telemedicine, telehealth, and mobile health applications that work: Opportunities and barriers. *American Journal of Medicine, 127*(3), 183–187. http://dx.doi.org/10.1016/j.amjmed.2013.09.032

Widman, J. (2019, April 30). *Fitness monitors, smartwatches are not medical devices.* Communications of the ACM. https://cacm.acm.org/news/236543-fitness-monitors-smartwatches-are-not-medical-devices/fulltext

Wood, C., Clements, S., McFann, K., Slover, R., Thomas, J., & Wadwa, P. (2016). Use of telemedicine to improve adherence to American Diabetes Association standards in pediatric type 1 diabetes. *Diabetes Technology & Therapeutics, 18*(1), 7–14. https://doi.org/10.1080/09638280802062553

World Health Organization. (2020). *Telehealth.* https://www.who.int/gho/goe/telehealth/en/

Wu, E., Torous, J., Hardaway, R., & Gutheil, T. (2017). Confidentiality and privacy for smartphone applications in child and adolescent psychiatry: Unmet needs and practical solutions. *Child Adolescent Psychiatric Clinics of North America, 26,* 117–124. http://dx.doi.org/10.1016/j.chc.2016.07.006

Wyatt, J. C. (2018). How can clinicians, specialty societies and others evaluate and improve the quality of apps for patient use? *BMC Medicine, 16*(1), 225. https://doi.org/10.1186/s12916-018-1211-7

Xu, T., Pujara, S., Sutton, S., & Rhee, M. (2018). Telemedicine in the management of type 1 diabetes. *Preventing Chronic Disease: Public Health Research, Practice and Policy, 15,* 170168. https://doi.org/10.5888/pcd15.170168

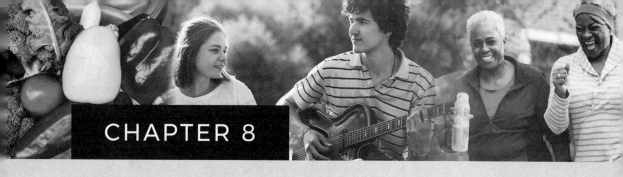

CHAPTER 8

Health Promotion Billing and Reimbursement

Alicia Craig-Rodriguez, DNP, MBA, APRN, FNP-BC, DipACLM
Lolita Melhado, PhD, MSN, APRN, FNP-BC, ACHPN

Nothing is more expensive than a missed opportunity.

H. Jackson Brown, Jr.

OBJECTIVES

This chapter will enable the reader to:

1. Discuss the economic impact of chronic disease and its burden on the current healthcare system.
2. Explain the economic and financial aspects of lifestyle and health promotion.
3. Describe the current trends of chronic disease management using evidence-informed, person-centered lifestyle prescriptive approaches used to promote health.
4. Differentiate among the various reimbursement and practice models for promoting healthy lifestyles.
5. Analyze different methods of maximizing reimbursement utilized in healthy lifestyle promotion practices.
6. Evaluate documentation requirements to maximize reimbursement.

Overview

Of the nation's $3.5 trillion healthcare expenditures, 80% to 90% are spent on individuals who suffer from preventable and reversible chronic and mental health conditions (Beckman, 2019; Bodai et al., 2017; National Center for Chronic Disease Prevention and Health Promotion, n.d.). Although research demonstrates that the economic benefits generated from lifestyle and health promotion interventions far outweigh the cost of administering the services, there is little financial incentive in the current healthcare system to focus on these evidence-informed interventions (Beckman, 2019). The traditional fee-for-service (FFS) payment model still dominates U.S. health care and is predicated on the efficient and rapid diagnosis and treatment of a high volume of patients and the

© Kathleen Gail/Shutterstock; © StoryTime Studio/Shutterstock; © kali9/Getty Images

prescribing of medications and treatments that may slow the trajectory of the illness but that fail to address the root cause (Benjamin et al., 2017; Jensen et al., 2019; National Center for Chronic Disease Prevention and Health Promotion, n.d.). Fifteen-minute appointments are commonplace, with an average of seven minutes spent between provider and patient (Lacagnina et al., 2018).

Treating the whole person (i.e., mental, emotional, social, environmental, and spiritual domains of the persons' health), not just the condition, is a fundamental concept of lifestyle and health promotion (Braman & Edison, 2017). Chronic conditions are highly related to unhealthy but modifiable lifestyle or behavioral factors, such as smoking, physical inactivity, poor diet, and resistant rates of obesity (Ma et al., 2016). The role of the lifestyle and health promotion provider is to educate and empower patients to reverse or manage their chronic disease through simple yet effective lifestyle and behavioral interventions. These interventions are often time intensive and require significant participant support to be successful.

Best treatment protocols involve evidence-informed therapeutic approaches and patient engagement strategies to promote healthy behaviors, delay disease, and improve quality of life. Patients treated with healthy lifestyle promotion approaches often do not need additional procedures, prescriptions, or office visits (Beckman, 2019). Despite generating substantial future cost savings to payers, most practitioners utilizing these approaches for their patients are not recognized for their efforts or reimbursed for providing these services (Beckman, 2019). The traditional FFS reimbursement model does not adequately reward lifestyle and health promotion approaches that include interventions such as education, counseling, and health coaching. Additionally, the current FFS model rewards the quantity over quality of care delivered and places a tremendous economic burden on the healthcare system (Blue, 2019). Ironically, reimbursement

rates for smoking cessation counseling and obesity counseling pay far less than other evaluation and management (E/M) services. This chapter will explore the economic and financial aspects of lifestyle and health promotion for the advanced practice provider (APP). It will examine practice models, reimbursement strategies, and future trends in the business of lifestyle and health promotion.

Overview of the Payer Landscape

The payer landscape comprises three participants involved in the process of healthcare reimbursement: the patient, the provider, and the payer (see **Figure 8.1**). A *provider* is a qualified healthcare professional or institution that delivers care to the patient and bills for services rendered; examples include physicians, nurse practitioners, physician associates, physical therapists, psychologists, hospitals, nursing homes, and medical practices (Reiter et al., 2021; Waxman, 2018). A *payer* can be a third-party organization, such as a commercial insurance company, private insurer, government agency, or managed care organization. When rendered services are not covered (or are only partially covered) by a third party, the patient becomes the payer and is responsible for any out-of-pocket costs (Reiter et al., 2021; Waxman, 2018). Third-party payers have their own fee schedules, and both the provider and the payer must negotiate agreeable terms of reimbursement before payment for services can be reimbursed (Buppert, 2021).

Prerequisites for Provider Reimbursement

A basic prerequisite for **provider reimbursement**, or billing, begins with providers obtaining a National Provider Identifier (NPI)

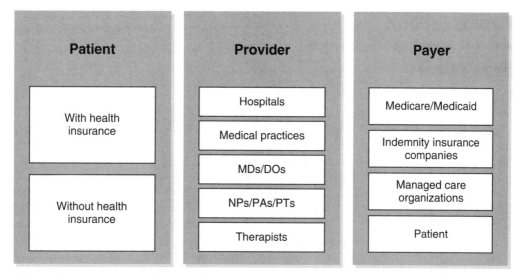

Figure 8.1 Healthcare participants.

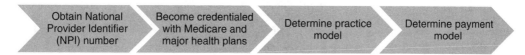

Figure 8.2 Prerequisites for provider reimbursement.

number from the National Plan and Provider Enumeration System (see **Figure 8.2**). The application can be completed online. Next, providers must be credentialed with Medicare, which requires completing a provider application to obtain a provider transaction access number. In addition, providers must be credentialed with the major health plans to receive reimbursement payments directly from them. The Council for Affordable Quality Healthcare ProView is an online credentialing service and database commonly used by insurance plans and organizations available at no cost to providers. The insurance plans will require providers to enter practice information, including their tax identification number, location, and practice affiliations.

Rules for insurance reimbursement vary by geographic location, provider contracts with insurers, and patient plans (Jensen et al., 2019). Investigating and understanding payer requirements can help prevent unwanted and costly mistakes (American College of Lifestyle Medicine [ACLM], 2019b). Insurance companies determine the reimbursement rates; if APPs are just starting or are an out-of-network provider, they will need to negotiate with insurance companies to become an in-network provider and negotiate a mutual contract. APPs are recommended to work in partnership with reimbursement experts. Working with an insurance specialist or a representative within an insurance company may help APPs navigate and negotiate contracts.

Practice Models and Reimbursement Structures

There are different practice models, each having its own unique reimbursement structure. These models are not mutually exclusive and may be combined within a single practice to create different operational opportunities to reduce barriers to reimbursement (ACLM, 2019). Payment models often include reimbursement for routine visits, ancillary counseling services, and behavioral modification as well as subscriptions and membership fees. Some providers may forgo billing to insurance companies entirely and use a cash-pay or membership model. The most common reimbursement practice models used by providers range from the most simple, such as direct primary care (DPC) and concierge medicine, to the more complex models, such as traditional FFS, time based, group visits (GVs), shared medical appointments, bundled, or a blended mix of the preceding models (see **Table 8.1**). In addition to the many lifestyle medicine (LM) delivery practice models, Gobble et al. (2022) described two common practice models that overlap with the previously discussed models, the independent or solo practice and the medical practice team approach. The team approach typically includes interprofessionals, such as a registered dietitian, physical therapist, and certified health

Table 8.1 Reimbursement Practice Models

Direct Primary Care	Concierge, or Membership, Medicine	Traditional FFS (Medical Decision-Making [MDM] vs. Time Based)	Bundled Payments	Group or Shared Medical Appointments
Flat fee charged monthly or annually. Office visits are free.	Personalized care, reduced patient panel A typical workflow is five days per week from 9:00 a.m. to 5:00 p.m. with one or two comprehensive exams and six regular visits. Annual membership fee, may vary by patient age Private insurance, Medicare accepted	Preventive, annual wellness visits, and E/M Select Current Procedural Terminology (CPT) code based on level of MDM or total time spent. (Total time spent includes all face-to-face and non–face-to-face time on the day of services for reviewing and completing records.) CPT codes 99202 to 99215. E/M visit includes medically appropriate history and examination.	Value-based reimbursement model designed to reduce costs associated with an FFS model. Providers are given a single payment for a defined episode of care (e.g., hip surgery).	90-minute time slots for a select group of diagnoses or conditions (established patients). Documentation reflects the individual services (usually a brief exam) provided to each patient and services provided to the group). CPT codes 99212 to 99214 are billed based on the level of MDM, not the face-to-face time with the patient

coach in addition to the primary care provider who work collaboratively to achieve healthy lifestyle behavior changes for patients. As the LM delivery practice models evolve, the value of lifestyle medicine will be recognized for its results, effectiveness, and patient and provider satisfaction.

Direct Primary Care

The DPC model is an alternative to the traditional FFS model and is not associated with billing an insurance plan (Braman & Edison, 2017; Jensen et al., 2019). The patient pays a monthly, quarterly, or annual retainer fee, and office visits are free. DPC visits cover basic labs and individualized primary care that includes services focused on health promotion and illness prevention—services typically missed in the traditional 15-minute encounter (Braman & Edison, 2017; Lamberts, 2019). Diagnostic services are usually contracted with other providers and are available at a significantly reduced cost. A typical DPC provider may have a panel of 500 patients and charge each $100 per month.

Concierge (Membership) Medicine

The concierge, or membership, medicine model is based on a significant reduction in the number of patients to ensure highly personalized care focused on prevention and wellness interventions. Unlike the DPC model, some concierge practices do not include primary care or urgent care services, and patients may have to continue with their primary care provider for those services (see **Table 8.2**). The concierge model is based on an annual membership fee that may vary by patient age. A predictable and steady income is derived from membership fees rather than from FFS reimbursement. Private insurance and Medicare can cover labs, imaging, and studies performed outside the office. As a rule

Table 8.2 Direct Primary Care Versus Concierge Care

Direct Primary Care	Concierge Care
Greater access to provider vs. traditional models	Greater access to provider vs. traditional models
Lower monthly subscription fees, ≤ $100	Higher monthly subscription fees, in addition to insurance
No insurance fees collected	Insurance fees collected
Larger panel of patients (400–800)	Smaller panel of patients (<300)
Focus on saving money vs. premium services	Focus on premium services (e.g., extended office visits)

Data from American College of Lifestyle Medicine. (2019a). *Literature review on medical payment models alignment with lifestyle medicine-physician incentives.* https://www.ardmoreinstituteofhealth.org/news/alignment-between-medical-payment-models-and-lifestyle-medicine-physician-incentives

of thumb, an average daily schedule for a concierge provider may consist of one to two comprehensive examinations and six regular visits in an eight-hour workday.

The concierge comprehensive annual health assessment visit is usually 90 minutes and lays the foundation for developing a personalized wellness or health promotion plan. This assessment includes a thorough history and physical examination and an array of screening tests (e.g., metabolic panels; lipid profiles; inflammation markers; blood counts; diabetes and thyroid screenings; and coordination of cancer screenings, colonoscopies, and mammograms) based on age, health status, and risk factors (Serna, 2019). Routine concierge visits are at least 30 to 60 minutes and may vary based on the patient's clinical condition, lifestyle goals, and level of health counseling needed to support progress and accountability.

Traditional Fee-for-Service Model

The traditional FFS model supports components of health promotion and lifestyle management, such as the initial preventive physical examination (IPPE) and the annual wellness visit (AWV). One hundred percent of preventive care is covered by most insurance plans and Medicare. If during the preventive service, the APP finds an acute or chronic condition that needs further evaluation and treatment, the patient will need to pay regular copays, coinsurance, and deductibles. Generally, insurance plans and commercial health plans follow the CMS rules, but they may have different conditions, modifying codes, or restrictions for their members. Therefore, it is advisable to check with the insurance plan to see what benefits will be covered for the individual member.

APPs need to be familiar with Medicare coverage and reimbursement for the three levels of services: IPPE, AWV, and routine preventive physical examination, as shown in **Figure 8.3**.

The CMS Medicare Preventive Services Quick Reference Chart is a helpful tool for providers (see Table 8.12 for a link). The chart includes codes and guidelines for all preventive services covered by Medicare and Medicare Advantage plans with no patient copay or coinsurance. Medicare provides guidelines and coverage for a variety of preventive services when specific statutory requirements are met. Sample codes and guidelines for IPPEs and AWVs for 2022 are shown in **Table 8.3**.

Initial Preventive Physical Examination

The IPPE, also known as the Welcome to Medicare visit, is for Medicare beneficiaries 65 years and older. It is intended to help keep Medicare beneficiaries healthy or help

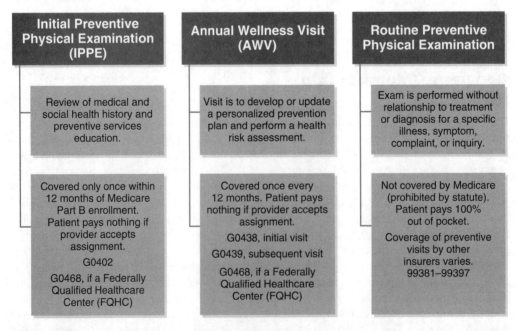

Figure 8.3 Medicare coverage of physical examination and annual wellness visit.

Adapted from Medicare Learning Network. (2022). *Medicare wellness visits.* Centers for Medicare and Medicaid Services. https://www.cms.gov/Outreach-and-Education/Medicare-Learning-Network-MLN/MLNProducts/preventive-services/medicare-wellness-visits.html

Table 8.3 CPT Codes and Guidelines for IPPE

CPT Codes	Guidelines for IPPE
G0402	Face-to-face visit, services limited to new beneficiaries during the first 12 months of Medicare enrollment
G0403	Electrocardiogram, routine ECG with 12 leads; performed as a screening for the IPPE with interpretation and report
G0404	Electrocardiogram, routine ECG with 12 leads; tracing only, without interpretation and report, performed as a screening for the IPPE
G0405	Electrocardiogram, routine ECG with 12 leads; interpretation and report only, performed as a screening for the IPPE
G0438 (first AWV) G0439 (subsequent AWV)	AWV; includes personalized prevention plan services, initial visit
G0468 (AWV in FQHC) G0469 (Subsequent AWV)	Federally Qualified Health Center (FQHC) IPPE or AWV; an FQHC visit that includes an IPPE or AWV and includes a typical bundle of Medicare-covered services that would be furnished per diem to a patient receiving an IPPE or AWV

Medicare Learning Network. (2022). *Medicare wellness visits.* Centers for Medicare and Medicaid Services. https://www.cms.gov/Outreach-and-Education /Medicare-Learning-Network-MLN/MLNProducts/preventive-services/medicare-wellness-visits.html

them become healthier by promoting positive health habits and a healthy lifestyle (Medicare Learning Network [MLN], 2022). The preventive visit includes a review of medical and social history, health education, and counseling about a preventive service. Typically, screenings for influenza and pneumococcal vaccines, simple vision tests, body mass index (BMI), and depression are discussed and documented (ACLM, 2019; MLN, 2022). The following box shows the components for a preventive visit.

Annual Wellness Visit

The AWV encourages individuals to take an active role in accurately assessing their health and improving their well-being and quality of life. The AWV is covered by Medicare Part B once every 12 months with no out-of-pocket copay or deductible. Medicare covers an AWV that provides personalized prevention plan services for beneficiaries. This visit is an excellent opportunity to identify all lifestyle-driven diseases that a patient has and discuss the lifestyle factors responsible for creating them (Braman & Edison, 2017). Components of the initial AWV include completing a health risk assessment, cognitive assessment, advanced care planning, activities of daily living, and instrumental activities of daily living (e.g., shopping, housekeeping, and handling finances).

Routine Preventive Physical Exam

The CPT codes 99381 through 99397 are for age-specific comprehensive preventive evaluations, or well visits, for new and established office patients. Unlike a problem-focused visit, the comprehensive preventive evaluation is meant for asymptomatic patients from infancy through adulthood with no chief complaint or present illness. This visit includes a comprehensive history and physical exam, age-appropriate counseling, screening labs and tests, and age-appropriate vaccines. Medicare does not cover these codes; the patient

Components of a Preventive Service Visit

- Review the patient's medical and social history.
- Review the patient's potential depression risk factors, including current or past experiences with depression or other mood disorders.
- Review the patient's functional ability and safety level.
- Perform an examination.
- Discuss end-of-life planning, on patient agreement.
- Review current opioid prescriptions.
- Screen for potential substance use disorders.
- Educate, counsel, and refer based on previous components.
- Educate, counsel, and refer for other preventive services.

Coverage of preventive visits varies by insurer, so it is important to be aware of the patient's health plan. Most plans limit the frequency of the preventive visit to once a year, and not all tests are covered.

Medicare Learning Network. (2022). *Medicare wellness visits.* Centers for Medicare and Medicaid Services. https://www.cms.gov/Outreach-and-Education/Medicare-Learning-Network-MLN/MLNProducts/preventive-services/medicare-wellness-visits.html

is responsible for 100% of the fees. Coverage of preventive visits by other insurers varies and may be limited to once yearly. The APP should be aware of the patient's health plan and which services are bundled (e.g., visual acuity testing) and which need to be billed separately (e.g., audiometry, Pap smear, and vaccines).

Traditional Fee-for-Service

APPs can choose either MDM or time-based reimbursement to determine the level of E/M services in a traditional FFS practice model. Commercial payers will waive the cost sharing by the patient when modifier 33 is included for services rated by the U.S. Preventive Services Task Force as A or B recommendations, (CodingIntel, n.d.). See Table 8.12 for a link

to the U.S. Preventive Services Task Force recommendations.

Medical Decision-Making

MDM refers to the complexity of establishing a diagnosis and selecting a management option (American Medical Association [AMA], 2021; MLN, 2021). The MDM associated with codes 99202 through 99215 consists of (a) the number and complexity of *problems* addressed, (b) the amount or complexity of *data* (e.g., medical records and diagnostic tests) reviewed or analyzed, and (c) the *risk* of complications and/or morbidity or mortality (MLN, 2021). To select a level of E/M service, two of the three elements must be met or exceeded. The overall visit level is determined by the highest level reached by at least two of the elements. For example, a visit in which there were multiple problems addressed that entailed limited data and low risk would be a *low* MDM visit overall. The APP would code the visit as a 99203 or 99213. **Table 8.4** shows the progression of elements required for each level of decision-making.

Time-Based Reimbursement

Total time spent face-to-face with the patient and non–face-to-face may be used to select the code level for the office or other outpatient services whether or not counseling or coordination of care dominates the service. Total time includes time spent on the day of the visit reviewing the chart, collaborating with other clinicians, and ordering tests before or after the face-to-face visit (AMA, 2021). Different categories of services use time differently, so it is imperative to be aware of this change. For example, time is not a billable code for the emergency department levels of E/M services because these services typically vary in intensity and often involve multiple encounters with several patients over an extended period of time (AMA, 2021). For other services, such as inpatient, time may only be used for selecting the level

Table 8.4 Elements for Each Level of Medical Decision-Making

Type of Decision-Making	Number of Diagnoses or Problems Addressed	Amount and/or Complexity of Data to Be Reviewed	Risk of Significant Complications, Morbidity, and/or Mortality
Straightforward (99202 and 99212)	Minimal	Minimal or none	Minimal
Low complexity (99203 and 99213)	Limited	Limited	Low
Moderate complexity (99204 and 99214)	Multiple	Moderate	Moderate
High complexity (99205 and 99215)	Extensive	Extensive	High

Adapted from Medicare Learning Network. (2021). *Evaluation and management services guide.* Centers for Medicare and Medicaid Services. https://www.cms.gov/Outreach-and-Education/Medicare-Learning-Network-MLN/MLNProducts/Downloads/eval-mgmt-serv-guide-ICN006764.pdf

of E/M services when counseling or coordination of care dominates the service.

When time is used to select the appropriate level for E/M service codes, time is defined by the service descriptors. The E/M services for which these guidelines apply require a face-to-face encounter with the qualified healthcare professional. Total time is measured as the precise time (in minutes) that the provider spent with the patient on the day of the encounter (see **Table 8.5**). This includes time spent preparing for the visit (e.g., reviewing prior lab results and diagnostic tests and obtaining and reviewing medical records), actual time spent during the visit, and time spent after the visit to finish documenting the encounter.

When using time-based billing, it is recommended that the provider document the actual time spent with the patient before, during, and after the encounter. For example, *"Total time spent was 30 minutes and included time spent before, during, and after the encounter on the day of the visit."* If during the encounter the provider performed additional time-based services (e.g., tobacco cessation counseling, nutrition counseling, or care planning), the

provider must document the precise time (not a range) spent on these unique services and should document the services separately. For example, when billing 99213 and 99406, the encounter note could read *"A total of 25 minutes was spent on this visit, with 20 minutes spent reviewing previous encounter notes, counseling the patient on type 2 diabetes and hypertension, ordering tests, refilling medications, and documenting the findings in the note. An additional five minutes were spent on tobacco cessation counseling, discussing the importance of quitting, options for medications, and a cessation plan"* (Mangoon, 2020). New reimbursement rules also stipulate that the provider sign the encounter note by midnight on the day of the encounter (Millette, 2020; Robeznieks, 2020).

Prolonged Services. When the total provider time on the date of the encounter exceeds the range of time listed for 99205 or 99215, a prolonged service code can be used (see Table 8.5). This time includes activities that require the provider but does not include time in activities normally performed by clinical staff. The total time should be documented in the medical record when used as the basis for code

Table 8.5 CPT Codes for Time-Based Billing

CPT Code	Time Range
99202	15–29 minutes
99203	30–44 minutes
99204	45–59 minutes
99205	60–74 minutes
99205 + 99417* (for each additional 15 min)	75+ minutes
99212	10–19 minutes
99213	20–29 minutes
99214	30–39 minutes
99215	40–54 minutes
99215 + 99417* (for each additional 15 min)	55+ minutes

* Use CPT G2212 for Medicare Advantage members because 99417 is invalid for Medicare.

Data from Magellan Health, Inc. (2020–2021). *2021 HIPAA coding changes for evaluation and management (E/M) office visits: Background and frequently asked questions.* https://www.magellanprovider.com/media/270100/2021_emcodingchanges_faq.pdf

selection (AMA, 2021). For coding purposes, the time for these services is the total time on the date of the encounter. It includes both the face-to-face and the non–face-to-face time personally spent by the provider on the day of the encounter. Qualified activities include preparing to see the patient (reviewing chart or test results); obtaining or reviewing separately obtained history; performing a medically appropriate examination or evaluation; counseling and educating the patient, family, or caregiver; ordering medications, tests, or procedures; referring and communicating with other healthcare professionals; documenting clinical information in the electronic or other health record; independently interpreting results (not separately reported) and communicating results to the patient, family, or caregiver; and

coordinating care (AMA, 2021). Waiting on hold for precertification authorization would not qualify; a peer-to-peer discussion with a qualified provider at an insurance company would qualify (CodingIntel, 2021). For prolonged billing codes, it is recommended that the provider consult with a billing expert.

Bundled Payments

Bundled payments are a good example of a value-based reimbursement model whereby a single payment is awarded for achieving patient outcomes for a specific and defined episode of care (Miller-Breslow & Raizman, 2020). These payments allow for services delivered by multiple providers to be combined into a single payment, which is then divided between the providers for the episode of care. Capitated plans differ from bundled plans because they are usually paid to a single healthcare organization and cover a wider array of services for a larger population over longer periods of time (Porter & Kaplan, 2016).

The bundled payments were developed to lower healthcare costs of the traditional FFS reimbursement model, shifting from a *volume-based* FFS approach to *value-based* care delivery. Instead of reimbursement of each element of care provided, a bundled payment includes a set amount for all of the services used in the care and treatment of the patient during that particular episode of care, including the visits, associated tests, and medications (Blue, 2019). Initially developed for acute care surgeries, such as coronary artery bypass grafting and hip replacement surgery, this model has demonstrated significant cost savings (Miller-Breslow & Raizman, 2020). While the bundled payment model is currently a more common reimbursement model in acute care, it has been used with success in the chronic care setting, such as with diabetes, with regular health checkups, including annual consultation and subsequent follow-up visits (e.g., dietary counseling, eye exams, and foot exams) (Struijs et al., 2020).

Group Shared Medical Appointments

A group visit (GV), also referred to as a shared medical appointment, drop-in group medical appointment, or group medical appointment, is an extended clinical encounter that allows a provider and patients to exchange valuable information regarding optimal chronic disease management within a supportive group format (Saxena, 2016). During the GV, patients can interact with the provider and have the added advantage of engaging with other participants while the provider leads the group and offers guidance (Frates et al., 2017). Studies show that social and educational support is linked to improved quality, access, efficiency, and patient and provider satisfaction and enhanced outcomes for low-acuity conditions that often require lifestyle change and education (Bartley & Haney, 2010; Braman & Edison, 2017). In most cases, a 90-minute time slot is scheduled for a selected group of patients (e.g., patients who share a diagnosis of obesity). The group size can vary depending on insurance or practice setting. The visit generally consists of a brief individual exam, 20 to 30 minutes of education, and 50 to 60 minutes for questions and answers and concludes with a reflection on self-management strategies to improve chronic conditions (Braman & Edison, 2017; Saxena, 2016). During GVs, providers avoid sharing the same information repeatedly in individual patient visits. They can also cover educational content that would otherwise be omitted due to the time constraints of a typical patient visit (Frates et al., 2017). Leading medical institutions, such as Harvard Vanguard, Kaiser Permanente, Cleveland Clinic, and Yale Health, have used the GV model for clinical, operational, and financial advantages (Saxena, 2016).

GV billing is described as a series of individual visits with other patients as observers in a supportive group setting (Saxena, 2016). Care is delivered in the same room, one by one, and documentation is done in the same manner as an individual (face-to-face) and standard office visit code. CPT codes such as 99212 through 99214 are billed on the level of MDM or face-to-face time spent with the patient. For example, appropriate MDM documentation with appropriate examination may qualify for 99213 or 99214 billing level. The time spent counseling the whole group is not billable, nor is it included in the face-to-face time.

Documentation for GVs should reflect the individual services provided to each patient as well as the services provided to the group during the encounter. The documentation reflects broad behavior modification strategies consisting of specific lifestyle or health promotion topics, primary therapeutic interventions, and personalized plans. In general, the patient completes the history of present illness, review of systems, past medical history, family history, and other appropriate sections of the visit form while waiting or during the group appointment time. Practical considerations for GVs include an adequately sized meeting space, such as a conference or waiting room, and a time that does not interfere with routine daily operations, such as the beginning or end of a clinic day (Saxena, 2016). The GV meeting location must be registered as a facility on record with the insurance company when billing insurance. If not restricted by health insurance, GVs may be done elsewhere, such as gyms, yoga studios, churches, or homes (Saxena, 2016).

Basic Principles of Evaluation and Management Documentation

Providers who bill CMS and commercial insurance companies must use a standard set of codes to bill and document services based on E/M guidelines. When a provider performs a billable patient service such as an office evaluation, the service is coded using the five-level

Health Promotion Research Study

Lifestyle Medicine Reimbursement

Background: Lifestyle medicine (LM) is a rapidly emerging clinical discipline that focuses on intensive therapeutic lifestyle changes to treat chronic disease, often producing dramatic health benefits. In spite of these well-documented benefits of LM approaches to provide evidence-informed care that follows current clinical guidelines, LM practitioners have found reimbursement challenging.

Methodology: The objective of this paper was to present the results of a 2019 online cross-sectional survey of LM practitioners regarding LM reimbursement and to propose policy priorities related to the ability of practitioners to implement and achieve reimbursement for these necessary services.

Results: A total of 857 respondents included dietitians, nurse practitioners, physician assistants, physical therapists, and physicians. The study sample was 58% female, with a median age of 51. A minority of the sample (17%) reported that all their practice was LM while 56% reported that some of their practice was LM. A total of 55% of the practitioners reported not being able to receive reimbursement for LM practice. Of those survey respondents who provided an answer to the question of what would make the practice of LM easier ($n = 471$), the following suggestions were offered: reimbursement overall (18%), reimbursement for more time spent with patients (17%), more support from leadership (16%), policy measures to incentivize health (13%), education in LM for practitioners (11%), LM-specific billing codes and billing knowledge along with better electronic medical record capabilities and streamlined reporting/paperwork (11%), and reimbursement for the extended care team (10%). Proposed policy changes focused on three areas: (1) support for the care process using an LM approach; (2) reimbursement emphasizing outcomes of health, patient experience, and delivering person-centered care; and (3) incentivizing treatment that produces disease remission/reversal. Rectifying reimbursement barriers to LM practice will require a sustained effort from health systems and policymakers.

Implications for Advanced Practice: If optimal health outcomes for chronic diseases truly are the goal, then significantly more resources need to be mobilized to best illuminate what types of lifestyle interventions are most effective and how to successfully implement them in a sustainable manner. Benchmarking for best LM practices and quantification of benefits of LM will help to support further reimbursement. Now is the time to acknowledge that chronic diseases, such as cardiovascular disease, diabetes, and obesity, are reversible; that remission is possible; and that LM practitioners who efficiently address the mitigating factors of disease to achieve these outcomes should be paid for their services in a manner that is commensurate with the value they provide, thereby further promoting the growth and accessibility of LM interventions.

Reference: Data from Freeman, K. J., Grega, M. L., Friedman, S. M., Patel, P. M., Stout, R. W., Campbell, T. M., Tollefson, M. L., Lianov, L. S., Pauly, K. R., Pollard, K. J., & Karlsen, M. C. (2021). Lifestyle medicine reimbursement: A proposal for policy priorities informed by a cross-sectional survey of lifestyle medicine practitioners. *International Journal of Environmental Research and Public Health, 18,* 11632. https://doi.org/10.3390/ijerph182111632

CPT coding system. CPT codes provide a standard method of coding procedures for insurance claims, medical records, and statistical tracking (Peters, 2020). These five-digit numerical codes describe actual services provided during new and established outpatient visits and reflect the actual work performed. The codes are used on the *superbill,* a detailed invoice that outlines the services a patient received and gives the insurer the information it needs to pay the claim. In most cases, billing for telemedicine visits is similar to billing for face-to-face E/M services, except that a modifier (GT or 95) is added to the claim. Rules vary by payer, so it is advisable to consult a medical coding specialist.

CMS and insurers require reasonable documentation to ensure that a service is consistent with the patient's insurance coverage and to validate the site of service, medical necessity, and appropriateness of the diagnostic or therapeutic services and that services furnished were accurately reported. The medical record should be clear and complete, including documentation of a reason for the encounter, relevant history, physical examination findings, prior diagnostic test results, assessment, clinical impression or diagnosis, and medical plan of care. The past and present diagnoses should be accessible to the treating and consulting provider and include relevant health risk factors as part of the documentation. The patient's progress, response to changes in treatment, and revisions to diagnoses, along with treatment codes reported on the health insurance claim or billing form, should be supported by documentation in the medical record (MLN, 2021).

The provider should use key descriptors when documenting the diagnoses or management options for patients presenting with an established diagnosis or without an established diagnosis. For example, when the patient has an established diagnosis, the record should reflect whether the problem is improved, well controlled, resolving, resolved, inadequately controlled, worsening, or failing to change as expected. For a new diagnosis, the assessment or clinical impression may be stated in the form of differential diagnoses or a possible, probable, or rule-out diagnosis (MLN, 2021).

Coding for Lifestyle Promotion

Coding for lifestyle promotion is much like coding for any other outpatient service. There are the standard outpatient E/M codes, which are for the typical new or established patient. However, there are additional billing codes that are used to report services for the purpose of promoting health and preventing illness (see **Table 8.6**). If these codes are used in addition

Table 8.6 Billable Codes for Lifestyle Promotion Services

Billable Lifestyle Promotion Services	Description	Code
Alcohol misuse/ abuse screening and counseling	Annual alcohol misuse screening, 15 minutes	G0442
	Brief face-to-face behavioral counseling for alcohol misuse, 15 minutes	G0443
	Alcohol and substance abuse screening, 15–30 minutes	99408
	Alcohol and/or substance abuse screening, >30 minutes	99409
Behavioral assessment	Brief emotional/behavioral assessment with scoring and documentation per standardized instrument	96127
Depression screening	Covered for patients when the service is provided in a primary care setting. Support staff is required to assist the provider in facilitating and coordinating referrals to mental health treatment providers.	G0444

(continues)

Table 8.6 **Billable Codes for Lifestyle Promotion Services** *(continued)*

Billable Lifestyle Promotion Services	Description	Code
Diabetes self-management training (DSMT)*	Diabetes outpatient self-management training services, individual, per 30 minutes	G0108
	Diabetes outpatient self-management training services, individual, group session (2 or more), per 30 minutes *Must be a certified DSMT provider	G0109
Intensive behavioral therapy for obesity*	Face-to-face behavioral counseling for obesity, 15 minutes Face-to-face, group (2–10), 30 minutes *The patient must have a BMI of ≥ 30 to be eligible for these services (International Classification of Diseases version 10 [ICD-10] codes Z68.30–Z68.39, Z68.41–Z68.45). There are frequency limits for this service.	G0447 G0473
Medical nutritional therapy*	Initial visit, 15 minutes	97802
	Follow-up visit, additional 15 minutes Group, 2 or more individuals, each 30 minutes *Available to registered dieticians or nutritional professionals who meet specific requirements as mandated by CMS	97803 97804
Medicare Diabetes Prevention Program*	Patient session attendance and weight loss *Must meet credentialing requirements and training to participate in this program	G9873–G9885 G9890–G9801
Preventive medicine, individual counseling services	Provider counseling related to subjects pertaining to prevention and risk factor reduction appropriate for the patient's family history, age, and other areas that might be of concern at an encounter separate from a preventive medicine visit, about 15 minutes	99401
	Provider counseling, about 30 minutes	99402
	Provider counseling, about 45 minutes	99403
	Provider counseling, about 60 minutes	99404
Preventive medicine, group counseling services	Provider advice on improving and maintaining health to a group of patients, about 30 minutes	99411
	Provider advice on improving and maintaining health to a group of patients, about 60 minutes	99412
Tobacco cessation counseling	Intermediate (3–10 min)	99406
	Intensive >10 minutes	99407

Data from 1) Medicare Learning Network. 2023. *Medicare preventive services*. https://www.cms.gov/Medicare/Prevention/PrevntionGenInfo/medicare-preventive-services/MPS-QuickReferenceChart-1.html#DIABETES_SELF 2); Centers for Medicare and Medicaid Services. (n.d.). *Medicare Diabetes Prevention Program (MDPP) Quick Reference Guide to Payment and Billing*. Retrieved May 1, 2023, from https://innovation.cms.gov/files/x/mdpp-billingpayment-refguide.pdf

to the standard E/M code, a 25 modifier to the E/M code should be applied to denote a separate service by the same provider on the same date of service. Both services should be documented in the medical record. Billing codes are updated annually, so it is advisable to work with a medical coding specialist. Additionally, it is important to contact payers to see what benefits will be covered.

Intensive Behavioral Therapy for Obesity

To deliver high-quality obesity care for Medicare beneficiaries, CMS introduced a regulatory coverage benefit in November 2011 to reimburse primary providers for delivering up to 22 visits of intensive behavioral therapy for weight loss within a primary care setting over a period of 12 months (CMS, 2011; MLN, 2012). Beneficiaries must have a BMI $\geq$30 kg/m^2 and are required to lose 3 kg of weight during the first six months to remain eligible. Intensive behavioral therapy for obesity includes screening for obesity, dietary assessment, and intensive counseling to promote weight loss through diet and exercise. Medicare requires the use and documentation of the 5As framework (assess, advise, agree, assist, and arrange) and measurement of height and weight at each visit.

Lifestyle Assessment and Counseling

Lifestyle assessment and counseling are often performed in the context of chronic disease or in health promotion and disease prevention management, yet APPs can overlook the importance of documenting these services and coding in a way that allows them to be reimbursed for counseling patients on diet, exercise, obesity, tobacco use, and other lifestyle habits related to health. For example, using appropriate physical activity assessment ICD-10 diagnoses and CPT codes to reflect time-based or MDM are reasonable strategies

Table 8.7 Physical Activity Assessment ICD-10 Codes

Description	ICD-10 Code
Lack of physical exercise	Z72.3
Exercise counseling	Z71.89
Obesity	E66.9
Physical deconditioning	R53.81
Sedentary lifestyle	Z91.89
Muscular deconditioning	R29.898

E codes (an external cause of injury), R codes (symptoms, signs, and abnormal clinical and laboratory findings), and Z codes (factors influencing health status) may not be allowed as a primary diagnosis. However, in most cases, physical activity assessment and counseling are performed within the context of another condition (e.g., high blood pressure, depression, obesity, or type 2 diabetes) or during a preventive health exam.

for many reimbursable office visits. A partial list of ICD-10 codes related to physical activity is shown in **Table 8.7**. Many offices have medical coding specialists who can review documentation and suggest appropriate coding to maximize reimbursement for lifestyle assessment and counseling provided.

Chronic Care Management

Chronic care management (CCM) services are monthly care coordination services that are expected to last at least 12 months or until the death of the patients and that are performed outside of the regular office visit for patients with multiple (two or more) chronic conditions that place them at significant risk of death, acute exacerbation/decompensation, or functional decline or for patients with psychosocial needs that require monitoring a care plan (Dacey, 2020). Requirements include patient consent, a comprehensive assessment and care plan, and 24/7 patient access to care. CCM services are usually conducted in a virtual environment (e.g., phone or telehealth visit), and eligible practitioners are permitted to bill the CCM code 99490 for at least 20 minutes

Table 8.8 Medicare Chronic Care Management Billing Codes

CPT Descriptor	CPT Codes
Initial care plan creation; billable once per patient per practice when setting up CCM	G0506 (add-on code to E/M)
Less than 20 minutes of noncomplex CCM services provided by clinical staff in a given month	Not reported separately
20–39 minutes of noncomplex CCM services provided by clinical staff in a given month	99490
40–59 minutes of noncomplex CCM services provided by clinical staff in a given month	99490 plus 99439 (add-on code for each additional 20 min)
60 minutes or more of noncomplex CCM services provided by clinical staff in a given month	99490 plus 99439 plus 99439 (add-on code can be used up to 2 times in a given month)

Data from Church, S. L., & Hughes, C. (2020). *Chronic care management coding updates for 2020.* https://www.aafp.org/journals/fpm/blogs/gettingpaid/entry/ccm_changes_2020.html

or more of non–face-to-face care coordination services provided by supervised clinical staff within a given month (MLN, 2019). **Table 8.8** provides the billing codes and descriptions for noncomplex CCM services. Additional codes are available for complex CCM by supervised clinical staff and for CCM provided by a qualified healthcare professional.

Best practices for CCM include having a template that allows the provider to track the monthly progress of the patients regarding their chronic conditions (Dacey, 2020). Examples of CCM activities include assessment and support for treatment regimen adherence, medication management, review of lab studies not previously reported as an E/M service, patient or caregiver education to support self-management, independent living and activities of daily living, communication with community agencies to facilitate access to care, and management of care transitions (Dacey, 2020).

Remote Physiologic Monitoring

Remote physiologic monitoring (RPM) (generally known as remote patient monitoring) involves the collection and analysis of patient physiologic data (e.g., weight, blood pressure, blood glucose, and oxygen saturation) in order to manage acute or chronic health conditions (Association of American Medical Colleges, n.d.). RPM allows patients to be monitored remotely while in their homes using medical devices that transmit data to providers for interpretation and implementation of treatment plan changes. Continuous monitoring is useful when promoting healthy lifestyle changes because it allows providers to monitor health behavior change outcomes and adjust medications without frequent or unnecessary office visits. **Table 8.9** provides the billing codes and descriptions for RPM.

Reimbursement Trends

With recent changes in health care and the push toward more value-based reimbursement, several trends are emerging that are promising for the APP seeking to empower patients to reverse or manage their chronic disease.

Health and Well-Being Coaching

Health and well-being coaching is a person-centered approach wherein patients are in complete charge of their health promotion

Table 8.9 Medicare Remote Physiologic Monitoring Billing Codes

CPT Descriptor	CPT Codes
Initial device setup and patient education on the use of equipment	99453
Device supply and recordings, each 30 days; requires a minimum of 16 days of readings	99454
Less than 20 minutes of RPM monitoring and data management in a given month	Not reported separately
20–39 minutes of RPM monitoring and data management in a given month	99457
40–59 minutes of RPM monitoring and data management in a given month	99457 plus 99458 (add-on code for each additional 20 min)
60 minutes or more of RPM monitoring and data management in a given month	99457 plus 99458 plus 99458 (add-on code can be used up to 2 times in a given month)

Data from Association of American Medical Colleges. (n.d.). *AAMC regulatory resource: 2021 Medicare coverage of remote physiologic monitoring (RPM)*. https://www.aamc.org/media/55306/download

Table 8.10 Category III Codes for Health and Well-Being Coaching

CPT Descriptor	CPT Codes
Health and well-being coaching face-to-face, individual, initial assessment	0591T
Health and well-being coaching face-to-face, individual, follow-up session, at least 30 minutes	0592T
Health and well-being coaching with group of 2 or more individuals, at least 30 minutes	0593T

Data from American Academy of Professional Coders. 2023. *Health And Well-Being Coaching CPT® Code range 0591T–0593T*. https://www.aapc.com/codes/cpt-codes-range/0591T-0593T

insurance payers typically wait until the codes are upgraded to a Category I approval before reimbursing for these services. Once sufficient evidence demonstrates that health coaching services are associated with improved clinical outcomes, Category I approval will occur. For this reason, it is imperative to include these codes in every applicable billing encounter to support and generate new evidence regarding the clinical efficacy of these interventions. Specific CPT codes for coaching are found in **Table 8.10**.

Social Determinants of Health and Health Equity

A study conducted by CMS highlighted the first analysis of Medicare FFS claims data for the utilization of Z codes associated with social determinants of health (Mathew et al., 2019). It identified 467,136 unique Medicare FFS beneficiaries with Z code claims in 2017, representing only 1.4% of the total FFS population. The findings of this study may underreport assessments of patient social needs. A recent study found that 24% of hospitals and 16% of physician practices screened for food

plan. With the support and guidance of a trained health coach, the patients design their health goals and monitor progress and behaviors, which increases accountability and creates positive and sustainable change (ACLM, 2019). The health coach is a nonphysician healthcare professional certified by either the National Board for Health and Wellness Coaching or the National Commission for Health Education Credentialing. While the AMA has acknowledged the importance of health and well-being coaching by giving these services a Category III approval,

Table 8.11 CPT Codes Related to Social Determinants of Health

CPT Descriptor	CPT Code
Problems related to education and literacy: Illiteracy/low level, schooling availability, failing school, underachievement, discord with teachers	Z55
Problems related to employment and unemployment: Changing of job, losing a job, no job, stressful work schedule, discord with boss/coworkers, poor working conditions	Z56
Occupational exposure to risk factors: Noise, radiation, dust, other air contaminants, tobacco, toxic agents in farming, extreme temperatures, vibration, others	Z57
Problems related to housing and economic circumstances: Homeless, inadequate housing, discord with neighbors/landlord, issues with residential living, lack of adequate food/safe drinking water, poverty, low income, insufficient social insurance/welfare support	Z59
Problems related to social environment: Adjustment to life cycle transitions, living alone, cultural differences, social exclusion and rejection, discrimination/persecution	Z60
Problems related to upbringing: Inadequate parental supervision/control, parental overprotection, upbringing away from parents, a child in custody, institutional upbringing (orphan or group home), hostility toward child, inappropriate/excessive parental pressure, child abuse including the history of (physical or sexual) abuse, neglect, forced labor, child–parent conflict	Z62
Other problems related to primary support group, include family circumstances: Spousal conflict, in-law conflict, absence of family member (death, divorce, deployment), dependent relative needing care, family alcoholism/drug addiction, isolated family	Z63
Problems related to certain psychosocial circumstances: Unwanted pregnancy, multiparity, discord with counselors	Z64
Problems related to other psychosocial circumstances: Civil/criminal convictions, incarceration, problems after release from prison, victim of crime, exposure to disaster/war, religious persecution	Z65

Data from American Hospital Association. (2022, January). *ICD-10-CM coding for social determinants of health.* https://www.aha.org/system/files/2018-04/value-initiative-icd-10-code-social-determinants-of-health.pdf

insecurity, housing instability, utilities, and transportation. While more screening may occur, it is less clear to what extent the needs are being documented and shared among providers to improve health equity (Mathew et al., 2019). Lifestyle and health promotion providers need to include screening for social determinants of health and to begin documenting the interventions and appropriate ICD-10 codes. Specific ICD-10 codes are found in **Table 8.11**.

The Business of Lifestyle Health Promotion

When opening a lifestyle health promotion–focused practice, it is essential to understand the business aspects of practice management. As previously noted, reimbursement is a vital component of any healthcare enterprise, and without steady, predictable income, no

---

Health Promotion Case Study Coding an Encounter for Lifestyle Medicine

---

Case Description: S.H. is a 40-year-old obese Hispanic male who presents to the office with high blood pressure. S.H. admits to occasional shortness of breath but has no other symptoms associated with high blood pressure. He states he is tired of being overweight and being told he has no willpower. He wants to change his lifestyle by eating less and exercising more, so he sought medical treatment to help him lose weight. S.H. has a family history of diabetes, and he is worried that if he does not get things under control, he will develop diabetes and associated complications.

- Past medical history: hypertension, hyperlipidemia, metabolic syndrome, sleep apnea
- Family history: diabetes
- Social history: married with two young children

Lifestyle Vital Signs: BMI 34 kg/m^2

The APP spent 45 minutes face-to-face with the patient and provided dietary and physical activity counseling. Diagnostic tests included 12-lead electrocardiogram, complete blood count, basic metabolic panel, and a hemoglobin A1C.

The ICD-10 codes for high blood pressure (I10), obesity (E66.9), and lack of physical exercise (Z72.3) were used.

Critical Thinking Questions

1. Determine the level or type of MDM used in S.H.'s case, considering the number of appropriate diagnoses or management codes; the amount and complexity of data to be reviewed; and the risk of significant complications, morbidity, and/or mortality.
2. What other CMS preventive services CPT codes might be useful with this encounter?
3. What might documentation look like if using time-based billing?

---

practice can survive long term. A practice must bring in more revenue than it spends to be viable. In other words, the revenue earned from patient visits must be adequate to cover the costs of operating the practice and generate enough revenue after expenses to drive the practice's future growth (e.g., hiring additional staff, purchasing new supplies and equipment, or expanding healthcare services).

Examples of standard practice expenses include equipment, medical and office supplies, employee labor, repairs and maintenance, insurance, licenses and permits, leasing, marketing expenses, and electronic medical record and billing software. Whether starting from scratch or creating a lifestyle health promotion practice within an existing outpatient office, building a sustainable practice requires a strong vision, careful thought, and creative business planning. Common questions to address include, "Where will the practice be located?" "How will the clinic operate?" "How will the care be delivered?" "How will the practice revenue and profit be generated?" and "How will the patients find the practice?" (Buppert, 2021). Important considerations include the type of practice model (e.g., virtual practice vs. brick-and-mortar practice), practice niche (e.g., cardiometabolic health, stress management, chronic pain, or mental health), and a reimbursement model (e.g., FFS, practice membership, or mixed payment methods). Many practices are grown on a smaller scale, often starting within an existing primary care practice (Motley, 2020). Sustainability over the long term will necessitate a working knowledge of practice reimbursement and revenue generation.

Revenue Generation

Revenue generated solely from the provision of patient care is known as patient service revenue (Reiter et al., 2021). An APP can plan or forecast revenue generation over time by calculating the average number of visits per day, per week, and per month and multiplying these visits by the average collection amount. For example, in an insurance-based FFS practice, if the average visit collection rate is $82 per visit and an average of 20 patients were seen each day, then $1,640 of revenue would be earned per day, or $8,200 per week. If the practice were open 48 weeks per year, the total revenue potential would be $393,600. Assuming an average of 40% deducted for overhead expenses and 10% deducted for uncollected fees (due to insurance denial), one could expect to have $196,000 remaining for provider salary and future growth. In a concierge or DPC practice, one can forecast revenue by simply multiplying the number of patients in the practice by the monthly membership fee to determine revenue potential.

When a practice has more than one provider on staff who can generate revenue and contribute to the payment of fixed practice expenses, it can leverage the revenue from each provider, resulting in economies of scale due to the proportionate saving in costs gained by the increased level of visit revenue. In other words, by spreading the fixed expenses across a greater volume of patients (and revenue), a practice can lower costs and yield greater profits. This is true in different practice models, including a concierge practice.

Practice expenses can run, on average, between 40% and 50% of revenue, depending on the type of practice (Buppert, 2021). Other revenue is often generated within a lifestyle promotion practice and can include consumer healthcare products, such as supplements, and additional funding, such as grants. While it may be highly beneficial to obtain outside funding to initially launch the clinical practice, these funds are not enough to sustain the practice on a long-term basis. For this reason, it is advisable to develop a robust number of patients to ensure a predictable source of income.

Community-Based Grants

Public and private funding sources are important options to explore before deciding on a course of action. The options may include grants or contracts. In general, grants involve funding for experimental, demonstration, or research projects in which success is uncertain. Most grants are awarded to nonprofit organizations. Contracts include money allocated to supply specific services to a funding agency. Contracts are usually awarded for programs that originate with the funding source. Public funds involve money raised through taxes and administered by federal, state, and local governments. Private funds involve money raised and administered by private organizations, such as corporations, foundations, and charities. Often available as grants, private funds are awarded for new or experimental projects (New York State Department of Health, 2012).

Foundation grants can be difficult to find and even more difficult to obtain. Typically, foundations have annual reports and funding guidelines available upon request. These documents should be studied and referred to when preparing a letter of intent or application. It is important to confirm that the program will be of interest to the funder and to follow the funding guidelines exactly. Many foundations specify what kind of projects will be funded. Most will not fund projects requesting 100% funding. Therefore, it is important to seek multiple funding sources for a project (New York State Department of Health, 2012).

Whether starting up a new community wellness program or looking to fund an existing program, potential funding sources include foundations; commercial payers; or government sources, such as the Health Resources and Services Administration. The Health Resources and Services Administration provides financial assistance in the form

Health Promotion Activity: Reflection on Reimbursement and Practice Models

Which of the various reimbursement and practice models for promoting healthy lifestyles discussed in this chapter have you experienced as a patient or provider? Describe your experiences. Which model resonates most with you? Why?

of grants to organizations to achieve specific purposes, such as providing primary health care to underserved people, getting lifesaving medications to uninsured people living with HIV/AIDS, or helping families of children with special healthcare needs access necessary services. Another resource is the Rural Health Information Hub (n.d.), which provides funding resources by type, sponsor, topic, and state for various initiatives in rural communities.

Summary

The goal of this chapter is to explore the economic and financial aspects of lifestyle and health promotion as well as the different practice models, methods of reimbursement, and current and future trends of chronic disease management using lifestyle approaches. While research demonstrates that evidence-informed, person-centered lifestyle prescriptive approaches improve health outcomes, these interventions are not entirely recognized in the current reimbursement paradigm, which rewards providers for medication-focused

disease management (ACLM, 2019; MLN, 2022). As a result, reimbursement can be a barrier for providers utilizing lifestyle approaches in their practice. For this reason, APPs must be highly competent in coding to maximize reimbursement.

There is much work to be done to provide financial incentives for billing lifestyle behavior interventions. Advocacy efforts from organizations such as the ACLM continue to push for new reimbursement models to reward providers for value-based care and to educate payers to recognize the tremendous economic and health benefits generated from lifestyle and health promotion interventions. APPs must have an astute understanding of how to successfully bill for lifestyle medicine services within each model of care. These models include FFS, concierge, telehealth, CCM, DPC, GVs, and bundled payments. New, innovative, value-based reimbursement models are being developed; until these models are fully adopted by payers, APPs must confidently and knowledgeably leverage existing models of care to maximize reimbursement and practice profitability.

TABLE 8.12	Evidence-Based Resources for Health Promotion Billing and Reimbursement
Resource	**URL**
Council for Affordable Quality Healthcare ProView	https://proview.caqh.org/pr/registration
National Plan and Provider Enumeration System	https://nppes.cms.hhs.gov/#

(continues)

TABLE 8.12	Evidence-Based Resources for Health Promotion Billing and Reimbursement *(continued)*

Resource	URL
Provider Transaction Access Number	https://verisys.com/what-is-a-ptan-number-2/#:~:text=The%20Provider%20Transaction%20Access%20Number,the%20location%20of%20the%20provider
Shared medical appointments and group visits	https://www.aafp.org/family-physician/practice-and-career/getting-paid/coding/group-visits.html
Time-based coding	https://codingintel.com/time-using-time-for-em-services-in-2021
U.S. Preventive Services Task Force A and B recommendations	https://www.uspreventiveservicestaskforce.org/uspstf/recommendation-topics/uspstf-and-b-recommendations
Coding for obesity	https://www.codingahead.com/cpt-codes-for-obesity-screening-counseling
Welcome to Medicare	https://www.cms.gov/Medicare/Prevention/PrevntionGenInfo/medicare-preventive-services/MPS-QuickReferenceChart-1.html#IPPE
CMS Preventive Services Quick Reference Chart	https://www.cms.gov/medicare/prevention/prevntiongeninfo/medicare-preventive-services/mps-quickreferencechart-1.html
Rural Health Information Hub	https://www.ruralhealthinfo.org/funding/topics/wellness-health-promotion-and-disease-prevention
Chronic Care Management Services	https://www.cms.gov/outreach-and-education/medicare-learning-network- mln/mlnproducts/downloads/chroniccaremanagement.pdf
Chronic care management FAQs	https://www.cms.gov/Medicare/Medicare-Fee-for-Service-Payment/PhysicianFeeSched/Downloads/Payment_for_CCM_Services_FAQ.pdf
CMS Physician Fee Schedule Look-Up Tool	https://www.cms.gov/Medicare/Medicare-Fee-for-Service-Payment/PFSlookup
CPT codes for psychiatry services	https://psychcentral.com/lib/cpt-codes-for-psychology-services
Health Behavior Assessment and Intervention Services	https://www.apaservices.org/practice/reimbursement/health-codes/health-behavior
Psychotherapy Codes for Psychologists	https://www.apaservices.org/practice/reimbursement/health-codes/psychotherapy
Medical nutrition therapy payment	https://www.eatrightpro.org/payment

American College of Lifestyle Medicine. (2019b). *Reimbursement roadmap.* www.lifestylemedicine.org

Acronyms

ACLM: American College of Lifestyle Medicine
APP: advanced practice provider
AWV: annual wellness visit
CCM: chronic care management
CMS: Centers for Medicare and Medicaid Services
CPT: Current Procedural Terminology
DPC: direct primary care
DSMT: diabetes self-management training
E/M: evaluation and management

FFS: fee-for-service
FQHC: Federally Qualified Healthcare Center
GV: group visit
ICD: International Classification of Diseases
IPPE: initial preventive physical examination
LM: lifestyle medicine
MDM: medical decision-making
MLN: Medicare Learning Network
NPI: National Provider Identifier
RPM: remote physiologic monitoring

References

American Academy of Professional Coders. (2023). *Health And Well-Being Coaching CPT® Code range 0591T–0593T.* https://www.aapc.com/codes/cpt-codes-range/0591T-0593T

American College of Lifestyle Medicine. (2019a). *Literature review on medical payment models alignment with lifestyle medicine-physician incentives.* https://www.ardmoreinstituteofhealth.org/news/alignment-between-medical-payment-models-and-lifestyle-medicine-physician-incentives

American College of Lifestyle Medicine. (2019b). *Reimbursement roadmap.* www.lifestylemedicine.org

American Hospital Association. (2022, January). *ICD-10-CM coding for social determinants of health.* https://www.aha.org/system/files/2018-04/value-initiative-icd-10-code-social-determinants-of-health.pdf

American Medical Association. (2021). *CPT® evaluation and management (E/M) office or other outpatient (99202-99215) and prolonged services (99354, 99355, 99356, 99XXX) code and guideline changes.* https://www.ama-assn.org/system/files/2019-06/cpt-office-prolonged-svs-code-changes.pdf

Association of American Medical Colleges. (n.d.). *AAMC regulatory resource: 2021 Medicare coverage of remote physiologic monitoring (RPM).* Retrieved May 1, 2023, from https://www.aamc.org/media/55306/download

Bartley, K. B., & Haney, R. (2010). Shared medical appointments: Improving access, outcomes, and satisfaction for patients with chronic cardiac diseases. *Journal of Cardiovascular Nursing, 25*(1), 13–19. https://doi.org/10.1097/JCN.0b013e3181b8e82e

Beckman, K. (2019). A new approach for lifestyle medicine payment. *American Journal of Lifestyle Medicine, 13*(1), 36–39. https://doi.org/10.1177/1559827618795410

Benjamin, E. J., Blaha, M. J., Chiuve, S. E., Cushman, M., Das, S. R., Deo, R., de Ferranti, S. D., Floyd, J., Fornage, M., Gillespie, C., Isasi, C. R., Jiménez, M. C.,

Jordan, L. C., Judd, S. E., Lackland, D., Lichtman, J. H., Lisabeth, L., Liu, S., Longenecker, C. T., . . . Muntner, P. (2017). Heart disease and stroke statistics—2017 update: A report from the American Heart Association. *Circulation, 135*(10). https://doi.org/10.1161/CIR.0000000000000485

Blue, T. (2019). How to package functional medicine for widespread adoption. *Integrative Medicine: A Clinician's Journal, 18*(2), 34–37.

Bodai, B. I., Nakata, T. E., Wong, W. T., Clark, D. R., Lawenda, S., Tsou, C., Liu, R., Shiue, L., Cooper, N., Rehbein, M., Ha, B. P., McKeirnan, A., Misquitta, R., Vij, P., Klonecke, A., Mejia, C. S., Dionysian, E., Hashmi, S., Greger, M., . . . Campbell, T. M. (2017). Lifestyle medicine: A brief review of its dramatic impact on health and survival. *The Permanente Journal.* https://doi.org/10.7812/TPP/17-025

Braman, M., & Edison, M. (2017). How to create a successful lifestyle medicine practice. *American Journal of Lifestyle Medicine, 11*(5), 404–407. https://doi.org/10.1177/1559827617696296

Buppert, C. (2021). *Nurse practitioner's business practice and legal guide* (7th ed.). Jones & Bartlett Learning.

Centers for Medicare and Medicaid Services. (n.d.). *Medicare Diabetes Prevention Program (MDPP) Quick Reference Guide to Payment and Billing.* Retrieved May 1, 2023, from https://innovation.cms.gov/files/x/mdpp-billingpayment-refguide.pdf

Centers for Medicare and Medicaid Services. (2011). *National coverage determination (NCD) for intensive behavioral therapy for obesity (210.12).* https://www.cms.gov/medicare-coverage-database/details/ncd-details.aspx?NCDId=353

Church, S. L., & Hughes, C. (2020). *Chronic care management coding updates for 2020.* https://www.aafp.org/journals/fpm/blogs/gettingpaid/entry/ccm_changes_2020.html

CodingIntel. (n.d.). *Using modifier 33: Quick reference.* Retrieved May 1, 2023, from https://codingintel.com/using-modifier-33-cheat-sheet

CodingIntel. (2021). *Prolonged services for 99202-99215: 99417, G2212.* https://codingintel.com/are-changes-coming-for-prolonged-services

Dacey, B. (2020). Chronic care management coding requirements. *Medical Economics, 97*(6), 7.

Frates, E. P., Morris, E. C., Sannidhi, D., & Dysinger, W. S. (2017). The art and science of group visits in lifestyle medicine. *American Journal of Lifestyle Medicine, 11*(5), 408–413. https://doi.org/10.1177/1559827617698091

Freeman, K. J., Grega, M. L., Friedman, S. M., Patel, P. M., Stout, R. W., Campbell, T. M., Tollefson, M. L., Lianov, L. S., Pauly, K. R., Pollard, K. J., & Karlsen, M. C. (2021). Lifestyle medicine reimbursement: A proposal for policy priorities informed by a cross-sectional survey of lifestyle medicine practitioners. *International Journal of Environmental Research and Public Health, 18,* 11632. https://doi.org/10.3390/ijerph182111632

Gobble, J., Donohue, D., & Grega, M. (2022). Reimbursement as a catalyst for advancing lifestyle medicine practices. *Supplement to the Journal of Family Practice. 71*(1), S105-S109. doi:10.12788/jfp.0255

Jensen, L. L., Drozek, D. S., Grega, M. L., & Gobble, J. (2019). Lifestyle medicine: Successful reimbursement methods and practice models. *American Journal of Lifestyle Medicine, 13*(3), 246–252. https://doi.org/10.1177/1559827618817294

Lacagnina, S., Moore, M., & Mitchell, S. (2018). The lifestyle medicine team: Health care that delivers value. *American Journal of Lifestyle Medicine, 12*(6), 479–483. https://doi.org/10.1177/1559827618792493

Lamberts, R. (2019, February 18). *Difference between concierge and direct care.* Medical Economics. https://www.medicaleconomics.com/view/difference-between-concierge-and-direct-care

Ma, J., Rosas, L. G., & Lv, N. (2016). Precision lifestyle medicine. *American Journal of Preventive Medicine, 50*(3), 395–397. https://doi.org/10.1016/j.amepre.2015.09.035

Magellan Health, Inc. (2020–2021). *2021 HIPAA coding changes for evaluation and management (E/M) office visits: Background and frequently asked questions.* https://www.magellanprovider.com/media/270100/2021_emcodingchanges_faq.pdf

Mangoon, V. (2020, November 6). 2021 Outpatient office E/M changes FAQ. *Family Practice Management Journal.* https://www.aafp.org/journals/fpm/blogs/inpractice/entry/em_changes_FAQ.html

Mathew, J., Hodge, C., & Khau, M. (2019). Z codes utilization among Medicare fee-for-service (FFS) beneficiaries in 2017. *CMS OMH Data Highlight No. 17.* CMS Office of Minority Health. https://www.cms.gov/files/document/cms-omh-january2020-zcode-data-

Medicare Learning Network. (2012). *Intensive behavioral therapy (IBT) for obesity.* Centers for Medicare and Medicaid Services. https://www.cigna.com/static/docs/medicare-2018/ibt-obesity.pdf

Medicare Learning Network. (2019). *Chronic care management services.* Centers for Medicare and Medicaid Services. https://www.cms.gov/outreach-and-education/medicare-learning-network-mln/mlnproducts/downloads/chroniccaremanagement.pdf

Medicare Learning Network. (2021). *Evaluation and management services guide.* Centers for Medicare and Medicaid Services. https://www.cms.gov/Outreach-and-Education/Medicare-Learning-Network-MLN/MLNProducts/Downloads/eval-mgmt-serv-guide-ICN006764.pdf

Medicare Learning Network. (2022). *Medicare wellness visits.* Centers for Medicare and Medicaid Services. https://www.cms.gov/Outreach-and-Education/Medicare-Learning-Network-MLN/MLNProducts/preventive-services/medicare-wellness-visits.html

Medicare Learning Network. (2023). *Medicare preventive services.* https://www.cms.gov/Medicare/Prevention/PrevntionGenInfo/medicare-preventive-services/MPS-QuickReferenceChart-1.html#DIABETES_SELF

Miller-Breslow, A. J., & Raizman, N. M. (2020). Physician reimbursement. *Hand Clinics, 36*(2), 189–195. https://doi.org/10.1016/j.hcl.2019.12.002

Millette, K. (2020). Countdown to the E/M coding changes. *Family Practice Management, 27*(5), 29–36.

Motley, E. (2020). Building a thriving lifestyle medicine practice within a primary care clinic: A model for aspiring lifestyle medicine practitioners. *American Journal of Lifestyle Medicine, 14*(2), 133–136. https://doi.org/10.1177/1559827620904868

National Center for Chronic Disease Prevention and Health Promotion. (n.d.). *How you can prevent chronic diseases.* Centers for Disease Control and Prevention. Retrieved May 1, 2023, from https://www.cdc.gov/chronicdisease/about/prevent/index.htm

New York State Department of Health. (2012). *Locating and applying for health promotion funds.* https://www.health.ny.gov/publications/4146.pdf

Peters, S. G. (2020). New billing rules for outpatient office visit codes. *Chest, 159*(1), 298–302. https://doi.org/10.1016/j.chest.2020.01.028

Porter, M., & Kaplan, R. (2016). How to pay for healthcare. *Harvard Business Review.* https://hbr.org/2016/07/how-to-pay-for-health-care

Reiter, K. L., Song, P. H., & Gapenski, L. C. (2021). *Gapenski's healthcare finance: An introduction to accounting and financial management* (7th ed.). Health Administration Press.

Robeznieks, A. (2020, November 6). *How 2021 E/M coding changes will reshape the physician note.* American Medical Association. https://www.ama-assn.org

/practice-management/cpt/how-2021-em-coding -changes-will-reshape-physician-note

Rural Health Information Hub. (n.d.). *Applying for grants to support rural health projects*. https://www.ruralhealth info.org/topics/grantwriting

Saxena, S. P. (2016). Leveraging time with lifestyle-based group visits. *American Journal of Lifestyle Medicine, 10*(5), 330–337. https://doi.org/10.1177/1559827 616638018

Serna, D. C. (2019). Lifestyle medicine in a concierge practice: My journey. *American Journal of Lifestyle Medicine, 13*(4), 367–370. https://doi.org/10.1177 /1559827618821865

Struijs, J. N., DeVries, E. F., Bean, C. A., van Gils, P. F., & Rosenthal, M. B. (2020). *Bundled-payment models around the world: How they work and what their impact has been*. https://www.commonwealthfund.org/sites /default/files/2020-04/Struijs_bundled_payment _models_around_world_ib.pdf

Waxman, K. T. (Ed.). (2018). *Financial and business management for the doctor of nursing practice* (2nd ed). Springer.

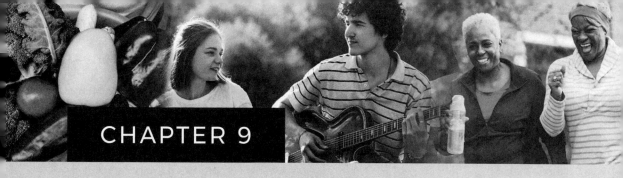

CHAPTER 9

Health Needs Assessment

Vicki L. Simpson, PhD, RN, CHES

Equality is giving everyone a shoe. Equity is giving everyone a shoe that fits.

Dr. Naheed Dosani

OBJECTIVES

This chapter will enable the reader to:

1. Discuss the interrelationships among the health of individuals, families, and communities.
2. Apply a holistic approach to the health needs assessment of individuals, families, and communities.
3. Identify theories and frameworks relevant to health needs assessment.
4. Evaluate the utility of health needs assessments in defining the health needs of individuals, families, and communities.
5. Utilize effective tools (approaches) to complete health needs assessments at multiple levels.
6. Identify strategies to incorporate comprehensive health needs assessments and the associated data into clinical practice.
7. Discuss the use of health needs assessments to enhance health equity.

Overview

Assessment of individuals and the environment surrounding them is vital to support healthy lifestyle behaviors. Individuals are influenced by and in turn influence the health of families and communities. It is necessary to understand this complex interrelationship's role in health outcomes. The health needs assessment (HNA) process is a systematic approach to the holistic identification of health and healthcare needs of a population, a subgroup, or an individual. Holistic provision of care requires healthcare professionals to conduct HNAs at each level to identify existing vulnerabilities and disparities that lead to poor health outcomes. Multilevel HNAs help individualize strategies to support healthy lifestyle behaviors. This chapter discusses the HNA process, which is used to identify all clinical and nonclinical factors that play a role in health outcomes (Cowley, 2021; Kawachi et al., 2020; Tobi, 2016).

© Kathleen Gail/Shutterstock; © StoryTime Studio/Shutterstock; © kali9/Getty Images

Relevance

Unmet health and healthcare needs must be systematically identified and addressed to improve population health. Efficient use of scarce healthcare resources requires a broader view of an individual's health beyond the narrow clinical perspective often played out in healthcare settings (Cantor & Thorpe, 2018). The capacity to achieve optimal health is affected by many factors that influence the ability to live a healthy lifestyle. The Robert Wood Johnson Foundation (RWJF, 2020) County Health Rankings model describes the estimated contribution of several interconnected factors (see **Figure 9.1**), including health behaviors, clinical care, social and economic factors, and the physical environment, to health outcomes. Estimates indicate that social and economic factors, commonly referred to as the social determinants of health (SDOH), account for 25% to 60% of deaths in the United States (Cantor & Thorpe, 2018; RWJF, 2020). Additionally, it is estimated that health issues cost $226 billion annually in loss of productivity (RWJF, 2021).

Addressing these nonmedical factors requires shifting focus from the healthcare system to individuals' broader social contexts, including the immediate family, household, neighborhood, and community (Cowley, 2021; Flowers & Evans, 2020; Fraze et al., 2016). While advanced practice providers (APPs) are generally aware of the role SDOH play, they are often unsure how to obtain the necessary data or how to intervene (Andermann, 2016). Countries such as New Zealand and the United Kingdom have standard practices to capture reliable data about SDOH, but they are not the norm. Similarly, screening for SDOH is not currently standard practice in most U.S. healthcare settings; when done, the assessment is limited, and strategies are generally not in place to address identified issues or needs (Billioux et al., 2017). Thus, this information, crucial to improving individual and population health outcomes, is not incorporated into clinical practice; resource allocation;

payment models; or evaluation of policies, strategies, and interventions to improve health (Graham & Bernot, 2017). Increased availability of data regarding SDOH in electronic health record (EHR) systems was advocated by the Institute of Medicine (2015) in a two-phased 2014 report. Easier availability of such data would help the APP better individualize specific interventions for patients, thus improving health outcomes and achieving health equity.

To understand needs and optimally allocate healthcare resources, the concept of equity must be central to all efforts to enhance health and health outcomes. Equity is the absence of avoidable, unfair, or remediable differences among groups of people, whether those groups are defined socially, economically, demographically, geographically, or by other means of stratification (World Health Organization [WHO], 2020). While awareness of equity may or may not be prominent in the minds of APPs as they go through their clinical day, inequities are readily apparent in the lives of the patients to whom care is provided. Inequities left unaddressed result in differences in length and quality of life, the severity of disease, and the ability to access resources (American Public Health Association, 2020; Centers for Disease Control and Prevention [CDC], 2016; WHO, 2020).

Equitable promotion of health and well-being requires efforts based on HNAs, which provide data that holistically reflect individuals and their environments. The National Quality Forum developed a national-level strategy to support the use of both clinical and nonclinical data, such as that reflecting the SDOH data into clinical practice (see **Figure 9.2**).

The data generated by these assessments enhance the ability of the provider to proactively guide care versus reacting as each patient arrives for a primary care appointment. One study found that providers who collected information regarding SDOH were more likely to report helping patients (Naz et al., 2016).

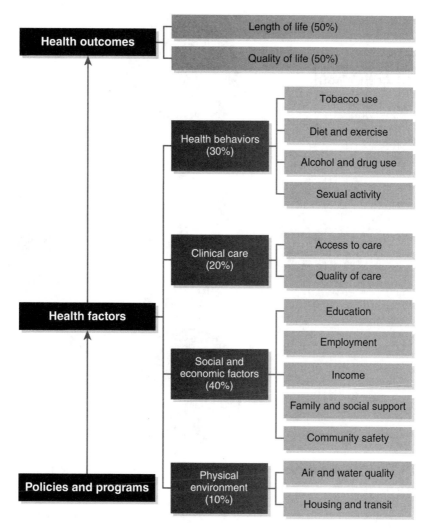

Figure 9.1 Robert Wood Johnson Foundation County Health Rankings model.
Reproduced with permission from The University of Wisconsin Population Health Institute. County Health Rankings & Roadmaps, 2023. www.countyhealthrankings.org

Enhanced understanding of social context aids collaboration with diverse stakeholders, including those within and outside the practice setting or the healthcare system, to support health and well-being. Linking efforts with other stakeholders who share responsibility for health addresses physical, mental, and social dimensions for individuals, families, and populations, thus helping to decrease fragmentation and improve health outcomes (Office of Disease Prevention and Health Promotion, 2020; Tobi, 2016; United Nations General Assembly, 2015).

Advanced practice competencies and guidelines developed by the American Association of Colleges of Nursing (2021) and the National Organization of Nurse Practitioner Faculties (2022) emphasize the need for holistic approaches to care, which include consideration of cultural, spiritual, and socioeconomic

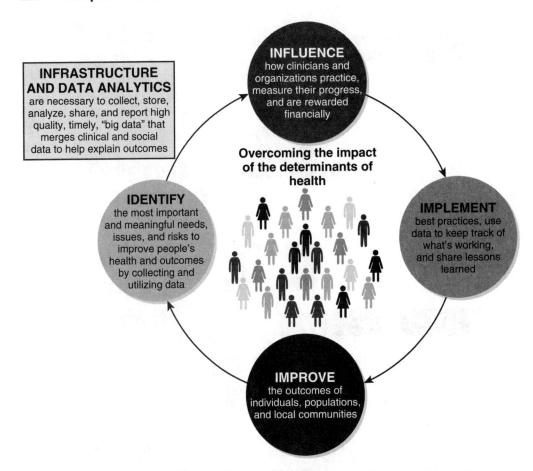

Figure 9.2 National Quality Forum approach to overcome the health effect of social determinants.
Reproduced from "An Evidence-Based Path Forward to Advance Social Determinants of Health Data," Health Affairs Blog, October 25, 2017

needs. Additionally, many other national and international organizations provide strong support, including the American Association of Nurse Practitioners (2019) and the American Academy of Physician Associates (2021). As healthcare organizations and APPs enhance their systems and processes to gather such data and work toward achieving *health for all*, a discussion of the HNA process is relevant.

Health Needs Assessment

An HNA is a systematic method for identifying health needs and health determinants for a specified population. Once identified, priorities are determined, and decisions are made about resource allocation to improve health (Cowley, 2021; Kawachi et al., 2020; Tobi, 2016). The holistic process acknowledges the effects of other factors besides biology, which must be addressed to increase APPs' understanding of the community they serve. Knowledge gained helps the APP leverage resources to support individual and population health while also identifying barriers to health.

A discussion of HNAs requires differentiation among the terms *health*, *healthcare needs*, and *health needs*. One of the most frequently used definitions of *health* was developed by the WHO in 1948 and is still used today.

According to the WHO (n.d., para. 1), health is "a state of complete physical, mental and social well-being and not merely the absence of disease or infirmity." While this definition does not directly acknowledge other factors that affect health and health outcomes, it does support the need to use a holistic approach when addressing health (Office of Disease Prevention and Health Promotion, 2020). *Healthcare needs* are described as those that can benefit from healthcare services and interventions, including both health promotion and disease management efforts, while *health needs* refer to demands that are often beyond the purview of medical care (Haughey, 2008). Health needs incorporate the SDOH and individual lifestyle behaviors, which affect health outcomes.

Needs can additionally be classified by type. Bradshaw (1972) described four types of needs: normative, comparative, felt, and expressed. *Normative needs* are those determined by expert opinion, generally based on the experience and consultation of experts. Recommended screenings such as mammograms or colonoscopies are examples of normative needs. Standardized assessment tools are often used at the individual level to identify normative needs. *Comparative needs* are identified by making comparisons between groups. For example, one community may have a larger population of older adults or a higher rate of a specific disease than a comparable community, thus having more significant needs for caregiving or palliative care resources. Comparative needs can be identified only if there is an objective standard on which to base comparisons. The distribution of resources at the population level is often based on comparative needs. Subjectivity characterizes *felt need*, defining need according to what individuals say they want or need. For example, a family with an autistic child may have a felt need for information and resources concerning the care and support of their child. Felt needs become *expressed needs* when vocalized or inferred from how individuals use services. In a community, there may be long wait times for individuals to see a mental health provider, thus indicating a potential need for more APPs. However, many factors may be responsible for the delays; they may not necessarily be due to a lack of resources. Expressed needs vary greatly from one area to another (Cowley, 2021; Tobi, 2016).

Health needs constantly change; many are not amenable to traditional medical approaches and are commonly referred to as a gap in what exists and what should be (Cowley, 2021; Kawachi et al., 2020). Incumbent in this definition is the concept of capacity to benefit. *Capacity to benefit* refers to the ability to intervene to meet identified needs effectively. According to this concept, resources and possible interventions should be available to address needs identified through the HNA process, thereby changing provider focus from treatment to development of health strategies (Tobi, 2016). At the community or population level, HNAs have traditionally been under the purview of public health professionals. However, in the United States and health systems worldwide, HNAs have become vital to planning accessible, effective health care for individuals, families, and communities. Assessments can be undertaken at each level, helping identify social and environmental context and acknowledge the complexity of influences across the life span on health promotion and disease prevention efforts. The process of HNA is not solely focused on the determination of needs; it also includes analysis of the collected data to identify resources necessary to address gaps efficiently and effectively. Throughout the HNA process, clinical, ethical, and economic considerations play a role. Multiple theories, frameworks, and approaches inform, guide, and support the HNA process. The most relevant theories and frameworks are discussed briefly in the next section to enhance understanding of the process.

Theories, Models, and Frameworks

The systems theory framework and the socioecological model are relevant to the HNA process. With a focus on the interactions and relationships of the parts that interact to achieve a specific goal, systems theory provides a framework from which phenomena can be investigated using a holistic approach (Plack et al., 2019). Systems are hierarchical, with each part affecting the whole. They contain super systems and subsystems that regularly interact, with each part of the system vital to achieving system aims (Plack et al., 2019). As applied to healthcare organizations, parts of the system may be tightly or loosely connected. These organizations have permeable boundaries, which support the exchange of resources or products. Both negative and positive feedback may occur during these exchanges, with positive feedback resulting in positive change or growth and negative feedback correcting errors to maintain the system in its current state. Systems are thus more than the sum of their parts (Lai & Lin, 2017). Understanding connections across social systems is vital to identifying health needs. Taking a systemic approach provides information needed to create measurable goals for improving health outcomes at all levels.

The socioecological model is derived from systems theory. This model "considers the complex interplay between individual, relational, community and societal factors" (CDC, 2020, para. 1). The model identifies four levels of influence on health behavior (see **Figure 9.3**).

Individual factors include age, education level, and income while relationship-level factors include close social circle friends and family members. Community-level factors include homes, neighborhoods, worksites, schools, and churches. Finally, at the societal level, norms and policies (e.g., health, economic, social, educational), which influence individuals and communities, play a substantial role. Reciprocal relationships exist among these levels of influence, reflecting the effect that public policies can have on individual behaviors as well as the influence that places where individuals live, work, and play can have on their health. For example, to address adult obesity in the practice population, the provider must first understand the policies, structures, behaviors, and norms that interact to promote obesity in the community. Individuals who live in areas designated as food deserts with limited physical activity options may have difficulty maintaining a healthy weight. This model encourages APPs to consider all factors contributing to the health needs to identify effective programs and resources.

Health Needs Assessment Process

Many types of information or data may have relevance to the care of individuals (see **Figure 9.4**). Epidemiological data that describe

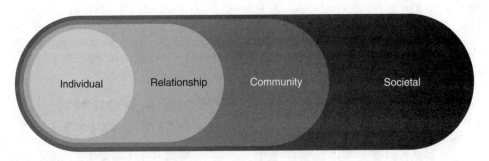

Figure 9.3 The socioecological model.

Source: Centers for Disease Control and Prevention, https://www.cdc.gov/violenceprevention/about/social-ecologicalmodel.html

Health Promotion Research Study

The HNA Process in Action

Background: This study was undertaken to identify the characteristics and health needs of individuals who inject drugs in Glasgow, Scotland.

Methodology: The HNA process included epidemiological, comparative, and corporate assessments. These included (1) secondary analysis of existing data from local sources in the community; (2) a rapid literature review; (3) a comparison of performance data for local addiction services to Scotland-wide surveillance data; and (4) stakeholder perspectives collected through semistructured interviews with six people who inject drugs in the city center, focus groups with individuals in recovery, and an online survey of staff from 33 relevant health services, community services, support organizations, and enforcement agencies.

Results: Findings indicated that priority health needs included addiction care, prevention and treatment of blood-borne illnesses and other injecting-related infections and injuries, and overdose and drug-related deaths. Stakeholders identified local facilitators and barriers to this issue. Support for safer injecting facilities was present across those providing services. This study offered support for plans to establish the world's first colocated safer injecting facility and treatment service.

Implications for Advanced Practice: Complex issues related to drug use require innovative approaches that consider the multiple factors at play. Colocation of these services can enhance clinical outreach and care to this population.

Reference: Data from Tweed, E. J., Rodgers, M., Priyadarshi, S., & Crighton, E. (2018). "Taking away the chaos": A health needs assessment for people who inject drugs in public places in Glasgow, Scotland. *BMC Public Health, 18*(1), 829. https://doi.org/10.1186/s12889-018-5718-9

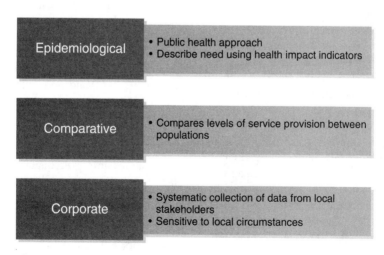

Figure 9.4 Types of health needs assessment data.

the incidence and prevalence of diseases in a population can help providers prioritize resources. Comparative data that reflect the effect of service provision in one population can inform the development of individualized strategies for a different population. Finally, corporate data that assess the perspectives of local stakeholders, including providers, community members, and policymakers, can help identify local circumstances that affect health (Tobi, 2016). For example, an APP desiring to address tobacco use disorder in adolescents in the community surrounding the health center where they practice might first seek epidemiological data from the county health department to assess tobacco use trends by, for example, age, race, and socioeconomic level. A comparative assessment of the outcomes of school-based tobacco prevention and cessation programs in the area would also be helpful information for identifying what is and what isn't working. The assessment process can also include a focus group of clinicians, educators, parents, and students to learn people's perceptions of the factors contributing to adolescent tobacco use.

Each type of data has advantages and drawbacks. The type utilized should be tailored to the needs of the organization conducting the assessment, including a consideration of the time and resources available to complete the HNA and the ability to integrate results into healthcare planning and services. Generally, most HNAs will include aspects of all three types to provide the most comprehensive assessment of need and promote health equity.

Elements and characteristics common to all HNAs include (a) purpose; (b) a structured, systematic approach; (c) a defined population; (d) collaboration/community engagement; (e) assessment; (f) analysis and prioritization; and (g) planning, intervention, and evaluation (Cowley, 2021; Tobi, 2016). Each is described separately next; descriptions are informed by the author's own experiences and the works of Cowley (2021), Kawachi et al. (2020), O'Shaughnessy et al. (2020), and Tobi (2016) and seminal work by Wright et al. (1998).

Purpose

Before undertaking an HNA, the APP must determine why the assessment will be done. Questions to consider relate to the principal concern and goal for the assessment. For example, does one community served by the practice appear to have higher infant and maternal mortality rates than nearby communities? Do the felt or comparative needs of the community require identification to help articulate a clear set of objectives and priorities to meet patient needs? The assessment could respond to a request from individuals in the community or evaluate possible community responses to services or programs being considered. Identifying the project's scope and goals will help determine whether resources and capacity are available to complete the assessment (Tobi, 2016).

Approach

Once the purpose of the HNA is determined and described, the resources necessary to complete the assessment must be identified. Questions to consider include the following: Is the time right to do the HNA now, or should it wait? Does the practice have the resources to conduct the HNA? Resources include money, personnel, time (which can be substantial), knowledge of the process, and the ability to complete an assessment that generates quality data. The identified population's leadership, support, and willingness to support HNAs are vital to success. Valid and reliable data take time to collect, often requiring focus groups, interviews, or survey development and distribution to collect comprehensive data. Failure to dedicate the resources needed for a thorough HNA may result in inadequate or biased data. Many factors affect the ability to collect data, including difficulty accessing current data, low response rates to surveys or focus groups, and lack of representativeness of the data. Often, data do not reflect the most vulnerable populations. It is essential to consider these factors and ameliorate them before beginning the HNA. A systematic, structured approach must be developed that describes and outlines the HNA process from start to finish, including a potential timeline to ensure success.

Defined Population

The purpose and goals of the HNA will help the clinician define the population for which data will be collected. Populations can be defined geographically, using existing boundaries or borders; by a specific setting such as a worksite, school, or correctional facility; or by a specific issue or medical condition such as being homeless or suffering from HIV. Population boundaries must be clearly identified to ensure the collection of relevant data. For example, the APP may be interested in lowering maternal and infant mortality secondary to substance use; thus, the population of interest would be pregnant women who use substances.

Collaboration and Engagement

The HNA process requires collaboration and engagement of those who will manage and conduct the HNA process and key stakeholders representing the target population and local community. An interprofessional team should be assembled to complete the needs assessment process. The actual number of individuals needed on the team should be determined by the scope of the project and the resources available to conduct it. For example, if the focus is a small, clearly defined population such as one worksite experiencing high lung cancer rates secondary to tobacco use behaviors, the resources required, including team members, would be less than for a larger-scale project. A larger-scale project such as one focused on the previous example of pregnant women who use substances would likely require a larger team due to the complexity of the issue. While consultants experienced in HNAs can be helpful, hiring an external individual or a group to conduct the assessment can be counterproductive to engaging stakeholders. However, it can be beneficial to collaborate with an academic partner from a nearby university. Academic researchers often engage with community entities to conduct research and provide extensive knowledge, support, and access to evidence-based resources through institutional repositories.

It is vital to engage community stakeholders, including those directly affected by the issue, concerned about addressing the problem and who have the power to affect the situation early in the process. This approach enhances stakeholders' diversity, contributing to a greater likelihood that data will be representative and stakeholders will support programs or strategies to address identified needs or gaps. Commonly referred to as community-based participatory or community-engaged research, several principles guide this approach and are readily apparent in the HNA process. These include the following:

- Focuses on the community as the unit of identity
- Builds on the community's strengths and resources
- Facilitates collaboration and equal partnership
- Promotes community capacity building
- Balances research and action
- Emphasizes local relevance of public health problems
- Attends to SDOH and causes of health inequities
- Collaborates with the community to disseminate findings
- Commits to sustainability (Israel et al., 2019).

Assessment

The assessment begins after the scope is defined, the population identified, and a team developed. Steps to complete the assessment include data collection, organization, and analysis, followed by prioritization of identified needs. Multiple methods of data collection can be used to collect quantitative and qualitative data from various sources, using methods appropriate to the data collected. Prior to data collection, decisions must be made concerning which data are needed specifically for this assessment, how much information is enough, and how the data will be organized and stored. Some data may be de-identified or not considered protected health information while other data may be protected or include data of a sensitive nature. Most institutions have guidelines concerning the storage of identifiable health data. Existing quantitative data are available at the local, state, and national levels regarding, for example, demographics, mortality and morbidity, risk factors, economics, health services use, infectious disease rates, substance use, and lifestyle behaviors. See **Table 9.1** for a list of possible sources.

It is best to start by reviewing available data. While readily available data may be easy to access through online databases or via published reports, it is important to note that such data may not be at the level needed or adequately reflect the population assessed. Additionally, there can be a lag time of one or more years between data collection and its publication for use by the public. Community HNAs, required by the Affordable Care Act of 2010, are examples of HNAs. Required of tax-exempt hospitals every three years, these assessments provide the basis for developing an implementation strategy to meet identified community health needs. These assessments, conducted in collaboration with a broad base of community stakeholders, aim to identify significant health needs, prioritize those needs, and identify resources in the community that can address identified needs (Internal Revenue Service, 2021).

Qualitative approaches best collect data that reflect the subjective experiences or perceptions of the target population's needs. These

Table 9.1 Sources of Quantitative Data

Data Source	Type of Data
International	
World Health Organization	Health profiles, infectious diseases, causes of mortality
Pan American Health Organization	Health profiles, infectious diseases, causes of mortality
National (United States)	
Behavioral Risk Factor Surveillance System (BRFSS)	Health-related risk behaviors, chronic health conditions, and use of preventive services
Centers for Disease Control and Prevention (CDC)	Health insurance, mortality and morbidity, injury prevention and control (WISQARS), infectious diseases, FastStats
State, Regional, County, and Local	
State and local health departments	Morbidity and mortality, infectious diseases, risk behaviors, injuries and fatalities, hospital discharges, maternal and child health, births, marriages
Community Health Needs Assessments (CHNAs)	Social determinants of health, local community needs, strategies for community improvement

often include the development of surveys or questionnaires distributed via mail or online to the entire population or identified subsets. Surveys can be specifically developed to meet the local assessment needs. Alternatively, freely available surveys from other entities may be found through national organizations or peer-reviewed literature (see **Table 9.2**).

Other approaches include the use of key informant interviews or focus groups. See **Table 9.3** for a description of qualitative approaches.

Table 9.2 Sources of Tools to Collect Specific Data

Screening Tool	Description
Protocol for Responding to and Assessing Patients' Assets, Risks, and Experiences (PRAPARE)	Standardized patient risk assessment tool; process and collection of resources to identify and act on the social determinants of health
Social Needs Screening Tool	Social determinants of health screening tool, available in short and long form (English and Spanish)
Health-Related Social Needs Screening Tool	Assesses for housing instability, food insecurity, transportation needs, utility needs, and interpersonal safety
Community Links Evidence to Action Research (CLEAR) Tool Kit	Clinical practice tool to better support disadvantaged patients and promote action on broader social determinants in the local context
Health Begins Upstream Risks Screening Tools	Includes multiple tools that assess economic stability, education, social and community contexts, neighborhood and physical environments, and food

Table 9.3 Qualitative Approaches to Data Collection

Approach	Description
Focus groups	Conducted with 8–10 people in one group; require a moderator and a notetaker; general questions are asked with follow-up questions as needed
Key informant interviews	Interviews of individuals selected for their knowledge or experience of the population or issue at hand; use a semistructured questionnaire with topics or open-ended probing questions
Public meetings	Open, advertised meetings; use structured or semistructured questions to guide the conversation
Direct observation	Document observations during meetings, program offerings, etc., using a form created explicitly for that purpose
Open-ended surveys	A survey is created with open-ended questions focused on the topic or issue at hand; distribute to the relevant population
Case studies	Collect information to create a detailed description of one person's experience

Sources of Data

Data collection beyond the clinical setting is necessary to provide a broader perspective. While some data related to mortality and morbidity are collected and reported routinely, other data are available less routinely. Some data will be available only at the community or population level while other data will provide more granular detail. Both governmental and nongovernmental entities collect and report population- or institution-based data. Population-based data are collected by censuses or other population-level surveys such as the Behavioral Risk Factor Surveillance System. Institution-level data are generally collected from individual health records at institutions (Chen et al., 2014). Both types are helpful when conducting an HNA. It is important to ensure that data obtained are valid and reliable and that data collected from different sources are comparable measures of health status. Table 9.1 includes a list of common sources that can provide access to data for HNAs. It is important to remember that there are many ways to learn about community needs. As discussed earlier in this section, interviews with community members, direct observation of behaviors, or a review of existing community, program, or EHRs can be used to collect data.

Due to the strengths and weaknesses of various types of data or differing data collection approaches, it is recommended that multiple sources and types of data be used to describe the population, a process referred to as triangulation. Triangulation uses multiple data types and sources to provide various views of the same issue or population. For example, data concerning the rates of substance use may be available from the local health department, which documents statistics through a needle syringe program. This information could be supplemented with data from the local emergency management system and mental health providers concerning the number of patients they see using substances. Further data may be obtained through interviews with community

Questions to Consider During Analysis and Prioritization

1. What information does the data provide?
2. What does the information mean for the practice?
3. Does it help to identify factors that may be contributing to inequities in the population?
4. How do different stakeholders perceive it?
5. What strategies might be helpful?
6. Can identified needs be addressed?

organizations providing services to those who use substances and focus groups or interviews with those who currently use substances or are recovering. This approach will provide a more comprehensive picture of the issue in the community. A thorough discussion of data and data collection methodology, including strengths and weaknesses, is beyond this chapter's scope. Refer to the evidence-based resources table (Table 9.7) at the end of this chapter to find resources for existing surveys. An example of a research study that used an existing survey to assess and better understand the needs of a specific population can be found at the end of the chapter (Health Promotion Case Study: Conducting a Health Needs Assessment).

Analysis and Prioritization

Once data have been collected, the provider will use the data to determine needs and gaps to identify health priorities. Questions to consider are listed in the preceding box.

It can be challenging to determine which gaps or needs to prioritize and how best to address them. When making these decisions, the APP must consider the capacity to benefit by considering whether resources are available to intervene effectively and meet identified needs. It is vital to continue to include identified stakeholders during prioritization. Multiple methods exist to prioritize data ranging from simple to complex. Simple approaches include the dot method, where stakeholders are given a limited number of slips of paper or dots to identify their three highest priorities, with prioritization based on the highest number of dots received. Stakeholders may also use multiple sessions to vote numerous times on the identified needs to reach a consensus on priorities. A nominal group process using small groups of stakeholders who select their top priorities through voting or ranking can also be used. Criteria for prioritization may also be developed, including the number of people affected or available resources. See **Table 9.4** for an example.

Table 9.5 includes web-based resources, descriptions of prioritization, and possible tools to support the process.

Analysis of data collected at the individual and family levels must also occur, with an intentional focus on social determinants during the prioritization process. Data collected at these levels may also be used to identify and prioritize community- or population-level health needs.

Table 9.4 Nominal Group Process

Identified Need	Stakeholder 1	Stakeholder 2	Stakeholder 3	Stakeholder 4
Housing	1	2	4	4
Health insurance	3	1	1	1
Social support	2	4	3	2
Primary care access	4	3	2	3

Table 9.5 Prioritization of Health Needs

Source	URL
American Hospital Association Community Health Assessment Toolkit	https://www.healthycommunities.org/resources/toolkit/files/step5-select-priority
Centers for Disease Control and Prevention	https://www.cdc.gov/chinav/tools/focus.html
Community Tool Box	https://ctb.ku.edu/en/table-of-contents/assessment/assessing-community-needs-and-resources/analyzing-community-problems/main
Association of State and Territorial Health Officials	https://www.astho.org
National Association of County and City Health Officials	https://naccho.org
Rural Health Information Hub	https://ruralhealthinfo.org
National Community Action Partnership	https://communityactionpartnership.com/publication_toolkit/community-needs-assessment-resource-guide
National Association for State Community Services Programs	https://nascsp.org

Planning, Intervention, and Evaluation

Once a decision has been made regarding which gaps or needs to address, the development of interventions and strategies can begin. Planning begins by prioritizing the identified gaps or needs for intervention and considering the processes and outcomes for evaluation. Methods described in the previous section can also be used to select and prioritize interventions. Multiple questions should be proposed and discussed. Some examples are provided in the following box.

Next, the best available evidence is used to develop new interventions or programs or to adapt existing practices to meet the prioritized need or gap. The issue will likely be multifactorial, including SDOH, health behaviors, clinical factors, and environmental factors, thus emphasizing the need to include not only all stakeholders who participated in the assessment but also those who can help address the problem (see the following box). Finally, an evaluation plan is developed to identify outcomes that reflect the intervention's effect.

Questions to Consider During Planning

1. Which gaps or needs are the most significant or severe?
2. Are there resources available to address the problem?
3. Should it be addressed, and if so, which individual, practice, or group is suitable to do it?
4. What are the potential outcomes of not addressing the problem?
5. What are the potential outcomes if it is addressed?
6. Will the identified interventions be acceptable and appropriate for the target population?
7. Which potential partners can help improve coordination and access to necessary services?

Questions to Consider When Selecting Interventions and Designing Evaluations

1. What are the advantages/disadvantages of each possible solution?
2. What are the goals of the interventions?
3. Who or what are the targets?
4. How will the effect of the interventions be evaluated?
5. Who will be doing the evaluation or be interested in the results?

Other Approaches to Assess Health Needs

While a thorough HNA such as described in this chapter provides the most valid, reliable, and representative data, APPs may not have the time or resources to conduct this level of assessment. APPs may use two other approaches, rapid appraisal and health profiling, to assess health needs. These approaches are less time consuming and resource intensive. Like a full HNA, these approaches identify needs at the practice, organization, school, specific population, or community level.

Rapid Appraisal

Rapid appraisals are helpful when timely insights are needed and resources are limited. However, it is important to note that this approach may generate less representative, reliable, and valid data, potentially contributing to bias. Despite these potential limitations, the data generated can be helpful. Generally, data for HNAs are systematically obtained from existing quantitative data sets and through key informant interviews or observations of the selected population on a more limited basis over a shorter time frame, with more substantial reliance on the information provided by key informants (Gilbeaux, 2012; Sparkes et al., 2017). For example, the practitioner may note that a large percentage of pregnant women using substances reside in areas around one location in the health system. Thus, a rapid appraisal might include interviewing maternal–child staff at this location and women who have experienced the issue first-hand. Other potential interviewees include community health workers focused on reducing infant mortality in the area and the local health department or other community entities and organizations providing services to address this issue. Local courts and children's services may also provide information that can supplement quantitative data, such as infant mortality rates, numbers of children born with neonatal abstinence syndrome, and numbers of pregnant women receiving medication-assisted treatment. This information can then be used by the provider to better individualize care for this population subset, including assessment for SDOH, which may be playing a role; identification of resources that are accessible; and interventions that meet the identified needs.

When using the rapid appraisal approach, it is important to use both quantitative and qualitative data to support triangulation as previously described to help strengthen the validity of the findings. If feasible, based on resources and time, multiple disciplines should also be involved to ensure a broad view of the population being studied. See the following box for an example of a rapid appraisal.

Health Profiling

Health profiling is another method used to quickly conduct an HNA (Cowley, 2021). This approach is generally more focused on quantitative data, although interviews with critical informants may also be completed if time and resources allow. Quantitative data typically collected in health profiling include demographics, descriptive community information, commonly available statistics regarding causes of morbidity and mortality, and those that capture lifestyle behavior and

Rapid Appraisal Research Study Abstract

This study used a rapid appraisal approach to conduct an HNA of African American breast cancer survivors. The researchers were interested in describing modifiable lifestyle risk factors. To complete the HNA in a shorter time frame, they conducted a literature review, secondary analysis of existing national-level data, and focus group discussions with African American breast cancer survivors. Findings were used to plan health promotion trials to develop community-engaged intervention approaches to increase adherence to cancer prevention guidelines.

Data from Smith, S. A., Claridy, M. D., Whitehead, M. S., Sheats, J. Q., Yoo, W., Alema-Mensah, E. A., Ansa, B. E-O., & Coughlin, S. S. (2015). Lifestyle modification experiences of African American breast cancer survivors: A needs assessment. *JMIR Cancer, 1*(2), e4892. https://doi.org/10.2196/cancer.4892

Health Profiling Research Study Abstract

This study used health profiling to describe health profiles, lifestyles, and health resource use by an immigrant population compared to the nonimmigrant population. The researchers analyzed existing quantitative secondary data collected by a national health survey. They found that the immigrant population was younger and displayed better lifestyle-related behaviors related to alcohol, smoking, and physical activity. While higher percentages of immigrants were hospitalized, use was found to be appropriate. This information helped identify healthcare needs and priorities for this population group.

Data from Carrasco-Garrido, P., De Miguel, A. G., Barrera, V. H., & Jiménez-García, R. (2007). Health profiles, lifestyles and use of health resources by the immigrant population resident in Spain. *European Journal of Public Health, 17*(5), 503–507. https://doi.org/10.1093/eurpub/ckl279

SDOH data (Cowley, 2021; Tobi, 2016). More limited than a full HNA or a rapid appraisal, health profiling can provide information about the population's common diseases, causes of death, and potential contributing factors. Using the previous example of pregnant women who use substances, the APP could gather the following data: (1) infant and maternal mortality, (2) drug use rates and treatment, (3) number of infants born with neonatal abstinence syndrome, and (4) characteristics of the geographic region where cases may be concentrated. Collectively, this data may help the provider to determine health needs. The preceding box provides an example of an HNA utilizing the health profiling method.

Family and Individual Health Needs Assessments

The previous section described the many characteristics and elements of population- or community-level HNAs. Individual- and family-level HNAs follow a similar pattern. Most APPs are experienced in collecting individual- and family-level data that identify strategies and interventions to enhance health promotion and disease prevention efforts. Initiatives are underway by federal- and state-level entities and multiple healthcare systems to gather data that support the ability to address lifestyle behaviors better and SDOH that affect care (Artiga & Hinton, 2018; Cantor & Thorpe, 2018). At the provider level, practices can adopt screening tools to collect SDOH data and adapt EHRs to support collection and usability. In the United States, these efforts are guided by two Institute of Medicine reports released in 2014 regarding the use of EHRs to collect data reflecting social and behavioral domains (Institute of Medicine, 2015). The ability to collect and use the power of an EHR to better understand lifestyle behaviors

and SDOH supports efforts to move beyond disease-oriented treatment.

Screening for data that reflect these domains should occur at every interaction with patients and families. This includes asking questions about transportation availability, access to healthy foods, physical activity options, employment, income, support systems, affordable day care, and accessible senior housing. While it seems that gathering such data will significantly affect the time needed for a visit, the collection of such data will streamline other visit aspects, such as anticipatory guidance and coordination of care (Andermann, 2016). The data can also be used to tailor interventions for individuals and families, using the resources and services available in their communities to support recommendations. In many cases, much of this data is likely already being shared and documented through conversations during provider visits. Unfortunately, APPs are often unsure how to address identified issues or may focus solely on the acute aspects of the disease process. Thus, the data go unnoticed and unused, resulting in poor health outcomes and return visits. Table 9.2 includes descriptions of existing tools available to use at the individual, family, and community levels.

Integration Into Clinical Practice

Efficient use of data collected through HNAs requires integration into clinical practice. EHRs provide an opportunity to manage population health by incorporating SDOH. Practice- and system-level changes such as workflow redesign and information technology assistance may be necessary to support the integration of SDOH data in clinical visits, health considerations, and decisions. Since the Institute of Medicine's 2014 reports, multiple initiatives have been undertaken in the United States to support the collection and integration of SDOH data (Artiga & Hinton, 2018; Billioux et al., 2017; Cantor & Thorpe, 2018). Federal-level payers and funding groups support these initiatives. Many EHR vendors have developed tools and applications to enhance interoperability of SDOH data, both publicly available data and data collected specifically from patients. Multiple tools have been developed for public use and are described in **Table 9.6**.

Health Promotion Case Study: Conducting a Health Needs Assessment

Case Description: A 65-year-old female is seen by the APP for an annual wellness visit. The patient has a history of arthritis and cardiac disease with a stroke one year prior. The patient is classified as overweight and prediabetic. During the wellness visit, the APP recommends that the patient increase her physical activity level. Water aerobic exercise is suggested due to the patient's arthritis. The APP also recommends a healthier, balanced diet to support weight loss and improve cardiovascular health.

Three months later, the APP is notified that the patient has suffered another stroke and is hospitalized. During a follow-up visit with the patient postrehabilitation, the APP assesses the patient's physical activity and diet prior to the stroke. The patient tearfully indicates there is a pool that she could use at a community center about two miles away but that she cannot afford the monthly fees nor has a way to get there. The patient also reports that she tries to eat a healthier diet but it is difficult due to her reliance on food banks for food access.

Based on this information, the APP decides to conduct a more detailed individual needs assessment, including collecting data that will reflect some of the SDOH that the patient has identified. During this assessment, which includes focusing on the patient's living environment and access to resources, the APP finds that the patient lives in subsidized housing with no access to transportation. Compounding these issues is a lack of access to the internet or up-to-date technology. Additionally, the patient tells the APP that she watches her granddaughter every day after school—something she enjoys immensely. Using this information, the APP works with the patient and a social worker to access the nearby pool for free and transportation through the local senior center. The APP connects the patient with a dietician to determine the best way to eat healthier given the food choices available to the patient.

Since many of the practice's patients live in the same subsidized housing, the APP decides to collaborate with other healthcare facilities to complete an HNA using a health profile approach. Together, they collect demographic data for the population that lives in the subsidized housing using locally available data. They capture information regarding common causes of morbidity and mortality and lifestyle behaviors for the patients from this area through the practice's EHR. Finally, with the help of local advocates, they collect information that describes the housing unit, the surrounding area, and the resources available in the nearby community, which can be used to support health. After completing both needs assessments, they believe that they will now be able to provide recommendations and care that may result in better adherence by the patient.

Critical Thinking Questions
1. How does the HNA approach address health disparities and support achievement of equitable care?
2. What are the benefits of this process beyond this individual patient?
3. How might you as an APP better integrate HNAs into daily practice?

Table 9.6 Tools and Resources to Support Health Needs Assessments at the Individual, Family, and Community Levels

Tool	Description	Level	URL
PRAPARE: Protocol for Responding to and Assessing Patients' Assets, Risks, and Experiences	Collects data needed to better understand and act on patients' social determinants of health	Individual (integrate into clinical workflow/ EHR)	https://prapare.org
Accountable Health Communities Health-Related Social Needs Screening Tool	Identifies unmet health-related social needs	Individual (integrate into clinical workflow/ EHR)	https://innovation.cms.gov/files /worksheets/ahcm -screeningtool.pdf
HealthBegins Upstream Risks Screening Tool	Includes 28 questions that assess five domains (economic stability, education, social and community context, neighborhood and physical environment, and food)	Individual (integrate into clinical workflow/EHR)	https://sdh-tools-review .kpwashingtonresearch.org /screening-tools/health-begins
Community Assessment for Public Health Emergency Response (CASPER) Toolkit (3rd ed.)	An epidemiological technique designed to provide public health leaders and emergency managers with household-based information about a community	Community	https://www.cdc.gov/nceh /casper/default.htm
Poverty: A Clinical Tool for Primary Care Providers	Identifies patients who may suffer health issues as a result of living in poverty	Individual	https://nbcfp.ca/health/poverty
Community Health Assessment Toolkit	A tool used by hospitals, public health departments, and other social service agencies to systematically identify, analyze, prioritize, and address key community health needs and concerns	Community	https://www.healthy communities.org/resources /community-health -assessment-toolkit
PRECEDE/ PROCEED	Provides a structure to assess health needs to support the development of programs to meet those needs	Community	https://ctb.ku.edu/en /table-contents/overview /other-models-promoting -community-health-and -development/preceder -proceder/main

Tool	Description	Level	URL
Social Needs Screening Tool	Tool for providers to screen for core health-related social needs, including housing, food, transportation, utilities, personal safety, employment, education, childcare, and financial strain	Individual, family	https://www.aafp.org/dam/AAFP /documents/patient_care /everyone_project/hops19 -physician-form-sdoh.pdf
Family Assessment Needs and Strengths (FANS 2.0)	Guides parents in identifying strengths and skills needed as parents; includes multiple domains	Family	https://www.nj.gov/dcf/about /divisions/dcsc/FANS-2.0 -Manual.docx

Clinical, Ethical, and Economic Considerations

HNAs often identify issues, concerns, and needs that are beyond the capacity of health entities or APPs. Additionally, despite using a systematic process or approach, subjectivity regarding identification and prioritization of needs cannot be totally eliminated. Determination of needs is not value-free, with decisions often based on time, resources, and expert opinion. Underresourced or poorly conducted HNAs may result in biased or nonrepresentative data, leading to the development of programs or resources that do not meet actual health needs. Often, APPs may feel conflicted about which needs to prioritize. It will not be possible for the practice or the provider to meet the full range of perceived unmet health needs. However, through an interprofessional team's involvement, needs could be addressed through improved service integration with the community and policies that support health. Clinical, ethical, and economic considerations are pervasive throughout the HNA process. Existing ethical models may be helpful as APPs and practices determine how to best use

and address HNA data to benefit individuals, families, populations, and communities. **Table 9.7** provides evidence-based resources to support the APP knowledge and development of the HNA.

Benefits and Barriers

HNAs can improve health outcomes through increased patient adherence to treatment recommendations, less fragmentation of care due to enhanced communication and coordination between APPs and community organizations, better use of resources, and development of policies and programs that address the SDOH.

There are also many barriers and challenges that the APP must consider before undertaking an HNA. The most-cited barriers include lack of knowledge regarding how to obtain information reflective of social and behavioral domains, lack of time and resources, and inability to address many of the needs that may be identified.

Several strategies can address the barriers and challenges associated with HNAs. First, the APP should select an assessment approach that aligns with the time and resources available. It may be that other providers or institutions in the community are also trying to identify needs. Thus, collaboration could

TABLE 9.7	Evidence-Based Resources for Health Needs Assessment

Resource	URL
National Library of Medicine	https://www.nlm.nih.gov/nichsr/stats_tutorial/cover.html
World Health Organization SCORE (Survey, Count, Optimize, Review, Enable) for Health Data Technical Package	https://www.who.int/data/data-collection-tools/score
Robert Wood Johnson Foundation Sentinel Communities	https://www.rwjf.org/en/about-rwjf/how-we-work/learning-and-evaluation/sentinel-communities.html
Guidelines for Conducting Rapid Participatory Appraisals of Community Health Needs in Developing Countries	https://doi.org/10.1177%2F10105395060180030801

Health Promotion Activity: Health Needs Assessment in Practice

Reflect on your current practice. How much do you know about the communities where your patients live? How often do you intentionally consider factors that affect your patients' ability to live a healthy lifestyle?

Review your EHR system for information that reflects the many factors discussed in this chapter, such as access to reliable transportation, food insecurity, and exposure to violence. Is data available that could be used to better individualize care and address SDOH? If not, are there ways such data could be incorporated? Do you think it would be helpful?

---

provide support and additional resources to the process. Academic institutions in the community may have faculty interested in collaborating on projects, lending expertise, and providing funding or personnel support. The time needed to complete an assessment can vary widely depending on the approach. A full-scale scientifically based survey might take a great deal of time to develop and distribute while a smaller survey could take only a few hours. Data can be collected from multiple individuals at a community-based meeting or gathering, maximizing numbers and minimizing time. Finally, just as with many health issues, there may be needs identified that the APP cannot directly address. However, knowledge of such issues enhances person-centered care and improves health equity.

Summary

This chapter provides an overview of HNAs. It is important to remember that HNAs need to be conducted routinely to reflect the environments' and communities' ever-changing nature. APPs are uniquely situated to obtain data to identify and address the many factors and determinants affecting the health of the individuals they serve. Understanding HNA principles and approaches can help APPs determine how they might best integrate the collection and use of HNA data into routine practice.

Acronyms

APP: advanced practice provider
EHR: electronic health record
HNA: health needs assessment

RWJF: Robert Wood Johnson Foundation
SDOH: social determinants of health
WHO: World Health Organization

References

American Academy of Physician Associates. (2021). *What is diversity, equity, and inclusion?* https://www.aapa.org/about/diversity-equity-and-inclusion-statement

American Association of Colleges of Nursing. (2021). *AACN essentials.* https://www.aacnnursing.org/AACN-Essentials

American Association of Nurse Practitioners. (2019). *Standards of practice for nurse practitioners.* https://www.aanp.org/advocacy/advocacy-resource/position-statements/standards-of-practice-for-nurse-practitioners

American Public Health Association. (2020). *Health equity.* https://www.apha.org/topics-and-issues/health-equity

Andermann, A. (2016). Taking action on the social determinants of health in clinical practice: A framework for health professionals. *Canadian Medical Association Journal, 188*(17–18), E474–E483. https://doi.org/10.1503/cmaj.160177

Artiga, S., & Hinton, E. (2018). Beyond health care: The role of social determinants in promoting health and health equity. *Health, 20*(10), 1–13.

Billioux, A., Verlander, K., Anthony, S., & Alley, D. (2017). Standardized screening for health-related social needs in clinical settings: The accountable health communities screening tool. *NAM Perspectives.* https://doi.org/10.31478/201705b

Bradshaw, J. (1972). The concept of social need. *New Society, 3*, 640–643. https://www.york.ac.uk/inst/spru/pubs/pdf/JRB.pdf

Cantor, M. N., & Thorpe, L. (2018). Integrating data on social determinants of health into electronic health records. *Health Affairs, 37*(4), 585–590. https://doi.org/10.1377/hlthaff.2017.1252

Carrasco-Garrido, P., De Miguel, A. G., Barrera, V. H., & Jiménez-García, R. (2007). Health profiles, lifestyles and use of health resources by the immigrant population resident in Spain. *European Journal of Public Health, 17*(5), 503–507. https://doi.org/10.1093/eurpub/ckl279

Centers for Disease Control and Prevention. (2016). *Health in all policies.* https://www.cdc.gov/policy/hiap/index.html

Centers for Disease Control and Prevention. (2020). *The socio-ecological model: A framework for prevention.* https://www.cdc.gov/violenceprevention/about/social-ecologicalmodel.html

Chen, H., Hailey, D., Wang, N., & Yu, P. (2014). A review of data quality assessment methods for public health information systems. *International Journal of Environmental Research and Public Health, 11*(5), 5170–5207. https://doi.org/10.3390/ijerph110505170

Cowley, S. (2021). Health needs assessment. In S. Cowley & K. Whittaker (Eds.), *Community public health in policy and practice e-book: A sourcebook.* Elsevier Health Sciences.

Flowers, J., & Evans, S. (2020). Assessing the health of populations. In I. Kawachi, I. Lang, & W. Ricciardi (Eds.), *Oxford handbook of public health practice* (4th ed.; pp. 9–42). Oxford University Press.

Fraze, T., Lewis, V. A., Rodriguez, H. P., & Fisher, E. S. (2016). Housing, transportation, and food: How ACOs seek to improve population health by addressing non-medical needs of patients. *Health Affairs, 35*(11), 2109–2115. https://doi.org/10.1377/hlthaff.2016.0727

Gilbeaux, K. (2012, February 21). *Rapid appraisal methods.* U.S. Resilience System. https://us.resiliencesystem.org/rapid-appraisal-methods

Graham, G., & Bernot, J. (2017). *An evidence-based path forward to advance social determinants of health data.* Connecticut Council for Philanthropy. https://www.ctphilanthropy.org/news/evidence-based-path-forward-advance-social-determinants-health-data

Haughey, F. (2008). Assessing and identifying health needs: Theories and frameworks in practice. In L. Coles & E. Porter (Eds.), *Public health skills: A practical guide for nurses and public health practitioners* (pp. 7–28). Wiley-Blackwell.

Institute of Medicine. (2015, January 8). *Capturing social and behavioral domains and measures in electronic health records: Phase 2.* Committee on the Recommended Social and Behavioral Domains and Measures for Electronic Health Records; Board on Population Health and Public Health Practice. https://doi.org/10.17226/18951

Internal Revenue Service. (2021). *Community health needs assessments for charitable hospital organizations – Section 501(r)(3).* https://www.irs.gov/charities-non-profits/community-health-needs-assessment-for-charitable-hospital-organizations-section-501r3

Israel, B. A., Schulz, A. J., Coombe, C. M., Parker, E. A., Reyes, A. G., Rowe, Z., & Lichtenstein, R. L. (2019). Community-based participatory research: An approach to research in the urban context. In S. Galea, C. Ettman, & D. Vlahov (Eds.), *Urban health* (pp. 272–284). Oxford University Press. https://doi.org/10.1093/oso/9780190915858.003.0029

Kawachi, I., Lang, I., & Ricciardi, W. (Eds.). (2020). *Oxford handbook of public health practice* (4th ed.). Oxford University Press.

Lai, C. H., & Lin, S. H. (2017). Systems theory. In C. Scott & L. Lewis (Eds.), *The international encyclopedia of organizational communication* (pp. 1–18). Wiley-Blackwell.

National Organization of Nurse Practitioner Faculties. (2022). *Nurse practitioner role core competencies.* https://www.nonpf.org/resource/resmgr/competencies/nonpf_np_role_core_competenc.pdf

Naz, A., Rosenberg, E., Andersson, N., Labonté, R., & Andermann, A. (2016). Health workers who ask about social determinants of health are more likely to report helping patients: Mixed-methods study. *Canadian Family Physician, 62*(11), e684–e693.

Office of Disease Prevention and Health Promotion. (2020). *Healthy People 2030.* https://www.healthypeople.gov/2020

O'Shaughnessy, A., Wright, J., & Cave, B. (2020). Assessing health needs. In I. Kawachi, I. Lang, & W. Ricciardi (Eds.), *Oxford handbook of public health practice* (4th ed.; pp. 9–42). Oxford University Press.

Plack, M. M., Goldman, E. F., Scott, A. R., & Brundage, S. B. (2019). *Systems thinking in the healthcare professions: A guide for educators and clinicians.* The George Washington University. https://hsrc.himmelfarb.gwu.edu/cgi/viewcontent.cgi?article=1000&context=educational_resources_teaching

Robert Wood Johnson Foundation. (2020). *County health rankings & roadmaps.* www.countyhealthrankings.org

Robert Wood Johnson Foundation. (2021). *Why build a culture of health?* https://www.rwjf.org/en/cultureofhealth/about/why-we-need-a-culture-of-health.html

Smith, S. A., Claridy, M. D., Whitehead, M. S., Sheats, J. Q., Yoo, W., Alema-Mensah, E. A., Ansa, B. E-O., & Coughlin, S. S. (2015). Lifestyle modification experiences of African American breast cancer survivors: A needs assessment. *JMIR Cancer, 1*(2), e4892. https://doi.org/10.2196/cancer.4892

Sparkes, S., Durán, A., & Kutzin, J. (2017). *A system-wide approach to analysing efficiency across health programmes.* World Health Organization. https://www.who.int/publications/i/item/9789241511964

Tobi, P. (2016). Health needs assessment. In K. Regmi & I. Gee (Eds.), *Public health intelligence* (pp. 169–186). Springer. https://doi.org/10.1007/978-3-319-28326-5_9

Tweed, E. J., Rodgers, M., Priyadarshi, S., & Crighton, E. (2018). "Taking away the chaos": A health needs assessment for people who inject drugs in public places in Glasgow, Scotland. *BMC Public Health, 18*(1), 829. https://doi.org/10.1186/s12889-018-5718-9

United Nations General Assembly. (2015, October 21). *Transforming our world: The 2030 Agenda for Sustainable Development.* https://www.refworld.org/docid/57b6e3e44.html

World Health Organization. (n.d.). *Constitution.* Retrieved May 12, 2023, from https://www.who.int/about/governance/constitution

World Health Organization. (2020). *Health equity.* https://www.who.int/health-topics/health-equity#tab=tab_1

Wright, J., Williams, R., & Wilkinson, J. R. (1998). Development and importance of health needs assessment. *BMJ, 316*(7140), 1310–1313. https://doi.org/10.1136/bmj.316.7140.1310

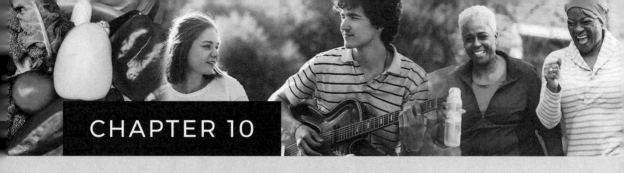

CHAPTER 10

Developing Interprofessional Community-Based Programs

Kendra Hoepper, DNP, APRN, PNP-BC
Carole Zarcone, DNP, APRN, ANP-C
Mary McCormack, DNP, APRN, FNP-C

Alone, we can do so little; together, we can do so much.

Helen Keller

OBJECTIVES

This chapter will enable the reader to:

1. Define Healthy Settings and varied settings for community health promotion programs.
2. Evaluate select conceptual and theoretical models for planning, implementing, and evaluating community health promotion programs.
3. Identify factors contributing to the successful implementation of community health promotion programs.
4. Compare selected community-based lifestyle change programs.
5. Explore the role of the advanced practice provider in community-led, collaborative solutions for advancing health equity and preventing chronic diseases.
6. Evaluate how patient outcomes can be affected by community interventions.

© Kathleen Gail/Shutterstock; © StoryTime Studio/Shutterstock; © kali9/Getty Images

Overview

According to the World Health Organization (WHO), "Health promotion is the process of enabling people to increase control over, and to improve, their health. It moves beyond a focus on individual behavior towards a wide range of social and environmental interventions. As a core function of public health, health promotion supports governments, communities, and individuals to cope with and address health challenges. This is accomplished by building healthy public policies, creating supportive environments, and strengthening community action and personal skills" (WHO, n.d.-a, para. 1–2).

The successful implementation of community health promotion programs depends on numerous factors, such as community engagement, assessment, funding, evidence-based programs, and interprofessional collaboration. Advanced practice providers (APPs) are well equipped to assist a community in performing community needs assessments, identifying vulnerable populations, influencing healthcare policy, and implementing programs that can positively affect community health outcomes. This chapter will discuss several evidence-based programs and frameworks for community health promotion and the factors affecting their success.

Community Health Priorities and Issues

Healthy People 2030 (U.S. Department of Health and Human Services [HHS], n.d.-a) has prioritized public health issues such as cardiovascular diseases, cancers, chronic respiratory diseases, and diabetes, which collectively are responsible for 74% of premature deaths from noncommunicable diseases worldwide (WHO, 2022). These diseases have been primarily driven by the following four major risk factors: tobacco use, physical inactivity, the harmful use of alcohol, and unhealthy diets.

The recent COVID-19 pandemic, in conjunction with these risk factors and the rise in chronic diseases among the aging population, has led to significant health consequences for individuals, families, and communities and has threatened to overwhelm health systems (HHS, n.d.-b). The pandemic has also increased awareness of and exacerbated other public health issues, including disparities in healthcare access and outcomes, social isolation, violence and trauma, and food insecurity (O'Connor, 2020).

The pandemic has also highlighted the importance of clinicians, public health officials, and policymakers to work together to address these issues before another public health disaster hits (Evans et al., 2020). The COVID-19 pandemic resulted in community health promotion initiatives focused on testing, distribution of supplies, and vaccination in a variety of settings, including health departments, clinics, pharmacies, mobile community vans, and college campuses. The pandemic also expanded the use of telehealth services and other innovative strategies to address the community's current and growing healthcare needs.

Healthy Settings for Community Health Promotion

The WHO initiated the Healthy Settings movement in 1980 as a component of its Health for All policy (Healthy Settings, n.d.). The approach was more clearly laid out in the 1986 Ottawa Charter for Health Promotion, which stated that "health is created and lived by people within the settings of their everyday life; where they learn, work, plan, and love" (WHO, 1986, p. 3) and emphasized the importance of health promotion to improve the overall health and well-being of individuals and communities. The charter also emphasized the need for a collaborative and coordinated approach by all stakeholders to improve access to resources and information, health equity, and health outcomes. In 1992, the Sundsvall Statement recommended focusing on settings for health (i.e., supportive environments) to enhance health promotion. The value of settings for comprehensive health promotion was again emphasized in the 1997 Jakarta Declaration (Healthy Settings, n.d.). The Healthy Cities program, which has been adopted by many cities worldwide, is an example of a successful Healthy Settings approach (WHO, n.d.-b).

The WHO defines a *Setting for Health* as "a place or social context in which people engage in daily activities in which environmental, organizational, and personal factors interact to affect their health and wellbeing" (Healthy Settings, n.d., para. 3). This definition broadens the context for health promotion from the clinical setting to include the settings of people's everyday lives. Community health promotion and disease prevention programs can be implemented in various settings, such as healthcare facilities, schools, faith communities, workplaces, community organizations, neighborhoods, and other settings where people live and interact regularly.

Many healthcare facilities, including hospitals, clinics, physician and dental offices, pharmacies, and other healthcare centers, have moved beyond the traditional roles of treating the sick to the role of improving the overall health of their patients and communities. These institutions have reoriented their health care to integrate health promotion and disease prevention. Hospitals have added community wellness programs, such as the AdventHealth Wellness Center and Spa in Celebration, Florida, which includes group fitness classes, personal training, and nutrition and counseling services. The American College of Lifestyle Medicine (www.lifestylemedicine.org) has developed competencies, education, and resources for healthcare providers to integrate a lifestyle medicine approach into their practice settings.

Health promotion in schools and communities is the most widespread settings-based approach with direct links between health and the environment. These settings facilitate the inclusion of best practices in the general community by identifying health issues, risks, and concerns, with a common goal and commitment to building a healthy living environment (WHO, n.d.-a). An example of a health promotion program implemented in a setting for health is an intimate partner violence (IPV) prevention program implemented in a school-based setting. Schools are uniquely positioned to promote the health and safety of the adolescent population and provide youth with interventions to prevent IPV and establish lifelong healthy behaviors. Schools provide a context in which such initiatives can be delivered on a large scale to a captive audience who have yet to experience or are just embarking on their intimate relationships (Stanley et al., 2015). IPV prevention programs are multifaceted due to the multiple factors contributing to the increased risk of IPV. These programs vary in curriculum content and age appropriateness and differentiate between middle school and high school use. A school-linked community program can involve all stakeholders, including parents, school systems, youth group agencies, and faith-based organizations, each of which plays a role in educating adolescents about healthy relationships (Li et al., 2015). Establishing programs in both the school and the community can be beneficial for a multifaceted approach to reducing the prevalence of IPV.

Other examples of health promotion implemented in settings for health include programs offered at college campuses, local community centers, and faith communities, which are often conducted in collaboration with healthcare facilities. Campus-based health promotion initiatives typically include fitness centers, healthy dining options, mental health counseling, and campus-based farmers markets. Informal learning activities focus on healthy eating, exercise, self-care, and self-defense. Community centers offer various health screening and health education programs to all age groups, including exercise, nutrition, and weight loss. In addition, community centers organize various health screenings (e.g., blood pressure, cholesterol), CPR training, and blood drives. In the faith-based setting, programs often include faith community nursing (Westberg Institute for Faith Community Nursing, n.d.), health screenings, blood drives, and food pantries.

The Healthy Settings movement also expands the focus from individual health behaviors to include determinants of health. The Healthy Settings model also works toward improving many risk factors in the community simultaneously. Therefore, it needs a collaborative approach to planning and implementing health promotion programs to achieve and sustain success.

Community Health Promotion Models

Various conceptual models offer guidance for community health promotion interventions. Selecting a community health promotion model that aligns well with the project population and setting can provide structure and insight into program planning, implementation, and evaluation.

Social–Ecological Model of Health

The social–ecological model (SEM) originally developed in 1977 theorized that environmental factors influence every facet of human development and that individuals are essential agents in creating the multiple dimensions of the dynamic environment in which they live (Bronfenbrenner, 1977). Subsequently the SEM has been applied to health, which describes the interactive characteristics of individuals and environments that underlie health outcomes and have been recommended to guide public health practice in implementing preventive strategies and community-based education programs (Golden & Earp, 2012). The SEM demonstrates the connection and interplay among the individual, relationships, community, and society (Bronfenbrenner, 1977). When applied in a health context, this model identifies the multifaceted factors associated with successfully implementing health promotion programs in a community. The overlapping of the rings in the model exemplifies the interconnection and how one component can influence another (see **Figure 10.1**). A thorough understanding of these relationships will be beneficial in developing community health promotion programs.

The characteristics of the *individual* in the SEM include age, gender, ethnicity, race, socioeconomic status, and attitudes and behaviors about health. Prevention strategies at this level include education and life skills training that promote attitudes and behaviors in developing healthy lifestyles. The *relationship* domain consists of formal and informal relationships, such as family, friends, and peers, which can

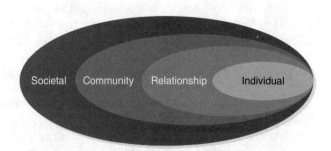

Figure 10.1 Social–ecological model of health.

positively and negatively affect our attitudes and behaviors. The *community* level evaluates environmental influences, including at school and in the workplace. *Societal* effects include cultural, gender, religious, and economic factors. Individuals' health beliefs, attitudes, and engagement in health promotion and disease prevention are influenced by all four domains of the SEM (Bronfenbrenner, 1977).

The SEM has been used to enhance understanding of the social and behavioral responses to infectious disease transmissions, such as HIV, AIDS, and the COVID-19 pandemic, and to guide the treatment and prevention of these diseases (Eaton & Kalichman, 2020). Eaton and Kalichman concluded that the public health approach to addressing COVID-19 is heavily dependent on social and behavioral change strategies to halt transmission. A multilevel intervention approach that includes interpersonal, intrapersonal, community, and societal factors is essential to combat and prevent the spread of disease. However, achieving behavioral change is challenging because individuals often rationalize their choices, whether good or bad, regarding health and are willing to accept some level of risk to continue living their lives (Eaton & Kalichman, 2020). Therefore, getting multiple sectors in society involved in addressing health and environmental issues is key to improving outcomes. Applying the lessons learned from previous public health issues and pandemics can guide the management of future ones. Preventing the worst-case effects of the COVID-19 pandemic can be achieved through intrapersonal, interpersonal, community, and societal levels of data-driven and well-coordinated interventions (Eaton & Kalichman, 2020).

A variation of the SEM, with a public policy domain, has been widely used for health promotion. McLeroy et al. (1998) suggested applying the ecological model for health promotion, which focuses on individual and social environmental factors, as a guide for health promotion interventions directed at changing interpersonal, organizational, community, and public policy. The assumption is that changes in the social environment will produce behavior changes in individuals and vice versa because the support of individual behavior change is essential for implementing environmental changes. Balcázar et al. (2012) used the ecological framework for their HEART Project, which addressed cardiovascular risk factors among Hispanics living near the United States–Mexico border. The outcome of their study acknowledged that a community model of prevention requires a comprehensive approach to community engagement. Moreover, the project's results validated the ecological model for preventing cardiovascular disease in the future of public health promotion.

PRECEDE-PROCEED Model

The principles of the PRECEDE–PROCEED model (PPM), developed for public health, can be applied to community health issues to guide planning, implementing, and evaluating community health promotion initiatives (Green & Kreuter, 1992, 2005). PRECEDE and PROCEED are acronyms used to describe the components of the model. PRECEDE guides the needs assessment and development of interventions and stands for predisposing, reinforcing, and enabling constructs in educational/environmental diagnosis and evaluation. Subsequently, PROCEED guides the implementation and evaluation of interventions and stands for policy, regulatory, and organizational constructs in educational and environmental development. Both have distinct phases that continue to build on one another to successfully implement a community-based intervention and focus on the outcome of the activity (see **Figure 10.2**).

In developing an intervention to address a health or community issue, one must consult with the community, understand and analyze community information, and understand the depth and context of the problem to create an intervention that will bring about the changes

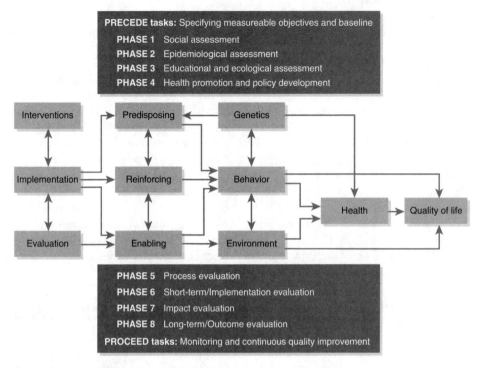

Figure 10.2 PRECEDE–PROCEED model.

the community wants and needs (Green & Kreuter, 2005). Health is more than just physical well-being or the absence of illness; it is a combination of economic, social, political, and physical factors that create a healthy status among individuals and communities. The PPM serves as a theoretical and ethical framework to guide practitioners through the various layers of a SEM of health and remains one of the most used approaches for promoting health (Porter, 2016). In addition to its use in the design, implementation, and evaluation of health promotion programs, the PPM can be used retrospectively in a community-based health program to identify how it can be improved (Johnson et al., 2018).

Social Cognitive Theory and Self-Efficacy

The social cognitive theory (SCT), originally known as the social learning theory, is based on the behavioral approach to social learning. In SCT, behavior is determined by four variables: self-efficacy (belief that a behavior is within one's control), outcome expectations (beliefs about the likely outcomes of the behavior), sociostructural factors (e.g., living conditions or health systems that facilitate or impede the performance of a behavior), and goals (intentions to perform the behavior) (Bandura, 1977) (see **Figure 10.3**). This approach includes both motivational and self-regulatory measures. Human actions result from a belief in one's capability to affect the environment and desired outcomes of their actions. Therefore, a triadic influence exists among the person, behavior, and environment.

An essential assumption of SCT is perceived self-efficacy. According to Bandura (2001), people have the ability or agency to influence their behavior and environment in a purposeful and goal-oriented fashion. Several studies have demonstrated that people with

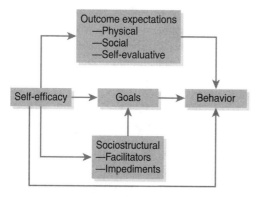

Figure 10.3 Social cognitive theory.

people's ability to transform observations into a usable form for future use. The *production* aspect is where people demonstrate their ability to perform what they have learned. The final aspect of observational learning is the *motivation* to use the new skills learned. For instance, if people perceive the consequences of learned behavior to be negative, they will most likely not be motivated to repeat the behavior (Denler et al., 2009). The SCT is an excellent framework for developing and implementing community-based health programs since it considers the social context of learning and behavior change.

a higher level of self-efficacy have more effective strategy use and better learning outcomes than those with lower perceived self-efficacy. Crapolicchio et al. (2021) identified self-efficacy as an important construct that community and social service organizations can use to develop intervention strategies for victims of IPV and a key to preventing posttraumatic stress disorder. McCarthy and Bianchi (2020) demonstrated that the IPV screening program at a university healthcare clinic was related to a positive change in healthcare providers' knowledge, attitudes, and self-efficacy of IPV screening. These studies underscore the importance of emphasizing self-efficacy in community health initiatives.

Observational learning is another crucial concept in the SCT. Bandura proposed a reciprocal relationship among observational learning/modeling, perceived self-efficacy, outcome expectations, goal setting, self-regulation, and health behavior change. In this process, learning or modeling results from observation of behavior and its consequences on the environment. The observations can be verbal, written, or video or audio recordings (Denler et al., 2009; Stajkovic & Luthans, 1979). The SCT suggests that observational learning depends on four factors: attention, retention, production, and motivation. Of these four factors, *attention* is the most critical; people must attend to the model and behaviors to learn. *Retention* is

Community Health Assessment

Most frameworks or models for community health promotion include an initial step of conducting a community health assessment. A community health assessment is a territorial health assessment that identifies critical health needs and issues through systematic and comprehensive data collection and analysis. The community health assessment focuses on evidence-based population-wide interventions with a targeted focus on addressing disparities, increasing community engagement, and improving health outcomes (Centers for Disease Control and Prevention [CDC], 2018b). The Public Health Accreditation Board (2011) defines *community health assessment* as "a systematic examination of the health status indicators for a given population that is used to identify key problems and assets in a community" (p. 8). The information from a community health assessment is used to identify the community's current health status and needs, develop effective strategies to address needs, and allocate resources (CDC, 2018b). Community health assessments use various tools and methods, but two essential components are community engagement and collaborative participation. APPs with expertise in health promotion and disease prevention are uniquely positioned to collaborate in the community health assessment process and facilitate strategic planning and implementation of interventions to improve the community's overall health.

Community Engagement

Community engagement is essential for all community-based health promotion programs. According to the WHO (2020, p. vii), community engagement is "a process of developing relationships that enable stakeholders to work together to address health-related issues and promote well-being to achieve positive health impact and outcomes." Community engagement begins during the planning phase of a health promotion program. When the purpose or goal of the health program is identified, the program development should be driven by an understanding of community culture; economic conditions; and government structures, values, and norms. It is important to consider what made earlier health promotion programs successful or not (WHO, 2020). Community trust is the building block of a successful health promotion program and community engagement. Community leaders can assist in improving community engagement, identifying resources, and making decisions to meet the community's needs.

The WHO recognizes five levels of community engagement, or participation: inform, consult, involve, collaborate, and empower. The purpose of *informing* is to disseminate information to the community while providing a communication channel (WHO, 2020). Community engagement is fostered by social mobilization through various venues such as health promotion posters, leaflets, and television and radio advertisements. It is also crucial to ensure that information shared is culturally appropriate. Increasing residents' awareness of the potential health issues and risks in their community and possible ways to mitigate these risks could influence them to act and participate in health promotion programs within their community.

Consulting is the next step to ensure community engagement. The community provides feedback on initial activities and develops connections between the community and the partner organizations during this level. Increased community participation in health promotion and community partnerships is established during the *involved* level. The partner organizations and the community work together to develop solutions at the *collaboration* level, and partnership trust is enforced. Finally, a strong partnership is formed between the community and the partner organizations in the *empowerment* process, and more extensive health promotion programs to improve community outcomes are developed (WHO, 2020).

Health Promotion Research Study

Community Engagement and the Diabetes Prevention Program

Background: Although it is well documented that the prevalence of type 2 diabetes is more prominent in minority communities, male participation in community lifestyle modification programs, such as the Diabetes Prevention Program (DPP), remains low.

Methodology: To increase the involvement of males residing in predominantly minority communities, the researchers of the Power Up for Health pilot study adapted the DPP to be more appealing. During the initial planning phase, researchers followed a community-based participatory research framework. They invited community leaders and experts in men's health to provide input into the proposed program. The next phase of the planning involved training laypersons to become DPP lifestyle coaches. Recruitment involved community outreach. Incentives such as a free six-month membership to the recreation center, calorie-counting books, pedometers, and measuring utensils were provided to participants.

Results: Twenty-nine participants enrolled in the Power Up for Health program, with 25 participants completing the 16-week program. Results revealed a modest overall weight loss at the 16-week evaluation (4% weight loss). Participants reported improved healthy eating habits, increased physical activity, and decreased depressive symptoms.

Implications for Advanced Practice: The DPP is a well-studied evidence-based lifestyle modification program. However, it is not a one-size-fits-all program. Repeated studies have indicated low enrollment in ethnic minority males. An adaptation of the program is needed to improve the participation of males residing in diverse communities. Many programs that professional organizations create have core components that may not be adapted. Nevertheless, there is often room for programs to be tailored to suit the needs of individual communities.

Reference: Gary-Webb, T. L., Walker, E. A., Realmuto, L., Kamler, A., Lukin, J., Tyson, W., Carrasquillo, O., & Weiss, L. (2018). Translation of the National Diabetes Prevention Program to engage men in disadvantaged neighborhoods in New York City: A description of Power Up for Health. *American Journal of Men's Health*, *12*(4), 998–1006. https://doi.org/10.1177/1557988318758788

Gary-Webb, T. L., Walker, E. A., Realmuto, L., Kamler, A., Lukin, J., Tyson, W., Carrasquillo, O., & Weiss, L. (2018). Translation of the National Diabetes Prevention Program to engage men in disadvantaged neighborhoods in New York City: A description of Power Up for Health. *American Journal of Men's Health*, *12*(4), 998–1006. https://doi.org/10.1177/1557988318758788

Community-Based Lifestyle Change Programs

Community-based lifestyle change programs are an effective strategy for improving individual and community health outcomes. *Lifestyle change programs* include wellness-focused interventions and information designed to help individuals learn the importance of a healthy lifestyle and strategies to reduce their health risks. Lifestyle change programs have been proven successful tools for improving individual and community health. In addition to improving health outcomes, these programs can be cost effective. A study conducted by Trust for America's Health (2009), titled Prevention for a Healthier America, found that investing $10 per person per year in proven community-based programs to increase physical activity, improve nutrition, and prevent smoking and other tobacco use could save the country more than $16 billion annually within five years. Out of the $16 billion in savings, Medicare could save more than $5 billion, Medicaid could save more than $1.9 billion, and private payers could save more than $9 billion.

Following is a description of a few selected government- and private-funded community-based lifestyle change programs and initiatives that have influenced health outcomes and reduced the burden of disease. APPs can refer at-risk patients to these programs and become involved in implementing these or similar programs in their communities.

Racial and Ethnic Approach to Community Health

A guiding principle in public health is that every person should reach their full health potential regardless of age, sex, race, or ethnicity (CDC, n.d.). The CDC developed the Racial and Ethnic Approaches to Community Health (REACH) in 1999 to remove healthcare barriers. Over the past 20 years, local and state health departments, universities, and other community organizations have been awarded funding to develop and support culturally appropriate programs to address racial and ethnic health disparities.

The REACH program focuses on chronic diseases such as hypertension, type 2 diabetes, heart disease, and obesity. Organizations utilize REACH funding to develop interventional programs to reduce chronic disease risk factors such as obesity, tobacco abuse, poor nutrition, and physical activity (CDC, n.d.). One example of a community REACH program is the Alabama REACH 2010 Breast and Cervical Cancer Coalition, which created a community action plan to address the barriers that prevent African American women aged 40 or older from receiving breast and cervical cancer screening services (CDC, 2007). The intervention outcomes included a decrease in disparity in mammography screening between African American and White women from 17% to 11%. Reducing risk factors and narrowing healthcare disparities gaps can significantly improve the overall health of minority communities (CDC, n.d.).

Wisewoman

Well-Integrated Screening and Evaluation for Women Across the Nation (WISEWOMAN) is a program developed by the CDC in 2008 to reduce women's risk of heart disease and stroke. The program provides risk screening for women ages 40 to 64 who are uninsured, underinsured, or low income. In addition to the screenings, women can receive counseling regarding their risk of heart disease and stroke and participate in evidence-based lifestyle modification programs that promote lifelong heart-healthy lifestyles (CDC, 2020).

An example of a WISEWOMAN program in Vermont is Ladies First, which provides participants with coupons to purchase locally grown fruits and vegetables (CDC, 2018a). During the program's first season, women were given coupons for use at local farmers markets. Women were also encouraged to start their own gardens. Seventy-five percent of participants reported eating more fresh fruits and vegetables during the growing season and planned to continue healthier eating all year round.

National Diabetes Prevention Program

To address the burden diabetes places on the healthcare system, the CDC (2021a) developed the Diabetes Prevention Program (DPP) in 2010. This program is a collaborative effort between the public and the private sectors, offering communities cost-effective, evidence-based lifestyle change programs geared toward reducing the incidence of type 2 diabetes. The goal of the DPP is to make quality, affordable, and effective lifestyle change programs available to the community. Interventions include individual case management, frequent contact over the entire trial, a structured 16-session initial core curriculum, and additional individualized maintenance programming. Hundreds of DPP programs teach participants to prevent or delay the progression of type 2 diabetes by eating healthier, increasing physical activity, and improving coping skills. To ensure high-quality programs, CDC-recognized lifestyle change programs need to meet three standards: an approved curriculum, facilitation by a trained lifestyle coach, and submission of data every six months to demonstrate that the program has a positive effect (CDC, 2021b).

The DPP has demonstrated effectiveness in preventing or delaying the onset of type 2 diabetes. The DPP Lifestyle Intervention Study found a 58% reduction in the incidence rate of diabetes with intensive lifestyle intervention and a 31% reduction with metformin compared with participants who took a placebo (Diabetes Prevention Program Research Group, 2002). The ongoing DPP Outcomes Study has found that prediabetes participants were still one-third less likely to develop type 2 diabetes 10 years later than individuals who took a placebo and those who developed type 2 diabetes delayed its onset by four years (Diabetes Prevention Program Research Group et al., 2009).

Complete Health Improvement Program

The Complete Health Improvement Program (CHIP) was developed in 1986 by Diehl to improve chronic disease outcomes and associated risk factors (Morton et al., 2016). The 12-week CHIP program (recently redesigned as Pivio) provides a comprehensive framework for participants to pivot away from chronic disease and toward optimal health. The CHIP program has been utilized over the past 35 years in many clinical, corporate, and community settings. Multiple large cohort-based implementation studies using the CHIP program in Rockford, Illinois, demonstrated significant reductions in participant body weight, improved lipid panels, and lower blood sugar levels. In addition to improved lifestyle choices and risk factor reduction, implementation of the CHIP program has been noted to decrease overall healthcare expenditures. A study conducted by Vanderbilt University revealed a 43% reduction in medical service use in type 2 diabetic employees enrolled in the CHIP program compared to a 13% increase in medical service utilization and a 10% increase in medication costs in those employees not enrolled in the program (Morton et al., 2016). In another cohort study, 44% of the diabetic participants taking oral diabetic medications and 42% of the insulin-dependent diabetic participants were instructed by their healthcare providers to decrease their daily medication dosages (Morton et al., 2016).

Measuring and Evaluating Health Outcomes

The process of measuring and evaluating community health outcomes is different from assessing patient-specific outcomes. Prior to implementing community health interventions, baseline metrics should be evaluated (Zaccagnini & White, 2011). Data regarding community health indices can be found in large population-based data sets accessed from governmental agencies and local health departments. To measure progress, benchmarking data from the outset of the project must be evaluated. *Healthy People 2030* (HHS, n.d.-a) and the National Health and Nutrition Examination Survey (NHANES) (CDC, 2022) are easy-to-access, evidence-based resources that provide benchmarking data on multiple key health indices.

Healthy People 2030 (HHS, n.d.-a) has created a list of objectives and goals to improve the nation's health over the next decade. The program provides key metrics related to disease prevalence and then strategically sets goals to achieve them. For example, diabetes prevention and management are areas in which community interventions can have a significant positive effect. Baseline metrics from *Healthy People 2030* indicate that 6.5 new cases of diabetes were diagnosed annually per 1,000 adults aged 18 to 84 during the years 2015 through 2018. The target is to reduce the incidence of new cases to 5.6 cases per 1,000 adults by 2030 (HHS, n.d.-c). There are multiple avenues available to attain this goal. One strategy would be implementing community-based primary prevention programs, such as the DPP, that emphasize the importance of lifestyle modifications to delay and prevent the onset of diabetes (Ely et al., 2017).

It is well documented in the literature that the rate of diabetes-associated complications increases significantly as hemoglobin A1C levels rise (Laiteerapong et al., 2017). Data from the NHANES report show that between 2013 and 2016, 18.7% of diabetics 18 years old and older had a hemoglobin A1C level >9% (CDC, 2022). The goal of *Healthy People 2030* is to reduce the percentage of individuals 18 years old and older with hemoglobin A1C levels >9% to 11.6% over the next decade (HHS, n.d.-d). Ethnic minorities are disproportionately affected by diabetes, and community interventions aimed at assisting individuals in obtaining glycemic control can be instrumental in achieving this goal (CDC, 2017). Secondary prevention programs offered through various professional organizations, such as the American Diabetes Association, emphasize diabetes self-management education and have been noted to help individuals obtain glycemic control and decrease the chance of developing long-term diabetes-associated complications.

Health Promotion Case Study Community Health Programs

Case Description: An APP employed at an urban university health center noticed an increase in students reporting IPV. The practitioner conducted a literature review to understand IPV better. The data revealed that one out of every four women and almost one out of every seven men had experienced some form of IPV, with an increased incidence noted in ethnic minorities (Smith et al., 2017). As the APP dove deeper into the literature, it was revealed that IPV occurs across the life span, often starting in early adolescence. Further inquiry revealed inconsistencies in practitioners' comfort level discussing IPV and varying screening processes. The literature also identified that proper education and training improve the healthcare providers' understanding of IPV, ability to recognize symptoms, and self-efficacy and comfort in screening. Liebschutz and Rothman (2012) suggested that all healthcare providers be alert to aspects of patients' histories or symptoms that could indicate IPV. Screening asymptomatic female patients may prove beneficial with minimal adverse effects. Implementing a comprehensive program would be most beneficial and should consist of effective screening tools, thorough initial and continuing education and training, and institutional support.

To understand the current screening practices at the health center, the APP met with the clinical staff and had an open discussion regarding the standard of care for IPV screening at the health center. The discussion revealed multiple inconsistencies in provider IPV screening practices, and it was then determined that a standardized IPV screening tool should be used with each patient encounter. Providers' use of a clinically focused assessment strategy could enhance consistency in screening for IPV. Davila et al. (2013) examined the use of RADAR, a clinically focused screening strategy utilized by APPs as part of routine care, and found that it enhanced the effectiveness in addressing IPV against women. RADAR consists of the following: routinely assessing every woman at every health encounter; asking directly about IPV; documenting positive suspected IPV; assessing immediate safety; and responding, reviewing options, and referring as needed.

After implementing the RADAR screening tool, multiple staff members expressed interest in obtaining additional IPV training and certification. Providing initial and ongoing training and education to all healthcare providers on the incidence and prevalence of IPV and implementing a universal screening and clinically focused tool like RADAR could benefit healthcare providers and patients. The next steps at this health center included further education and training on IPV.

Soon after becoming certified IPV educators, the health center clinicians felt compelled to do more and decided to expand their efforts to increase awareness of IPV in the community. They researched several evidence-based community education programs, decided on the Katie Brown Educational Program (KBEP), and completed additional training specific to this program. After obtaining permission from the program director, they began offering community education and training on IPV at local high schools, college campuses, community centers, and faith-based outreach programs using the Katie Brown Educational Program. They plan to conduct a research study on the effectiveness of the program.

Katie Brown Educational Program (KBEP): This program started in 2001 and is a brief four-session program using a group-based curriculum that has been implemented with success in Massachusetts and Rhode Island. The sessions are designed to deliver information in a classroom setting, with 50–60 minutes for each session, and to accommodate up to 35 students at one time (Joppa et al., 2016). The philosophy behind the program is that all young people could benefit from age-appropriate relationship violence prevention education to help them understand and build healthy relationships from childhood into adulthood.

The KBEP curriculum uses the social cognitive theory as its framework. Lessons are aimed at modifying cognitions (dating attitudes, expectations, and knowledge) and behaviors (conflict resolution and communication skills) to assist students in developing healthy relationships (Joppa et al., 2016). The curriculum employs various teaching methods, including lectures, group discussions, individual activities, handouts, self-reflection exercises, videos, and PowerPoint presentations. The school KBEPs are age appropriate and designed for students in fourth grade through high school. There are several additional or affiliated programs: summer camps, college Relationship and Sexual Violence Prevention Program (RSVP), professional development workshops, parent workshops, and adult programs.

The KBEP is a primary prevention program designed to serve as a resource for school districts and community organizations with the main goal of improving awareness, attitudes, and beliefs among adolescents and adults. Several concepts in the KBEP are like other evidence-based programs, such as Safe Dates. However, the KBEP age-appropriate, skill-based curriculum was developed in the community, is brief, and provides the tools and information to develop and sustain healthy relationships (Joppa et al., 2016).

Critical Thinking Questions

- How can resources available in your community improve outcomes for victims of IPV?
- Evaluate the research and evidence to support using a standardized screening tool in your practice and the positive effect it can have on patient outcomes.
- Identify the key stakeholders for designing and implementing a successful IPV educational program in the community.
- What are the important aspects of the KBEP that contribute to its effectiveness?

References

Davila, Y., Mendias, E. P., & Juneau, C. (2013). Under the RADAR: Assessing and interviewing intimate partner violence. *Journal of Nurse Practitioners, 9*(9), 594–599. https://doi.org/10.1016/j.nurpra.2013.05.022

Joppa, M. C., Rizzo, C. J., Nieves, A. V., & Brown, L. K. (2016). Pilot investigation of the Katie Brown Educational Program: A school-community partnership. *Journal of School Health, 86*(4), 288–297. https://doi.org/10.1111/josh.12378

Liebschutz, J., & Rothman, E. F. (2012). Intimate-partner violence: What physicians can do. *New England Journal of Medicine, 367*(22), 2071–2073. https://doi.org//10.1056/NEJMp1204278

Smith, S. G., Chen, J., Basile, K. C., Gilbert, L. K., Merrick, M. T., Patel, N., Walling, M., & Jain, A. (2017). *The National Intimate Partner and Sexual Violence Survey (NISVS): 2010–2012 state report.* Centers for Disease Control and Prevention. https://www.cdc.gov/violenceprevention/pdf/nisvs-statereportbook.pdf

Interprofessional Collaboration for Community Health Promotion

The *Healthy People 2030* initiative has created various health improvement goals to improve the overall health of U.S. citizens over the next decade. However, these goals cannot be accomplished by any individual or group. An effective means of achieving these goals is via the collective impact approach. *Collective impact* refers to the process in which a network of community members, organizations, and institutions collaborate to achieve population- and systems-level change (Collective Impact Forum, n.d.).

One example of collective impact is the shift over the past decade toward interprofessional education and collaborative practice (WHO, 2010). Interprofessional collaboration is commonly described within the healthcare setting as a team-based approach to patient care. Traditionally, primary care providers refer their patients to members of other healthcare disciplines (e.g., physicians, medical specialists, behavioral health practitioners, APPs, pharmacists, dietitians, exercise specialists, and social workers) to prevent and address patient health concerns. These healthcare professionals, with diverse knowledge and skills see patients through their unique perspectives. The team delivers high-quality care through data sharing and effective communication, improving the patients' health and well-being.

Interprofessional collaboration is also key to delivering effective community health promotion. The collaboration may look different depending on the demographics of the community, the health needs to be addressed, and the scope of the initiative. The WHO (2010, p. 7) defined *interprofessional collaborative practice* as when "workers from different professional backgrounds provide comprehensive services by working with patients, their families, careers, and communities to deliver the highest quality of care across settings." Although written in the context of healthcare delivery, this definition can be applied to community health promotion. Without the unique knowledge base, skill set, and perspectives of various individuals and community entities, it is impossible to fully understand or address the broader health needs of individuals and communities. Interprofessional community-based programs can improve coordination between different sectors and access to health interventions for individuals and their families (World Health Professions Alliance, n.d.). APP academic programs have started to emphasize interprofessional education, preparing future clinicians to collaborate effectively with other professions to achieve a common goal: improve the health of patients, families, and communities.

Across the country, numerous grassroots organizations share that goal. Many of these organizations are spearheaded by local healthcare workers, faith community leaders, and community advocates. The structures of these organizations vary, with many of them having medical advisory boards composed of medical experts and leading researchers. Their collaborative efforts are geared toward improving the overall health of communities by providing education, health fairs, and screening programs. The Healthiest Cities and Counties Challenge (www.healthiestcities.org) provides examples of community-led, collaborative solutions for advancing health equity and preventing chronic diseases. The APP's knowledge of community health promotion models, assessment and evaluation methods, and evidence-based programs enables them to engage with their community and collaborate toward implementing healthcare policy changes at the local, state, and national levels.

Health Promotion Activity: Effect of Community Interventions on Health Outcomes

Identify a health issue in your patient population or community. Then review the National Center for Chronic Disease Prevention and Health Promotion Success Stories Library at https://nccd.cdc .gov/nccdsuccessstories/searchstories.aspx for creative ways that communities have addressed this issue. How did the community apply concepts in this chapter to improve health outcomes? How might a similar intervention in your community affect patient outcomes?

Summary

Lifestyle-driven chronic disease, disparities in healthcare access and outcomes, social isolation, violence, and food insecurity are priorities for public health initiatives. These can often be best addressed in healthy community settings where people live and interact regularly. Conceptual models such as the social–ecological model, PRECEDE–PROCEED, and social cognitive theory can guide community health promotion initiatives. Selecting a model that aligns well with the population, setting, and goals can provide structure and insight into the program.

Several factors can affect the success of community health promotion programs. Successful health promotion programs are formed through community engagement and collaboration. The program's goals should reflect the community's needs and provide evidence-based solutions tailored to its resources, values, and norms. Various evidence-based lifestyle change programs successfully implemented across the country are available via the CDC and WHO websites. See **Table 10.1** for additional

TABLE 10.1	Evidence-Based Resources for Community Health Promotion
Resource	**URL**
Community Tool Box	https://ctb.ku.edu/en
Community Health Assessment and Group Evaluation (CHANGE) Tool	https://www.cdc.gov/nccdphp/dnpao/state-local-programs/change-tool/index.html
National Diabetes Prevention Program (DPP)	https://www.cdc.gov/diabetes/prevention/index.html
Healthiest Cities and Counties Challenge	http://www.healthiestcities.org
Healthy People 2030	https://health.gov/healthypeople
Katie Brown Educational Program	https://kbep.org/program
National Center for Chronic Disease Prevention and Health Promotion Success Stories Library	https://nccd.cdc.gov/nccdsuccessstories/searchstories.aspx
National Health and Nutrition Examination Survey	https://www.cdc.gov/nchs/nhanes/index.htm
Pivio (was Complete Health Improvement Program)	https://piviohealth.com
Racial and Ethnic Approaches to Community Health (REACH)	https://www.cdc.gov/nccdphp/dnpao/state-local-programs/reach/index.htm
WISEWOMAN	https://www.cdc.gov/wisewoman/index.htm
World Economic Forum Healthy Cities and Communities Playbook	https://www.weforum.org/whitepapers/healthy-cities-and-communities-playbook
World Health Professions Alliance	https://www.whpa.org

community health promotion resources. Interprofessional collaboration with a collective impact approach is integral to achieving common goals. APPs are experts in translational research and are well suited to applying the most up-to-date evidence to improve individual, community, and population health.

Acronyms

APP: advanced practice provider
CDC: Centers for Disease Control and Prevention
CHIP: Complete Health Improvement Program
DPP: Diabetes Prevention Program
IPV: intimate partner violence
KBEP: Katie Brown Educational Program
NHANES: National Health and Nutrition Examination Survey

PPM: PRECEDE–PROCEED model
REACH: Racial and Ethnic Approaches to Community Health
SCT: social cognitive theory
SEM: social–ecological model
WHO: World Health Organization
WISEWOMAN: Well-Integrated Screening and Evaluation for Women Across the Nation

References

Balcázar H., Wise, S., Rosenthal, E. L., Ochoa, C., Rodriguez, J., Hastings, D., Flores, L., Hernandez, L., & Duarte-Gardea, M. (2012). An ecological model using promotores de salud to prevent cardiovascular disease on the US-Mexico border: The HEART Project. *Preventing Chronic Disease, 9*, 110. http://dx.doi.org/10.5888/pcd9.110100

Bandura, A. (1977). Self-efficacy: Toward a unifying theory of behavioral change. *Psychological Review, 84*, 191–215. https://doi.org/10.1037/0033-295X.84.2.191

Bandura, A. (2001). Social cognitive theory: An agentic perspective. *Annual Review of Psychology, 52*, 1–26. https://doi.org/10.1146/annurev.psych.52.1.1

Bronfenbrenner, U. (1977). Toward an experimental ecology of human development. *American Psychologist, 32*, 513–531. https://doi.org/10.1037/0003-066X.32.7.513

Centers for Disease Control and Prevention. (n.d.). *REACH.* Retrieved May 15, 2022, from https://www.cdc.gov/chronicdisease/resources/publications/factsheets/reach.htm

Centers for Disease Control and Prevention. (2007). *The power to reduce health disparities: Voices from REACH communities.* https://stacks.cdc.gov/view/cdc/12109/cdc_12109_DS1.pdf

Centers for Disease Control and Prevention. (2017). *Communities succeed at creating healthier environments.* https://www.cdc.gov/nccdphp/dch/programs/healthycommunitiesprogram/evaluation-innovation/successes.htm

Centers for Disease Control and Prevention. (2018a). *Access to fresh fruits and vegetables for better nutrition.* https://www.cdc.gov/wisewoman/vermont-farmers-markets.htm

Centers for Disease Control and Prevention. (2018b). *Community health assessments and health improvement plans.* https://www.cdc.gov/publichealthgateway/cha/plan.html

Centers for Disease Control and Prevention. (2020). *WISEWOMAN.* https://www.cdc.gov/wisewoman/index.htm

Centers for Disease Control and Prevention. (2021a). *About the National DPP.* https://www.cdc.gov/diabetes/prevention/about.htm

Centers for Disease Control and Prevention. (2021b). *Requirements for CDC recognition.* https://www.cdc.gov/diabetes/prevention/requirements-recognition.htm

Centers for Disease Control and Prevention. (2022). *National Health and Nutrition Examination Survey.* http://www.cdc.gov/nchs/nhanes.htm

Collective Impact Forum. (n.d.). *What is collective impact?* Retrieved May 15, 2022, from https://collectiveimpactforum.org/what-is-collective-impact

Crapolicchio, E., Vezzali, L., & Regalia, C. (2021). "I forgive myself": The association between self-criticism, self-acceptance, and PTSD in women victims of IPV, and the buffering role of self-efficacy. *Journal of Community Psychology, 49*(2), 252–265. https://doi.org/10.1002/jcop.22454

Davila, Y., Mendias, E. P., & Juneau, C. (2013). Under the RADAR: Assessing and intervening for intimate partner violence. *Journal of Nurse Practitioners, 9*(9), 594–599. https://doi.org/10.1016/j.nurpra.2013.05.022

Denler, H., Wolters, C., & Benzon, M. (2009). *Social cognitive theory.* https://project542.weebly.com/uploads/1/7/1/0/17108470/social_cognitive_theory__education.com.pdf

Diabetes Prevention Program Research Group. (2002). The Diabetes Prevention Program (DPP): Description of lifestyle intervention. *Diabetes Care*, 25(12), 2165–2171. https://doi.org/10.2337/diacare.25.12.2165

Diabetes Prevention Program Research Group, Knowler, W. C., Fowler, S. E., Hamman, R. F., Christophi, C. A., Hoffman, H. J., Brenneman, A. T., Brown-Friday, J. O., Goldberg, R., Venditti, E., & Nathan, D. M. (2009). 10-Year follow-up of diabetes incidence and weight loss in the Diabetes Prevention Program Outcomes Study. *The Lancet*, 374(9702), 1677–1686. https://doi.org/10.1016/S0140-6736(09)61457-4

Eaton, L. A., & Kalichman, S. C. (2020). Social and behavioral health responses to COVID-19: Lessons learned from four decades of an HIV pandemic. *Journal of Behavioral Medicine*, 43, 341–345. https://doi.org/10.1007/s10865-020-00157-y

Ely, E. K., Gruss, S. M., Luman, E. T., Gregg, E. W., Ali, M. K., Nhim, K., Rolka, D. B., & Albright, A. L. (2017). A national effort to prevent type 2 diabetes: Participant-level evaluation of CDC's National Diabetes Prevention Program. *Diabetes Care*, 40(10), 1331–1341. https://doi.org/10.2337/dc16-2099

Evans, M. L., Lindauer, M., & Farrell, M. E. (2020). A pandemic within a pandemic—Intimate partner violence during Covid-19. *New England Journal of Medicine*, 383, 2302–2304. https://www.nejm.org/doi/full/10.1056/NEJMp2024046

French, D. P., & Wright, J. D. (2015). Self-efficacy and health. In International encyclopedia of the social and behavioral sciences (pp. 509-514). Elsevier BV.

Gary-Webb, T. L., Walker, E. A., Realmuto, L., Kamler, A., Lukin, J., Tyson, W., Carrasquillo, O., & Weiss, L. (2018). Translation of the National Diabetes Prevention Program to engage men in disadvantaged neighborhoods in New York City: A description of Power Up for Health. *American Journal of Men's Health*, 12(4), 998–1006. https://doi.org/10.1177/1557988318758788

Golden, S. D., & Earp, J. E. (2012). Social ecological approaches to individuals and their contexts: Twenty years of health education and behavior health promotion interventions. *Health Education & Behavior*, 39(3), 364–372. https://doi.org/10.1177/1090198111418634

Green, L. W., & Kreuter, M. W. (1992). CDC's planned approach to community health as an application of PRECEED and an inspiration for PROCEED. *Journal of Health Education*, 23(3), 140–147. https://doi.org/10.1080/10556699.1992.10616277

Green, L. W., & Kreuter, M. W. (2005). *Health program planning: An educational and ecological approach* (4th ed.). McGraw-Hill Higher Education.

Healthy Settings. (n.d.). *Settings-based health promotion. Retrieved May 31, 2023, from* http://www.healthysettings.org

Johnson, O., Pintauro, S., Brock, D., & Bertmann, F. (2018). Application of the PRECEDE-PROCEED model for community program evaluation. *Journal of the Academy of Nutrition and Dietetics*, 118(9), Supplement A66. https://doi.org/10.1016/j.jand.2018.06.028

Joppa, M. C., Rizzo, C. J., Nieves, A. V., & Brown, L. K. (2016). Pilot investigation of the Katie Brown Educational Program: A school-community partnership. *Journal of School Health*, 86(4), 288–297. https://doi.org/10.1111/josh.12378

Laiteerapong, N., Karter, A., Moffet, H., Cooper, J., Gibbons, R., Liu, J., Gao, Y., & Huang, E. S. (2017). Ten-year hemoglobin A1c trajectories and outcomes in type 2 diabetes mellitus: The Diabetes and Aging Study. *Journal of Diabetes and Its Complications*, 31(1), 94–100. https://doi.org/10.1016/j.jdiacomp.2016.07.023

Li, E., Freedman, L. R., Fernandez, E., Garcia, Y., & Miller, E. (2015). Exploring the role of faith-based organizations and addressing adolescent relationship abuse. *Violence Against Women*, 22(5), 609–624. https://doi.org/10.1177/1077801215608702

Liebschutz, J., & Rothman, E. F. (2012). Intimate-partner violence: What physicians can do. *New England Journal of Medicine*, 367(22), 2071–2073. https://doi.org/10.1056/NEJMp1204278

McCarthy, J., & Bianchi, A. (2020). Implementation of an intimate partner violence screening program in a university health care clinic. *Journal of American College Health*, 68(4), 444–452. https://doi.org/10.1080/07448481.2019.1577864

McLeroy, K. R., Bibeau, D., Steckler, A., & Glanz, K. (1998). An ecological perspective on health promotion programs. *Health Education Quarterly*, 15(4), 351–377. https://doi.org/10.1177/109019818801500401

Morton, D., Rankin, P., Kent, L., & Dysinger, W. (2016). The Complete Health Improvement Program (CHIP): History, evaluation, and outcomes. *American Journal of Lifestyle Medicine*, 10(1), 64–73. https://doi.org/10.1177/1559827614531391

O'Connor, S. W. (2020). *4 key public health issues in 2020*. Northeastern University. https://www.northeastern.edu/graduate/blog/public-health-issues

Porter, C. M. (2016). Revisiting Precede–Proceed: A leading model for ecological and ethical health promotion. *Health Education Journal*, 75(6), 753–764. https://doi.org/10.1177/0017896915619645

Public Health Accreditation Board. (2011). *Acronyms and glossary of terms* (Version 1.0). https://www.phaboard.org/wp-content/uploads/PHAB-Acronyms-and-Glossary-of-Terms-Version-1.02.pdf

Smith, S. G., Chen, J., Basile, K. C., Gilbert, L. K., Merrick, M. T., Patel, N., Walling, M., & Jain, A. (2017). *The National Intimate Partner and Sexual Violence Survey (NISVS): 2010-2012 state report*. Centers for Disease Control and Prevention. https://www.cdc.gov/violenceprevention/pdf/nisvs-statereportbook.pdf

Stajkovic, A. D., & Luthans, F. (1979). Social cognitive theory and self-efficacy: Implications for motivation theory and practice. In R. M. Steers, L. W. Porter, & G. A. Bigley (Eds.), *Motivation and work behavior* (7th ed., pp. 126–140). McGraw-Hill.

Stanley, N., Ellis, J., Farrelly, N., Hollinghurst, S., & Downe, S. (2015). Preventing domestic abuse for children and young people: A review of school-based interventions. *Children and Youth Services Review, 59*, 120–131. https://doi.org/10.1016/j.childyouth.2015.10.018

Trust for America's Health. (2009). *Prevention for a healthier America: Investments in disease prevention yield significant savings, stronger communities.* https://www.tfah.org/report-details/prevention-for-a-healthier-america

U.S. Department of Health and Human Services. (n.d.-a). *Healthy People 2030: Building a healthier future for all.* Retrieved May 15, 2022, from https://health.gov/healthypeople

U.S. Department of Health and Human Services. (n.d.-b). *Healthy People 2030: Emergency preparedness.* Retrieved May 15, 2022, from https://health.gov/healthypeople/objectives-and-data/browse-objectives/emergency-preparedness

U.S. Department of Health and Human Services. (n.d.-c). *Reduce the number of diabetes cases diagnosed yearly— D-01.* Retrieved May 15, 2022, from https://health.gov/healthypeople/objectives-and-data/browse-objectives/diabetes/reduce-number-diabetes-cases-diagnosed-yearly-d-01

U.S. Department of Health and Human Services. (n.d.-d). *Reduce the proportion of adults with diabetes who have an A1c value above 9 percent—D-03.* Retrieved May 15, 2022, from https://health.gov/healthypeople/objectives-and-data/browse-objectives/diabetes/reduce-proportion-adults-diabetes-who-have-a1c-value-above-9-percent-d-03

Westberg Institute for Faith Community Nursing. (n.d.). *What is faith community nursing?* Retrieved May 11, 2022, from https://westberginstitute.org/faith-community-nursing

World Health Organization. (n.d.-a). *Health promotion.* Retrieved March 26, 2022, from https://www.who.int/westernpacific/about/how-we-work/programmes/health-promotion

World Health Organization. (n.d.-b). *Creating healthy cities.* Retrieved May 15, 2022, from https://www.who.int/activities/creating-healthy-cities

World Health Organization. (1986). *Ottawa Charter for Health Promotion: First International Conference on Health Promotion Ottawa, 21 November 1986.* https://www.healthpromotion.org.au/images/ottawa_charter_hp.pdf

World Health Organization. (2010). *Framework for action on interprofessional education and collaborative practice.* https://www.who.int/publications/i/item/framework-for-action-on-interprofessional-education-collaborative-practice

World Health Organization. (2020). *Community engagement: A health promotion guide for universal health coverage in the hands of the people.* https://www.who.int/publications/i/item/9789240010529

World Health Organization. (2022, September 16). *Noncommunicable diseases.* https://www.who.int/news-room/fact-sheets/detail/noncommunicable-diseases

World Health Professions Alliance. (n.d.). *Interprofessional collaborative practice.* Retrieved May 31, 2023, from https://www.whpa.org/activities/interprofessional-collaborative-practice#_ftn1

Zaccagnini, M. E., & White, K. W. (2011). *The doctor of nursing practice essentials: A new model for advanced practice nursing.* Jones & Bartlett Learning.

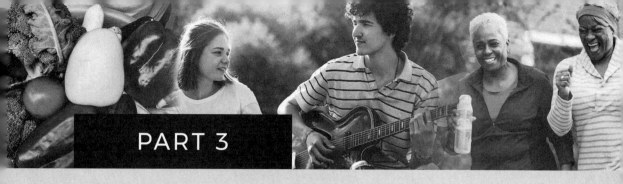

PART 3

A-SMART Lifestyle Prescriptions for Health Promotion

© Kathleen Gail/Shutterstock; © StoryTime Studio/Shutterstock; © kali9/Getty Images

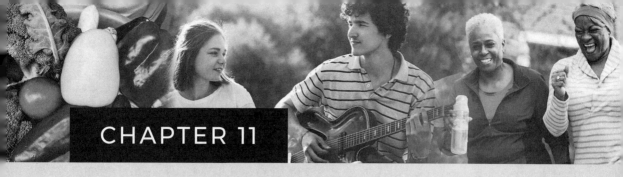

CHAPTER 11

Adopt Healthy Eating

Loureen Downes, PhD, APRN, FNP-BC, DipACLM, FAANP, NBC-HWC
Lilly Tryon, DNP, FNP-BC, DipACLM, NBC-HWC

Let food be thy medicine and medicine be thy food.

Hippocrates

OBJECTIVES

This chapter will enable the reader to:

1. Explain the significance of nutrition assessment and summarize its components.
2. Describe the dietary spectrum and the plant-predominant dietary pattern recommended for health promotion and disease prevention.
3. Synthesize the evidence for a plant-predominant dietary pattern to prevent, manage, and treat diet-related chronic disease.
4. Compose nutrition prescriptions for improved health outcomes.
5. Identify strategies to empower patients to change dietary habits.
6. Summarize the role of interprofessional collaboration in addressing the nutritional needs of patients.

Overview

Poor dietary habits are one of the foremost lifestyle behaviors contributing to the leading causes of death and noncommunicable diseases (NCDs). Worldwide, inadequate nutrition and nutrition-related disorders such as heart disease, type 2 diabetes, and obesity have contributed to one in five deaths (Afshin et al., 2019). Approximately 60% of Americans have at least one or more preventable, nutrition-related chronic diseases (U.S. Department of Health and Human Services & U.S. Department of Agriculture [HHS & USDA], 2020). Moreover, nearly 90% of Americans do not consume recommended amounts of fruits and vegetables as part of an overall healthy diet known to reduce the risk of leading causes of chronic illnesses (Lee-Kwan et al., 2017). Furthermore, excessive intake of processed foods and sweetened beverages compounds poor dietary habits to increase diet-related disorders (HHS & USDA, 2020).

© Kathleen Gail/Shutterstock; © StoryTime Studio/Shutterstock; © kali9/Getty Images

This chapter describes evidence-informed strategies for assessing and managing malnutrition. The focus is to provide a foundation for the advanced practice provider (APP) to (a) understand current research and basic guidelines for a healthy diet to prevent and manage dietary-related chronic diseases, (b) assess nutrition deficiency or excess, (c) prescribe nutritional interventions, (d) offer resources for patient nutrition education, and (e) use an interprofessional approach for managing nutrition in the plan of care.

Effect of Malnutrition

Malnutrition is defined as deficiencies, excesses, or imbalances in an individual's intake of calories or nutrients (World Health Organization [WHO], 2021). Malnutrition is a term for three overarching concepts: undernutrition, overnutrition, and micronutrient-related malnutrition. Undernutrition is a deficiency of calories or essential nutrients that results in stunted growth, wasting, and being underweight. Conversely, overnutrition is an overconsumption of nutrients that adversely affects health and contributes to overweight and obesity. Micronutrient-related malnutrition refers to micronutrient deficiencies, such as a lack of essential vitamins and minerals or an excess of micronutrients (WHO, 2021).

Globally in 2020, nearly 2 billion (30%) adults suffered from overnutrition while 462 million were underweight. Over 41 million children under the age of 5 years were overweight or obese while some 144 million were stunted (too short for age) and 45 million were wasted (too thin for height) (WHO, 2021). Additionally, nearly one-third of women of reproductive age and over 40% of children under 5 years are affected by anemia, most commonly caused by nutritional deficiencies (WHO, n.d.).

Poor nutrition or malnutrition affects individuals in every country (WHO, 2020). Children and the elderly are more vulnerable than adults to poor health outcomes due to undernutrition or micronutrient deficiencies. Minorities and individuals of lower socioeconomic status are more likely to experience food insecurity and limited access to nutritious foods such as fresh fruit, vegetables, and legumes (Lee-Kwan et al., 2017; HHS & USDA, 2020). In contrast, foods and drinks high in fat, sugar, and salt are more readily available and perceived to be cheaper, leading to an epidemic of children and adults who are overweight and obese. It is not unusual to find undernutrition and overweight in the same person. For example, it is conceivable to be both overweight and micronutrient deficient.

Diet and Disease

There is substantial evidence that suboptimal nutrition contributes to the leading causes of mortality and disability globally and nationally (Afshin et al., 2019; Mokdad et al., 2018). The Global Burden of Disease Study evaluated the population intake of foods and nutrients in 195 countries to determine the effect of suboptimal diets on adult health outcomes aged 25 or older (Afshin et al., 2019). Researchers found that dietary risk factors were associated with 11 million deaths and 225 years of healthy life lost due to disability (YLD) in 2017. Specifically, elevated sodium intake (3 million deaths and 70 million YLD), inadequate intake of whole grains (3 million deaths and 82 million YLD), and insufficient fruit intake (2 million deaths and 65 million YLD) were among the leading diet risk factors for death and YLD globally and in several countries. They concluded that a suboptimal diet high in sodium and low in whole grains, fruits, nuts, seeds, vegetables, and omega fats had a greater influence on deaths than all the risk factors, including tobacco smoke.

Approximately 60% of Americans have one or more preventable diet-related chronic diseases, such as cardiovascular disease (CVD), type 2 diabetes (T2D), overweight and obesity, and some cancers (HHS & USDA,

2020). Dietary choices may also affect neurological diseases, inflammatory and rheumatic diseases, mental health, and athletic performance (Mitrou, 2022) as well as COVID-19 infection and mortality rates (Abdulah & Hassan, 2020). Furthermore, the body's response to medical therapies is affected by its nutritional status. APPs should consider implementing individual and population health interventions to improve diet and collaborate with policymakers to influence the availability of healthy foods for the populations served.

In a U.S. study, researchers used a comparative risk assessment model to assess the dietary factors associated with heart disease, stroke, and T2D mortality and identified that the highest proportion of deaths was attributed to excess sodium intake; inadequate intake of vegetables, fruits, nuts, and seeds; high intake of processed meats; low intake of seafood omega-3 fats; and sugar-sweetened beverages (Micha et al., 2017). These findings are sobering in light of other findings that only 5% of Americans eat the recommended amount of fiber (Quagliani & Felt-Gunderson, 2017), just 10% of adults eat fruits and vegetables as recommended (Lee-Kwan et al., 2017), and youth intake of recommended amounts of vegetables is a dismal 2%, with only 9% meeting the recommended amount of fruit intake (Moore et al., 2017). Income inequality also compounds poor dietary habits. Seven percent of adults who live at or below the poverty level eat the recommended amounts of vegetables, compared to 11.4% with the highest income level (Lee-Kwan et al., 2017). Consequently, improving diet quality is essential in health promotion and disease prevention.

Diet, Inflammation, and Dysbiosis

According to the American Society for Nutrition, inflammation and diet play an important role in overall health (Marx et al., 2021). Inflammation in and of itself is not bad because it is merely the response of the body's immune system to a trigger that may be harmful. A small amount of inflammation is necessary to maintain an intact immune system. However, chronic low-grade inflammation that persists over time may cause pathologies such as metabolic syndrome, T2D, nonalcoholic fatty liver disease, hypertension (HTN), CVD, chronic kidney disease, various types of cancer, depression, neurodegenerative and autoimmune diseases, osteoporosis, and sarcopenia (Furman et al., 2019). The high-fat diet typical in the Western-style diet has been associated with both low-grade inflammation and dysbiosis (see **Figure 11.1**), two closely interrelated mechanisms (Malesza et al., 2021).

APP's Role in Nutrition

In light of the current nutritional crisis, the recent 50th Anniversary White House Conference on Food, Nutrition, and Health Report made a priority recommendation that health professionals receive an improved knowledge of nutrition and be adequately prepared to provide appropriate nutrition intervention (Mande et al., 2020). Moreover, one of the objectives of *Healthy People 2030* is to increase the proportion of healthcare visits in which clinicians include nutrition counseling (Office of Disease Prevention and Health Promotion [ODPHP], n.d.-c). The goals of *Healthy People 2030* extend the objective of *Healthy People 2020* to promote healthy behaviors and well-being across the life span (ODPHP, n.d.-c). Several objectives relate specifically to healthy eating (ODPHP, n.d.-b). Nutrition should be essential in healthcare delivery, allowing healthcare providers to individualize evidence-informed nutrition interventions to improve diet-related health concerns and positively affect the cost of health care.

According to a recent Gallup poll (Reinhart, 2020), healthcare providers in general are regarded as the most trustworthy among a variety of professionals. As such, APPs should provide the utmost care to those who rely on them

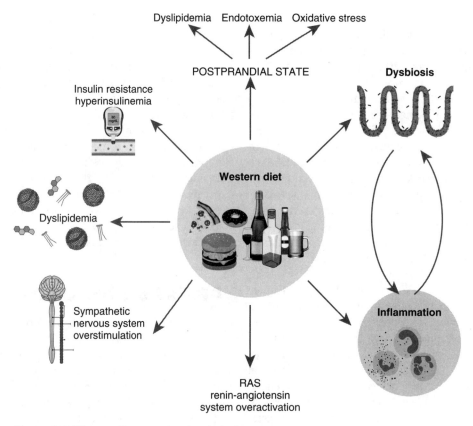

Figure 11.1 Western diet–associated pathologies.

Malesza, I. J., Malesza, M., Walkowiak, J., Mussin, N., Walkowiak, D., Aringazina, R., Bartkowiak-Wieczorek, J., & Mądry, E. (2021). High-fat, Western-style diet, systemic inflammation, and gut microbiota: A narrative review. *Cells, 10*(11), 3164. https://doi.org/10.3390/cells10113164

for information and advice to promote health and prevent disease. APPs are well positioned to conduct nutrition screening, assessment, dietary counseling, and nutrition education in a variety of healthcare settings, particularly primary care and community settings. APPs can translate skills in prescribing medications to nutrition prescriptions for diet-related diseases to transform health care from *sick* care to *health* care. Furthermore, by providing nutrition counseling, APPs can proactively prevent disease and promote health, which may ultimately decrease the cost of health care and the incidences of NCDs, the primary causes of mortality in the United States.

APPs are not required to be nutrition experts or provide comprehensive nutrition counseling. But just as clinicians need to know when to order a diagnostic test or how to develop a plan of care, they also need to know how to screen, assess, determine when a nutrition intervention is relevant, and recommend dietary changes (Barnard, 2018). They must also translate current research on healthy eating patterns into meaningful, actionable messages that patients can put into practice. Furthermore, APPs must recognize the role of the registered dietitian nutritionist (RDN) as a member of the interprofessional team and refer patients when needed.

Health Promotion Research Study

Community-Based Nutrition Intervention

Background: Chronic diseases such as heart disease, T2D, and obesity disproportionately affect minority adults, including African Americans. Engaging in lifestyle changes such as improving dietary habits and increasing physical activity can decrease the incidence and severity of these chronic diseases. This research study aimed to explore the effect of a nutrition education program on health behaviors, lifestyle barriers, emotional eating, and body mass index (BMI) in a community-based setting with a minority sample.

Methodology: A convenience sample of 47 primarily African American adults participated in two similar Full Plate Diet nutrition interventions for 6 weeks (group I) and 8 weeks (group II). Participants completed pre-assessment and post-assessment of fruit, vegetable, and fat intake as well as pre-assessment and post-assessment on physical activity, healthy lifestyle barriers, emotional eating, and BMI.

Results: After the intervention, there was a significant increase in the intake of fruits and vegetables and decreased fat intake. No significant differences were found in physical activity, healthy lifestyle barriers, emotional eating, or BMI after the intervention.

Implication for Advanced Practice: A structured, community-based nutrition education program may improve African Americans' dietary habits.

Reference: Downes, L. S., Buchholz, S. W., Bruster, B., Girimurugan, S. B., Fogg, L. F., & Frock, M. S. (2019). Delivery of a community-based nutrition education program for minority adults. *Journal of the American Association of Nurse Practitioners, 31*(4), 267–277. https://doi.org/10.1097/JXX.00000000000 00144

Nutrients

Food contains macronutrients and micronutrients essential for the optimal function of the body and immune system and the prevention and treatment of diet-related chronic diseases. Macronutrients are nutrients the body uses in relatively large (macro) amounts every day. Micronutrients are nutrients needed in smaller (micro) amounts, such as vitamins, minerals, and antioxidants. Although this chapter cannot cover these nutrients in detail, salient concepts will be addressed. Moreover, it should be noted that a healthy dietary pattern is more reflective of the totality of what a person eats and drinks than of individual components based on food groups or nutrients. Furthermore, parts of an eating pattern may act synergistically and can potentially have cumulative health outcomes (HHS & USDA, 2020).

However, for clarification purposes, this chapter will review individual components to provide the APP with the foundational knowledge to be used in practice.

Macronutrients

There are three primary macronutrients: carbohydrate, protein, and fat. Most foods are a combination of all three in varying amounts. Each macronutrient has a different role in promoting health. These nutrients provide energy in the form of kilocalories, commonly referred to as calories. A kilocalorie (kcal) is the unit of food energy supplied by macronutrients (carbohydrate, protein, fat). Carbohydrate and protein each have 4 kcal/g, whereas fat has 9 kcal/g. Though alcohol is not a macronutrient, it is another source of energy with 7 kcal/g. Although alcohol and fat contain more calories than protein and carbohydrate, they do not provide the nutritional value required for optimal health. This information can help patients shift from high-calorie foods, such as foods high in fat, to lower-calorie whole-plant carbohydrate and plant-based protein to decrease calories and improve nutrient intake.

Carbohydrate

Carbohydrate, in the form of sugar and starch, provides the primary energy source for human physical activity and brain function and is responsible for more than 50% of the calories in the diet. Additionally, it spares protein to preserve muscle mass during physical activity. Many individuals avoid carbohydrates due to the misconception that they cause weight gain. However, nutrition science confirms that not only are carbohydrates essential for a healthy diet but also the type of carbohydrate may be of more concern than the amount (Ludwig et al., 2018). The clinical importance of identifying the different types of carbohydrates is underscored by evidence that processed foods, added sugars, and refined foods are implicated as the primary contributors to the mounting epidemic of CVD, T2D, and high blood pressure (Bhardwaj et al., 2016). Carbohydrates are found in a variety of healthy and unhealthy foods and are the only macronutrient with no required minimum amount. Healthy carbohydrates are also known as complex, minimally processed, or unprocessed. In contrast, unhealthy carbohydrates are called simple or processed.

Healthy carbohydrate foods are nutrient dense and support good health by providing the body with vitamins, minerals, fiber, and many phytonutrients. Besides the overall health benefits of eating carbohydrates from whole foods, the higher fiber content provides greater satiety and the capacity to eat more food while at the same time consuming fewer calories. Broccoli, beans, and whole grains, such as oats, barley, and quinoa, are examples

of healthy carbohydrates. Carbohydrates are more likely to retain their nutritional value if unprocessed or minimally processed. For example, brown rice is processed when the outer bran is removed to make white rice. Likewise, wheat is processed when the outer bran and germ are removed during milling, leaving the center endosperm from which white flour is made. Due to removing the outer bran, white rice and white flour have less fiber and nutrients than brown rice and whole wheat flour.

Because healthy carbohydrates are high in fiber and low in processed fats and sugars, many also have a lower glycemic index, which is a measure of how quickly a food raises blood sugar levels. Food is assessed for glycemic index by eating 50 grams of carbohydrate of a specific food without the fiber and then measuring the glucose levels after 2 hours. High glycemic index foods digest and absorb quickly, resulting in a spike in blood sugar levels. Examples include simple carbohydrates such as cookies and sweetened beverages. These foods tend to be high in sugar and processed fat and low in fiber content. Low glycemic index foods help decrease blood sugar levels and are recommended for adequate diabetes management. Eating foods high in fiber or combining fiber-rich foods with low-fiber foods can help slow the digestion and absorption of foods, resulting in a decreased spike in glucose levels.

Protein

Protein is another essential macronutrient, providing the building blocks (amino acids) needed to synthesize and maintain body tissue, including deoxyribonucleic acid (DNA) and ribonucleic acid (RNA), cell membranes, hormones, neurotransmitters, and plasma proteins. Protein is also used to meet energy needs when glycogen stores are depleted.

The Institute of Medicine (IOM, 2005a) recommends that adults consume 0.8 g of protein per kg of body weight per day, with higher intake during periods of growth (e.g., pregnancy, lactation, vigorous physical activity) and specific conditions (e.g., acute illness, burns, end-stage renal disease). This equates to about 46 g of protein per day for the average woman and about 56 g per day for the average man. However, protein deficiency is rarely a problem. Most Americans consume far more protein than they need (Berryman et al., 2018), which increases the risk for kidney stones, chronic kidney disease, osteoporosis, T2D, certain cancers, and overall mortality (Barnard, 2018). These concerns have caused considerable debate over the usefulness of a high-protein diet for weight loss and enhanced athletic performance.

Another concern is the quality of protein consumed. Proteins consist of 22 amino acids, nine of which are considered essential because the human body cannot synthesize them. Animal-based proteins are good sources of complete protein because they contain all of the amino acids. Plant-based foods often lack one or more essential amino acids, leading many to favor animal protein over plant sources of protein. However, although there are a few plant-based sources of complete protein (e.g., soy, quinoa, chia seeds), a person doesn't need to obtain all amino acids from one food source. Neither is it crucial to combine plant foods in every meal to maximize amino acid intake. By eating a variety of plant-based foods daily, an individual can obtain all the amino acids needed for optimal health without eating animal-based protein (Physicians Committee for Responsible Medicine [PCRM], n.d.).

The protein "package," or the other nutrients packaged with the protein, is more critical than the amount or quality of protein. The different kinds and amounts of fats, carbohydrates, and micronutrients that come with protein can promote health or contribute to disease. **Table 11.1** lists several familiar

Table 11.1 Comparing Protein Packages

Food	PRO (g)	SFA (g)	MUFA (g)	PUFA (g)	ALA (g)	Marine Omega-3 Fats (g)	Fiber (g)	Na (mg)
Sirloin steak, broiled (4 oz)	33	4.6	4.9	0.4	0.4	0	0	66
Sockeye salmon, grilled (4 oz)	30	1.1	2.1	1.5	0.3	1.0	0	104
Chicken thigh, no skin (4 oz)	28	2.7	3.9	2.0	0.1	0.1	0	200
Ham steak (4 oz)	22	1.6	2.2	0.5	0.5	0	0	1,439
Lentils, cooked (1 c)	18	0.1	0.1	0.3	0.3	0	15	4
Milk (8 oz)	8	3.1	1.4	0.2	0.3	0	0	115
Almonds, dry roasted, unsalted (1 oz)	6	1.2	9.4	3.4	0	0	3.1	1

PRO = protein; SFA = saturated fatty acids; MUFA = monounsaturated fatty acids; PUFA = polyunsaturated fatty acids; ALA = alpha-Linolenic acid; Na = sodium

Data from Harvard T. H. Chan School of Public Health. (n.d.). *Protein*. The Nutrition Source. Retrieved January 18, 2023, from https://www.hsph.harvard.edu/nutritionsource/what-should-you-eat/protein

sources of protein, sorted by the amount of protein in a serving. At first glance, sirloin steak is a good protein choice. However, its protein package contains 4.6 g of saturated fat. Ham steak provides 22 g of protein in a 4 oz serving. But it also delivers 1.6 g of saturated fat and 1,439 mg of sodium. On the other hand, a 1 cup serving of cooked lentils provides a similar amount of protein with no cholesterol, low saturated fat, and low sodium. It also has the added advantage of being a rich source of fiber. Equally as crucial as choosing nutrient-dense carbohydrates, the U.S. Dietary Guidelines maintain that a healthy dietary pattern also includes protein sources from nutrient-dense foods (HHS & USDA, 2020).

A healthy vegetarian dietary pattern can be achieved by incorporating protein foods from plant sources (HHS & USDA, 2020). Nutrient-dense choices include legumes (e.g., beans, peas, and lentils), nuts, seeds, and soy products such as tofu. It is important to note that these protein sources, being plant based, are also high in fiber and low in saturated fat.

Fats. Dietary fats provide energy (containing more than twice as many calories per gram as proteins or carbohydrates), help the body absorb vitamins, and influence cholesterol levels. The recommended amount of dietary fat ranges widely from 20% to 35% of total calories for individuals older than 19 years of age. The literature is filled with much debate about healthy and unhealthy fats. According to the U.S. Dietary Guidelines, what is most important is the type of fat eaten because more recent research indicates that healthy fats are necessary and beneficial to health (HHS & USDA, 2020).

There are four different types of fats with varying effects on the body: polyunsaturated fatty acid (PUFA), monounsaturated fatty acid (MUFA), trans-fatty acid (TFA), and saturated fatty acid (SFA) (Hever & Cronise, 2017). The unsaturated fats, PUFA and MUFA, are considered "good," or healthy, fats due to scientific evidence that they lower the risk for CVD,

T2D, cancer, and autoimmune diseases (Liu et al., 2017). The only essential fats in the diet are PUFA, particularly omega-3 and omega-6 (Hever & Cronise, 2017). These are essential because the body needs them for health, including decreased inflammation, improved heart health, and brain function. However, the human body cannot synthesize them; they must be obtained from food. Omega-3 deficiency is related to decreased intelligence, depression, cardiac disease, arthritic problems, and cancer. In general, healthy fats eaten in moderation do not need to be limited for any individual. In particular, children need healthy fats in sufficient quantity for healthy brain development. For a more detailed discussion of dietary fats, review Liu et al. (2017).

There is evidence that omega-3 fats have anti-inflammatory effects, whereas omega-6 fats may have proinflammatory effects (Saini & Keum, 2018). Omega-6 fats, also known as linoleic acid, are commonly available in the food supply. In the Western diet, the consumption of omega-6 fats is often excessive due to the high intake of processed foods, which tend to be low in omega-3 fats (Saini & Keum, 2018). However, when omega-3 intake is balanced with the intake of omega-6, inflammation is reduced.

Omega-3 fats include both long-chain and short-chain fatty acids. The long-chain omega-3 fats, eicosapentaenoic acid (EPA) and docosahexaenoic acid (DHA), are more readily absorbed and used by the body. EPA and DHA are found in fatty fish, such as salmon and tuna. The fish accumulate EPA and DHA in their tissues because they consume phytoplankton, also known as microalgae. Seaweed and algae are some of the few plant foods that contain EPA and DHA and can be important sources of omega-3 for people on a vegetarian or vegan diet. The shorter chain of omega-3 fats found in plant sources is available as alpha-Linolenic acid (ALA), which is converted primarily by the liver in limited amounts to the longer-chain fatty acids EPA and DHA. Plant sources of ALA are found in flax seeds, hemp hearts, chia seeds, leafy green vegetables, walnuts, and wheat germ (Hever & Cronise, 2017).

Though animal foods have the best sources of EPA and DHA, obtaining nutrients from animal sources is fraught with health concerns. Animals are mostly fed grains, including soy and corn; therefore, the PUFAs in meat from grain-fed animals are primarily omega-6. Grass-fed animals, on the other hand, have higher amounts of omega-3 fatty acids. Other sources of omega-3 are fish, available in varying amounts. Cold-water fatty fish, such as salmon and tuna, contain higher amounts than lower-fat fish, such as bass, tilapia, and shellfish (Office of Dietary Supplements [ODS], 2021b). Plant sources of PUFAs may be healthier due to contaminants such as mercury, lead, cadmium, pollutants from factories (e.g., dichlorodiphenyltrichloroethane, polychlorinated biphenyls), and other impurities sometimes found in fish (Domingo, 2016). The adequate intake for omega-3s is 1.1 g for females 14 years and older and 1.6 g for males 14 years and older; lower amounts are recommended for those 13 years or younger. One tablespoon of flaxseed oil provides 7.26 g of ALA, and 1 oz of chia seeds provides 5.96 g ALA, whereas 3 oz of cooked wild Atlantic salmon provides 1.23 g of DHA and 0.35 g of EPA.

TFA and SFA are generally considered "bad," or unhealthy, fats. Most TFAs are found in processed foods made with partially hydrogenated vegetable oils or produced through heating (e.g., frying). Due to evidence that the intake of TFAs increases chronic disease risk, the recommendation is to avoid them (Pipoyan et al. 2021). Furthermore, in 2015, the U.S. Food and Drug Administration (FDA) determined that partially hydrogenated oils, the primary source of TFAs, are unsafe, and food manufacturers were banned from adding them to food as of June 18, 2018 (FDA, 2018). For a more detailed discussion of the effects of TFAs on health, consult the review article by Pipoyan and colleagues (2021).

Compared to unsaturated fats, SFAs have negative health consequences and may be best avoided or eaten in limited amounts of less than 10% of the daily calorie intake, based on the U.S. dietary guidelines (HHS & USDA, 2020). The American Heart Association (2021) recommends aiming for 5% to 6% of daily calorie intake. SFAs are primarily found in animal-based foods, such as meat and dairy, and tropical fats, such as coconut and palm oils. There is limited research evidence that coconut oil may have health benefits, but more rigorous studies are needed to make general recommendations (Forouhi et al., 2018).

Alcohol

Although alcohol provides energy, it is not considered a nutrient. When viewed from a nutritional perspective, alcohol interferes with the nutritional process by affecting digestion, storage, utilization, and excretion of nutrients. There is much conflicting research around alcohol, showing potential for being both beneficial and detrimental. Findings from the Nurses' Health Study suggest that modest alcohol intake is associated with a lower risk of HTN, myocardial infarction, stroke, sudden cardiac death, gallstones, cognitive decline, and all-cause mortality. On the other hand, it also increases the risk of breast cancer, bone fractures, colon polyps, and colon cancer (Mostofsky et al., 2016). A recent study found that alcohol increased the risk of cancer even at low levels of consumption (Rumgay et al., 2021). Alcohol consumption is not recommended in the U.S. Dietary Guidelines for Americans. If consumed, it should only be in moderation—up to one drink per day for women and two drinks per day for men on days when alcohol is consumed (HHS & USDA, 2020).

Micronutrients

Micronutrients, such as vitamins and minerals, are essential dietary elements required in minute amounts. Still, they play a vital role in growth and development, disease prevention, and well-being and are essential for the metabolism of protein, carbohydrate, and fat. Minerals include selenium, sodium, iodine, copper, zinc, and fluoride. Vitamins include A, B, C, D, E, and K. There are 28 essential micronutrients that are not produced in the body, and most can be obtained from nutrient-dense whole foods if a well-balanced, healthy diet is consumed. Another key point is that micronutrient supplementation in amounts that exceed the recommended dietary allowance may be harmful (Rautiainen et al., 2016).

Several micronutrients are significant antioxidants, including beta-carotene, vitamin C, and vitamin E. Antioxidants are known to counteract the oxidative stress that may promote cell damage and diseases such as cancer, heart disease, T2D, Alzheimer's disease, Parkinson's disease, cataracts, and macular degeneration (National Center for Complementary and Integrative Health [NCCIH], 2013). Vegetables and fruits are excellent sources of antioxidants. Governmental organizations strongly encourage people to eat fruits and vegetables (NCCIH, 2013). There are no known concerns about the safety of obtaining excess amounts of antioxidants from food. However, there is evidence that high doses of antioxidant supplements may result in adverse health outcomes. For instance, high doses of beta-carotene supplements are associated with an increased risk of lung cancer in smokers, and vitamin E supplements are implicated in hemorrhagic stroke risk (NCCIH, 2013). Furthermore, patients should be advised to inform their APPs of supplement use to avoid medication interactions (NCCIH, 2013).

Micronutrient deficiencies can have harmful effects on health, resulting in congenital disabilities, impaired cognitive ability, and reduced productivity (Centers for Disease Control and Prevention [CDC], 2021). Common micronutrient deficiencies include iron, vitamin B12, and vitamin D. Therefore, APPs need to consider micronutrient deficiencies and their effect on health. For a more detailed description of the 28 essential micronutrients, their function in the body, deficiency or toxicity, symptoms, and the USDA daily recommended amounts, see **Table 11.16** for the online resource *Nutrition Guide for Clinicians* (PCRM, 2022).

Iron

Iron deficiency is the most common micronutrient deficiency, affecting approximately 25% of people worldwide (Warner & Kamran, 2021). Although iron deficiency is more prevalent in developing countries, low-income families in the United States are at increased risk of iron deficiency as well as children and pregnant women (Warner & Kamran, 2021). In neonates and infants, breastfeeding is protective against iron deficiency due to the bioavailability of iron in breast milk compared to cow's milk (Warner & Kamran, 2021).

Most individuals get enough iron from food. There are two types of dietary iron: heme (found only in animal sources and well absorbed) and nonheme (found in plant sources and not as well absorbed as heme iron). The most common food source of iron in the United States is meat. Nevertheless, individuals who eat little or no meat can get adequate iron from eating a variety of iron-rich plant foods such as leafy greens, legumes, whole grains, and mushrooms (Bjarnadottir, 2019). Three ounces of ground beef provides nearly 30% of the daily recommended amount of iron, similar to half a cup of cooked kidney beans, which provides 33% of the recommended amounts of nonheme iron (Bjarnadottir, 2019). Eating iron-rich foods with vitamin C enhances the body's absorption of iron. When prescribing iron supplementation, APPs should monitor iron levels because the body does not excrete iron rapidly, causing iron to build up over time and lead to iron toxicity in some people.

Vitamin B12

Cobalamin, referred to as vitamin B12, is an essential nutrient for the development of the nervous system, brain function, and red blood cell production. A deficiency in vitamin B12 can lead to neurological problems and anemia. However, the complications related to vitamin B12 deficiency can be reversed if addressed early in the process. Although APPs should assess for symptoms and potential contributors to vitamin B12 deficiency, there are currently no guidelines or recommendations regarding routine testing for vitamin B12 deficiency.

Older adults are more prone to vitamin B12 deficiency due to malnutrition, malabsorption, and medications, such as metformin and gastric acid inhibitors, that can decrease the absorption of vitamin B12 (ODS, 2021a). The IOM Food and Nutrition Board recommends that adults older than 50 years eat foods fortified with vitamin B12 or take a vitamin B12 supplement to meet the recommended dietary allowance.

Another population to assess for vitamin B12 deficiency is those who eat a completely plant-based diet since vitamin B12 is only found naturally in animal foods. Furthermore, the human body only has a long-term storage capacity for vitamin B12 for up to four years. Therefore, vitamin B12 is one of the few nutrients that must be supplemented in individuals who predominantly eat plant-based foods. The recommended dietary allowance (RDA) for vitamin B12 varies depending on age and gender. For individuals 14 years and older, the RDA is 2.4 mcg for males and females.

Vitamin D

Vitamin D is a fat-soluble hormone that promotes calcium absorption and maintains calcium and phosphate blood levels to support healthy bone development and prevent osteoporosis in adulthood. Additionally, vitamin D modulates cell growth, neuromuscular and immune system function, and the inflammatory response (ODS, 2021c). Vitamin D deficiency is associated with brittle bones, rickets in children, and osteomalacia in adults. Food sources of vitamin D include oily fish, beef liver, egg yolks, and fortified foods. It is also produced when ultraviolet radiation from sun exposure triggers vitamin D synthesis in the skin (ODS, 2021c).

The serum concentration of 25-hydroxyvitamin D3, the primary circulating form of vitamin D, is the best indicator of an individual's vitamin D levels. The RDA for vitamin D is 600 IU for males and females between 1 and 70 years old and 800 IU for adults over 70. Vitamin D supplements are available in two forms, D2 and D3. Both vitamin D2 and D3 increase the blood level, but vitamin D3 is more effective at sustaining blood levels (ODS, 2021c).

Water

Water is not a nutrient but is very important for aiding digestion, delivering nutrients to cells, promoting bowel movements, replacing fluids used during metabolism, and other body functions (CDC, 2020). Recently, researchers determined the relationship between optimal hydration and the aging process in humans in a cohort analysis of 15,752 middle-aged (45–66 years) individuals over 25 years of follow-up (Dmitrieva et al., 2023). In this study, sodium level was used as a marker for hydration status. The findings revealed that serum sodium levels in the upper normal range (135–146 mmol/l) predicted a faster rate of biological aging and increased incidences of chronic diseases or NCDs in advanced age. Additionally, the results indicated that a serum sodium limit of 142 mmol/l is a benchmark that can be used in clinical practice to ascertain individuals at risk. APPs should conduct a more thorough assessment of hydration status in patients with serum sodium levels of 142 mmol/l or greater. The researchers concluded that more research is needed to assess the likelihood of the anti-aging effects of improved hydration status (Dmitrieva et al., 2023).

Daily fluid intake (total water) is the amount consumed from foods, plain drinking water, and other beverages (CDC, 2020).

Many factors determine individual water needs, including age, sex, weight, pregnancy, breastfeeding, exercise, exposure to extreme temperatures, fever, and underlying health conditions. A general rule of thumb to determine whether water intake is adequate is voiding colorless or pale yellow urine several times daily. While there is no recommendation for the amount of plain drinking water an individual should consume daily, the IOM (2005b) recommends about 13 cups daily for healthy men and about 9 cups daily for healthy women of total water intake from a variety of beverages and foods. Although all fluids count toward total water intake, plain water has many benefits as opposed to sweetened beverages because it does not have calories and may aid in weight loss (CDC, 2020).

Nutrient Recommendations

The IOM (2006) Food and Nutrition Board establishes dietary reference intakes (DRIs) for nutrient intakes of healthy individuals. The DRI includes three measures: recommended dietary allowance (RDA), adequate intake (AI), and tolerable upper intake level (UL). RDA is the average daily level sufficient to meet the nutrient requirements of most (97–98%) healthy people. However, even healthy individuals will vary in nutritional needs based on age, gender, and activity (Kesari & Noel, 2022). AI is determined when insufficient evidence is available to develop an RDA. The UL is the highest amount that can be consumed without adverse health effects. **Table 11.2**

Table 11.2 Daily Nutritional Goals for Age–Gender Groups Based on DRIs and Dietary Guidelines

Nutrient	Source Goal	Child 1–3 y	Child 4–8 y	Female 9–13 y	Male 9–13 y	F/M 14–18 y	F/M 19–50 y	F/M 50–70+ y
CHO g/day	RDA	130	130	130	130	130	130	130
CHO% kcal	AMDR	45–65	45–65	45–65	45–65	45–65	45–65	45–65
PRO	RDA	13	19	34	34	46/52	46/46	56
Linoleic acid (g/d) omega-6	AI	7	10	10	12	11/16	12/17	11/14
ALA (g/d) omega-3	AI	0.7	0.9	1.0	1.2	1.1/1.6	1.1/1.6	1.1/1.6
Vitamin B12 µg/d	RDA	0.9	1.2	1.8	1.8	2.4	2.4	2.4
Vitamin D µg/d	RDA	15	15	15	15	15	15	20
Fiber g/day	AI	19	25	26	31	26/38	25/38	21/30
Water L/day	AI	1.3	1.7	2.1	2.4	2.3/3.3	2.7/3.7	2.7/3.7

CHO = carbohydrate; PRO = protein; AMDR = acceptable macronutrient distribution range. Total water includes all water contained in food, beverages, and drinking water. Calciferol 1 µg = 40 IU vitamin D.
Data from Institute of Medicine. 2005b. *Dietary reference intakes for water, potassium, sodium, chloride, and sulfate.* National Academies Press and Institute of Medicine. (2011). *Dietary reference intakes (DRIs): Recommended dietary allowances and adequate intakes, vitamins.* https://www.ncbi.nlm.nih.gov/books/NBK56068/table/summarytables.t2/?report=objectonly

provides daily nutritional goals based on DRIs. For a comprehensive list of DRI requirements, please refer to *Dietary Reference Intakes: The Essential Guide to Nutrient Requirements* (IOM, 2006).

Dietary Patterns

In practice, people do not eat nutrients in isolation. Therefore, a patient's overall dietary pattern is more important than individual nutrients or foods. Dietary patterns are defined as "the quantities, proportions, variety, or combination of different foods, drinks, and nutrients (when available) in diets, and the frequency with which they are habitually consumed" (Boushey et al., 2020, p. 9). As a result, dietary patterns are more closely associated with overall health status and disease risk than is the consumption (or lack) of individual foods or nutrients. They also provide the opportunity to individualize the nutrition prescription to meet the nutrition and lifestyle needs of the patient.

A relatively broad dietary spectrum of eating patterns exists in the United States (see **Figure 11.2**). The typical Western diet, often referred to as the standard American diet, is characterized by high intakes of refined sugars, animal fats, processed meats, refined grains, high-fat dairy products, and salt with low intakes of unprocessed fruits, vegetables, whole grains, grass-fed animal products, fish, nuts, and seeds (Malesza et al., 2021). Additionally, the eating pattern consists of large portions and frequent eating. This calorie-rich, nutrient-poor Western diet is closely related to the Western lifestyle of low physical activity, insufficient sleep, and increased stress.

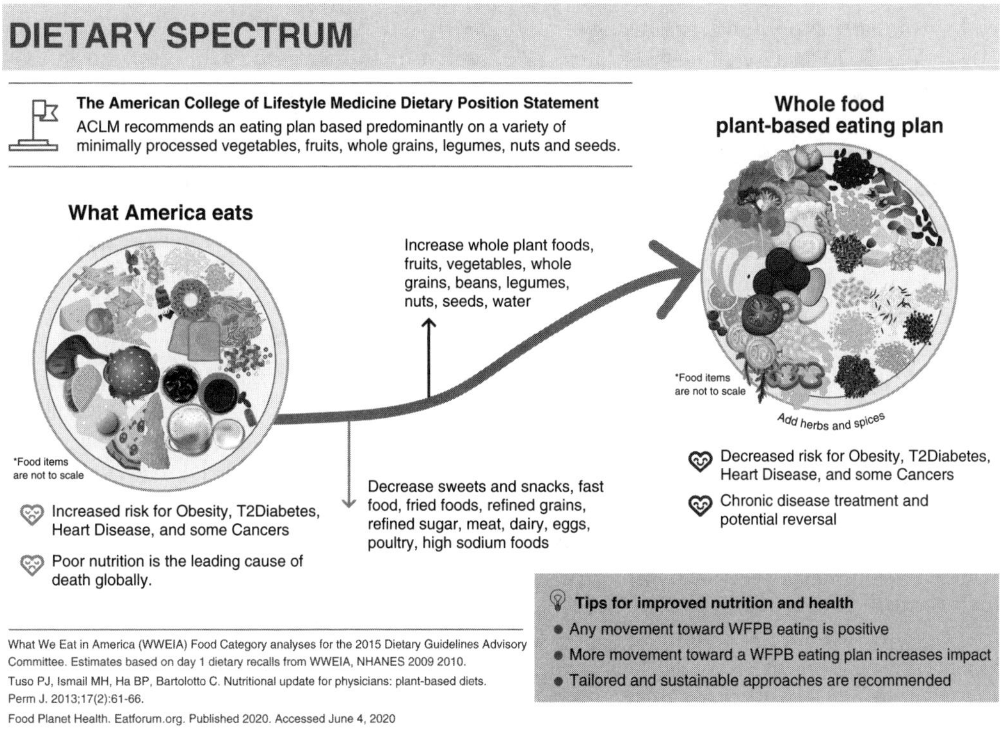

DIETARY SPECTRUM

The American College of Lifestyle Medicine Dietary Position Statement
ACLM recommends an eating plan based predominantly on a variety of minimally processed vegetables, fruits, whole grains, legumes, nuts and seeds.

Whole food plant-based eating plan

What America eats

Increase whole plant foods, fruits, vegetables, whole grains, beans, legumes, nuts, seeds, water

*Food items are not to scale

*Food items are not to scale

Add herbs and spices

Decreased risk for Obesity, T2Diabetes, Heart Disease, and some Cancers

Chronic disease treatment and potential reversal

Increased risk for Obesity, T2Diabetes, Heart Disease, and some Cancers

Poor nutrition is the leading cause of death globally.

Decrease sweets and snacks, fast food, fried foods, refined grains, refined sugar, meat, dairy, eggs, poultry, high sodium foods

💡 **Tips for improved nutrition and health**
- Any movement toward WFPB eating is positive
- More movement toward a WFPB eating plan increases impact
- Tailored and sustainable approaches are recommended

What We Eat in America (WWEIA) Food Category analyses for the 2015 Dietary Guidelines Advisory Committee. Estimates based on day 1 dietary recalls from WWEIA, NHANES 2009 2010.
Tuso PJ, Ismail MH, Ha BP, Bartolotto C. Nutritional update for physicians: plant-based diets. Perm J. 2013;17(2):61-66.
Food Planet Health. Eatforum.org. Published 2020. Accessed June 4, 2020

Figure 11.2 Dietary spectrum.

American College of Lifestyle Medicine. (2020). *Dietary spectrum.* https://lifestylemedicine.org/wp-content/uploads/2022/07/ACLM-Dietary-Spectrum-8.5x11.pdf

On the other end of the spectrum are plant-predominant eating patterns, which promote health by increasing the intake of minimally processed nutrient-dense plant foods that provide fiber, water, antioxidants, and healthy fats. Other terms used for this focus on increasing plant foods in the diet include plant based, plant forward, plant exclusive, plant focused, plant slant, plant shift, and plant rich. Dietary patterns that are plant predominant include the whole-food plant-based (WFPB) dietary pattern (Tuso et al., 2013), the Mediterranean diet (Davis et al., 2015), the DASH diet (Sacks et al., 1999), the MIND diet (Morris et al., 2015), Blue Zones (n.d.), and vegan/vegetarian eating patterns (Clem & Barthel, 2021).

Plant-based diets have demonstrated improved weight control and cardiometabolic outcomes compared to usual diets and some health-oriented diets (Craig et al., 2021; Remde et al., 2022). They also provide a preventive and therapeutic role in cancer, gut microbiome, and anti-inflammatory functions (Craig et al., 2021). The 2020 Dietary Guidelines Advisory Committee, Dietary Patterns Subcommittee conducted a systematic review to determine the relationship between dietary patterns consumed and all-cause mortality (Boushey et al., 2020). The committee concluded that "strong evidence demonstrates that dietary patterns in adults and older adults characterized by vegetables, fruits, legumes, nuts, whole grains, unsaturated vegetable oils, and fish, lean meat or poultry when meat was included, are associated with decreased risk of all-cause mortality. These patterns were also relatively low in red and processed meat, high-fat dairy, and refined carbohydrates or sweets" (p. 9). In addition to health benefits, plant-based diets use fewer natural resources to produce and are more environmentally friendly (Craig et al., 2021).

It is beyond the scope of this chapter to review the plethora of diets that lie between the Western diet and plant-predominant eating patterns on the spectrum of dietary patterns. The APP should assess where the patient is on the dietary spectrum and encourage the intake of fruits, vegetables, whole grains, beans, legumes, nuts, seeds, and water, recognizing that any movement toward a plant-predominant eating pattern will result in better health outcomes.

Food Preparation

Food preparation methods can affect the nutritional value of foods and should be considered when assessing the diet. Although cooking food can improve the digestion and absorption of nutrients, it can also contribute to the loss of nutrients. Furthermore, cooking at high temperatures can generate products of oxidation that are harmful to human health and that accelerate the aging process. One of the most common is advanced glycation end products (AGEs). AGEs are proteins or lipids that become glycated as a result of exposure to sugar, known as the Maillard reaction (browning of food that occurs when sugar combines with amino acids; Davis, 2019). Factors contributing to increased AGE formation in food include animal-derived foods, high dry-heat cooking methods (e.g., grilling), and frying for an extended time. Other sources of AGEs are roasted nuts. AGEs are associated with oxidative stress and inflammation, the processes implicated in the cause and progression of chronic diseases, including atherosclerosis, T2D, chronic kidney diseases, and Alzheimer's disease (Uribarri et al., 2015). In a recent study, with a large sample of over 100,000, one in three who ate red meat or chicken cooked on an open flame more than 15 times per month were more likely to develop diabetes than those who ate it less than four times per month (Liu et al., 2018).

Starting the Conversation

A positive conversation about nutrition will help to inspire patients to adopt healthier eating habits. Furthermore, patients will care more about their diet if they know that their healthcare provider prioritizes nutrition and addresses it routinely. An opener for starting the conversation about diet is for the APP to express the importance of nutrition and its role in promoting health. For example, "Nutrition is one of the primary pillars for good health. While medication is useful for treating [high blood pressure, diabetes, chronic disease, etc.], it can't replace what a healthy diet can do."

A person-centered conversation strategy is to use a nondirective, partner approach. Instead of advising dietary change, the APP should ask permission to have a conversation on nutrition: "If it's all right with you, can we talk about how food choices can improve your triglyceride level?" or "As part of your annual wellness visit today, would it be okay if we spent a few minutes talking about nutrition and how eating habits affect your health?" If the patient agrees, the APP can transition into nutrition screening and assessment.

To initiate the discussion with a patient, the 2015–2020 dietary guidelines provide suggestions for conversation starters. See **Table 11.3** for additional questions to start the conversation.

Nutrition Screening and Assessment

Nutrition screening and assessment allow the APP to screen and assess a patient's nutritional status to do the following:

- Determine whether a patient is undernourished, overnourished, underweight, overweight, or obese for intervention or referral
- Identify the risk of undernutrition or overnutrition for early intervention or referral
- Track child growth
- Identify complications that affect the ability of the body to metabolize nutrients
- Inform nutrition education and counseling
- Provide a baseline measure to assess the effectiveness of dietary changes

Table 11.3 Dietary Pattern Conversation Starters

Question	Clinician Tips
What is your family's favorite dinner?	Meet patients where they are. Once you establish a baseline of eating habits, you can make suggestions for shifts or substitutions using the evidence for best dietary practices, as suggested in the dietary guidelines.
Who does the grocery shopping in your home? Who cooks?	Determine what patients are buying and how much they are cooking. You might be able to suggest new food to try or set goals for cooking at home more often or packing a lunch.
What are some of your family's favorite food routines and traditions?	Are patients eating together at dinner or eating separately? Discuss how healthy eating patterns may be adaptable to traditions or customs.
When you're thirsty, what kind of drink do you reach for?	Nearly 50% of added sugar in the American diet comes from sodas, fruit drinks, and other sweetened beverages. Suggest healthier options, such as water or infusion water.
Does eating healthier seem difficult or unrealistic?	Identify if there are barriers and suggest work-arounds.

Data from U.S. Department of Health and Human Services and U.S. Department of Agriculture. (2015, December). *2015 – 2020 dietary guidelines for Americans* (8th ed.). https://health.gov/our-work/food-nutrition/previous-dietary-guidelines/2015

Table 11.4 **Factors Affecting Nutritional Status**

Physiological	Pathological	Psychosocial
Age	Genetics	Socioeconomic conditions
Sex	Infections	Calamities
Growth	Inflammation	Cultural norms
Pregnancy	Chronic disease	Religious beliefs
Physical activity	Malignancies	Eating disorders
Dentition	Surgery	Mental illness
Mental status	Trauma	Alcohol
	Medication adverse effects	Substance use

Data from Kesari, A., & Noel, J. Y. (2022, April 16). *Nutritional assessment*. StatPearls [Internet]. https://www.ncbi.nlm.nih.gov/books/NBK580496

Nutrition is not just the food one eats; it is complex and is associated with culture, policy, and religious beliefs. Many physiological, pathological, and psychosocial factors also affect nutritional status (see **Table 11.4**). These factors can also be interdependent. Therefore, nutrition assessment should be comprehensive and include medical history, clinical findings, diet history, and social history to determine individualized nutrition needs and the most appropriate dietary prescription within a cultural and familial context.

Nutrition Screening

Nutrition screening is the initial step in determining whether patients are appropriately nourished or at risk of being malnourished (overnourished or undernourished). It allows for the prevention of diet-related health conditions when the risk of disease is identified and for early treatment when health problems are diagnosed. Early detection and treatment across the life span may decrease healthcare costs and ultimately improve health outcomes and quality of life. A recent scientific statement from the American Heart Association recommends incorporating a rapid diet screening tool and discussion of dietary patterns with the patient into routine primary care visits (Vadiveloo et al., 2020). Nutrition screening should be included in every encounter as a

component of the lifestyle vital signs to help patients achieve optimum eating habits.

Nutrition screening can be provided in various settings and is a quick and straightforward way to identify people who may be malnourished or at risk of being malnourished to determine the need for a more comprehensive assessment. Simple nutrition screening includes measuring weight and height to determine BMI or scores on a growth chart, measuring mid-upper arm circumference (MUAC), checking for pitting edema, and asking about appetite and recent health problems (Cashin & Oot, 2018). The Malnutrition Universal Screening Tool (MUST) is a five-step screening tool to identify adults who are malnourished, at risk of malnutrition (undernutrition), or obese. This tool produces a risk score based on BMI, unplanned weight loss, and acute disease effects on nutritional intake (Stratton et al., 2004).

Several brief, validated dietary screening tools are useful for clinical practice. The simplest, based on the Dietary Guidelines for Americans and the WHO Healthy Diet, asks only two questions: (a) How often per week do you eat ≥5 fruits and vegetables? (0–1 days/week = 3 points; 2–3 days/week = 2 points; 4–5 days/week = 1 point; 6–7 days/week = 0 points) and (b) How often do you consume sugary food/drinks (juice, sweeteners in coffee or tea, sugary sodas)? (0–1 days/week = 0 points; 2–3 days/week = 1 point;

4–5 days/week = 2 points; 6–7 days/week = 3 points). A combined score of 3 or higher prompts further assessment and counseling (Powell & Greenberg, 2019).

Other dietary screening tools include the 8-item Starting the Conversation (STC) tool (Paxton et al., 2011), the 16-item Rapid Eating Assessment for Participants Short Form (REAP-S) (Segal-Isaacson et al., 2004), the 14-item Mediterranean Diet Adherence Screener (MEDAS) used in the PREVIMED study (Schröder et al., 2011), and the 26-item Dietary Screener Questionnaire (DSQ) used by the National Health and Nutrition Examination Survey 2009–2010 (National Cancer Institute, 2021). The Mini-Nutritional Assessment Short Form (MNA-SF) is a validated nutrition screening and assessment tool for the elderly (Kaiser et al., 2009). If a patient screens positive for nutrition risk, further assessment, dietary counseling, and referral may be considered.

Food insecurity should also be assessed. The USDA defines food insecurity as a household-level economic and social condition of limited or uncertain access to adequate food (Economic Research Service, n.d.). Socioeconomic factors (e.g., low income, unemployment, lack of education, ethnicity, and disability) and neighborhood conditions (e.g., few grocery stores, limited transportation options) can affect a person's diet by contributing to a reliance on high-calorie, low-cost foods or a lack of food. Food insecurity can lead to malnourishment, weight gain, and other adverse health outcomes (ODPHP, n.d.-a). The two-question Hunger Vital Sign is a universal screening tool to identify food insecurity (Hager et al., 2010). An individual or family is at risk if either or both of the following statements is "often true" or "sometimes true":

- "Within the past 12 months, we worried whether our food would run out before we got money to buy more."
- "Within the past 12 months, the food we bought just didn't last, and we didn't have money to get more."

ABCDs of Nutrition Assessment

The nutrition assessment is a more detailed evaluation of the patient's nutritional status and related risk factors and morbidities. It creates a framework for treatment and identifies if a referral to a nutrition specialist is needed. APPs should be proficient in conducting a basic nutritional assessment, which includes four areas: (1) anthropometric data, (2) biochemical data, (3) clinical assessment, and (4) dietary assessment (see **Table 11.5**). These

Table 11.5 ABCDs of Nutrition Assessment

Anthropometric Assessment	Biochemical Assessment	Clinical Assessment	Dietary Assessment
Weight	Lab tests	Age	Daily intake of solids/liquids
Height		Gender	24-hour recall
BMI		Medical history	3-day food intake
Waist circumference		Surgical history	Meal schedule
MUAC		Weight history	Social history
Growth pattern indices		Nutritional history	Family structure
Body composition		Vital signs	Psychosocial stressors
		Physical exam	Cultural beliefs

Data from Food and Nutrition Technical Assistance III Project. (2016). *Module 2. Nutrition assessment and classification* (Version 2, p. 5). https://www.fantaproject.org/sites/default/files/resources/NACS-Users-Guide-Module2-May2016.pdf areas are referred to as the ABCDs of nutrition assessment. Complex patients should be referred to an RDN for a more comprehensive nutrition assessment.

Anthropometric Assessment

Anthropometric assessment includes measurements of the body and body composition. The most common body measurements are height, weight, BMI, waist circumference, MUAC, and weight-for-height z-score (WHZ). Body composition can be measured by calipers or a handheld bioelectrical impedance device. For accuracy, it is essential to get measured data instead of estimated or self-reported data.

Body Mass Index. BMI may be used as an indicator of overall nutritional status in adults and children older than 6 years. Once an accurate height and weight are obtained, the BMI is easily calculated using an online BMI calculator or the following formula: weight (kg) ÷ [height (m)]^2. If height has been measured in centimeters, divide by 100 to convert to meters. When using English measurements, the BMI formula is 703 x weight (lb) ÷ [height (in.)]^2. **Table 11.6** provides the classification of weight using BMI. Weight and BMI cannot differentiate between muscle mass and adipose tissue, nor may they represent the accurate nutritional status of pregnant women and individuals with edema or dehydration.

Waist Circumference. The waist circumference (WC) is taken with a tape measure in a horizontal plane around the abdomen at the level of the iliac crest. The tape should be snug but should not compress the skin. The measurement is made at the end of expiration. Although WC and BMI are interrelated, WC is an independent predictor of the risk of health conditions above and beyond the BMI (National Heart, Lung, and Blood Institute [NHLBI], 2000) (see **Table 11.7**). The WC is useful for patients with normal or overweight BMI scores ranging from 25 to 34.9 kg/m^2. Excess abdominal fat, as determined by WC, increases the risk for obesity-related health concerns, such as T2D, HTN, and heart disease. In special populations, such as Asian Americans or individuals of Asian descent, WC is more indicative of disease risk than BMI (NHLBI, 2000).

Middle-Upper Arm Circumference. In addition to BMI and WC measures to determine nutritional status, there is evidence supporting that MUAC is an appropriate measure for assessing malnutrition (Benítez Brito et al., 2016), particularly in community settings and low-resource areas. MUAC is determined by measuring the circumference of the upper arm at the midpoint between the elbow and

Table 11.6 Classification of Weight Using BMI

Pre-Pregnancy Nutritional Status	Pre-Pregnancy BMI
Underweight	Less than 18.5
Normal weight	18.5–24.9
Overweight	25.0–29.9
Obese	30 or greater

Food and Nutrition Technical Assistance III Project. (2016). *Module 2. Nutrition assessment and classification* (Version 2, p. 5). https://www.fantaproject.org/sites/default/files/resources/NACS-Users-Guide-Module2-May2016.pdf

Table 11.7 High-Risk Waist Circumference

High Risk
Men: >102 cm (>40 in.) Women: >88 cm (>35 in.)

National Heart, Lung, and Blood Institute. (2000). *The practical guide: Identification, evaluation, and treatment of overweight and obesity in adults* (NIH Publication No. 00-4084). U.S. Department of Health and Human Services, National Institutes of Health. https://www.nhlbi.nih.gov/files/docs/guidelines/prctgd_c.pdf

the shoulder using a measuring tape. Measurements in millimeters are more precise than measurements in centimeters. MUAC is a surrogate measure of muscle mass (which indicates protein status; Kesari & Noel, 2022). It is not deterred by pregnancy and is independent of height (Food and Nutrition Technical Assistance III Project [FANTA], 2016). MUAC is appropriate for individuals who cannot stand for weight and height measurements, infants, pregnant women, and postpartum women for 6 months (Benítez Brito et al., 2016). **Table 11.8** and **Table 11.9** provide MUAC cutoffs to classify nutritional status. MUAC is not recommended for infants under 6 months and should not be used to determine nutritional status in people with edema (FANTA, 2016).

Growth Pattern Indices. Nutrition screening to identify risks in children is based on standardized child growth references established by the CDC and the WHO (CDC, n.d.). According to the CDC, the WHO growth charts are more suited to monitor growth in infants and children ages 0 to 2 years of age, and in the United States, the CDC growth charts are suited to monitor growth for children ages 2 and older. Growth charts may not reflect ideal growth patterns due to the limitations in growth charts reflecting how children should grow when provided with ideal conditions. Clinicians often use the CDC growth charts as standards. However, the CDC and WHO growth charts are merely references indicating how typical children grow during a specific period under ideal conditions. Serial measurements are essential for tracking changes over time. The APP should also consider other factors that may affect growth patterns, such as ethnicity and breastfeeding. It is important

Table 11.8 MUAC Cutoff to Classify Nutritional Status in Children 6 Months to 14 Years of Age

Age	Normal Nutritional Status	Severe Acute Malnutrition	Moderate Acute Malnutrition
6–59 months	≥125	<115 mm	≥115 to <125
5–9 years	≥145	<135 mm	≥135 to <145
10–14 years	≥185	<160 mm	≥160 to <185

Food and Nutrition Technical Assistance III Project. (2016). *Module 2. Nutrition assessment and classification* (Version 2, p. 6). https://www.fantaproject.org/sites/default/files/resources/NACS-Users-Guide-Module2-May2016.pdf

Table 11.9 Recommended MUAC Cutoffs to Classify Nutritional Status in Adults

Nonpregnant/Nonpostpartum	Pregnant/Postpartum	Nutritional Status
<185 mm	<190	Severe acute malnutrition
≥185 to <220 mm	≥190 to <230 mm	Moderate malnutrition
≥220 mm	≥230 mm	Normal nutritional status

Food and Nutrition Technical Assistance III Project. (2016). *Module 2. Nutrition assessment and classification* (Version 2, p. 7). https://www.fantaproject.org/sites/default/files/resources/NACS-Users-Guide-Module2-May2016.pdf to note that the WHO growth standards are based on breastfed infants (CDC, n.d.).

Body Composition. Less common anthropometric measurements include body composition studies, which analyze the body's composition of water, air, muscle, bones, and fat mass (Kesari & Noel, 2022). Bioelectrical impedance analysis (BIA) uses the variation of electrical conduction in different body tissues to analyze body composition. Tissues with more water and electrolytes conduct more electricity than adipose and bone tissues. BIA devices are low cost, and the technology has been integrated into many home use weight scales. It is important to note that the results are affected by hydration status, extremely high BMI, fluid overload, and pregnancy (Kesari & Noel, 2022).

Skinfold thickness measurements are an indication of energy stores (more specifically, fat stores). A skinfold caliper measures the skinfold thickness at several body sites. The values are then input into an equation to calculate the overall body fat percentage (Elsey et al., 2021). Although convenient, simple, and low cost, the accuracy of results depends on the tester's expertise and the equation used. Furthermore, use in obese patients may be limited because most skinfold calipers have an upper limit of 45 to 60 mm (Elsey et al., 2021).

Biochemical Assessment

No single laboratory test or group of tests can determine nutritional status. Therefore, the APP should evaluate all laboratory results in the context of clinical presentation, hydration status, and underlying diseases. Several routine laboratory tests may be used to assess nutritional status, including complete blood count, blood glucose level, serum electrolytes, blood urea nitrogen, creatinine, liver enzymes, and lipid profile (see **Table 11.10**). Individual micronutrient levels such as 25-hydroxy vitamin D, vitamin B12, calcium, magnesium, zinc, selenium, and iron can be measured if specific micronutrient deficiencies are suspected. C-reactive protein can be evaluated for the presence of inflammation (Kesari & Noel, 2022).

Clinical Assessment

The clinical assessment is similar to the traditional assessment. It includes a review of the medical history relevant to nutrition status, such as age, gender, activity level, and weight history. A review of medications should ask about the use of dietary supplements. The review of systems (ROS) should include questions about recent weight changes, gastrointestinal system, factors affecting food intake (e.g., appetite, dentition, swallowing difficulty), symptoms suggestive of malnutrition (e.g., poor wound healing, skin rashes or dryness, edema, hair loss, mouth sores, bleeding gums, loss of night vision, and paresthesia), menstruation, physical activity, use of tobacco and alcohol, and socioeconomic conditions that could affect nutritional status (Kesari & Noel, 2022). The physical exam should be based on medical history and ROS; include vital signs; and assess the condition of the skin, hair, nails, eyes, oral cavity, extremities (e.g., muscle weakness, edema, bowing of limbs), and function.

Dietary Assessment

Traditional methods for determining the quantity and quality of food intake include the 24-hour diet recall, food record, and food frequency questionnaire (Bailey, 2021). The *24-hour diet recall* is a simple strategy in which the APP can assess typical food and fluid intake by asking the patient to recall all foods and beverages consumed on the previous day. Although fast, convenient, and not dependent on patient literacy, the limitations to the 24-hour diet recall include patient forgetfulness and inability to capture daily variations in food intake. The *food record* is a comprehensive recording of all food and beverage intake over a designated period. The APP can ask the

Table 11.10 Laboratory Tests Used to Diagnose Nutritional and Medical Problems

Test	Possible Reason for Why Low	Possible Reason for Why High
Glucose	Hypoglycemia, liver disease, adrenal insufficiency, excess insulin	Hyperglycemia, certain types of diabetes, prediabetes, pancreatitis, hyperthyroidism
Blood urea nitrogen (BUN)	Malnutrition	Liver or kidney disease, heart failure
Creatinine	Low muscle mass, malnutrition	Chronic or temporary decrease in kidney function
Protein	Liver or kidney disease, malnutrition	Dehydration, liver or kidney disease, multiple myeloma
Albumin	Liver or kidney disease, malnutrition	Dehydration
Alkaline phosphate (ALP)	Malnutrition	Paget's disease or certain cancers that spread to the bone, bile duct obstruction, liver cancer
Alanine aminotransferase (ALT)	Generally not a concern	Certain toxins such as excess acetaminophen or alcohol, hepatitis
White blood cell count	Autoimmune illness, bone marrow failure, viral infections	Infection, inflammation, cancer, stress, intense exercise
Red blood cell count	Iron, vitamin B12, or folate deficiency, bone marrow damage	Dehydration, renal problems, pulmonary or congenital heart disease
Hemoglobin	Iron, vitamin B12, or folate deficiency, bone marrow damage	Dehydration, renal problems, pulmonary or congenital heart disease
Hematocrit	Iron, vitamin B12, or folate deficiency, bone marrow damage	Dehydration, renal problems, pulmonary or congenital heart disease
Mean corpuscular volume (MCV)	Iron deficiency	Vitamin B12 or folate deficiency
Mean corpuscular hemoglobin (MCH)	Iron deficiency	Vitamin B12 or folate deficiency
Platelet count	Viral infections, lupus, pernicious anemia	Leukemia, inflammatory conditions

Data from Food and Nutrition Technical Assistance III Project. (2016). *Module 2. Nutrition assessment and classification* (Version 2, p. 9). https://www.fantaproject.org/sites/default/files/resources/NACS-Users-Guide-Module2-May2016.pdf

patient to record two workdays and one day off and bring the record to the next appointment. Mobile dietary applications are also available for patients to track dietary intake (Scarry et al., 2022). A limitation of the food record is that it depends on the patient's literacy and diligence in recording. *Food frequency questionnaires* (FFQs) assess how often the patient consumes specific foods or food groups and help determine overall dietary intake, dietary patterns, or changes over time. *Food habit questionnaires* assess food intake habits, such as the timing of meals, food preferences, meal preparation methods, and the circumstances around eating. Many rapid dietary screening tools are available for the APP short on time. In addition, assessment tools can be completed by patients while in the waiting room and quickly reviewed during the patient encounter.

Additional dietary assessment can be conducted through an interview format in which the APP asks the patients about their dietary habits. These questions should be open ended to obtain the most data. Examples of diet interview questions include "Tell me about your current diet and eating habits," "Who does the grocery shopping in your family?" "Who prepares the meals?" and "What does a typical lunch/snack/dinner look like?"

Assessing dietary intake is an essential component of a nutritional assessment, providing the APP with a clear picture of patients' food intake, food preferences, food allergies and intolerances, meal preparation, eating habits, schedule, religious and cultural practices related to food, and other factors contributing to their dietary pattern. The dietary assessment also enables the APP to make nutritional recommendations, identify patient knowledge gaps and challenges, and prioritize nutrition counseling. A referral to an RDN should be made for a more thorough dietary assessment and nutrition analysis.

Nutrition Recommendations

Nutrition prescriptions are based on the assessment of the patient's nutritional status and are grounded in evidence-based clinical practice guidelines. However, there are several important considerations to avoiding a one-size-fits-all dietary approach. The plan for improving nutrition should be tailored to the patient's specific health issues, life stage, readiness to change, personality, resources, and lifestyle needs. Diet is a fundamental component of culture, family, and one's identity (Hever & Cronise, 2017). Therefore, APPs also need to consider how cultural norms may affect the delivery of the nutrition intervention and the patient's reception.

Evidence-Based Clinical Practice Guidelines

An emphasis on an overall healthy eating pattern is an important concept to convey to patients because often their understanding is focused on individual nutrients, single foods, or food groups to consume or avoid, for example, eating dairy for calcium and meat for protein or limiting carbohydrate-rich foods such as pasta and potatoes. However, what matters most for promoting health is fostering a healthy eating pattern that emphasizes various nutrient-dense foods and that follows evidence-based recommendations.

The *2020–2025 Dietary Guidelines for Americans* provides basic recommendations for a healthy eating pattern, including (1) follow a healthy eating pattern across the life span; (2) focus on variety, nutrient density, and amount; (3) limit calories from added sugars and saturated fats and reduce sodium intake; (4) shift to healthier food and beverage choices; and (5) consider cultural and personal preferences to make these shifts easier to accomplish and maintain (HHS & USDA, 2020). The Dietary Guidelines Advisory Committee (2020) concluded that "dietary patterns associated with positive health outcomes include higher intake of vegetables, fruits, legumes, whole grains, low- or non-fat dairy, lean meat and poultry, seafood, nuts, and unsaturated vegetable oils and low consumption of red and processed meats, sugar-sweetened foods and drinks, and refined grains" (p. 8). Similarly, the American College of Lifestyle Medicine's (ACLM) Dietary Lifestyle Position Statement for Treatment and Potential Reversal of Disease states that "For the treatment, reversal,

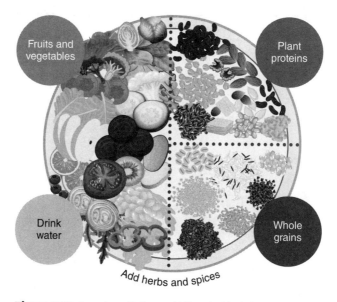

Figure 11.3 American College of Lifestyle Medicine whole-food plant-based plate.

American College of Lifestyle Medicine. (2019). *Adult whole food, plant-based plate.* www.lifestylemedicine.org

and prevention of lifestyle-related chronic disease, an eating plan based predominantly on a variety of minimally processed vegetables, fruits, whole grains, legumes, nuts and seeds is recommended" (PRWeb, 2018). **Figure 11.3** depicts a visual image of this WFPB plate.

Lifestyle behavior modification, including nutrition, is identified in several clinical practice recommendations as an essential first line in the prevention and management of chronic diseases, such as obesity (Garvey et al., 2016), T2D (American Diabetes Association [ADA], 2023; Garber et al., 2020), CVD (Arnett et al., 2019), chronic coronary syndromes (Knuuti et al., 2020), HTN (Unger et al., 2020), dyslipidemia (Reiter-Brennan et al., 2020), and cancer (World Cancer Research Fund & American Institute for Cancer Research, 2018). PCRM compiled evidence-informed dietary interventions for these and many more common conditions in their *Nutrition Guide for Clinicians* as well as best practices for discussing dietary changes with patients (Barnard, 2018). A few are summarized in **Table 11.11**. Although each health issue has specific considerations regarding nutritional guidance, the consensus among position statements and practice recommendations is that eating more unrefined plant-based foods is an essential strategy in health promotion and the prevention and management of chronic diseases.

Though patients with more advanced disease states may need a more focused nutrition prescription, a closer look at the nutrition considerations for preventing and treating the most common chronic conditions reveals that the same prescriptions can often help multiple diseases. The recommendation to eat more unrefined plant foods is reinforced by guidelines and position statements of many leading organizations, including the American Cancer Society, the ADA, the American Heart Association, and the Endocrine Society, among others (ACLM, n.d.). Although a significant trend in recent research is an emphasis on plant-based diets, it is noteworthy that the focus on optimizing nutrition for promoting health and healing disease was advocated in the first century by the Greek

Table 11.11 Nutritional Considerations by Condition

Condition	Nutritional Consideration

Coronary heart disease	Avoid hydrogenated and partially hydrogenated oils
	    Increase fiber-containing whole-plant foods
	    Consume soy and other legumes
	    Increase fruits, vegetables, and whole grains

Breast cancer	High-fiber, low-fat diet
	    Limit or avoid meat
	    Consume more vegetables and legumes (including soy products)

Colorectal cancer	Avoid red and processed meats Consume more fruits, vegetables, and whole grains

Constipation	Increase high-fiber foods
	    Increase fluid intake
	    Avoid cow's milk

T2D	Low-fat plant-based dietary pattern emphasizing low-glycemic index foods

Dyslipidemia	Plant-based dietary patterns rich in soluble fiber from vegetables, fruits, grains, and legumes
	    Minimize saturated and trans fats; emphasize monounsaturated and polyunsaturated fats
	    Consume more soy products, nuts, and foods rich in plant sterols

Gastroesophageal reflux disease	Increase fiber (fruit, whole grains)
	    Reduce fat
	    Avoid coffee, alcohol, and irritating foods

HTN	Diet rich in fruits and vegetables
	    Reduce saturated fat
	    Restrict sodium intake

Obesity	Consume foods lower in energy density and higher in water and fiber (e.g., salads, soups, vegetables, and fruits)
	    Reduce dietary fat intake
	    Minimize sugars

Data from Barnard, N. D. (Ed.). (2018). *Nutrition guide for clinicians* (3rd ed.). Physicians Committee for Responsible Medicine. https://nutritionguide.pcrm.org /nutritionguide /view/Nutrition_Guide_for_Clinicians/1342054/all /Nutrition_Guide_for_Clinicians

physician Hippocrates: "Let food be thy medicine, and let medicine be thy food."

Determining Caloric Needs

To provide nutrition counseling for maintaining a healthy weight, APPs need a basic understanding of estimating a patient's energy (calorie) needs. The recommended daily calorie intake depends on age, gender, height, weight, overall health, and physical activity level. Calorie consumption, even of healthy foods, that is consistently higher or lower than a person's energy needs can lead to poor health outcomes.

Basal metabolic rate (BMR) is the least amount of calories an individual needs when in a neutral environmental temperature during a fasting state. Although BMR is impractical to measure, resting energy expenditure (REE) is

Table 11.12 Mifflin-St Jeor Equation to Estimate Resting Energy Expenditure

Gender	Formula
Men	10 x weight (kg) + 6.25 x height (cm) – 5 x age (y) + 5
Women	10 x weight (kg) + 6.25 x height (cm) – 5 x age (y) - 161

Data from Mifflin, M. D., St Jeor, S. T., Hill, L. A., Scott, B. J., Daugherty, S. A., & Koh, Y. O. (1990). A new predictive equation for resting energy expenditure in healthy individuals. *The American Journal of Clinical Nutrition, 51*(2), 241–247. https://doi.org/10.1093/AJCN/51.2.241

Table 11.13 Physical Activity Level Multipliers

Physical Activity Level (PAL)	Multiplier
Little/no exercise (sedentary lifestyle)	1.2
Light exercise 1–2 times/week	1.375
Moderate exercise 2–3 times/week	1.55
Hard exercise 4–5 times/week	1.725
Physical job or hard exercise 6–7 times/week	1.9
Professional athlete	2.4

Data from Michałowska, J., & Zaborowska, L. (2023). *TDEE calculator - Total daily energy expenditure*. Omni Calculator. https://www.omnicalculator.com/health/tdee

used as a proxy since it is approximately 10% greater than BMR. REE is the energy (calories) required to maintain vital organ activity in a resting state over 24 hours. An estimated 65% of calorie expenditure is needed for REE, with variations based on height, weight, age, gender, and body composition. Lean body mass significantly correlates with REE. Regular physical activity, particularly weight-bearing exercises such as walking, increases lean muscle mass and as such increases REE. Aging decreases REE due to lean muscle mass decline over time; however, older adults who remain physically active can positively affect REE (Hark et al., 2014). REE can be determined by the Mifflin-St Jeor equation (see **Table 11.12**) or an online calculator such as the MyPlate Plan online calculator on the USDA MyPlate .gov website.

Once the REE is established, a physical activity level (PAL) multiplier is used to determine total daily energy expenditure (TDEE) for maintaining weight (see **Table 11.13**). TDEE is the total number of calories the body expends in 24 hours, including all activities. The formula for calculating TDEE is TDEE (kcal/day) = REE * PAL. If the patient's goal is to lose weight, the TDEE can be adjusted by no more than 20% to obtain a calorie deficit. It is important to note that whole-plant foods are naturally low in calories while at the same time providing satiety due to their high fiber

and water content. As a result, people who include more plant foods in their diet may find that they can lose weight without counting calories.

Writing the Nutrition Prescription

Once the APP assesses the patient's nutritional status and makes appropriate dietary recommendations, the APP should write an individualized nutrition prescription to include specific instructions for the patient to translate the recommendation into action. Nutrition prescriptions need to be written with the same level of detail as prescriptions for medication. The typical medication prescription includes the drug name, strength, dosage, route, frequency, and amount prescribed. Likewise, a nutrition prescription outlining the details of what to eat, how much, and how often is more likely to be followed than merely receiving vague advice to "Eat more fruits and vegetables" or "Increase intake of healthy fats."

After discussing the benefits of moving toward a plant-predominant dietary pattern and reviewing recommendations about the patients' health risks related to diet, the APP should use a partner approach to identify the actions patients are willing and ready to take. A key to helping patients be successful is to start with small action steps. For example, patients can begin by adding one plant-based meal each week. Once they succeed with one habit change, they will be motivated to add another. Likewise, too many nutrition prescriptions at once can overwhelm them. Prescriptions that focus on adding a food (e.g., "Eat ½ cup of beans once daily") rather than cutting back (e.g., "Limit eggs to 3 per week") are generally more acceptable to the patients and an excellent place to start.

The mnemonic TAF is a guideline to consider when writing a nutrition prescription (Kelly & Clayton, 2021):

- Type of food, as specific as possible (e.g., "Cruciferous vegetables, such as broccoli, cabbage, and kale"). Focus on specific foods or food groups (e.g., berries) instead of nutritional categories (e.g., fiber, unsaturated fats), which are harder to track and measure.
- Amount of food to be eaten, as exact as possible (e.g., "1 serving, which is 1 cup raw or ½ cup cooked").
- Frequency food should be eaten (e.g., "Once daily"). This may also be time limited (e.g., "Once daily for 2 weeks").

Appropriate "dosing" of the nutrition prescription is essential: patients with existing diseases will require more intensive nutrition therapy than the healthy individual whose goal is to minimize risk (Kelly & Clayton, 2021). Nutrition prescriptions should also consider the patient's readiness to change, circumstances, access to nutritious foods, and personal preferences. In addition, each element of SMART (specific, measurable, attainable, relevant, and time-bound) should be considered.

Dietary Counseling and Nutrition Education

The U.S. Preventive Services Task Force (2020) recommends dietary counseling for individuals with risk factors for cardiac disease, such as overweight and obesity, T2D, elevated blood pressure or HTN, dyslipidemia, and unhealthy diet. Dietary counseling is the process of helping patients make healthy food choices and form healthy eating habits (National Cancer Institute, n.d.). A nutritional coaching approach, in which the APP uses motivational interviewing to guide patients to develop a vision for healthy eating, set specific short-term goals, create a realistic action plan, and find solutions to challenges, will empower patients to take responsibility for their health and achieve better outcomes (Lancha et al., 2018).

Health Promotion Case Example: Nutrition Coaching for Weight Loss

Case Description: A 42-year-old businessman with obesity had tried numerous diets over the previous 7 years to modify his body composition and blood biochemistry. Although successful at losing weight many times, each attempt was followed by weight regain within 2–6 months. One likely reason for this is that his dietary modifications were not sustainable. In fact, after finishing a diet, he reported that he felt "free to eat everything that had been prohibited during the dieting period."

Intervention: Nutrition assessment included anthropometric measurements of weight, body composition, skinfold measurements, and WC. In addition, the patient was interviewed to evaluate daily nutritional routines. A 24-hour recall assessed nutritional intake.

Rather than prescribing another diet, the clinician offered a nutritional coaching approach consisting of 12 weekly nutritional coaching sessions, scheduled for 45 minutes each. Half of the sessions were conducted face-to-face, and half were electronic (using the Skype platform). Regular communication between the coach and patient occurred between sessions via email and text message.

Using motivational interviewing, the patient's strengths, values, and desires were determined; a vision was formed; and specific short-term goals were set. Following is an example of a nutritional goal-setting coaching conversation:

Coach: *What would you like to change about your eating habits?*

Patient: *I would like to reduce the amount of fried food I eat.*

Coach: *Okay, what is your intake today, and what would you want it to become?*

Patient: *Nowadays, I have some fried food once a day, and I would like to reduce it to twice a week.*

Coach: *Okay, on a scale of 0 to 10, how confident are you that you can reduce your fried food intake from daily to twice a week?*

Patient: *Seven to 8, because it is really important to me and I have already done this in the past. So I know that I can.*

Results: After 12 nutritional coaching sessions, reductions in body fat mass (30.9% down to 26%) and total body weight (111.0 kg down to 102.2 kg) were attained. WC dropped from 107 cm to 99.3 cm. Nutritional habits also improved as the patient showed decreased total energy intake (2,200 to 1,500 kcal/day), reduced fat intake (41% of energy intake to 17%), and increased fiber ingestion (8 to 30 g/day). The patient also increased daily physical activity and energy expenditure.

Implications for Advanced Practice: The nutritional coaching strategy was effective at helping the patient develop new eating patterns that were sustainable. Subsequently, related health parameters were improved. By using a nutritional coaching approach that keeps patients at the core of promoting their lifestyle changes, APPs may be able to induce immediate health benefits and improved dietary habits.

Reference: Lancha, A. H., Jr., Sforzo, G. A., & Pereira-Lancha, L. O. (2018). Improving nutritional habits with no diet prescription: Details of a nutritional coaching process. *American Journal of Lifestyle Medicine, 12*(2), 160–165. https://doi.org/10.1177/1559827616636616

When communicating nutrition education, the Elicit-Provide-Elicit technique allows the APP to share information in a neutral, nonjudgmental fashion that supports patients' autonomy (Miller & Rollnick, 2012). First, assess the patients' knowledge on the topic to avoid sharing information they already know and uncover any misunderstandings or gaps in knowledge. Then elicit the patients' permission to provide information, for example, "May I share some strategies others have used to lower cholesterol successfully?" If patients express interest, the APP can briefly provide the information. The APP follows the information by eliciting the patients' thoughts on what was shared, for example, "Do any of those strategies stand out for you?"

The focus of nutrition education should be on overall dietary patterns, diet quality, and nutrient-dense foods rather than on single nutrients (Forouhi et al., 2018). The APP should condense complex information into actionable messages that are meaningful to patients and easy to understand and visualize (Liu et al., 2017). A simple photo or instruction on using the hand to estimate portion size can help patients quickly visualize the "dose" of foods in the nutrition prescription. Images such as ACLM's WFPB plate (see Figure 11.3) depict the variety of foods to be consumed. Another simplistic way to guide patients concerning healthy foods is to advise them to eat a rainbow of colorful fruits, vegetables, legumes, grains, nuts, and seeds (Blumfield et al., 2022).

Food Density

Understanding the energy density of foods is integral to maintaining a healthy weight (Stelmach-Mardas et al., 2016). Food energy density, or calorie density, is the number of kilocalories (energy) in a unit measure (typically in grams) of food. Most plant foods (except for plant oils and nuts) have low energy density and high fiber and water content. The fiber and water increase the food's volume, so a person can eat more and feel fuller while consuming fewer calories. On the other hand, animal and processed foods have high energy density and low fiber and water content. Even small amounts of these foods can carry a lot of calories. Dietary patterns that contain high amounts of low energy density foods are associated with decreased body weight (Stelmach-Mardas et al., 2016).

Another way to compare foods is by nutrient density. Foods with high nutrient density have a lot of nutritional value (e.g., micronutrients, fiber, omega-3 fats) in proportion to their energy (or calories). Foods with low nutrient density and high calories are referred to as empty calorie foods. The plant-predominant dietary patterns are made up of foods that have the highest nutrient density and the lowest energy density. Charts comparing the energy density of foods and images comparing the volume of low energy density foods with that of high energy density foods can help patients visualize these concepts and make healthier food choices.

Food Labels

In general, patients should be advised to eat foods that do not have a label by selecting foods from the produce section of a grocery store or shopping at the local farmers market. However, due to the current fast-paced style of living and busy lifestyles, many people purchase convenience foods packaged with labels. Therefore, patients must understand how to read food labels to make healthier food choices.

In 2016, the FDA introduced a new food label reflective of the most recent scientific evidence and the link between food and chronic diseases (FDA, 2022). **Figure 11.4** depicts the revised nutrition facts label. Additionally, the FDA has provided resources for health professionals to teach individuals about the nutrition facts label and how to utilize the information to select healthier foods (see Table 11.16). It is essential that patients understand the number of servings in a package and that the package size does not reflect the typical portion size that a person might eat or determine serving sizes. Some items packaged in small containers may contain several servings. For example, in Figure 11.4, there are 230 calories in each two-thirds cup serving. Furthermore, it is also important for patients to understand that the nutrition facts label is based on an intake of 2,000 calories, which may not be the appropriate calorie level for the patient.

Food labels also alert patients to the nutrients within a food item, which can be helpful when deciding the quantity of a particular food to consume. See **Table 11.14** for the recommended amount of foods to be consumed daily based on desired daily calorie intake.

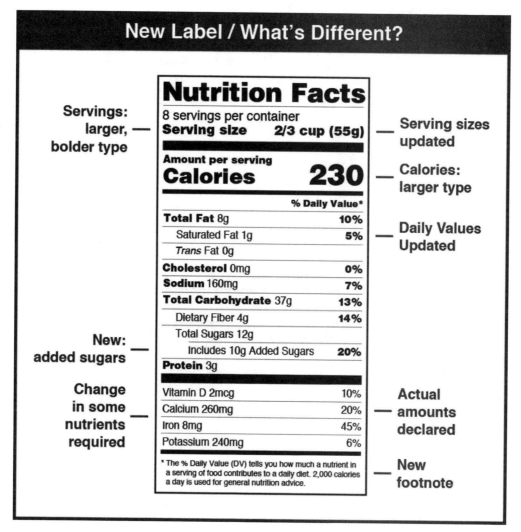

Figure 11.4 Revised nutrition facts food label.

U.S. Food and Drug Administration. (2022, March 7). *Changes to the nutrition facts label*. Department of Health and Human Services. https://www.fda.gov/food/food-labeling-nutrition/changes-nutrition-facts-label

Plant-Predominant Diet Questions Answered

Changing well-established dietary patterns can be daunting, and patients may have questions and concerns about the recommendation to move toward a plant-predominant diet. **Table 11.15** lists some of these questions and possible answers that an APP can provide. An informed patient can safely transition to eating more plant foods without concern for nutrient deficiency (Craig et al., 2021). The role of the APP for these patients is to be a trusted source of information and to provide ongoing follow-up for nutritional assessment and education support.

Table 11.14 General Recommendations for Categories of Food That Should Be Included in the Daily Eating Pattern

Daily Calories	Vegetables (cups)	Fruits (cups)	Grains (ounces)	Protein (ounces)	Dairy or Dairy Substitute (cups)	Limit Sodium, Saturated Fat, and Added Sugar
1,000	1	1	3	2	2	Sodium 1,500 mg Saturated fat 11 g Added sugar 25 g
1,600	2	1½	5	5	3	Sodium 2,300 mg Saturated fat 18 g Added sugar 40 g
2,000	2½	2	6	5½	3	Sodium ≤2,300 mg Fats 22 g Added sugars 50 g

Adapted from ChooseMyPlate.gov.

Table 11.15 Answers for Frequently Asked Patient Questions About Nutrition

Patient Questions	Answers
Are gluten-free foods healthier?	Gluten-free foods are not healthier unless you have celiac disease or are gluten sensitive. If you choose to avoid gluten without a health reason, you may not get adequate vitamins, fiber, and minerals. A gluten-free diet is not intended for weight loss.
Should I avoid all fats if I am trying to eat healthier and lose weight?	You do not need to avoid all fats if you are trying to eat healthier or lose weight. Fats from specific food sources provide essential PUFAs or omega-3s that must be consumed by food or supplemented. Since fats have more calories per gram than protein or carbohydrates, you may want to limit refined oils to avoid extra calories. Healthy fats can be obtained from avocados, olives, walnuts, and almonds. Only a handful, or 1 oz, serving of nuts is needed per day. Avoid fats from saturated sources, such as whole-fat cheese or milk, and replace them with lower-fat or nondairy alternatives.
Do I have to purchase organic foods to eat healthfully?	No, you do not need to purchase organic foods to eat healthfully. The USDA has reported that they have not found detectable harmful pesticides on more than 99% of products sampled annually.
Do I need to drink milk or dairy to get enough calcium?	No, plants are the original sources of calcium absorbed from the soil. Plants can supply adequate amounts of calcium. For example, 2 c of cooked broccoli contains 125 mg of calcium, 1 c of cooked collards has 260 mg, and 1 c of almond milk has 450 mg.
Are carbohydrates bad for me?	No, carbohydrates are the brain's only source of energy and the body's preferred energy source. The type of carbohydrate is important, however. Carbohydrates from whole-plant foods (vegetables, whole grains, beans, legumes) are the best choices.

Patient Questions	Answers
Will I get enough protein if I don't eat meat, eggs, or cheese?	Plants such as beans, legumes, nuts, and vegetables provide adequate protein, including additional fiber, antioxidants, and essential nutrients not found in animal foods. For example, 1 c of red lentils contains 18 g of protein, and 3 oz of salmon contains 20 g.
Does it cost more to eat healthfully?	It is possible to eat healthy foods on a budget. For example, packaged processed foods and meat cost more than beans and whole grains. Planning and preparing meals at home will cost less than eating out.
What does GMO mean, and is it healthy to eat genetically modified (GMO) foods?	GMO stands for genetically modified organisms. Foods are genetically modified by changing their DNA using genes from other plants or animals. The gene for the desired trait in one plant or animal is inserted into another plant or animal. The FDA evaluates all GMO foods for safety before they are sold. Furthermore, other governmental agencies, including the Environmental Protection Agency and the U.S. Department of Agriculture, regulate genetically modified or bioengineered foods. The benefits of GMO foods are that they can be modified to be more nutritious, tastier, resistant to diseases, and resistant to pests requiring fewer pesticides, increasing the shelf life of food. Concerns regarding GMO foods causing allergic reactions, harmful genetic changes, and decreased nutrients in food are unfounded (MedlinePlus, n.d.).

Adapted from the National Institute of Diabetes and Digestive and Kidney Diseases. (2017). *Some myths about nutrition and physical activity.* U.S. Department of Health and Human Services. https://www.niddk.nih.gov/health-information/weight-management/myths-nutrition-physical-activity and MedlinePlus. (n.d.). *Genetically engineered foods.* National Library of Medicine. Retrieved January 17, 2023, from https://medlineplus.gov/ency/article/002432.htm

Educational Resources

The APP who prioritizes nutrition education will want to build a collection of evidence-based handouts to save time during the patient visit and aid in the retention and recall of the information provided. Since the internet abounds with conflicting nutrition information, it is also helpful to guide patients to reliable online information sources and web-based resources (see **Table 11.16**). Numerous mobile apps are also available to support patients in nutrition education and dietary change.

Health Promotion Case Study: Suboptimal Nutrition

Case Description: B.T., a 35-year-old female, visits the clinic for a physical required for admission to graduate school in 1 month. She denies any chronic health problems except occasional "indigestion," which she describes as upper abdominal or mid-chest burning for about 60 minutes after eating fast food. Her 24-hour diet recall reveals that she does not eat breakfast most days but instead has two cups of coffee. For lunch, she has two Mountain Dews and a green salad and for dinner, a burger and fries with a milkshake.

- Past medical history: Unremarkable.
- Medications: None.
- Allergies: No known allergies.

(continues)

Health Promotion Case Study: Suboptimal Nutrition   *(continued)*

- Social history: Single, works full-time as a nurse.
- Vital signs: BP 114/70 mmHg left arm, heart rate 66 bpm, respirations 16 bpm, temperature 98.6°F, O_2 saturation 98% on room air, weight 135 lb, height 63 in., BMI 24.7 kg/m^2.
- Review of systems: Occasional indigestion or upper abdominal or mid-chest burning after eating fast food. All other systems are negative.
- Physical exam: The physical exam was unremarkable.
- Labs: Not available.

Lifestyle Vital Signs

- Adopt healthy eating: Occasionally eats fruit and usually has a green salad from the cafeteria when she is at work 3–4 days per week. She drinks about 2 c of coffee and two sodas daily. Dinner is usually fast food or a frozen dinner cooked in the microwave.
- Stress less: Does not feel stressed but is concerned that graduate school will be stressful.
- Move often: She usually walks for 30 minutes most days.
- Avoid alcohol: She denies drinking alcohol except for one glass of wine during social events once or twice a year.
- Rest more: Sleeps 8–9 hours each night.
- Treat tobacco use: She has never smoked.

Assessment: Suboptimal nutrition.

Critical Thinking Questions

- Considering the ABCDs of nutrition assessment, what additional information do you want to obtain, and why?
- Based on the U.S. dietary guidelines, what are B.T.'s estimated calories needed per day for her age, sex, and physical activity?
- What is your plan for improving B.T.'s nutrition?
- Using the TAF prescription formula, write three appropriate nutrition prescriptions based on the 2020–2025 dietary guidelines. Provide a rationale for your prescriptions.

Reference: U.S. Department of Health and Human Services & U.S. Department of Agriculture. (2020). *Dietary guidelines for Americans, 2020–2025* (9th ed.). https://www.dietaryguidelines.gov

TABLE 11.16	Evidence-Based Resources for Adopting Healthy Eating	
Organization	**Resource**	**URL**
Afro-Vegan Society	Resources, recipes, *African American Vegan Starter Guide*	https://www.afrovegansociety.org
American Association of Clinical Endocrinology and The Obesity Society	*Clinical Practice Guidelines for Healthy Eating for the Prevention and Treatment of Metabolic and Endocrine Diseases in Adults*	https://www.endocrinepractice.org/article/S1530-891X(20)43460-3/fulltext

Organization	Resource	URL
American College of Lifestyle Medicine (ACLM)	*The Benefits of Plant-Based Nutrition* white paper series	https://lifestylemedicine.org/articles/benefits-plant-based-nutrition/
CulinaryMedicine.org (Tulane University)	Culinary medicine, Continuing Medical Education (CME), conferences, certification, resources	https://culinarymedicine.org
CulinaryRx	Online nutrition and cooking course for patients and providers	https://plantricianproject.org/culinary-rx
Esselstyn Foundation	Resources, videos, recipes	https://esselstynfamilyfoundation.org
Forks Over Knives	Documentary, cooking course, recipes, meal planner, success stories, articles	https://www.forksoverknives.com
Full Plate Living	Online and group resources on increasing intake of whole, plant-based foods	https://www.fullplateliving.org/resources-physicians
International Plant-Based Nutrition Healthcare Conference	Annual conference and online CME focusing on scientific research for using whole food, plant-based nutrition for preventing and treating chronic disease	https://pbnhc.com
National Institutes of Health (NIH) Office of Dietary Supplements	Databases and tools for DRIs, daily values, and nutrient recommendations	https://ods.od.nih.gov/Health Information/nutrient recommendations.aspx
NutritionCME.org	Online nutrition-related CME on the role of nutrition in brain health, heart health, diabetes, obesity, and more, free of commercial sponsorship	www.NutritionCME.org
NutritionFacts.org	Videos and articles on the latest science about foods. Provides the *Daily Dozen* app.	https://nutritionfacts.org
Omni Calculator	Free health calculators for body measurement, BMI, dietary, etc.	https://www.omnicalculator.com/health
Physicians Committee for Responsible Medicine (PCRM)	*Nutrition Guide for Clinicians* (free mobile app), *Food for Life* cooking and nutrition class, nutrition education, patient resources, research articles, recipes, fact sheets, free 21-Day Vegan Kickstart	https://www.pcrm.org/good-nutrition

(continues)

TABLE 11.16	Evidence-Based Resources for Adopting Healthy Eating *(continued)*

Organization	Resource	URL
Plant-Based Prevention of Disease (P-POD)	Continuing education conferences	https://www.preventionof disease.org
PlantBasedResearch.org	Collection of peer-reviewed scientific research papers and educational resources relevant to plant-based nutrition	http://www.plantbased research.org
Swich	Free online plant-based cooking education	https://thebigswich.com
T. Colin Campbell Center for Nutrition Studies (CNS)	CME, recipes, resources	https://nutritionstudies.org
T. Colin Campbell Center for Nutrition Studies (CNS)	Free *Plant-Based Health* mini course	https://nutritionstudies.org /plant-based-health-mini -course
The Plantrician Project	*International Journal of Disease Reversal and Prevention*; information and resources for healthcare providers on whole-food plant-based nutrition; *Plant-Based Nutrition Quick Start Guide*	https://plantricianproject.org
The Vegetarian Resource Group	*Vegetarian Journal* and other educational resources	https://www.vrg.org
U.S. Food and Drug Administration (FDA)	Health Educator's Nutrition Toolkit	https://www.fda.gov /food/nutrition-education -resources-materials/health -educators-nutrition-toolkit -setting-table-healthy-eating
U.S. Food and Drug Administration (FDA)	Nutrition and food safety information and resources	https://www.fda.gov/food /resources-you-food /healthcare-professionals
U.S. Food and Drug Administration (FDA)	Nutrition facts label CME	https://www.fda.gov/food /healthcare-professionals /nutrition-facts-label -continuing-medical -education-program -physicians
HHS and USDA	*Dietary Guidelines for Americans, 2020–2025*	https://www.dietaryguidelines .gov

Organization	Resource	URL
Vegan Health	Evidence-based nutrient recommendations	https://veganhealth.org
Websites of plant-based documentaries	Viewing information, resources	www.codebluedoc.com www.forksoverknives.com/the-film https://gamechangersmovie.com www.adventhealth.com/plantwise-documentary
Websites of plant-based dietitians	Evidence-based information, resources, recipes	www.brendadavisrd.com https://plantbaseddietitian.com https://www.theveganrd.com

Interprofessional Collaboration

Helping patients change their dietary patterns and establish new habits around eating takes time and can be challenging. A team approach of several professionals with different perspectives and expertise can support the APP in this endeavor. A referral to an RDN for medical nutrition therapy (MNT) is important to consider in the plan of care, especially for patients with obesity, diabetes, digestive issues, and kidney disease. MNT includes more in-depth nutrition assessment, diagnosis, intervention, counseling, monitoring, and evaluation. It is cost effective for improving many nutrition-related health outcomes (Academy of Nutrition and Dietetics, 2022). MNT is covered by Medicare and many other insurance providers for T2D and kidney disease. Certified diabetes educators specialize in educating, supporting, and promoting self-management of diabetes. Certified health coaches have additional training in the science of behavior change and can provide frequent and ongoing support to patients as they develop healthier behaviors and attitudes around food. Patients with food insecurity should be referred to licensed social workers, local community resources (e.g., food pantry), and federal food assistance programs such as the National School Lunch Program (NSLP); the Women, Infants, and Children (WIC) program; and the Supplemental Nutrition Assistance Program (SNAP).

Health Promotion Activity: Food Record

Complete a food record of all food and beverage you consume over 3 days. Include two workdays (or school days) and one day off. In addition, explore mobile apps for recording food intake.

What did you learn about your food intake and habits?

Based on your experience, what challenges might your patients face in completing a food record? What tips or tools might you recommend?

What did you learn from this experience? How will you apply these insights to advanced practice?

Summary

There is strong evidence that suboptimal nutritional status contributes to a leading cause of mortality and disability nationally and globally. Current research strongly supports a plant-predominant diet consisting of a variety of colorful fruits and vegetables, whole grains, legumes, nuts, and seeds to prevent and treat diet-related chronic disease. Accordingly, improving dietary quality is an essential health promotion and disease prevention skill for the APP.

Foods contain macronutrients (e.g., carbohydrates, fats, proteins) and micronutrients (e.g., vitamins, minerals), which are essential for the optimal functioning of the body and immune system and the prevention and treatment of diet-related chronic diseases. The IOM Food and Nutrition Board establishes DRIs for nutrient intake in healthy individuals. While it is important for the APP to understand these nutrients and recommended intakes, the patients' overall dietary pattern is more important than any individual nutrient or food.

There is a relatively wide range of diets in the United States, from the typical Western diet on one end of the spectrum to plant-predominant diets on the other. The former includes high intakes of refined sugars, animal fats, processed meats, refined grains, high-fat dairy, and salt; the latter prioritizes minimally processed, nutritious plant-based foods that provide fiber, water, antioxidants, and healthy fats. Any movement toward a plant-predominant eating pattern will result in better health outcomes.

The APP is well positioned to start the conversation with patients about nutrition and articulate its importance in improving their health. The APP–patient relationship provides the context for conducting nutritional screening and comprehensive nutritional assessments, including anthropometric, biochemical, clinical, and dietary. The APP's plan of care for patients' nutritional needs is based on evidence-based clinical practice guidelines and should be tailored to patients' needs and preferences. APPs can translate skills in prescribing medications to nutrition prescriptions, using the TAF mnemonic as a guide: (a) type of food, (b) quantity of food, and (c) frequency. In addition, each element of SMART must be considered.

The focus should be on overall dietary patterns, dietary quality, and nutrient-dense foods rather than on individual nutrients. The APP is encouraged to use a nutritional coaching approach to provide dietary counseling and the Elicit-Provide-Elicit technique in communicating nutrition education.

Helping patients adopt healthy eating and establish new dietary patterns can be time consuming and difficult. A team approach that includes RDNs, certified diabetes educators, certified health coaches, licensed social workers, and community resources can support APPs in this endeavor.

Acronyms

ABCDs: anthropometric, biochemical, clinical, and dietary assessment
ACLM: American College of Lifestyle Medicine
ADA: American Diabetes Association
AGEs: advanced glycation end products
AI: adequate intake
ALA: alpha-Linolenic acid

AMDR: acceptable macronutrient distribution range
APP: advanced practice provider
BIA: bioelectrical impedance analysis
BMI: body mass index
BMR: basal metabolic rate
CDC: Centers for Disease Control and Prevention

CVD: cardiovascular disease
DHA: docosahexaenoic acid
DNA: deoxyribonucleic acid
DRI: dietary reference intake
DSQ: Dietary Screener Questionnaire
EPA: eicosapentaenoic acid
FANTA: Food and Nutrition Technical Assistance III Project
FDA: U.S. Food and Drug Administration
FFQ: food frequency questionnaire
GMO: genetically modified organism
HHS: U.S. Department of Health and Human Services
HTN: hypertension
MEDAS: Mediterranean Diet Adherence Screener
MNA-SF: Mini-Nutritional Assessment Short Form
MNT: medical nutrition therapy
MUAC: mid-upper arm circumference
MUFA: monounsaturated fatty acid
MUST: Malnutrition Universal Screening Tool
Na: sodium
NCCIH: National Center for Complementary and Integrative Health
NCD: noncommunicable disease
NHLBI: National Heart, Lung, and Blood Institute

ODPHP: Office of Disease Prevention and Health Promotion
ODS: Office of Dietary Supplements
PAL: physical activity level
PCRM: Physicians Committee for Responsible Medicine
PRO: protein
PUFA: polyunsaturated fatty acid
RDA: recommended dietary allowance
RDN: registered dietitian nutritionist
REAP-S: Rapid Eating Assessment for Participants Short Form
REE resting energy expenditure
RNA: ribonucleic acid
ROS: review of systems
SFA: saturated fatty acid
STC: Starting the Conversation tool
T2D: type 2 diabetes
TDEE: total daily energy expenditure
TFA: trans-fatty acid
UL: tolerable upper intake level
USDA: U.S. Department of Agriculture
WC: waist circumference
WFPB whole food plant based
WHO: World Health Organization
WHZ: weight-for-height z-score
YLD: years of healthy life lost due to disability

References

Abdulah, D. M., & Hassan, A. B. (2020). Relation of dietary factors with infection and mortality rates of COVID-19 across the world. *Journal of Nutrition, Health and Aging, 24*(9), 1011. https://doi.org/10.1007/S12603-020-1512-3

Academy of Nutrition and Dietetics. (2022, June 2). *Medical nutrition therapy.* https://www.andeal.org/topic.cfm?menu=5284

Afshin, A., Sur, P. J., Fay, K. A., Cornaby, L., Ferrara, G., Salama, J. S., Mullany, E. C., Abate, K. H., Abbafati, C., Abebe, Z., Afarideh, M., Aggarwal, A., Agrawal, S., Akinyemiju, T., Alahdab, F., Bacha, U., Bachman, V. F., Badali, H., Badawi, A., . . . Murray, C. J. L. (2019, May 11). Health effects of dietary risks in 195 countries, 1990–2017: A systematic analysis for the Global Burden of Disease Study 2017. *Lancet, 393*(10184), 1958–1972. https://doi.org/10.1016/S0140-6736(19)30041-8

American College of Lifestyle Medicine. (n.d.). *The benefits of plant-based nutrition* [White paper]. https://lifestylemedicine.org/articles/benefits-plant-based-nutrition

American College of Lifestyle Medicine. (2020). Dietary spectrum. https://lifestylemedicine.org/wp-content/uploads/2022/07/ACLM-Dietary-Spectrum-8.5x11.pdf

American Diabetes Association. (2023). Standards of care in diabetes—2023 abridged for primary care providers. *Clinical Diabetes, 41*(1), 4–31. https://doi.org/10.2337/cd23-as01

American Heart Association. (2021). *Saturated fat.* https://www.heart.org/en/healthy-living/healthy-eating/eat-smart/fats/saturated-fats

Arnett, D. K., Khera, A., & Blumenthal, R. S. (2019). 2019 ACC/AHA guideline on the primary prevention of cardiovascular disease: Part 1, lifestyle and behavioral factors. *Journal of the American Medical Association (JAMA) Cardiology, 4*(10), 1043–1044. https://doi.org/10.1001/jamacardio.2019.2604

Bailey R. L. (2021). Overview of dietary assessment methods for measuring intakes of foods, beverages, and dietary supplements in research studies. *Current Opinion in Biotechnology, 70,* 91–96. https://doi.org/10.1016/j.copbio.2021.02.007

Barnard, N. D. (Ed.). (2018). *Nutrition guide for clinicians* (3rd ed.). Physicians Committee for Responsible Medicine. https://nutritionguide.pcrm.org/nutritionguide/view/Nutrition_Guide_for_Clinicians/1342054/all/Nutrition_Guide_for_Clinicians

Berryman, C. E., Lieberman, H. R., Fulgoni, V. L., & Pasiakos, S. M. (2018). Protein intake trends and conformity with the dietary reference intakes in the United States: Analysis of the National Health and Nutrition Examination Survey, 2001–2014. *American Journal of Clinical Nutrition, 108*(2), 405–413. https://doi.org/10.1093/ajcn/nqy088

Bhardwaj, B., O'Keefe, E., & O'Keefe, J. (2016). Death by carbs: Added sugars and refined carbohydrates cause diabetes and cardiovascular disease in Asian Indians. *Missouri Medicine, 113*(5), 395–400.

Bjarnadottir, A. (2019, May 21). *7 nutrient deficiencies that are incredibly common.* Healthline. https://www.healthline.com/nutrition/7-common-nutrient-deficiencies

Blue Zones. (n.d.). *Food guidelines.* Retrieved January 18, 2023, from https://www.bluezones.com/recipes/food-guidelines

Blumfield, M., Mayr, H., De Vlieger, N., Abbott, K., Starck, C., Fayet-Moore, F., & Marshall, S. (2022). Should we "eat a rainbow"? An umbrella review of the health effects of colorful bioactive pigments in fruits and vegetables. *Molecules, 27*(13), 4061. https://doi.org/10.3390/molecules27134061

Boushey, C., Ard, J., Bazzano, L., Heymsfield, S., Mayer-Davis, E., Sabaté, J., Snetselaar, L., Van Horn, L., Schneeman, B., English, L. K., Bates, M., Callahan, E., Venkatramanan, S., Butera, G., Terry, N., & Obbagy, J. (2020). *Dietary patterns and all-cause mortality: A systematic review.* USDA Nutrition Evidence Systematic Review. https://www.ncbi.nlm.nih.gov/books/NBK578477

Benítez Brito, N., Suárez Llanos, J. P., Fuentes Ferrer, M., Oliva García, J. G., Delgado Brito, I., Pereyra-García Castro, F., Caracena Castellanos, N., Acevedo Rodríguez, C. X., & Palacio Abizanda, E. (2016). Relationship between mid-upper arm circumference and body mass index in inpatients. *PloS ONE, 11*(8), e0160480. https://doi.org/10.1371/journal.pone.0160480

Cashin, K., & Oot, L. (2018). *Guide to anthropometry: A practical tool for program planners, managers, and implementers.* FHI 360, Food and Nutrition Technical Assistance III Project. https://www.fantaproject.org/sites/default/files/resources/FANTA-Anthropometry-Guide-May2018.pdf

Centers for Disease Control and Prevention. (n.d.). *Growth charts.* Retrieved June 11, 2023, from https://www.cdc.gov/growthcharts/index.htm

Centers for Disease Control and Prevention. (2020). *Get the facts: Drinking water and intake.* https://www.cdc.gov/nutrition/data-statistics/plain-water-the-healthier-choice.html

Centers for Disease Control and Prevention. (2021). *Micronutrients.* https://www.cdc.gov/nutrition/micronutrient-malnutrition/index.html

Clem, J., & Barthel, B. (2021). A look at plant-based diets. *Missouri Medicine, 118*(3), 233–238.

Craig, W. J., Mangels, A. R., Fresán, U., Marsh, K., Miles, F. L., Saunders, A. V., Haddad, E. H., Heskey, C. E., Johnston, P., Larson-Meyer, E., & Orlich, M. (2021). The safe and effective use of plant-based diets with guidelines for health professionals. *Nutrients, 13*(11), 4144. https://doi.org/10.3390/nu13114144

Davis, B. (2019). *Kick diabetes essentials: The diet and lifestyle guide.* Healthy Living.

Davis, C., Bryan, J., Hodgson, J., & Murphy, K. (2015). Definition of the Mediterranean diet: A literature review. *Nutrients, 7*(11), 9139–9153. https://doi.org/10.3390/nu7115459

Dietary Guidelines Advisory Committee. (2020, July). *Scientific report of the 2020 Dietary Guidelines Advisory Committee: Advisory report to the Secretary of Agriculture and the Secretary of Health and Human Services.* https://www.dietaryguidelines.gov/sites/default/files/2020-07/ScientificReport_of_the_2020Dietary GuidelinesAdvisoryCommittee_first-print.pdf

Dmitrieva, N. I., Gagarin, A., Liu, D., Wu, C. O., & Boehm, M. (2023). Middle-age high normal serum sodium as a risk factor for accelerated biological aging, chronic diseases, and premature mortality. *EBioMedicine, 87*(104404). https://doi.org/10.1016/j.ebiom.2022.104404

Domingo, J. L. (2016). Nutrients and chemical pollutants in fish and shellfish. Balancing health benefits and risks of regular fish consumption. *Critical Reviews in Food Science and Nutrition, 56*(6), 979–988. https://doi.org/10.1080/10408398.2012.742985

Downes, L. S., Buchholz, S. W., Bruster, B., Girimurugan, S. B., Fogg, L. F., & Frock, M. S. (2019). Delivery of a community-based nutrition education program for minority adults. *Journal of the American Association of Nurse Practitioners, 31*(4), 267–277. https://doi.org/10.1097/JXX.0000000000000144

Economic Research Service. (n.d.). *Definitions of food security.* Retrieved January 17, 2023, from https://www.ers.usda.gov/topics/food-nutrition-assistance/food-security-in-the-u-s/definitions-of-food-security

Elsey, A. M., Lowe, A. K., Cornell, A. N., Whitehead, P. N., & Conners, R. T. (2021). Comparison of the three-site and seven-site measurements in female collegiate athletes using BodyMetrix™. *International Journal of Exercise Science, 14*(4), 230–238.

Food and Nutrition Technical Assistance III Project. (2016). *Module 2: Nutrition assessment and classification* (Version 2, p. 5). https://www.fantaproject.org /sites/default/files/resources/NACS-Users-Guide -Module2-May2016.pdf

Forouhi, N. G., Krauss, R. M., Taubes, G., & Willett, W. (2018). Dietary fat and cardiometabolic health: Evidence, controversies, and consensus for guidance. *British Medical Journal, 361*, k2139. https://doi.org /10.1136/bmj.k2139

Furman, D., Campisi, J., Verdin, E., Carrera-Bastos, P., Targ, S., Franceschi, C., Ferrucci, L., Gilroy, D. W., Fasano, A., Miller, G. W., Miller, A. H., Mantovani, A., Weyand, C. M., Barzilai, N., Goronzy, J. J., Rando, T. A., Effros, R. B., Lucia, A., Kleinstreuer, N., & Slavich, G. M. (2019). Chronic inflammation in the etiology of disease across the life span. *Nature Medicine, 25*(12), 1822–1832. https://doi.org/10.1038/s 41591-019-0675-0

Garber, A. J., Handelsman, Y., Grunberger, G., Einhorn, D., Abrahamson, M. J., Barzilay, J. I., Blonde, L., Bush, M. A., DeFronzo, R. A., Garber, J. R., Garvey, W. T., Hirsch, I. B., Jellinger, P. S., McGill, J. B., Mechanick, J. I., Perreault, L., Rosenblit, P. D., Samson, S., & Umpierrez, G. E. (2020). Consensus statement by the American Association of Clinical Endocrinologists and American College of Endocrinology on the comprehensive type 2 diabetes management algorithm - 2020 executive summary. *Endocrine Practice, 26*(1), 107–139. https://doi.org/10.4158/CS -2019-0472

Garvey, W. T., Mechanick, J. I., Brett, E. M., Garber, A. J., Hurley, D. L., Jastreboff, A. M., Nadolsky, K., Pessah-Pollack, R., & Plodkowski, R. (2016). American Association of Clinical Endocrinologists and American College of Endocrinology comprehensive clinical practice guidelines for medical care of patients with obesity. *Endocrine Practice, 22*, 1–203. https://doi .org/10.4158/EP161365.GL

Hager, E. R., Quigg, A. M., Black, M. M., Coleman, S. M., Heeren, T., Rose-Jacobs, R., Cook, J. T., Ettinger de Cuba, S. E., Casey, P. H., Chilton, M., Cutts, D. B., Meyers A. F., & Frank, D. A. (2010). Development and validity of a 2-item screen to identify families at risk for food insecurity. *Pediatrics, 126*(1), 26–32. https://doi.org10.1542/peds.2009-3146.

Hark, L., Deen, D., & Morrison, G. (2014). *Medical nutrition and disease: A case-based approach* (5th ed.). Wiley-Blackwell.

Harvard T. H. Chan School of Public Health. (n.d.). *Protein.* The Nutrition Source. Retrieved January 18, 2023, from https://www.hsph.harvard.edu/nutritionsource /what-should-you-eat/protein

Hever, J., & Cronise, R. (2017). Plant-based nutrition for healthcare professionals: Implementing diet as a primary modality in the prevention and treatment of chronic disease. *Journal of Geriatric Cardiology, 14*(5), 355–368. https://doi.org/10.11909/j.issn.1671-5411 .2017.05.012

Institute of Medicine. (2005a). *Dietary reference intakes for energy, carbohydrate, fiber, fat, fatty acids, cholesterol, protein, and amino acids.* National Academies Press. https://doi.org/10.17226/10490

Institute of Medicine. (2005b). *Dietary reference intakes for water, potassium, sodium, chloride, and sulfate.* National Academies Press. https://doi.org/10.17226/10925

Institute of Medicine. (2006). *Dietary reference intakes: The essential guide to nutrient requirements.* National Academies Press. https://doi.org/10.17226/11537

Kaiser, M. J., Bauer, J. M., Ramsch, C., Uter, W., Guigoz, Y., Cederholm, T., Thomas, D. R., Anthony, P., Charlton, K. E., Maggio, M., Tsai, A. C., Grathwohl, D., Vellas, B., Sieber, C. C., & MNA-International Group. (2009). Validation of the Mini Nutritional Assessment Short-Form (MNA-SF): A practical tool for identification of nutritional status. *Journal of Nutrition, Health and Aging, 13*(9), 782–788. https://doi.org/10.1007/s 12603-009-0214-7

Kelly, J., & Clayton, J. S. (2021). *Foundations of lifestyle medicine: Board review manual* (3rd ed.). American College of Lifestyle Medicine.

Kesari, A., & Noel, J. Y. (2022, April 16). *Nutritional assessment.* StatPearls [Internet]. https://www.ncbi.nlm .nih.gov/books/NBK580496

Knuuti, J., Wijns, W., Saraste, A., Capodanno, D., Barbato, E., Funck-Brentano, C., Prescott, E., Storey, R. F., Deaton, C., Cuisset, T., Agewall, S., Dickstein, K., Edvardsen, T., Escaned, J., Gersh, B. J., Svitil, P., Gilard, M., Hasdai, D., Hatala, R., ... Bax, J. J. (2020). 2019 ESC Guidelines for the diagnosis and management of chronic coronary syndromes: The task force for the diagnosis and management of chronic coronary syndromes of the European Society of Cardiology (ESC). *European Heart Journal, 41*(3), 407–477. https://doi.org/10.1093 /eurheartj/ehz425

Lancha, A. H., Jr., Sforzo, G. A., & Pereira-Lancha, L. O. (2018). Improving nutritional habits with no diet prescription: Details of a nutritional coaching process. *American Journal of Lifestyle Medicine, 12*(2), 160–165. https://doi.org/10.1177/1559827616636616

Lee-Kwan, S., Moore, L., Blanck, H., Harris, D., & Galuska, D. (2017). Disparities in state-specific adult fruit and vegetable consumption—United States, 2015. *Morbidity and Mortality Weekly Report, 66*(45), 1241–1247. https://www.cdc.gov/mmwr/volumes/66 /wr/mm6645a1.htm

Liu, A. G., Ford, N. A., Hu, F. B., Zelman, K. M., Mozaffarian, D., & Kris-Etherton, P. M. (2017). A healthy approach to dietary fats: Understanding the science and taking action to reduce consumer confusion. *Nutrition Journal, 16*, 53. https://doi.org/10.1186/s12937 -017-0271-4

Liu, G., Zong, G., Wu, K., Hu, Y., Li, Y., Willett, W. C., Eisenberg, D. M., Hu, F. B., & Sun, Q. (2018). Meat cooking methods and risk of type 2 diabetes: Results from three prospective cohort studies. *Diabetes Care*, *41*(5), 1049–1060. https://doi.org/10.2337/dc17-1992

Ludwig, D. S., Hu, F. B., Tappy, L., & Brand-Miller, J. (2018, June 13). Dietary carbohydrates: Role of quality and quantity in chronic disease. *British Medical Journal*, *361*, k2340. https://doi.org/10.1136/bmj.k2340

Malesza, I. J., Malesza, M., Walkowiak, J., Mussin, N., Walkowiak, D., Aringazina, R., Bartkowiak-Wieczorek, J., & Mądry, E. (2021). High-fat, Western-style diet, systemic inflammation, and gut microbiota: A narrative review. *Cells*, *10*(11), 3164. https://doi.org/10.3390/cells10113164

Mande, J., Willet, W., Auerbach, J., Bleich, S., Economos, C., Griffin, T., Grumbly, T., Hu, F., Koh, H., Mozaffarian, D., Pérez-Escamilla, R., Seligman, H., Story, M., Wilde, P., & Woteki, C. (2020). *Report of the 50th anniversary of the White House Conference on Food, Nutrition, and Health: Honoring the past, taking actions for our future.* Tufts University. https://sites.tufts.edu/foodnutritionandhealth2019

Marx, W., Veronese, N., Kelly, J. T., Smith, L., Hockey, M., Collins, S., Trakman, G. L., Hoare, E., Teasdale, S. B., Wade, A., Lane, M., Aslam, H., Davis, J. A., O'Neil, A., Shivappa, N., Hebert, J. R., Blekkenhorst, L. C., Berk, M., Segasby, T., & Jacka, F. (2021). The dietary inflammatory index and human health: An umbrella review of meta-analyses of observational studies. *Advances in Nutrition*, *12*, 1681–1690. https://doi.org/10.1093/advances/nmab037

MedlinePlus. (n.d.). *Genetically engineered foods.* Retrieved January 17, 2023, from https://medlineplus.gov/ency/article/002432.htm

Micha, R., Peñalvo, J. L., Cudhea, F., Imamura, F., Rehm, C. D., & Mozaffarian, D. (2017). Association between dietary factors and mortality from heart disease, stroke, and type 2 diabetes in the United States. *Journal of the American Medical Association*, *317*(9), 912–924. https://doi.org/10.1001/jama.2017.0947

Michałowska, J., & Zaborowska, L. (2023). *TDEE calculator - Total daily energy expenditure.* Omni Calculator. https://www.omnicalculator.com/health/tdee

Mifflin, M. D., St Jeor, S. T., Hill, L. A., Scott, B. J., Daugherty, S. A., & Koh, Y. O. (1990). A new predictive equation for resting energy expenditure in healthy individuals. *The American Journal of Clinical Nutrition*, *51*(2), 241–247. https://doi.org/10.1093/AJCN/51.2.241

Miller, W. R., & Rollnick, S. (2012). *Motivational interviewing: Helping people change* (3rd ed.). Guilford Press.

Mitrou, P. (2022). Is lifestyle modification the key to counter chronic diseases? *Nutrients*, *14*(15), 3007. https://doi.org/10.3390/nu14153007

Mokdad, A. H., Ballestros, K., Echko, M., Glenn, S., Olsen, H. E., Mullany, E., Lee, A., Khan, A. R., Ahmadi, A., Ferrari, A. J., Kasaeian, A., Werdecker, A., Carter, A., Zipkin, B., Sartorius, B., Serdar, B., Sykes, B. L., Troeger, C., Fitzmaurice, C., . . . Rehm, C. D. (2018). The state of US health, 1990–2016: Burden of diseases, injuries, and risk factors among US states. *Journal of the American Medical Association*, *319*(14), 1444–1472. https://doi.org/10.1001/jama.2018.0158

Moore, L. V., Thompson, F. E., & Demissie, Z. (2017). Percentage of youth meeting federal fruit and vegetable intake recommendations, Youth Risk Behavior Surveillance System, United States and 33 states, 2013. *Journal of the Academy of Nutrition and Dietetics*, *117*(4), 545–553. https://doi.org/10.1016/j.jand.2016.10.012

Morris, M. C., Tangney, C. C., Wang, Y., Sacks, F. M., Barnes, L. L., Bennett, D. A., & Aggarwal, N. T. (2015). MIND diet slows cognitive decline with aging. *Alzheimer's & Dementia*, *11*(9), 1015–1022. https://doi.org/10.1016/j.jalz.2015.04.011

Mostofsky, E., Mukamal, K. J., Giovannucci, E. L., Stampfer, M. J., & Rimm, E. B. (2016). Key findings on alcohol consumption and a variety of health outcomes from the Nurses' Health Study. *American Journal of Public Health*, *106*(9), 1586–1591. https://doi.org/10.2105/AJPH.2016.303336

National Academies Press and Institute of Medicine. (2011). *Dietary reference intakes (DRIs): Recommended dietary allowances and adequate intakes, vitamins.* https://www.ncbi.nlm.nih.gov/books/NBK56068/table/summarytables.t2/?report=objectonly

National Cancer Institute. (n.d.). *NCI dictionary of cancer terms: Dietary counseling.* Retrieved June 11, 2023, from https://www.cancer.gov/publications/dictionaries/cancer-terms/def/dietary-counseling

National Cancer Institute. (2021). *Dietary screener questionnaires (DSQ) in the NHANES 2009–10: DSQ.* https://epi.grants.cancer.gov/nhanes/dietscreen/questionnaires.html

National Center for Complementary and Integrative Health. (2013). *Antioxidants: In depth.* https://www.nccih.nih.gov/health/antioxidants-in-depth

National Heart, Lung, and Blood Institute. (2000). *The practical guide: Identification, evaluation, and treatment of overweight and obesity in adults.* https://www.nhlbi.nih.gov/files/docs/guidelines/prctgd_c.pdf

National Institute of Diabetes and Digestive and Kidney Diseases. (2017). *Some myths about nutrition and physical activity.* U.S. Department of Health and Human Services. https://www.niddk.nih.gov/health-information/weight-management/myths-nutrition-physical-activity

Office of Dietary Supplements. (2021a, April 6). *Vitamin B12: Fact sheet for health professionals.* https://ods.od.nih.gov/factsheets/VitaminB12-HealthProfessional

Office of Dietary Supplements. (2021b, August 4). *Omega-3 fatty acids: Fact sheet for health professionals.*

https://ods.od.nih.gov/factsheets/Omega3FattyAcids-HealthProfessional/#en3

Office of Dietary Supplements. (2021c, August 17). *Vitamin D: Fact sheet for health professionals.* https://ods.od.nih.gov/factsheets/VitaminD-HealthProfessional/#en1

Office of Disease Prevention and Health Promotion. (n.d.-a). *Healthy People 2030: Food insecurity.* https://health.gov/healthypeople/priority-areas/social-determinants-health/literature-summaries/food-insecurity#cit1

Office of Disease Prevention and Health Promotion. (n.d.-b). *Healthy People 2030: Nutrition and healthy eating.* https://health.gov/healthypeople/objectives-and-data/browse-objectives/nutrition-and-healthy-eating

Office of Disease Prevention and Health Promotion. (n.d.-c). *Healthy People 2030: Overweight and obesity.* https://health.gov/healthypeople/objectives-and-data/browse-objectives/overweight-and-obesity

Paxton, A. E., Strycker, L. A., Toobert, D. J., Ammerman, A. S., & Glasgow, R. E. (2011). Starting the conversation: Performance of a brief dietary assessment and intervention tool for health professionals. *American Journal of Preventive Medicine, 40,* 67–71. https://doi.org/10.1016/j.amepre.2010.10.009

Physicians Committee for Responsible Medicine. (n.d.). *Protein: Power up with plant-based protein.* Retrieved June 11, 2023, from https://www.pcrm.org/good-nutrition/nutrition-information/protein

Physicians Committee for Responsible Medicine. (2022). *Nutrition guide for clinicians* (3rd ed.) [Mobile app]. Unbound Medicine. Google Play Store. App Store. https://nutritionguide.pcrm.org/nutritionguide/mobile

Pipoyan, D., Stepanyan, S., Stepanyan, S., Beglaryan, M., Costantini, L., Molinari, R., & Merendino, N. (2021). The effect of trans fatty acids on human health: Regulation and consumption patterns. *Foods, 10*(10), 2452. https://doi.org/10.3390/foods10102452

Powell, H. S., & Greenberg, D. L. (2019). Screening for unhealthy diet and exercise habits: The electronic health record and a healthier population. *Preventive Medicine Reports, 14,* 100816. https://doi.org/10.1016/j.pmedr.2019.01.020

PRWeb. (2018, September 25). *American College of Lifestyle Medicine announces dietary lifestyle position statement for treatment and potential reversal of disease.* https://www.prweb.com/pdfdownload/15786205.pdf

Quagliani, D., & Felt-Gunderson, P. (2017). Closing America's fiber intake gap: Communication strategies from a food and fiber summit. *American Journal of Lifestyle Medicine, 11*(1), 80–87. https://doi.org/10.1177/1559827615588079

Rautiainen, S., Manson, J. E., Lichtenstein, A. H., & Sesso, H. D. (2016). Dietary supplements and disease prevention: A global overview. *Nature Reviews Endocrinology, 12*(7), 407–420. https://doi.org/10.1038/nrendo.2016.54

Reinhart, R. J. (2020, January 6). *Nurses continue to rate highest in honesty, ethics.* https://news.gallup.com/poll/274673/nurses-continue-rate-highest-honesty-ethics.aspx

Reiter-Brennan, C., Osei, A. D., Iftekhar Uddin, S. M., Orimoloye, O. A., Obisesan, O. H., Mirbolouk, M., Blaha, M. J., & Dzaye, O. (2020). ACC/AHA lipid guidelines: Personalized care to prevent cardiovascular disease. *Cleveland Clinic Journal of Medicine, 87*(4), 231–239. https://doi.org/10.3949/ccjm.87a.19078

Remde, A., DeTurk, S. N., Almardini, A., Steiner, L., & Wojda, T. (2022). Plant-predominant eating patterns: How effective are they for treating obesity and related cardiometabolic health outcomes? A systematic review. *Nutrition Reviews, 80*(5), 1094–1104. https://doi.org/10.1093/nutrit/nuab060

Rumgay, H., Shield, K., Charvat, H., Ferrari, P., Sornpaisarn, B., Obot, I., Islami, F., Lemmens, V., Rehm, J., & Soerjomataram, I. (2021). Global burden of cancer in 2020 attributable to alcohol consumption: A population-based study. *The Lancet Oncology, 22*(8), 1071–1080. https://doi.org/ https://doi.org/10.1016/S1470-2045(21)00279-5

Sacks, F. M., Appel, L. J., Moore, T. J., Obarzanek, E., Vollmer, W. M., Svetkey, L. P., Bray, G. A., Vogt, T. M., Cutler, J. A., Windhauser, M. M., Lin, P. H., & Karanja, N. (1999). A dietary approach to prevent hypertension: A review of the Dietary Approaches to Stop Hypertension (DASH) Study. *Clinical Cardiology, 22*(7 Suppl), III6–III10. https://doi.org/10.1002/clc.4960221503

Saini, R. K., & Keum, Y. (2018). Omega-3 and omega-6 polyunsaturated fatty acids: Dietary sources, metabolism, and significance: A review. *Life Sciences, 203,* 255–267. https://doi.org/ 10.1016/j.lfs.2018.04.049

Scarry, A., Rice, J., O'Connor, E. M., & Tierney, A. C. (2022). Usage of mobile applications or mobile health technology to improve diet quality in adults. *Nutrients, 14*(12), 2437. https://doi.org/10.3390/nu14122437

Schröder, H., Fitó, M., Estruch, R., Martínez-González, M. A., Corella, D., Salas-Salvadó, J., Lamuela-Raventós, R., Ros, E., Salaverría, I., Fiol, M., Lapetra, J., Vinyoles, E., Gómez-Gracia, E., Lahoz, C., Serra-Majem, L., Pintó, X., Ruiz-Gutierrez, V., & Covas, M. I. (2011). A short screener is valid for assessing Mediterranean diet adherence among older Spanish men and women. *Journal of Nutrition, 141*(6), 1140–1145. https://doi.org/10.3945/jn.110.135566

Segal-Isaacson, C. J., Wylie-Rosett, J., & Gans, K. M. (2004). Validation of a short dietary assessment questionnaire: The Rapid Eating and Activity Assessment for Participants short version (REAP-S). *The Diabetes Educator, 30*(5). https://doi.org/10.1177/014572170403000512

Stelmach-Mardas, M., Rodacki, T., Dobrowolska-Iwanek, J., Brzozowska, A., Walkowiak, J., Wojtanowska-Krosniak, A., Zagrodzki, P., Bechthold, A., Mardas, M., & Boeing, H. (2016). Link between food energy density and body weight changes in obese adults. *Nutrients, 8*(4), 229. https://doi.org/10.3390/nu8040229

Stratton, R. J., Hackston, A., Longmore, D., Dixon, R., Price, S., Stroud, M., King, C., & Elia, M. (2004). Malnutrition in hospital outpatients and inpatients: Prevalence, concurrent validity and ease of use of the "malnutrition universal screening tool" ("MUST") for adults. *British Journal of Nutrition, 92*(5), 799–808. https://doi.org/10.1079/bjn20041258

Tuso, P. J., Ismail, M. H., Ha, B. P., & Bartolotto, C. (2013). Nutritional update for physicians: Plant-based diets. *The Permanente Journal, 17*(2), 61–66. https://doi.org/10.7812/TPP/12-085

Unger, T., Borghi, C., Charchar, F., Khan, N. A., Poulter, N. R., Prabhakaran, D., Ramirez, A., Schlaich, M., Stergiou, G. S., Tomaszewski, M., Wainford, R. D., Williams, B., & Schutte, A. E. (2020). 2020 International Society of Hypertension global hypertension practice guidelines. *Hypertension*, 1334–1357. https://doi.org/10.1161/HYPERTENSIONAHA.120.15026

Uribarri, J., del Castillo, M. D., de la Maza, M. P., Filip, R., Gugliucci, A., Luevano-Contreras, C., Macías-Cervantes, M. H., Markowicz Bastos, D. H., Medrano, A., Menini, T., Portero-Otin, M., Rojas, A., Sampaio, G. R., Wrobel, K., Wrobel, K., & Garay-Sevilla, M. E. (2015). Dietary advanced glycation end products and their role in health and disease. *Advances in Nutrition, 6*(4), 461–473. https://doi.org/10.3945/an.115.008433

U.S. Department of Health and Human Services & U.S. Department of Agriculture. (2015, December). *2015 – 2020 dietary guidelines for Americans* (8th ed.). https://health.gov/our-work/food-nutrition/previous-dietary-guidelines/2015

U.S. Department of Health and Human Services & U.S. Department of Agriculture. (2020). *Dietary guidelines for Americans, 2020–2025* (9th ed.). https://www.dietaryguidelines.gov

U.S. Food and Drug Administration. (2018, May 18). *Trans fat*. https://www.fda.gov/food/food-additives-petitions/trans-fat

U.S. Food and Drug Administration. (2022, March 7). *Changes to the nutrition facts label*. https://www.fda.gov/food/food-labeling-nutrition/changes-nutrition-facts-label

U.S. Preventive Services Task Force. (2020, November 14). *Final recommendation statement: Healthy diet and physical activity for cardiovascular disease prevention in adults with cardiovascular risk factors: Behavioral counseling interventions*. https://www.uspreventiveservicestaskforce.org/uspstf/recommendation/healthy-diet-and-physical-activity-counseling-adults-with-high-risk-of-cvd

Vadiveloo, M., Lichtenstein, A. H., Anderson, C., Aspry, K., Foraker, R., Griggs, S., Hayman, L. L., Johnston, E., Stone, N. J., & Thorndike, A. N. (2020). Rapid diet assessment screening tools for cardiovascular disease risk reduction across healthcare settings: A scientific statement from the American Heart Association. *Circulation, 13*(9), e000094. https://doi.org/10.1161/HCQ.0000000000000094

Warner, M. J., & Kamran, M. T. (2021). *Iron deficiency anemia*. StatPearls.

World Cancer Research Fund & American Institute for Cancer Research. (2018). *Diet, nutrition, physical activity, and cancer: A global perspective. Continuous Update Project Expert Report 2018*. https://www.wcrf.org/diet-activity-and-cancer

World Health Organization. (n.d.). *Anaemia*. Retrieved June 11, 2023, from http://www.who.int/nutrition/topics/ida/en

World Health Organization. (2020). *2020 Global nutrition report: Action on equity to end malnutrition*. https://globalnutritionreport.org

World Health Organization. (2021, June 9). *Malnutrition*. https://www.who.int/news-room/fact-sheets/detail/malnutrition

CHAPTER 12

Stress Less

Roberta Christopher, EdD, MSN, ARNP, NE-BC, CAIF
Lila de Tantillo, PhD, MS, APRN, FNP-BC

Be thankful for everything; gratitude is an antidote to stress.

Dr. Loureen Downes

OBJECTIVES

This chapter will enable the reader to:

1. Differentiate between eustress and distress along the stress continuum using conceptual and theoretical approaches.
2. Discuss stress implications across the life span.
3. Describe three approaches to assessing stress, including (1) psychological, (2) environmental/epidemiological, and (3) biological.
4. Apply interprofessional evidence-informed lifestyle prescription approaches to stress prevention and management.
5. Employ conversation starters and evidence-informed resources for stress prevention and management in clinical practice.

Overview

This chapter will provide the advanced practice provider (APP) a foundation for managing patient stress and mental health concerns from a health promotion perspective in the advanced practice setting. Psychological and physical health are inextricably related, yet the connections between these two are not well understood (Ohrnberger et al., 2017). Despite this challenge, clinicians must consider the relationship when caring for their patients.

The definitions of stress, types of stressors, and the theoretical underpinnings of our modern understanding of stress theory will be reviewed. Additionally, key stressors that may affect patient populations throughout their life span will be discussed. This chapter will also explore tools for assessing stress and specific recommendations for promoting stress management and well-being applicable to patients and APPs.

© Kathleen Gail/Shutterstock; © StoryTime Studio/Shutterstock; © kali9/Getty Images

What Is Stress?

The Stress Curve

The National Institute of Mental Health (n.d.) defines stress as the way an individual emotionally and physically responds to any demand. The word *stress* derives from the Latin *strictus*, meaning to bind or pull tightly. In the popular lexicon, *stress* generally carries a negative connotation associated with an unpleasant event. One analysis of the concept of stress noted its characteristics as an overwhelming pressure and the inability of an organism to

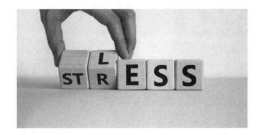

Figure 12.1 Stress less.

© Dmitry Demidovich/Shutterstock

meet the challenge posed by the stimulus (Goodnite, 2014). In the clinical setting, distress is generally used to describe a patient whose physical status may be compromised. In contrast, psychological distress is more specifically an emotional state that results in harm (Ridner, 2004).

However, not all stress is toxic or unhealthy. The existence of stress is considered an inherent aspect of life. APPs can play a role in helping patients identify and respond to stressors in their lives. In their groundbreaking work, Yerkes and Dodson (1908) proposed a U-shaped dose-response continuum regarding stress. As stress increased, performance increased. However, excess stress led to rapid performance decreases. Too little stress may lead to apathy, boredom, or indifference while too much may lead to anxiety, worry, and failure. Stress can affect activities at all levels of acuity and importance. Ideal stress levels vary for each person. Therefore, individualized stress management is essential in clinical care to sustain the delicate balance of the stress curve, as noted in **Figure 12.2**.

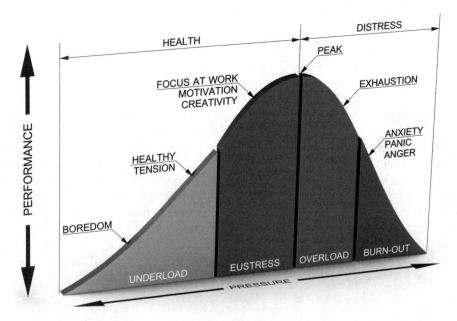

Figure 12.2 The stress curve.

© Olivier Le Moal/Shutterstock

General Adaptation Syndrome

The modern understanding of stress was advanced by Hans Selye, who examined stress and its effect on the individual. In his germinal works, Selye (1950, 1959, 1976, 1980) described a living being exposed to stress as experiencing a three-stage progression, which he termed general adaptation syndrome (GAS). This triphasic response consists of the alarm reaction, stage of resistance, and stage of exhaustion (see **Table 12.1**). The alarm reaction is marked by a strong adrenal response that can provide mechanisms the individual needs for survival. This reaction was conceptualized as the fight-or-flight response by Cannon (1929). However, it is impossible to exist continuously in a state of alarm. If the individual survives and remains under stress, the next phase is the resistance stage. The body will continue to adapt in response to stress but may eventually be driven to the stage of exhaustion. Selye (1950) noted that GAS might be frequently accompanied by hormonal derangements resulting from maladaptation to stress.

Selye (1976) is also credited with identifying types of stress, describing eustress as associated with desirable results and distress with that which impairs function. Generally, a positive and welcoming event, such as receiving a promotion or getting married, can motivate the individual. However, if not appropriately managed, the psychological toll of eustress on an individual may still resemble that of negative stressors or distress, such as losing a job or getting a divorce. Selye noted that both eustress and distress might cause the same nonspecific response; however, eustress causes less damage and more desirable effects (see Figure 12.2).

The Stress Response, Coping, and Resilience

Stress Response

The stress-as-transaction framework has categorized stress as acute, episodic, intermittent, and chronic. One especially concerning aspect of stress is its effect on the body over an extended period, known as chronic stress. Chronic stress is a significant national and global problem. One study found that 59% of primary care patients reported stress levels

Table 12.1 Stages of General Adaptation Syndrome

Stage	Stress Response	Physiological Response	Psychological Response
Alarm reaction	▪ Low resistance ▪ Excessive response to stimulus	▪ Tachycardia ▪ Loss of muscle tone ▪ Decreased temperature ▪ Hypotension	▪ Emotional arousal
Stage of resistance	▪ Adaptation observed ▪ Resistance increased	▪ Reversal of physical symptoms of stress	▪ Sensitization to additional stressors
Stage of exhaustion	▪ Loss of adaptability ▪ Eventual exhaustion	▪ Symptoms reemerge ▪ Life may be endangered	▪ Potential for depression and frustration

Data from Selye, H. (1950). Stress and the general adaptation syndrome. *British Medical Journal, 1*(4667), 1383–1392. https://doi.org/10.1136/bmj.1.4667.1383

to be higher than "a little" (Wiegner et al., 2015). In addition, recent indications are that levels of stress may be increasing. According to the American Psychological Association's (2020) *Stress in America 2020: A National Mental Health Crisis* report, Americans have been highly affected by the COVID-19 pandemic. This national survey included 1,026 participants ages 13 to 17 and 3,409 participants 18+ years of age. Survey findings noted that approximately 80% of adult participants reported a significant increase in stress related to the pandemic. About 20% of those indicated their stress and mental health were worse than the previous (prepandemic) year. During pandemic peaks, limited access to health care resulted in a delay in preventive and follow-up visits, negatively affecting physical and mental health. Disruption in access to education and childcare further exacerbated perceived levels of stress. Additionally, two out of three adults in the study reported significant financial stress related to employment disruption, job stability, and reduced work hours.

Another study (Morneau Shepell Ltd., 2017) noted that 47% of employees reported that stress negatively affected their work performance, including difficulty concentrating, absenteeism, poor work quality, and disciplinary action. Chronic stress has been implicated in disease progression, including cancer, Alzheimer's, and cardiovascular diseases (Bisht et al., 2018; Yao et al., 2019). There is also growing evidence that chronic stress can negatively affect the immune system and contribute to low-grade inflammation (Gouin, 2011). Stress can negatively affect sleep patterns and is strongly associated with increased energy intake and obesity (Geiker et al., 2018). There are also indications that chronic stress can interfere with effective decision-making capability and memory (Friedman et al., 2017; Tran et al., 2011). Further, chronic stress may have a negative effect on fertility, as associations have been found between stressors and decreased semen quality and reduced ovarian reserve (Li et al., 2011; Pal et al., 2010).

Therefore, coping and resilience skill development may be indicated to prevent and reduce the longitudinal negative effect of chronic stress (Dooley et al., 2017).

Coping

Lazarus and Cohen (1977) and Lazarus and Folkman (1984) developed a theory of stress that described stress as a transaction between the individual and the environment. The theory presented coping as a response to the experience of stress. According to Lazarus and Folkman, coping includes employing conscious or subconscious mental energy to reduce stress levels. The goal of coping is to resolve the problem that stimulates the stress response and return to homeostasis. Coping strategies may be positive (adaptive) or negative (maladaptive) and therefore increase or decrease an individual's mental well-being. Coping is derived through an individual's perception of the experience and may depend on personality patterns. Thus, coping strategies, or modes of coping, selected to adapt to stress are highly individualized and situational. Understanding and engaging with how individuals cope can provide an opportunity for APPs to promote adaptive behavior and provide guidance regarding maladaptive behavior. Further, APPs may refer individuals with maladaptive coping who may be at risk for anxiety or depression for behavioral health counseling and further evaluation.

Resilience

Werner (1982) described resilience as an individual's capacity to cope effectively with internal and external stressors. Thus, according to Werner, coping protective processes that promote resilience may mitigate maladaptive responses to stress. Rutter's (2006) germinal work in resilience takes a life span approach. According to Rutter, resilience is "an interactive concept that refers to a relative resistance to environmental risk experiences, or the overcoming of stress or adversity" (p. 1). Further, Rutter noted that resilience might be higher or lower depending on the circumstances, the risks, and the environment at a particular time. Individual differences like genetics or environmental conditions may yield dissimilarities among risk (vulnerability) and protective factors. Rutter asserted that positive coping and social relationships might mediate risk, whereas the right resources may bolster an individual's ability to adapt to stress at the right time despite adversity. Thus, the APP may include social assessment as part of the health promotion planning process to understand better the individual's social support system and environmental risk and protective factors.

Shean (2015) recommended a strengths-based approach to supporting resiliency skills in a comprehensive review of resilience theory and literature. These skills included problem-solving, self-efficacy, social skills, and accessing resources. Thus, APPs may refer individuals to culturally and community-appropriate programs and resources. One example is The Resilience Program, which strengthens mentalization skills via a flexible web-based program (Bak et al., 2015). Bak et al. define mentalization as "the skills involved in understanding mental states, not only in others but also one's mental states as well as their connections with behavior" (p. 1). Such understanding provides context for identifying risk factors and vulnerabilities in which the APP may further employ evidence-informed interventions to address the individual's unique needs.

Stress Across the Life Span

A holistic approach to understanding developmental stressors provides an essential context for prescribing health promotion and lifestyle strategies for stress prevention and management. Stress levels and potential causes are known to change throughout the life span. Researchers have examined these patterns, and APPs should be aware of specific stressors that patients may be more likely to encounter at each stage of growth and development (Lupien et al., 2018).

Life stages inherently include stressors unique to each life stage (**Figure 12.3**) encountered across the life span. Erikson's (1950) initial stages of the psychosocial development model included eight stages. Joan Erikson (1997) extended her husband's work to include the elements of a ninth life cycle stage experienced when one is older than 80. The Stress and Wellbeing Life Stage model (Panchal et al., 2017) adds further context to key stressors and life events experienced within each stage noted by Erikson. The case of the González family, in the following box, provides an example of family members in different life stages experiencing various developmental conflicts and unique life stage stressors. Framing stress within a life stage perspective provides insight into potential causes and lifestyle treatment of stress based on the respective life stage of the individual.

Table 12.2 highlights key life events that occur within each developmental stage and

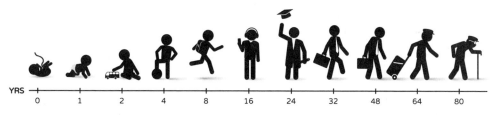

YRS 0 1 2 4 8 16 24 32 48 64 80

Figure 12.3 Life stages.
© Radoma/Shutterstock

Table 12.2 Stress Across Life Stages

Age	Life Events (Erikson, 1997)	Developmental Stage Conflicts (Erikson, 1997)	Stressors (Panchal et al. 2017)
0–1 year	Feeding, comfort	Basic trust vs. mistrust	Parental separation
1–3 years	Toileting, dressing	Autonomy vs. shame	
3–6 years	Exploration, play	Initiative vs. guilt	
6–12 years	School, activities, social relationships, identity	Industry vs. inferiority	Academic pressure; peer pressure; bullying
12–18 years		Identity vs. confusion	Sexual concerns; illicit drug and alcohol use; perceptions of others, particularly through social media forums
18–40 years	Intimate relationships, work, parenthood	Intimacy vs. isolation	Establishing and developing a career; social pressure; romantic relationships; fertility; financial pressures and responsibilities; parenthood; time constraints; practical responsibilities
40–64 years	Work, parenthood	Generativity vs. stagnation	Caring for both children and parents; divorce; health concerns; mortality
65+ years	Life reflection, death	Integrity vs. despair; hope and faith vs. despair (80 years to death)	Retirement; empty nest phenomenon; health concerns; loss of loved ones; reduced mobility; mortality

Data from Erikson, J. M. (1997). *Erik H. Erikson: The life cycle completed.* W. W. Norton & Company. Panchal, S., Palmer, S., O'Riordan, S., & Kelly, A. (2017). Stress and well-being: A life stage model. *International Journal of Stress Prevention and Wellbeing, 1*(5), 1–3.

Case Example of Life Stage Stressors

During the past year, every member of the González family has reported elevated stress levels but not for the same reason. Grandmother Adela is experiencing isolation and loneliness, exacerbated by not seeing her family during the COVID-19 pandemic and losing her best friend to the virus. Her middle-aged son, Martin, is stressed because he lost his job while his wife, Becky, is stressed due to taking on extra hours at the family business. Meanwhile, their adolescent son, Albert, is experiencing stress because of interactions with a bully online.

particular stressors the APP should consider during the assessment, prevention, and treatment of stress across the life span.

Nature Versus Nurture

The way individuals respond to stress is based on many factors. For decades, research has indicated that the magnitude of stress in the parent–child relationship can affect the child's psychological outcomes (Berry & Jones, 1995; Hattangadi et al., 2020; Webster-Stratton, 1990). Extensive research has continued to explore the factors as to why some individuals exposed to stressful or traumatic experiences develop posttraumatic stress disorder (PTSD) or other chronic mental health disorders while some do not (Howie et al., 2019). Evidence indicates a genetic predisposition may influence an individual's capacity to demonstrate resilience in a stressful situation (Maul et al., 2020). One study found that suicide attempts after stressful life events appeared to be regulated via a gene–environment interaction (Ben-Efraim et al., 2011).

An emerging field of study is epigenetics and how stress interacts with genes from a macro physiological level to a microcellular level, as stress may be internally or externally induced (Lee et al., 2020). The Centers for Disease Control and Prevention (2020) defined epigenetics as a field of study focused on how environments and behaviors affect or change the way genes function. Lee et al. (2020) noted in a review of the literature that biochemical reactions are fluid and affected by lifestyle choices, such as tobacco use, obesity, alcohol or drug use, poor nutrition, sleep deficits, and stress. The authors also found evidence suggesting that social determinants of health (e.g., access to health care, socioeconomic status, education level) serve as leading external influences of the epigenome. Furthermore, health-promoting lifestyles may positively affect the epigenome through choices such as engaging in social support networks, relaxation, physical activity, and meditation. These findings suggest that a more comprehensive approach by the APP is needed for stress prevention and management.

Health Promotion Research Study

Relationship of Stress and Mortality

Background: In recent years, an increase in all-cause mortality has been observed in the United States, which varies by race and ethnicity. Specifically, non-Hispanic Blacks have experienced higher mortality rates than other groups while women and Hispanics have had lower mortality. It is hypothesized that the cumulative experiences of racism and structural inequality contribute to a theory of physiological change known as weathering. During the process of repeated stress, the body is exposed to multisystem risk, known as an allostatic load, that has been associated with increased mortality.

Methodology: A secondary data analysis of the National Health and Nutrition Examination Survey (NHANES) III and the 2015 Linked Mortality File (LMF) for adults 25 years or older ($n = 13,673$ with 6,026 deaths) was conducted to examine whether the allostatic load was associated with all-cause and cardiovascular mortality within specific racial/ethnic groups in the United States.

Findings: As in previous studies, high allostatic load was linked with mortality rates in U.S. adults. Increased allostatic scores were found in populations of older age, with less education and low income, and Black or Mexican Americans. In addition, the analysis found specific associations for cardiovascular mortality.

Implications for Advanced Practice: The APP should be aware of and screen for the role social inequities play in causing chronic stress, cardiovascular disease, and risk factors for increased mortality across racial/ethnic, gender, and age groups.

Reference: Data from Borrell, L. N., Rodríguez-Álvarez, E., & Dallo, F. J. (2020). Racial/ethnic inequities in the associations of allostatic load with all-cause and cardiovascular-specific mortality risk in U.S. adults. *PLOS One, 15*(2), e0228336. https://doi.org/10.1371/journal.pone.0228336

Assessing and Evaluating Stress

When the APP is assessing a patient for stress, it is helpful to consider the primary, secondary, and tertiary levels of health promotion. According to Katz and Ali (2009), primary prevention fosters wellness and may prevent chronic or maladaptive stress from becoming established. Thus, the assessment of a patient aims to prevent or reduce the stressor(s). In secondary prevention, the APP uses screening to detect and alter an individual's response to the stressor(s). Finally, during the tertiary stage, the APP treats stress-related illness or disease.

The APP may use clinical strategies and lifestyle management approaches to care for mental health at stages that could affect a patient's lived experience of stress. Cohen et al. (2016) noted three traditional approaches to assessing stress: (1) psychological, (2) environmental and epidemiological, and (3) biological. The following tools may be used among diverse clinical settings and populations to measure aspects of stress on a continuum from eustress to distress and assist in developing an evidence-informed lifestyle prescription for stress. **Table 12.3** provides a listing of available instruments and indications.

Wellness-Specific Tool for Assessing for Stress

The Substance Abuse and Mental Health Services Administration (SAMHSA, 2017a) proposed using a wellness, strength-based, and whole-person method to promote optimal health. Swarbrick and Yudof (2017) developed an eight-dimensional wellness self-assessment tool called the Wellness Inventory (WI) that aligns with the SAMHSA framework. Addressing stress assessment from a wellness and lifestyle approach allows APPs to glean holistic insights into the lived experience of stress for patients, families, and communities.

The WI provides the APP a foundational tool for developing a comprehensive lifestyle prescription for stress that can be used in all settings. Additionally, the following screening tools may serve to identify those at risk and in need of further evaluation by a mental or behavioral health professional.

Psychological Tools

There are several tools an APP can use to assess stress throughout the life span. Crosswell and Lockwood (2020) noted that the period of latency between stress exposure and its measurement is critical when evaluating the subsequent stress response. Further, psychological instruments and tools measure various aspects of stress, such as behavioral and cognitive responses and appraisal of the stressor. Therefore, selecting a tool should be built on factors including the patient's potential stress exposure, appraisal, and response. For example, in a primary care setting, during a routine initial wellness visit, the APP might select a shorter screening tool, such as the Perceived Stress Scale, to establish a baseline for current stress and to serve as a conversation starter for health promotion. If the patient presents for a stress-related encounter, the APP might select the longer Perceived Stress Questionnaire (PSQ) to screen for comorbid conditions such as depression or anxiety. Therefore, APPs may consider psychological instruments incorporating different theoretical and conceptual approaches to measuring stress in practice based on the individual or population health promotion needs. The following instruments might be used to inform treatment and management of stress in practice.

The Perceived Stress Scale (PSS), developed by Cohen et al. (1983, 1988, 2012), is one of the most used stress scales. The tool measures individuals' appraisal of stressful situations in their lives. They are asked to rate feelings and thoughts related to stress during the last month. The 10-item PSS is anchored by a 5-point Likert scale from 0 = *never* to 4 = *very often*.

Table 12.3 Tools for Assessing and Evaluating Stress

Tool	Authors	Indication	URL
Wellness Inventory (WI)	Swarbrick and Yudof (2017)	High-level eight-dimensional wellness inventory to identify dimensions of strength or opportunity	https://www.center4healthandsdc .org/uploads/7/1/1/4/71142589 /wellness_in_8_dimensions _booklet_with_daily_plan.pdf
Perceived Stress Scale (PSS)	Cohen et al. (1983, 1988, 2012)	10-item appraisal of stressful situations; score indicates low to high perceived stress	https://www.sprc.org/system/files /private/event-training/Penn%20 College%20-%20Perceived%20 Stress%20Scale.pdf
COVID Stress Scales	Taylor et al. (2020)	Appraisal of COVID-19–related stressors	https://www.sciencedirect.com /science/article/pii /S0887618520300463
Perceived Stress Questionnaire (PSQ)	Levenstein et al. (1993)	Assesses stressful life events that may trigger or worsen disease symptoms	https://www.med.upenn.edu/cbti /assets/user-content/documents /Perceived%20Stress%20 Questionnaire%20(PSQ).pdf
Life Stressor Checklist-Revised (LSC-R)	Wolfe et al. (1997)	Measures 30 stressful and traumatic life events	https://www.ptsd.va.gov/professional /assessment/te-measures/lsc-r.asp
Life Events Checklist for DSM-5 (LEC-5)	Weathers et al. (2013)	Screens for 16 life event exposures that may result in PTSD or distress	https://www.ptsd.va.gov/professional /assessment/te-measures/life _events_checklist.asp

The PSS provides insights into how often people experience negative feelings of upset, lack of control and coping, anger, and positive feelings of self-efficacy, positive outlook, and maintaining control. Scores may total up to 40, with 0 to 13 indicating low stress, 14 to 26 indicating moderate stress, and 24 to 40 indicating high perceived stress. The PSS is strongly validated and has been used across diverse populations. A shorter PSS-4 scale is available and focuses on how often, during the last month, individuals felt (1) able to control important things in their lives, (2) confidence in their ability to manage personal problems, (3) that things were going their way, and (4) that difficulties were piling up so high that they could not overcome them.

In pandemic times, a stress screening tool that distinguishes COVID-19–related stress from other causes may guide a more individualized treatment plan. APPs may use the instrument to assess individuals at high risk of COVID stress syndrome and the resulting distress. A systematic review and meta-analysis by Salari et al. (2020) found that individuals who frequently monitored COVID-19 news suffered more anxiety. Disparities in COVID-19–related stress were reported in vulnerable populations with less access to healthcare services, financial resources, and mental health resources. Findings also indicated that women are at higher risk for COVID-19–related stress, depression, and anxiety, as well as any gender, ages 21 to 40 years, and those with higher levels of education. The COVID Stress Scales (CSS), developed by Taylor et al. (2020), measure COVID-19–specific distress and anxiety. The CSS were developed from extant literature and expert feedback. The final CSS are comprised of 36 self-report items and rated on a 5-point Likert scale from 0 = *not at all* to 4 = *extremely or almost always*. When completing the instrument, the individual is asked to recall the last seven days. An example of an item of the CSS includes "I am worried about catching the virus." The measure demonstrates good to excellent reliability.

Environmental and Epidemiological Stress Tools

According to the American Psychiatric Association (2020), the environmental or epidemiological approach centers on significant life events, daily events, and chronic stress. Traumatic life events include those in which an individual experiences a threatened death or severe injury. Examples include natural disasters, military combat, physical assault, terrorist attack, and automobile accident. These differ from life changes or major life events that may also lead to stress but are considered transitions as part of the life cycle. Examples of major life events include marriage, divorce, death of a loved one, change in job, personal injury or illness (e.g., COVID-19), or change in finances. The following tools are a sampling that APPs may use to assess the effect of environmental stressors and the need for referral or intervention.

One of the most common tools used in practice is the Life Events Checklist for DSM-5 (LEC-5) by Weathers et al. (2013). The checklist screens for 16 life event exposures that may result in PTSD or distress as well as item 17, which asks for any other incredibly stressful events or experiences. The LEC-5 comes in a standard and an extended self-report instrument. The extended version includes eight additional probing questions for any affirmative responses noted in items 1 through 17.

The PSQ, created by Levenstein et al. (1993), is a 30-item self-report tool that assesses stressful life events that may trigger or worsen disease symptoms. This tool focuses on sleep disturbances and may be used in a variety of clinical settings. Levenstein et al. reported an excellent internal consistency. The PSQ has been used to measure stress during the previous year or two or in the previous month.

Another option for APPs evaluating environmental stress over a more extended period is the Life Stressor Checklist-Revised (LSC-R) by Wolfe et al. (1997). This self-report tool measures 30 stressful and traumatic life events, including sexual or physical assault, natural disasters, the death of a relative, and other events. Patients are asked to think back over their lives when responding to items. The responses are dichotomic in a nominal yes-or-no format. The LSC-R has good criterion and convergent validity as well as test-retest reliability (Choi et al., 2017). Table 12.3 provides a listing of commonly used tools and instruments for assessing psychological and environmental stress.

Biological Measurement of Stress

According to Cohen et al. (2016), biological measurement of stress centers on physiological responses to stress and ranges from homeostatic to maladaptive levels. Biological measurement of stress is deeply rooted in Selye's (1950, 1959, 1976, 1980) research and theory. Godoy et al. (2018) extended Selye's work by examining stress processing and resulting coping strategies from a neurobiology perspective. According to Godoy et al., the stress system begins with psychological and/or physical stressors, which activate a stress response through the hypothalamus-pituitary-adrenal (HPA) and the sympathetic-adreno-medullar (SAM) axes. The stress response has immediate and longer-term effects before returning to healthy homeostasis (equilibrium) or causing a maladaptive chronic imbalance. Overall, body receptors induce repression of digestion, metabolic alterations, energy deployment, immune system stimulation, and reproduction cessation. Brain receptors stimulate genomic and nongenomic effects, epigenetic programming, and immune reactivity. Next, corresponding altered cellular mechanisms yield cellular excitability as well as the ability of neurons and synapses to strengthen or weaken over time (plasticity). Both body and brain receptor activation result in behavioral and physiological changes, which produce complex and dynamic adaptation or maladaptation. APPs should be attuned to the maladaptive biological and physiological changes resulting from stress that underpin chronic disease processes.

Adaptation is not linear but rather regulated to achieve physiological equilibrium or allostasis. Koolhaas et al. (2010, 2011) described this state of allostasis as a set point and the ability to achieve homeostasis through change and adaptation (Sterling & Eyer, 1988). The cumulative effects of stress from daily to major life events and the resulting physiological consequences generate what is called allostatic load or allostatic overload if pathological (Godoy et al., 2018; Guidi et al., 2021).

Guidi et al. (2021) outlined two clinical criteria for diagnosing allostatic overload through a systematic review. Criterion A requires the presence of distress that has an identifiable source and has surpassed the individual's coping skills. Criterion B examines the previous 6 months for symptoms (e.g., sleep impairment, sadness, irritability, anxiety, dizziness, demoralization) or impairment in functioning (e.g., social, occupational, environmental).

APPs may utilize biological markers to assist in quantifying allostatic load or overload and identifying appropriate strategies for stress prevention and management. Frequent biological and physiological measures of adaptive and maladaptive stress that APPs may consider evaluating include the following:

- Biological: cholesterol, body mass index, resting systolic and diastolic blood pressure, waist–hip ratio, dehydroepiandrosterone (DHEA), cortisol, norepinephrine, epinephrine, and glycosylated hemoglobin
- Functioning: metabolic, cardiovascular, immune, brain, and respiratory functioning
- Allostatic processes: neuroendocrine, sleep (chrono-disruption), metabolism and dysmetabolic consequences, inflammation levels, and immune cells (Cohen et al., 2016; Godoy et al., 2018; Guidi et al., 2021; Mathur et al., 2015; Seeman et al., 1997; Seeman et al., 2001).

A Wellness Approach to Stress Prevention and Management

APPs are encouraged to provide their patients with an evidence-informed and theoretically informed wellness approach to stress prevention and management strategies. Swarbrick and Yudof's (2017) eight-dimensional wellness approach was adopted by SAMHSA (2017a) as a multifaceted model for integrating behavioral and physical health. As stress has both psychological and physiological aspects, the eight dimensions provide a useful and empowering model for assessing, preventing, and reducing stress in a variety of populations. The eight dimensions address the (1) emotional, (2) environmental, (3) financial, (4) intellectual, (5) occupational, (6) physical, (7) social, and (8) spiritual aspects of wellness (see **Figure 12.4**). SAMHSA noted that wellness extends beyond the absence of stress and disease to include happiness, positive relationships, satisfying work and play, purposeful life, and a healthy body and living environment. Thus, health promotion strategies and techniques

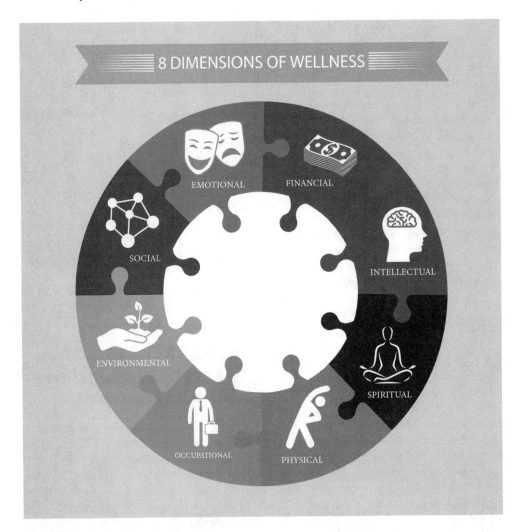

Figure 12.4 Dimensions of wellness.

© Nazrul Iznan/Shutterstock

aimed at preventing or mitigating pathological stress and distress within the eight dimensions of wellness assist APPs in prescribing effective lifestyle modalities for being well in a positive sense (Dunn, 1961).

Conversation Starters

Assessing a patient's wellness and stress levels can be incorporated as a routine aspect of care. The APP can begin by engaging in conversations with patients about their well-being,

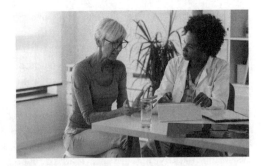

Figure 12.5 Starting the conversation.

Lordin/Shutterstock.

remaining alert to cues regarding stress and other mental health concerns (Thombs et al., 2021). In all cases, APPs should offer a welcoming, nonjudgmental environment in which the patient can express feelings. Some individuals feel embarrassed or ashamed that they are not managing their lives as stress-free as they perceive others around them. The APP plays a critical role by starting the conversation with the patient. The questions in **Table 12.4** can be used as a guide. The APP should adhere to local guidelines and make an informed decision as to when to implement and interpret person-centered validated measures that evaluate mental health (Kilbourne et al., 2018). The use of these measures is necessary to provide referrals to quality resources. The APP should ensure all ideas for addressing stress are delivered with sensitivity, which demonstrates a human connection and caring presence (Christopher et al., 2020).

Emotional Dimension and Lifestyle Prescription for Stress

SAMHSA (2017a, 2017b) conceptualized emotional wellness as the ability to cope effectively and sustain meaningful relationships. Stoewen (2017) further elaborated the emotional dimension of appreciating the feelings of others; constructive management of emotions; respect and understanding of values, feelings, and attitudes; and a positive mindset about life. Finally, Swarbrick and Yudof (2017) added the elements of enjoyment of life and the ability to adjust to emotional challenges. SAMHSA (2017a, 2017b) suggests the following evidence-informed strategies to support emotional wellness.

First, APPs may have patients keep a daily journal to reflect candidly and privately on their emotions, how they expressed or did not

Table 12.4 Conversation Starters

Dimension	Questions	APP Tips
Emotional wellness	▪ How would you describe your current level of stress? ▪ How does stress affect your daily life?	▪ Conduct an initial evaluation of stress and its effect on your patient's life.
	▪ What causes you stress? ▪ How do you recognize stress in your life and your body?	▪ Use this opportunity to establish rapport and learn about your patient's stressors in a nonjudgmental manner.
	▪ How do you relieve stress? ▪ What are your current approaches to managing stress? ▪ How do you feel emotionally and physically?	▪ Determine whether your patient's current approaches to managing stress are unhealthy or even dangerous. ▪ Evaluate for potential barriers to coping and use of stress management approaches to address them in the lifestyle prescription for stress.
	▪ Do you think your current stress levels are sustainable over time? ▪ How capable are you of relieving your stress, or do you need help?	▪ Identify patients who may require a referral for additional support.

(continues)

Table 12.4 Conversation Starters   (continued)

Dimension	Questions	APP Tips
Physical wellness	■ What routines do you have for physical activity?	■ Use this opportunity to explore other areas of physical wellness such as nutrition; sleep; alcohol, drug, and tobacco use; medication safety; and preventive visits. ■ Identify patients who may require a referral for additional support, such as physical therapy.
Intellectual wellness	■ What activities do you find intellectually stimulating (e.g., personal interests, education, brain exercises, conversations)?	■ Identify patients who may require a referral for additional support, such as community groups or organizations.
Financial wellness	■ How satisfied are you with your current and future financial situation?	■ Identify patients who may require a referral for community resources, such as Temporary Assistance for Needy Families (TANF), Low Income Home Energy Assistance Program (LIHEAP), or the Housing Choice Voucher Program (Section 8).
Environmental wellness	■ Thinking about where you live, how safe do you feel? ■ What is the outdoor environment like where you live?	■ Identify patients who may require a referral for additional support, such as parks and recreation centers in their local communities.
Spiritual wellness	■ How satisfied are you with your spiritual practices? ■ How do you take time each day to reflect or meditate on your spirituality?	■ Identify patients who may require a referral for additional support, such as community groups or organizations.
Social wellness	■ How often do you socialize with friends or family? ■ How do you make time to go to places where you can meet new people or visit new locations?	■ Identify patients who may require a referral for additional support, such as local or online support groups.
Occupational wellness	■ How satisfied are you with your current job or work? ■ If retired, how satisfied are you in your planning to do something every day?	■ Identify patients who may require a referral for additional support, such as community groups or organizations and their state's job resources website.

express them, and what they learned from their experiences. Self-honesty and privacy are essential to the journaling process for the patient to gain maximum benefit. Journaling may help identify stress triggers and provide patients with the opportunity to step back from stress-causing situations and identify healthy coping strategies preemptively (Caragol et al., 2021;

SAMHSA, 2017a, 2017b). Next, APPs can encourage patients to develop regular routines and habits to help them effectively process their feelings to fulfill their emotional needs. For example, APPs may teach patients deep breathing exercises, such as diaphragmatic breathing, which may serve as an effective, nonpharmacological intervention to reduce stress (Hopper et al., 2019). Such mindful pauses promote relaxation and mental clarity for coping with stressful events. Finally, APPs may ask patients to identify a comfortable and quiet space where they can go for psychological and physical safety during emotionally challenging events.

For self-care within the emotional dimension, SAMHSA (2017a, 2017b) promotes support groups to provide patients with opportunities to share feelings; strengthen coping skills; and reduce feelings of isolation, loneliness, and judgment. During the COVID-19 pandemic, support groups and individual mental healthcare services were offered via telehealth and videoconferencing platforms (Viswanathan et al., 2020). Peer support groups significantly improved the perception of resilience, coping self-efficacy, and perceived support (Jao et al., 2016).

As APPs encourage different practices to help manage stress, patients can be advised to create their wellness toolbox (Fessell & Cherniss, 2020). Promotion of daily routines such as yoga, meditation, mindful eating, restorative sleep, and physical fitness are encouraged lifestyle prescriptions for stress reduction and prevention. Another essential element within daily habits is time for self beyond obligations and work. Patients should be encouraged to identify renewing activities that bring them joy and self-fulfillment. One strategy demonstrated to be particularly beneficial is Three Good Things, which involves the daily recording of three items that were positive or went well (Seligman et al., 2005). Daily positive affirmations may help patients reframe negative thoughts and emotions and cultivate empowering thoughts and emotions.

Environmental Dimension and Lifestyle Prescription for Stress

SAMHSA (2017a, 2017b) focuses on the environmental dimension of being and feeling safe. Access to clean air, food, water, and safe living spaces is essential to the environmental dimension. The APP should assess for risks or hazards in or near the home. For example, if a home was built before 1978, patients may be exposed to lead-based paint (United States Environmental Protection Agency, 2021). Based on the risk assessment, the APP may refer patients to community resources and agencies for guidance and assistance, such as the local health department.

Furthermore, preservation of green and natural spaces for life, work, and learning, which are stimulating and pleasant, is noted by SAMHSA (2017a, 2017b) to support well-being, reduce stress, and promote relaxation. The lifestyle prescription for stress in this dimension may concentrate on green living, change of scenery, and the home and work environments. APPs can guide patients to spend more time outdoors, visit a public park or attend an outdoor sporting event, and take a walk break outdoors during work hours.

Chevalier et al. (2012) conceptualized earthing or grounding as the direct physical contact of the human body with the earth, such as walking barefoot. Emerging research suggests earthing may produce positive health benefits (Chevalier et al., 2012; Menigoz et al., 2020). A study by Chevalier et al. (2019) found that grounding significantly improved quality of life, physical function, energy, pain, depressed mood, and tiredness. A review of 20 research studies by Menigoz et al. (2020) provides further support for earthing as an integrative lifestyle approach to stress.

One recommendation for home and work environments is to declutter the spaces and schedule routine cleaning and organizing.

Having patients cultivate aesthetically appealing spaces through style, textures, and music can further promote stress reduction. The APP can also advise the patient to consider reducing or eliminating potentially stressful environmental inputs, such as excessive news coverage of distressing events. Viewership of this kind generally rises during mass trauma and can have a particularly insidious effect on those individuals with prior existing PTSD (Solomon et al., 2021). The APP can help patients develop individualized strategies for staying informed while limiting practices detrimental to well-being.

Financial Dimension and Lifestyle Prescription for Stress

According to SAMHSA (2017a, 2017b), the financial dimension involves an individual's contentment with their current and future financial situation. White et al. (2019) reported that individuals under financial stress are more likely to smoke, consume alcohol, overspend, eat a poor diet, and reduce exercise. Furthermore, White et al. noted that financial education and coaching help to improve self-control, perceived control, and perceived quality of life. SAMHSA (2017a, 2017b) reported that knowledge of financial processes and resources affects one's ability to manage money via income generation, savings, retirement, and manageable debt. APPs may refer patients to community courses on financial life skills, such as balancing their accounts (checkbook), developing a savings and retirement plan, budgeting for vacations and homeownership, and planning for unforeseen events like short- or long-term disabilities. Patients can identify their life goals and develop a budget for their finances. Free classes and resources through the local library or the patient's bank may further aid in financial planning and reduce stress and distress resulting from the lack of a manageable plan.

Intellectual Dimension and Lifestyle Prescription for Stress

For the intellectual dimension, SAMHSA (2017a, 2017b) emphasizes four key areas that may be incorporated into a lifestyle prescription for stress, including personal interests, education, brain exercise, and stimulating conversation. Examples of strategies APPs might recommend for personal interests include engagement in community groups or public events. Participation in cultural activities has been associated with reduced mortality of cancer and cardiovascular causes, potentially due to its effect on stress reduction (Løkken et al., 2021). Patients may be encouraged to explore public events, debates, or other community organizations to expand their perspectives and foster diverse thinking. For education, a host of free or low-cost community courses may be available focused on skills training, such as blogging, sign language, writing, or public speaking. Brain exercises that may be prescribed include crossword puzzles, mind teasers, memory games, and Sudoku. Rehman (2015) noted that mentorship promotes intellectual wellness through analytical thinking, problem-solving, and the use of higher-order cognitive skills.

Occupational Dimension and Lifestyle Prescription for Stress

Occupational wellness concerns career, volunteer work, and employment. According to SAMHSA (2017a, 2017b), such endeavors should align with an individual's beliefs, values, and interests and provide purpose and meaning. Areas of emphasis within this dimension include work relationships, balance, and accomplishment. APPs may explore the patient's satisfaction with employment, lack of employment, or retirement. Next, SAMHSA (2017a, 2017b) recommends assessing for balance between career demands and access to leisure time.

Patients may be prescribed the use of a calendar to schedule leisure time and to track workload. Reflection on their sense of accomplishment provides meaning and purpose to their career and work. Other evidence-informed strategies for mitigating occupational stress reported by Clough et al. (2017) included mental imagery, relaxation, attention techniques, breathing exercises, and biofeedback interventions focused on heart rhythm patterns. Clough et al. also noted that occupational stress that has reached burnout or beyond may warrant referral for cognitive or behavioral therapy.

Physical Dimension and Lifestyle Prescription for Stress

Physical wellness is central to stress prevention and management. SAMHSA (2017a, 2017b) notes that good physical health habits, such as healthy eating, physical activity, sleep, and preventive health care, are vital to the physical wellness domain. SAMHSA (2017a, 2017b) emphasizes evaluating access to healthy and fresh food and having patients track what they eat. In addition to lifestyle prescriptions for stress focused on a health-promoting diet, the APP might consider referral to local food co-ops, a registered dietician, or self-help support groups, such as Overeaters Anonymous or Take Off Pounds Sensibly.

Individuals who participate in regular physical activity, as appropriate, may benefit from increased resilience to acute stress (Childs & de Wit, 2014; Xu et al., 2021). Wilson et al. (2021) found that starting or sustaining physical activity mitigated psychological distress related to the COVID-19 pandemic. Smith et al. (2022) found that moderate to vigorous physical activity buffers the effect of negative emotions, including stress, and may directly affect eating regulation. Thus, assessing the frequency and intensity of physical activity informs the need for supportive resources, including yoga and fitness, through local gyms such as the YMCA. Referral to a certified personal trainer or physical therapist may assist patients in meeting their unique physical wellness needs.

Sleep disruption and loss of circadian rhythmicity affect homeostatic regulating systems within the body that may yield an individual more susceptible to acute and chronic stress (Agorastos & Olff, 2021). Blaxton et al. (2017) found that daily increases in sleep quality predicted higher levels of positive affect and reductions in stress. Therefore, assessment of sleep patterns and practices before bed provides valuable insights into needed patient education, such as reducing screen time before bed, decreasing caffeine intake after lunch, and avoiding large meals in the evening to foster restorative sleep.

SAMHSA (2017a, 2017b) recommends evaluating tobacco, alcohol, and drug use as part of a comprehensive stress assessment. Based on the assessment findings, the lifestyle prescription for stress could include community smoking cessation programs, support groups, Alcoholics Anonymous, Narcotics Anonymous, or other free resources to enhance coping, self-efficacy, and social support. Taylor et al. (2014), in their meta-analysis of 26 studies, found that smoking cessation significantly improved mental health, including stress reduction. Finally, as part of a comprehensive wellness approach to stress, SAMHSA (2017a, 2017b) recommends routine preventive healthcare visits, including those for other disciplines, such as dentistry.

Social Dimension and Lifestyle Prescription for Stress

SAMHSA (2017a, 2017b) focuses the social dimension on community, healthy relationships, and social time. COVID-19 has significantly affected the safety and availability of social activities (Benfante et al., 2020; Williams et al., 2021). The APP may suggest creative ways for the patient to interact with family and friends, such as using video communication tools (e.g., FaceTime, Zoom, Skype) or meeting outdoors in small groups. Other methods for interacting socially include playing multiplayer video games or outdoor tai chi and yoga. For some, social media may provide an option for broadening one's community and potential for interaction, as research has indicated that the number of contacts on online platforms such as Facebook can serve as a predictor of social support (Nabi et al., 2013). Spending time with animals can provide a beneficial social experience and is particularly valuable when a human experience is not available (Ein et al., 2018). SAMHSA (2017b) also suggests volunteering and engagement with one's spiritual community as potential prescription strategies. A social calendar can help patients plan to connect and spend quality time with others. Key elements of the lifestyle prescription for

stress might include referral to support groups or community groups related to the patient's unique interests and needs.

Spiritual Dimension and Lifestyle Prescription for Stress

Within the spiritual dimension, SAMHSA (2017a, 2017b) emphasizes resources focused on beliefs, involvement, and time. An essential component of the spiritual dimension is the need to have balance, purpose, meaning, peace, and a deep appreciation for life. Spiritual practices, such as prayer, and involvement in faith communities, further support connection to others and deepen spiritual understanding (Achour et al., 2019). Meditation

---

Health Promotion Case Study Self-Care for Health Professionals

Case Description: Self-care is vital for well-being and stress prevention. The work of health professionals (HPs) can be emotionally challenging, demanding, and stressful. The following case study describes the experience of HPs during the COVID-19 pandemic.

    Since the beginning of the COVID-19 pandemic, HPs working in a busy outpatient clinic have been skipping lunch and binge eating later in the evening in front of the television. Though the HPs were around people all day at the clinic, they have been experiencing increased feelings of isolation from friends and family, as most of their time is dedicated to long hours at work. Many of the HPs used to exercise four or five days per week but have not participated in any routine physical activity for the past 6 months. Several also used to cycle each weekend as a group at a local trail but have stopped this practice as well. The HPs cherished this time outdoors and in nature.

    Two of the HPs reported that they have not been sleeping well for some time and have been using alcohol each night to fall asleep. These HPs have experienced increased agitation, tiredness, low energy levels, and spiritual detachment. Most HPs have skipped routine preventive visits for dental hygiene and annual physicals. Some HPs reported that they have stopped reading or engaging in activities outside of work with close colleagues. Finally, several HPs noted that coping with work and family stress is increasingly difficult. Many are considering leaving their HP roles for other industries.

    As an APP, what issues would you consider when caring for members of this HP group? Use the following reflection questions in developing your plan of care.

Critical Thinking Questions

1. Which SAMHSA (2017a) wellness dimensions are out of balance and contributing to their stress?

2. Which screening tools might aid in the assessment of stress and wellness for the HPs?

3. Why might HPs forgo their own stress prevention and management habits and routines?

4. What evidence-informed self-care strategies might the HPs use or be prescribed for stress?

5. If you were the clinic's manager or leader, what might you put into place to support occupational wellness?

Health Promotion Activity: Assessing and Addressing Stress

---

1. Conduct a stress screening assessment of a classmate (or as directed by your course faculty) using one of the instruments discussed in this chapter.
2. Develop a comprehensive lifestyle prescription for stress and plan of care based on the assessment findings.

---

may be prescribed to assist patients in exploring their values, principles, and beliefs as well as discovering how spirituality affects their actions. The practice of mindfulness-based stress reduction, which includes meditation and associated exercises involving focus and relaxation, is strongly established as an evidence-informed method of stress reduction (Grossman et al., 2004; Khoury et al., 2015). Many patients may benefit from guarded time each day to reflect and engage in spiritual practices that support their search for meaning and purpose in life.

Summary

Stress is understood to be the way an individual responds emotionally and physically to any demand. It is considered a normal aspect of life and plays an integral role in the well-being of an individual. APPs are essential in helping their patients identify and manage stressors in their lives. When managed appropriately, everyday stress does not necessarily

detract from quality of life. However, severe stress can have dire consequences for mental health, including anxiety, depression, and burnout. Stress can also have enduring effects on physical health. APPs should be alert for signs of excessive, extreme, or chronic stress in patients and screen for stress in all stages of the life span. When evaluating a patient's stress and coping, it is recommended to initiate open dialogue in a nonjudgmental manner. It is essential to be alert for potential self-harm signs and follow appropriate protocols when identified. The APP may also consider using validated psychometric tools to gather additional information about the patient's needs and to guide referrals. To support their patients in addressing stress as part of overall mental health, APPs should consider addressing the eight dimensions of wellness described by the SAMHSA framework: (1) emotional, (2) environmental, (3) financial, (4) intellectual, (5) occupational, (6) physical, (7) social, and (8) spiritual. See **Table 12.5** for additional evidence-based resources on stress.

TABLE 12.5	Evidence-Based Resources for Stress
Resource	**URL**
American Psychiatric Association	https://www.psychiatry.org
Centers for Disease Control and Prevention: Coping With Stress (good for patients)	https://www.cdc.gov/violenceprevention/about/copingwith-stresstips.html
Centers for Disease Control and Prevention: Healthcare Personnel and First Responders: How to Cope with Stress and Build Resilience During the COVID-19 Pandemic	https://www.cdc.gov/coronavirus/2019-ncov/hcp/mental-health-healthcare.html

(continues)

TABLE 12.5	Evidence-Based Resources for Stress	[continued]

Resource	URL
Cleveland Clinic: Stress Overview (good for patients)	https://my.clevelandclinic.org/health/articles/11874-stress
Institute of Lifestyle Medicine: Stress Tools and Resources	https://www.instituteoflifestylemedicine.org/?page_id=12
Mayo Clinic: Healthy Lifestyle: Stress Management (good for patients)	https://www.mayoclinic.org/healthy-lifestyle/stress-management/in-depth/stress-symptoms/art-20050987
National Alliance on Mental Illness	https://www.nami.org
National Institute of Mental Health: I'm So Stressed Out! Fact Sheet (good for patients)	https://www.nimh.nih.gov/health/publications/stress
Substance Abuse and Mental Health Services Administration	https://www.samhsa.gov
Suicide Prevention Resource Center	https://www.sprc.org
U.S. Department of Health and Human Services: COVID-19 Behavioral Health Resources	https://asprtracie.hhs.gov/technical-resources/115/covid-19-behavioral-health-resources/99
U.S. Department of Health and Human Services: *Healthy People 2030*	https://health.gov/healthypeople
U.S. Department of Veterans Affairs: Veteran Crisis Line	https://www.veteranscrisisline.net

Acronyms

APP: advanced practice provider
CSS: COVID Stress Scales
DHEA: dehydroepiandrosterone
GAS: general adaptation syndrome
HPA: hypothalamus-pituitary-adrenal axis
LEC-5: Life Events Checklist for DSM-5
LSC-R: Life Stressor Checklist-Revised

PSQ: Perceived Stress Questionnaire
PSS: Perceived Stress Scale
SAM: sympathetic-adreno-medullar axis
SAMHSA: Substance Abuse and Mental Health Services Administration
WI: Wellness Inventory

References

Achour, M., Azmi, B. A. G. I., Isahak, M. B., Nor, M. R. M., & Yusoff, M. Y. Z. M. (2019). Job stress and nurses well-being: Prayer and age as moderators. *Community Mental Health Journal, 55*(7), 1226–1235. https://doi.org/10.1007/s10597-019-00410-y

Agorastos, A., & Olff, M. (2021). Sleep, circadian system and traumatic stress. *European Journal of Psychotraumatology, 12*(1), 1–7. https://doi.org/10.1080/20008198.2021.1956746

American Psychiatric Association. (2020). *What is post-traumatic stress disorder?* https://www.psychiatry.org/patients-families/ptsd/what-is-ptsd

American Psychological Association. (2020). *Stress in America 2020: A national mental health crisis.* https://www.apa.org/news/press/releases/stress/2020/report-october

Bak, P. L., Midgley, N., Zhu, J. L., Wistoft, K., & Obel, C. (2015). The Resilience Program: Preliminary evaluation of a mentalization-based education program. *Frontiers in Psychology, 6,* 1–6. https://doi.org/10.3389/fpsyg.2015.00753

Ben-Efrain, Y. J., Wasserman, D., Wasserman, J., & Sokolowski, M. (2011). Gene-environment interactions between *CRHR1* variants and physical assault in suicide attempts. *Genes, Brain and Behavior, 10,* 663–672. https://doi.org/10.1111/j.1601-183X.2011.00703.x

Benfante, A., Di Tella, M., Romeo, A., & Castelli, L. (2020). Traumatic stress in healthcare workers during COVID-19 pandemic: A review of the immediate impact. *Frontiers in Psychology, 11,* 2816. https://doi.org/10.3389/fpsyg.2020.569935

Berry, J. O., & Jones, W. H. (1995). The parental stress scale: Initial psychometric evidence. *Journal of Social and Personal Relationships, 12*(3), 463–472. https://doi.org/10.1177/0265407595123009

Bisht, K., Sharma, K., & Tremblay, M. È. (2018). Chronic stress as a risk factor for Alzheimer's disease: Roles of microglia-mediated synaptic remodeling, inflammation, and oxidative stress. *Neurobiology of Stress, 9,* 9–21. https://doi.org/10.1016/j.ynstr.2018.05.003

Blaxton, J. M., Bergeman, C. S., Whitehead, B. R., Braun, M. E., & Payne, J. D. (2017). Relationships among nightly sleep quality, daily stress, and daily affect. *The Journals of Gerontology, Series B Psychological Sciences and Social Sciences, 72*(3), 363–372. https://doi.org10.1093/geronb/gbv060

Borrell, L. N., Rodríguez-Álvarez, E., & Dallo, F. J. (2020). Racial/ethnic inequities in the associations of allostatic load with all-cause and cardiovascular-specific mortality risk in U.S. adults. *PLOS One, 15*(2), e0228336. https://doi.org/10.1371/journal.pone.0228336

Cannon, W. B. (1929). *Bodily changes in pain, hunger, fear and rage.* Appleton, Century, Crofts.

Caragol, J. A., Johnson, A. R., & Kwan, B. M. (2021). A gratitude intervention to improve clinician stress and professional satisfaction: A pilot and feasibility trial. *International Journal of Psychiatry Medicine.* Advance online publication. https://doi.org/10.1177/0091217420982112

Centers for Disease Control and Prevention. (2020). *What is epigenetics?* https://www.cdc.gov/genomics/disease/epigenetics.htm

Chevalier, G., Patel, S., Weiss, L., Chopra, D., & Mills, P. J. (2019). The effects of grounding (earthing) on bodyworkers' pain and overall quality of life: A randomized controlled trial. *Explore* (NY), *15*(3), 181–190. https://doi.org/10.1016/j.explore.2018.10.001

Chevalier, G., Sinatra, S. T., Oschman, J. L., Sokal, K., & Sokal, P. (2012). Earthing: Health implications of reconnecting the human body to the earth's surface electrons. *Journal of Environmental and Public Health, 2012,* 1–8. https://doi.org/10.1155/2012/291541

Childs, E., & de Wit, H. (2014). Regular exercise is associated with emotional resilience to acute stress in healthy adults. *Frontiers in Physiology, 5,* 161. https://doi.org/10.3389/fphys.2014.00161

Choi, K. R., Kim, D., Jang, E. Y., Bae, H., & Kim, S. H. (2017). Reliability and validity of the Korean version of the lifetime stressor checklist-revised in psychiatric outpatients with anxiety or depressive disorders. *Yonsei Medical Journal, 58*(1), 226–233. https://doi.org/10.3349/ymj.2017.58.1.226

Christopher, R., de Tantillo, L., & Watson, J. (2020). Academic caring pedagogy, presence, and Communitas in nursing education during the COVID-19 pandemic. *Nursing Outlook, 68*(6), 822–829. https://doi.org/10.1016/j.outlook.2020.08.006

Clough, B. A., March, S., Chan, R. J., Casey, L. M., Philips, R., & Ireland, M. J. (2017). Psychosocial interventions for managing occupational stress and burnout among medical doctors: A systematic review. *Systematic Reviews, 6*(144), 1–19. https://doi.org/10.1186/s13643-017-0526-3

Cohen, S., Gianaros, P. J., & Manuck, S. B. (2016). A stage model of stress and disease. *Perspectives on Psychological Science, 11*(4), 456–463. https://doi.org/10.1177/1745691616646305

Cohen, S., & Janicki-Deverts, D. (2012). Who's stressed? Distributions of psychological stress in the United States in probability samples from 1983, 2006 and 2009. *Journal of Applied Social Psychology, 42*(6), 1320–1334. https://doi.org/10.1111/j.1559-1816.2012.00900.x

Cohen, S., Kamarck, T., & Mermelstein, R. (1983). A global measure of perceived stress. *Journal of Health and Social Behavior, 24,* 385–396.

Cohen, S., & Williamson, G. (1988). Perceived stress in a probability sample of the United States. In S. Spacapan & S. Oskamp (Eds.), *The social psychology of health* (pp. 31–67). SAGE.

Crosswell, A. D., & Lockwood, K. G. (2020). Best practices for stress measurement: How to measure psychological stress in health research. *Health Psychology Open, 7*(2), 1–12. https://doi.org/10.1177/2055102920933072

Dooley, L. N., Slavich, G. M., Moreno, P. I., & Bower, J. E. (2017). Strength through adversity: Moderate lifetime stress exposure is associated with psychological resilience in breast cancer survivors. *Stress Health, 33*(5), 549–557. https://doi.org/10.1002/smi.2739

Dunn, H. L. (1961). *High-level wellness: A collection of twenty-nine short talks on different aspects of the theme "high-level wellness for man and society."* R. W. Beatty.

Ein, N., Li, L., & Vickers, K. (2018). The effect of pet therapy on the physiological and subjective stress response: A meta-analysis. Stress and health. *Journal* of the International Society for the Investigation of Stress, 34(4), 477–489. https://doi.org/10.1002/smi.2812

Erikson, E. H. (1950). *Childhood & society.* W. W. Norton & Company.

Erikson, J. M. (1997). *Erik H. Erikson: The life cycle completed.* W. W. Norton & Company.

Fessell, D., & Cherniss, C. (2020). Coronavirus disease 2019 (COVID-19) and beyond: Micropractices for burnout prevention and emotional wellness. *Journal of the American College of Radiology,* 17(6), 746. https://doi.org/10.1016/j.jacr.2020.03.013

Friedman, A., Homma, D., Bloem, B., Gibb, L. G., Ammemori, K. I., Hu, D., Delcasso, S., Truong, T. F., Yang, J., Hood, A. S., Mikofalvy, K. A., Beck, D. W., Nguyen, N., Nelson, E. D., Toro Arana, S. E., Vorder Bruegge, R. H., Goosens, K. A., & Graybiel, A. M. (2017). Chronic stress alters striosome-circuit dynamics, leading to aberrant decision-making. *Cell,* 171(5), 1191–1205. https://doi.org/10.1016/j.cell.2017.10.017

Geiker, N. R. W., Astrup, A., Hjorth, M. F., Sjödin, A., Pijls, L., & Markus, C. R. (2018). Does stress influence sleep patterns, food intake, weight gain, abdominal obesity and weight loss interventions and vice versa? *Obesity Reviews,* 19(1), 81–97. https://doi.org/10.1111/obr.12603

Godoy, L. D., Rossignoli, M. T., Delfino-Pereira, P., Garcia-Cairasco, N., & de Lima Umeoka, E. H. (2018). A comprehensive overview on stress neurobiology: Basic concepts and clinical implications. *Frontiers in Behavioral Neuroscience,* 12(127). https://doi.org/10.3389/fnbeh.2018.00127

Goodnite, P. M. (2014). Stress: A concept analysis. *Nursing Forum,* 49(1), 71–74. https://doi.org/10.1111/nuf.1204

Gouin, J. P. (2011). Chronic stress, immune dysregulation, and health. *American Journal of Lifestyle Medicine,* 5(6), 476–485. https://doi.org/10.1177/1559827610395467

Grossman, P., Niemann, L., Schmidt, S., & Walach, H. (2004). Mindfulness-based stress reduction and health benefits: A meta-analysis. *Journal of Psychosomatic Research,* 57(1), 35–43. https://doi.org/10.1016/S0022-3999(03)00573-7

Guidi, J., Lucente, M., Sonino, N., & Fava, G. A. (2021). Allostatic load and its impact on health: A systematic review. *Psychotherapy and Psychosomatics,* 90(1), 11–27. https://doi.org/10.1159/000510696

Hattangadi, N., Cost, K. T., Birken, C. S., Borkhoff, C. M., Maguire, J. L., Szatmari, P., & Charach, A. (2020). Parenting stress during infancy is a risk factor for mental health problems in 3-year-old children. *BMC Public Health,* 20(1726), 1–7. https://doi.org/10.1186/s12889-020-09861-5

Hopper, S. I., Murray, S. L., Ferrara, L. R., & Singleton, J. K. (2019). Effectiveness of diaphragmatic breathing for reducing physiological and psychological stress in adults: A quantitative systematic review. *JBI Evidence Synthesis,* 17(9), 1855–1876. https://doi.org/10.11124/JBISRIR-2017-003848

Howie, H., Rijal, C. M., & Ressler, K. J. (2019). A review of epigenetic contributions to post-traumatic stress disorder. *Dialogues in Clinical Neuroscience,* 21(4), 417–428. https://doi.org/10.31887/DCNS.2019.21.4/kressler

Jao, Y. L., Epps, F., McDermott, C., Rose, K. M., & Specht, J. K. (2016). Effects of support groups for individuals with early-stage dementia and mild cognitive impairment: An integrative review. *Research in Gerontological Nursing,* 10(1), 35–51. https://doi.org/10.3928/19404921-20160726-01

Katz, D. L., & Ali, A. (2009). *Preventive medicine, integrative medicine and the health of the public. A paper commissioned for the IOM Summit on Integrative Medicine and the Health of the Public.* https://www.researchgate.net/publication/237429179_Preventive_medicine_integrative_medicine_and_the_health_of_the_public

Khoury, B., Sharma, M., Rush, S. E., & Fournier, C. (2015). Mindfulness-based stress reduction for healthy individuals: A meta-analysis. *Journal of Psychosomatic Research,* 78(6), 519–528. https://doi.org/10.1016/j.jpsychores.2015.03.009

Kilbourne, A. M., Beck, K., Spaeth-Rublee, B., Ramanuj, P., O'Brien, R. W., Tomoyasu, N., & Pincus, H. A. (2018). Measuring and improving the quality of mental health care: A global perspective. *World Psychiatry,* 17(1), 30–38. https://doi.org/ 10.1002/wps.20482

Koolhaas, J. M., Bartolomucci, A., Buwalda, B., de Boer, S. F., Flügge, G., Korte, S. M., Meerlo, P., Murison, R., Oliver, B., Palanza, P., Richter-Levin, G., Sgoifo, A., Steimer, T., Stiedl, O., van Dijk, G., Wöhr, M., & Fuchs, E. (2011). Stress revisited: A critical evaluation of the stress concept. *Neuroscience & Biobehavioral Reviews,* 35(5), 1291–1301. https://doi.org/10.1016/j.neubiorev.2011.02.003

Koolhaas, J. M., de Boer, S. F., Coppens, C. M., and Buwalda, B. (2010). Neuroendocrinology of coping styles: Towards understanding the biology of individual variation. *Frontiers in Neuroendocrinology,* 31, 307–321. https://doi.org/10.1016/j.yfrne.2010.04.001

Lazarus, R. S., & Cohen, J. B. (1977). Environmental stress. In I. Altman & J. F. Wohlwill (Eds.), *Human behavior and environment* (pp. 89–127). Springer.

Lazarus, R. S., & Folkman, S. (1984). *Stress, appraisal, and coping.* Springer.

Lee, J., Papa, F., Atu Jani, P., Alpini, S., & Kenny, M. (2020). An epigenetics-based, lifestyle medicine–driven approach to stress management for primary patient care: Implications for medical education. *American Journal of Lifestyle Medicine,* 14(3), 294–303. https://doi.org/10.1177/1559827619847436

Levenstein, S., Prantera, C., Varvo, V., Scribano, M. L., Berto, E., Luzi, C., & Andreoli, A. (1993). Development of the perceived stress questionnaire: A new tool for psychosomatic research. *Journal of Psychosomatic Research,* 37(1), 19–32. https://doi.org/10.1016/0022-3999(93)90120-5

Li, Y., Lin, H., Li, Y., & Cao, J. (2011). Association between socio-psycho-behavioral factors and male semen quality: Systematic review and meta-analyses. *Fertility and Sterility*, *95*(1), 116–123. https://doi.org/10.1016/j.fertnstert.2010.06.031

Løkken, B. I., Merom, D., Sund, E. R., Krokstad, S., & Rangul, V. (2021). Association of engagement in cultural activities with cause-specific mortality determined through an eight-year follow up: The HUNT Study, Norway. *PLoS One*, *16*(3), e0248332. https://doi.org/10.1371/journal.pone.0248332

Lupien, S. J., Juster, R. P., Raymond, C., & Marin, M. F. (2018). The effects of chronic stress on the human brain: From neurotoxicity, to vulnerability, to opportunity. *Frontiers in Neuroendocrinology*, *49*, 91–105. https://doi.org/ 10.1016/j.yfrne.2018.02.001

Mathur, M. B., Epel, E., Kind, S., Desai, M., Parks, C. G., Sandler, D. P., & Nayer, K. (2015). Perceived stress and telomere length: A systematic review, meta-analysis, and methodologic considerations for advancing the field. *Brain, Behavior, and Immunity*, *54*, 158–169. https://doi.org/ 10.1016/j.bbi.2016.02.002

Maul, S., Giegling, I., Fabbri, C., Corponi, F., Serretti, A., & Rujescu, D. (2020). Genetics of resilience: Implications from genome-wide association studies and candidate genes of the stress response system in posttraumatic stress disorder and depression. *American Journal of Medical Genetics Part B Neuropsychiatry Genetics*, *183*(2), 77–94. https://doi.org/10.1002/ajmg.b.32763

Menigoz, W., Latz, T. T., Ely, R. A., Kamei, C., Melvin, G., & Sinatra, D. (2020). Integrative and lifestyle medicine strategies should include earthing (grounding): Review of research evidence and clinical observations. *Explore* (NY), *16*(3), 152–160. https://doi.org/ 10.1016/j.explore.2019.10.005

Morneau Shepell Ltd. (2017). *Stress at work: What we can learn from EAP utilization*. https://us.lifeworks.com/sites/default/files/assets/downloads/Whitepaper_MorneauShepell_Stress_at_work_E-US_0417.pdf

Nabi, R. L., Prestin, A., & So, J. (2013). Facebook friends with (health) benefits? Exploring social network site use and perceptions of social support, stress, and well-being. *Cyberpsychology, Behavior, and Social Networking*, *16*(10), 721–727. https://doi.org/10.1089/cyber.2012.0521

National Institute of Mental Health. (n.d.). *I'm so stressed out! Fact sheet*. https://www.nimh.nih.gov/health/publications/stress

Ohrnberger, J., Fichera, E., & Sutton, M. (2017). The relationship between physical and mental health: A mediation analysis. *Social Science & Medicine*, *195*, 42–49. https://doi.org/ 10.1016/j.socscimed.2017.11.008

Pal, L., Bevilacqua, K., & Santoro, N. F. (2010). Chronic psychosocial stressors are detrimental to ovarian reserve: A study of infertile women. *Journal of Psychosomatic Obstetrics & Gynecology*, *31*(3), 130–139. https://doi.org/10.3109/0167482X.2010.485258

Panchal, S., Palmer, S., O'Riordan, S., & Kelly, A. (2017). Stress and well-being: A life stage model. *International Journal of Stress Prevention and Wellbeing*, *1*(5), 1–3.

Rehman, R. (2015). Intellectual wellness, medical students and mentorship. *International Journal of Emergency Mental Health and Human Resilience*, *17*(3), 608.

Ridner, S. H. (2004). Psychological distress: Concept analysis. *Journal of Advanced Nursing*, *45*(5), 536–545. https://doi.org/10.1046/j.1365-2648.2003.02938.x

Rutter, M. (2006). Implications of resilience concepts for scientific understanding. *Annals of the New York Academy of Science*, *1094*, 1–12. https://doi.org/10.1196/annals.1376.002

Salari, N., Hosseinian-Far, A., Jalali, R., Vaisi-Raygani, A., Rasoulpoor, S., Mohammadi, M., Rasoulpoor, S., & Khaledi-Paveh, B. (2020). Prevalence of stress, anxiety, depression among the general population during the COVID-19 pandemic: A systematic review and meta-analysis. *Globalization and Health*, *16*(57), 1–11. https://doi.org/10.1186/s12992020-00589-w

Seeman, T. E., McEwen, B. S., Rowe, J. W., & Singer, B. H. (2001). Allostatic load as a marker of cumulative biological risk: MacArthur studies of successful aging. *Proceedings of the National Academy of Sciences*, *98*(8), 4770–4775. https://doi.org/10.1073/pnas.081072698

Seeman, T. E., Singer, B. H., Rowe, J. W., Horwitz, R. I., & McEwen, B. S. (1997). Price of adaptation—Allostatic load and its health consequences: MacArthur studies of successful aging. *The Archives of Internal Medicine*, *157*(19), 2259–2268. https://doi.org/10.1001/archinte.1997.00440400111013

Seligman, M. E. P., Steen, T. A., Park, N., & Peterson, C. (2005). Positive psychology progress: Empirical validation of interventions. *American Psychologist*, *60*, 410–421. https://doi.org/10.1037/0003-066X.60.5.410

Selye, H. (1950). Stress and the general adaptation syndrome. *British Medical Journal*, *1*(4667), 1383–1392. https://doi.org/10.1136/bmj.1.4667.1383

Selye, H. (1959). Perspectives in stress research. *Perspectives in Biology and Medicine*, *2*(4), 403–416. https://doi.org/10.1353/pbm.1959.0000

Selye, H. (1976). Stress without distress. In G. Serban (Ed.), *Psychopathology of human adaptation*. Springer. https://doi.org/10.1007/978-1-4684-2238-2_9

Selye, H. (1980). Stress, aging and retirement. *The Journal of Mind and Behavior*, *1*(1), 93–110.

Shean, M. (2015). *Current theories relating to resilience and young people: A literature review*. https://evidenceforlearning.org.au/assets/Grant-Round-II-Resilience/Current-theories-relating-to-resilience-and-young-people.pdf

Smith, K. E., Mason, T. B., Wang, W. L., Schumacher, L. M., Pellegrini, C. A., Goldschmidt, A. B., & Unick, J. L. (2022). Dynamic associations between anxiety, stress, physical activity, and eating regulation over the course of a behavioral weight loss intervention. *Appetite, 168.* https://doi.org/10.1016/j.appet.2021.105706

Solomon, Z., Ginzburg, K., Ohry, A., & Mikulincer, M. (2021). Overwhelmed by the news: A longitudinal study of prior trauma, posttraumatic stress disorder trajectories, and news watching during the COVID-19 pandemic. *Social Science & Medicine, 278,* 113956. https://doi.org/10.1016/j.socscimed.2021.113956

Sterling, P., & Eyer, J. (1988). Allostasis: A new paradigm to explain arousal pathology. In S. Fisher & J. Reason (Eds.), *Handbook of life stress, cognition and health* (pp. 629–649). Wiley.

Stoewen, D. L. (2017). Dimensions of wellness: Change your habits, change your life. *Canadian Veterinary Journal, 58*(8), 861–862.

Substance Abuse and Mental Health Services Administration. (2017a). *Creating a healthier life: A step-by-step guide to wellness.* https://store.samhsa.gov/sites/default/files/d7/priv/sma16-4958.pdf

Substance Abuse and Mental Health Services Administration. (2017b). *What individuals in recovery need to know about wellness.* https://store.samhsa.gov/sites/default/files/d7/priv/sma16-4950.pdf

Swarbrick, M., & Yudof, J. (2017). *Wellness in eight dimensions.* https://www.researchgate.net/publication/299127407_Wellness_in_the_8_Dimensions

Taylor, G., McNeill, A., Girling, A., Farley, A., Lindson-Hawley, N., & Aveyard, P. (2014). Change in mental health after smoking cessation: Systematic review and meta-analysis. *BMJ, 348:g1141,* 1–22. https://doi.org/10.1136/bmj.g1151

Taylor, S., Landry, C. A., Paluszek, M. M., Fergus, T. A., McKay, D., & Asmundson, G. J. G. (2020). Development and initial validation of the COVID Stress Scales. *Journal of Anxiety Disorders, 72,* 1–7. https://doi.org/10.1016/j.janxdis.2020.102232

Thombs, B. D., Markham, S., Rice, D. B., & Ziegelstein, R. C. (2021). Does depression screening in primary care improve mental health outcomes? *BMJ, 374.* https://doi.org/10.1136/bmj.n1661

Tran, T. T., Srivareerat, M., & Alkadhi, K. A. (2011). Chronic psychosocial stress accelerates impairment of long-term memory and late-phase long-term potentiation in an at-risk model of Alzheimer's disease. *Hippocampus, 21*(7), 724–732. https://doi.org/10.1002/hipo.20790

United States Environmental Protection Agency. (2021). *Protect your family from lead in your home—Real estate disclosure.* https://www.epa.gov/lead/protect-your-family-lead-your-home-real-estate-disclosure

Viswanathan, R., Myers, M. F., & Fanous, A. H. (2020). Support groups and individual mental health care via video conferencing for frontline clinicians during the COVID-19 pandemic. *Psychosomatics, 61*(5), 538–543. https://doi.org/10.1016/j.psym.2020.06.014.

Weathers, F. W., Blake, D. D., Schnurr, P. P., Kaloupek, D. G., Marx, B. P., & Keane, T. M. (2013). *The Life Events Checklist for DSM-5 (LEC-5).* National Center for PTSD. www.ptsd.va.gov

Webster-Stratton, C. (1990). Stress: A potential disruptor of parent perceptions and family interactions. *Journal of Clinical Child Psychology, 19*(4), 302–312. https://doi.org/10.1207/s15374424jccp1904_2

Werner, E. E. (1982). Vulnerable, but invincible: A longitudinal study of resilient children and youth. *American Journal of Orthopsychiatric Association, 59.*

White, N. D., Packard, K., & Kalkowski, J. (2019). Financial education and coaching: A lifestyle medicine approach to addressing financial stress. *American Journal of Lifestyle Medicine, 13*(6), 540–543. https://doi.org/10.1177/1559827619865439

Wiegner, L., Hange, D., Björkelund, C., & Ahlborg, G. (2015). Prevalence of perceived stress and associations to symptoms of exhaustion, depression and anxiety in a working age population seeking primary care—An observational study. *BMC Family Practice, 16*(1), 1–8. https://doi.org/10.1186/s12875-015-0252-7

Williams, C. Y. K., Townson, A. T., Kapur, M., Ferreira, A. F., Nunn, R., Galante, J., Phillips, V., Gentry, S., & Usher-Smith, J. A. (2021). Interventions to reduce social isolation and loneliness during COVID-19 physical distancing measures: A rapid systematic review. *PLoS One, 16*(2), 1–28. https://doi.org/10.1371/journal.pone.0247139

Wilson, K. E., Corbett, A., Van Horn, A., Beltran, D. G., Ayers, J. D., Alcock, J., & Aktipis, A. (2021). Associations between change over time in pandemic-related stress and change in physical activity. *Journal of Physical Activity and Health, 18*(11), 1419–1426. https://doi.org/10.1123/jpah.2021-0276

Wolfe, J., Kimerling, R., Brown, P., Chrestman, K., & Levin, K. (1997). *The Life Stressor Checklist-Revised (LSC-R).* http://www.ptsd.va.gov/professional/assessment/te-measures/lsc-r.asp

Xu, S., Liu, Z., Tian, S., Ma, Z., Jia, C., & Sun, G. (2021). Physical activity and resilience among college students: The mediating effects of basic psychological needs. *International Journal of Environmental Research and Public Health, 18*(7), 1–11. https://doi.org/10.3390/ijerph18073722

Yao, B. C., Meng, L. B., Hao, M. L., Zhang, Y. M., Gong, T., & Guo, Z. G. (2019). Chronic stress: A critical risk factor for atherosclerosis. *Journal of International Medical Research, 47*(4), 1429–1440. https://doi.org/10.1177/0300060519826820

Yerkes, R. M., & Dodson, J. D. (1908). The relation of strength of stimulus to rapidity of habit formation. *Journal of Comparative and Neurological Psychology, 18*(5), 459–482. https://doi.org/10.1002/cne.920180503

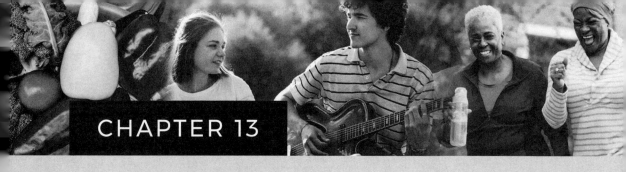

CHAPTER 13

Move Often

Jeff Young, BS, CSCS, ACSM-EIM
Sheila Hautbois, PA-C, MPAS, MPH, CHES®, DipACLM
Nanette Morales, DNP, NP-C, DipACLM

Lack of activity destroys the good condition of every human being, while movement and physical exercise save and preserve it.

Plato

Walking is man's best medicine.

Hippocrates

OBJECTIVES

This chapter will enable the reader to:

1. Define terminology related to physical activity and exercise.
2. Explain exercise science principles.
3. Describe exercise guidelines.
4. Discuss patient education and counseling specific to physical activity and exercise.
5. Identify interprofessional collaboration opportunities to enable patients to exercise safely.
6. Consider practical applications and benefits of exercise.

Overview

Move often. This short phrase is the antidote for the problems associated with a sedentary lifestyle. The risk of death increases by 20% to 30% for people who are insufficiently active (World Health Organization, 2020). This chapter provides inspiration for moving often, a detailed discussion of the benefits of exercise on every system in the body, and the science behind how to start exercise and progress to continue reaping optimal benefits. The focus is on foundational physical activity and exercise science definitions, principles, and guidelines that all advanced practice providers (APPs) and others giving movement advice should understand. It also illustrates the best ways to discuss this topic and apply clinical guidelines with patients, including a combination of education, person-centered counseling,

© Kathleen Gail/Shutterstock; © StoryTime Studio/Shutterstock; © kali9/Getty Images

and goal setting. Finally, it describes patient assessments, including those that can be done in the clinic and those that should be referred to qualified exercise professionals.

APPs who implement the principles from this chapter into their own life will experience the power of regular movement and structured exercise to benefit many aspects of personal health. That personal experience will enable APPs to share authentic enthusiasm for exercise with patients. When a patient is ready to add exercise, doing so will frequently elicit improvements in other lifestyle behaviors. Sleep and stress management can improve quickly after increasing exercise, in contrast to nutrition, which often improves over time as a person realizes how important good nutrition is for exercise performance. Social connections can increase with group exercise or by doing physical activity with family, friends, or a personal trainer. Risky substance use often decreases as exercise increases. Exercise can truly work synergistically with other lifestyle behaviors to optimize whole health.

Effect of Physical Activity on Health and Disease

Societies across the globe are being negatively affected by increasing physical inactivity, which correlates with increasing chronic disease. Chronic diseases are prevalent in all age groups, genders, and ethnicities. Not only is the health of populations suffering but also healthcare expenditures are rising while workforce attendance and productivity are declining (Raghupathi & Raghupathi, 2020).

Physical inactivity contributes to many of the leading causes of death in the United States and as such is an important health risk factor. According to the 2018 National Health Interview Survey, physical inactivity caused an overall 8.3% increase in premature deaths in adults aged 40 and over (Carlson et al., 2018). In the United States, only 25% of adults and 20% of adolescents meet physical activity guidelines for both aerobic and strengthening activities (Centers for Disease Control and Prevention, 2019).

Since exercise is a cornerstone in the primary prevention of dozens of chronic conditions, physical inactivity should be specifically addressed on a population level and with individual patients. Cardiovascular and muscle-strengthening exercises positively affect every major system in the human body. Examples include improved or increased strength, cardiorespiratory fitness, blood flow, oxygen consumption, body composition, bone density, gut health, neural drive, and neuroplasticity (Nay et al., 2021). Exercise may also increase the likelihood of tobacco cessation; improve cognitive function; and improve mental health by reducing stress, anxiety, and depression (Schuch et al., 2018). Exercise has a positive effect on balance and coordination, reduces the risk of falls and other injuries, mitigates joint pain, and makes activities of daily living easier. Additionally, exercise helps reduce chronic systemic inflammation, thereby improving immune function (Buresh & Berg, 2014). Because of its powerful effects, exercise should be considered a first-line intervention in the prevention, management, and reversal of medical maladies, including but not limited to cardiovascular, metabolic, pulmonary, neural, and musculoskeletal conditions (Pedersen & Saltin, 2006).

Definitions Every APP Should Know

Physical activity and exercise are not necessarily interchangeable, but they are sometimes used interchangeably. *Physical activity* is any movement that increases energy expenditure above the resting baseline. Movement of any type counts toward daily physical activity, whether occupational, household, leisure time, or transportation. Physical activity can be categorized by level of intensity. This term has positive connotations and is acceptable to most patients. *Exercise* refers to structured

Health Promotion Research Study

Effect of Resistance Training for Seniors

Background: In 1985, the first of two landmark studies occurred where frail, institutionalized subjects were put on high-intensity resistance training programs using exercise protocols developed by Dr. Bill Evans, who is widely considered one of the premier researchers on fitness and aging.

Methodology: Ten subjects were recruited, and nine completed the study; they ranged in age from 86 to 96 years. All subjects were considered extremely sedentary. Seven of the nine required a cane to walk, eight had fallen at least once in the previous year, and four had evidence of undernutrition. Their most prevalent chronic conditions included arthritis, coronary artery disease, osteoporotic fractures, and hypertension. The intervention consisted of one exercise—the seated knee extension (considered by some as a *nonfunctional* exercise, which increases the risk of a knee injury). The subjects performed this exercise at 80% of their one-repetition maximum for three sets of eight repetitions (i.e., each set was taken to momentary muscle failure) three times per week. The weight lifted increased each week.

Results: At the study's completion, just two months later, the average increase in strength was 174%. Lean muscle tissue increased by 10% in five of the subjects, five subjects improved tandem gait speed by 48%, two subjects no longer needed to use a cane, and one subject no longer needed sit-to-stand assistance.

Implications for Advanced Practice: This research shows the importance of resistance training across the life span and dispels the following five common myths:

1. Resistance training is unsafe for seniors.
2. Resistance training for seniors should always be light in intensity.
3. High-intensity resistance training is unsafe when performed in the presence of disease or orthopedic issues.
4. Seniors, especially the oldest of the old, cannot make meaningful gains in strength or lean muscle tissue.
5. Only functional exercises can improve function.

Since the completion of this landmark study, a large body of similar research has been conducted with seniors, consistently showing that resistance training (including in the high-intensity domain) is well tolerated and safe when supervised and appropriately designed. The corresponding increases in strength and lean muscle tissue can reverse osteopenia, osteoporosis, and sarcopenia. Additionally, they reduce the risk of falls and increase the ease of activities of daily living. Studies such as these also show that a significant transfer effect occurs from general strengthening, even through the use of nonfunctional exercises such as the leg press and seated knee extension, to functional activities such as sitting to standing, walking, and stair-climbing.

As people age, it becomes increasingly important to engage in muscle strengthening exercises. Supervision by qualified exercise specialists is critical during the early stages of program design to provide proper guidance and safe progression. A recent position statement on resistance training for older adults published by the National Strength and Conditioning Association offers detailed information and guidelines concerning the benefits of strength exercise for seniors as well as suggestions for exercise prescription (Fragala et al., 2019). It is recommended that APPs familiarize themselves with this information, counsel all patients on the importance of muscle strengthening, and provide referrals to qualified exercise specialists whenever possible.

Reference: Data from Fiatarone, M. A. (1990). High-intensity strength training in nonagenarians. *JAMA, 263*(22), 3029. https://doi.org/10.1001/jama.1990.03440220053029

physical activity intended to improve one or more of the following areas: cardiorespiratory endurance, muscular strength, muscular endurance, flexibility, and body composition (National Center for Health Statistics, 2019). Sometimes a patient may have a negative feeling toward the word *exercise*.

Physical activity and exercise are both important. Becoming more physically active (e.g., parking farther away, taking the stairs, using sit–stand desks, doing active chores, and gardening and other leisure activities) prevents adverse effects of a sedentary lifestyle and contributes to overall health and well-being. But structured, planned, intentional exercise that improves physical fitness is also essential and often overlooked. Even when exercise is encouraged, sometimes the piece that is overlooked is that exercise must continue to progress over time to keep the body challenged and achieve and maintain optimal physical fitness. The APP should encourage patients to become more physically active throughout the day as well as encourage them to include purposeful exercise during the week to increase fitness and improve overall health. Ideally, APPs will support patients in achieving the recommendations for both physical activity and exercise.

Physical Activity Guidelines

In 2018, the Physical Activity Guidelines Committee (PAGC) published updated physical activity guidelines (Piercy et al., 2018). The guidelines listed in **Table 13.1** serve as a foundation for exercise prescription in healthy adults. In addition, the PAGC recommends the following:

- Preschool-aged children aged 3 to 5 years should be physically active throughout the day to enhance growth and development.
- Children and adolescents aged 6 to 17 years should perform 60 minutes or

Table 13.1 Summary of U.S. Department of Health and Human Services Physical Activity Guidelines (PAG) for Healthy Adults

General PAG	Specific PAG
Inactivity should be avoided.	150–300 minutes of moderate-intensity aerobic physical activity per week.
Aerobic activity should be spread throughout the week.	OR 75–150 minutes of vigorous-intensity aerobic physical activity per week.
Strength training should be of moderate or greater intensity.	An equivalent combination of moderate and vigorous activity can be conducted to meet the recommended time duration.
Health benefits can be achieved by adults who sit less and do any amount of moderate to vigorous physical activity.	Additional health benefits can be achieved by doing more than 300 minutes of moderate-intensity physical activity per week.
	Strength training exercises should be done for all major muscle groups two or more days per week.

Data from Piercy, K. L., Troiano, R. P., Ballard, R. M., Carlson, S. A., Fulton, J. E., Galuska, D. A., George, S. M., & Olson, R. D. (2018). The Physical Activity Guidelines for Americans. *JAMA, 320*(19), 2020. https://doi.org/10.1001/jama.2018.14854

more of moderate to vigorous physical activity daily.

- Older adults should perform multicomponent physical activity that includes balance training as well as aerobic and muscle-strengthening activities.
- Pregnant and postpartum women should perform at least 150 minutes of moderate-intensity aerobic activity a week. The American College of Obstetricians and Gynecologists (2022) recommends that women who had a cesarean birth or physical complications discuss with their providers when it would be safe to begin exercising after pregnancy.
- Adults with chronic conditions or disabilities, who are able, should follow the key guidelines for adults and do both aerobic and muscle-strengthening activities.

The PAGC's recommendations emphasize that moving more and sitting less will benefit nearly everyone. The most sedentary individuals benefit the most, even with modest increases in moderate to vigorous physical activity. Additionally, the American College of Sports Medicine (ACSM) recommends that both general and special populations *start low, go (or progress) slow* (Liguori et al., 2021).

While it is important to keep these guidelines in mind, it is also vital to meet the patients where they are. Often, exercise frequency is determined by the patients' time constraints and desire or motivation. The APP can help determine appropriate starting points for each patient and counsel on the importance of progression in small, tolerable increments. Able-bodied patients with no known disease or orthopedic conditions can follow the ACSM exercise guidelines for aerobic, strengthening, flexibility, and balance training. For special populations or deconditioned patients, it may be prudent to begin with a volume and an intensity that mimic their activities of daily living, at least as an initial starting point.

The appropriate selection of exercises is also an important consideration. Setting patients up for success and establishing self-efficacy are critical factors leading to long-term exercise adherence (Collado-Mateo et al., 2021). For example, a patient who suffers from metabolic syndrome who typically walks no more than a block and finds a set of five air squats (bodyweight sit-to-stand) challenging could begin with those exercises and progress from there. Conversely, to counsel the same patient to start a generic program of walking a mile, five days per week, and performing multiple sets of 10 air squats may be too challenging and increase the risk of injury or cause the patient to give up. Exercise advice should be personalized to each patient to improve adherence and reduce the risk of injury.

The Role of the APP in Promoting Physical Activity and Exercise

Two foundational roles of the APP in promoting physical activity and exercise are that of educator and counselor. As an educator, the APP shares information with the patients to help them understand how a sedentary lifestyle relates to health and recommends appropriate exercises and progression for improving health. As a counselor, the APP assesses the patients' readiness to change and guides them in the process of behavior change.

The Transtheoretical Model

The transtheoretical model (TTM) has fostered much success in promoting physical activity (Freitas et al., 2020; Kirk et al., 2010; Menezes et al., 2016; Mostafavi et al., 2015). APPs should be familiar with how each stage of change is defined and the unique patient behaviors related to each stage (see **Table 13.2**). The TTM guides the APP's interaction to create an alliance that sets the tone for behavioral change and ensures a patient-driven

Table 13.2 Action Plan for Physical Activity Using the Transtheoretical Model (TTM)

TTM Stage	Precontemplation	Contemplation	Planning	Action	Maintenance	Termination	Relapse
Description	No plan for change in the area of physical activity. Not ready for change in the area of physical activity.	Considering change in the area of physical activity. Ambivalent about change.	Ready to change but has not done so yet.	Began changed behavior but has not reached physical activity goal.	Physical activity goal behavior met and maintained.	Physical activity goal behavior achieved without risk of relapse into nonaction.	Physical activity goal behavior is no longer being met.
Patient action statement	"I don't have time to exercise." "I'm too old to start exercising now."	"I've always wanted to train for a marathon. Can you show me how?"	"My local gym is running a special, so my friends and I decided to start yoga twice per week."	"I started running, but my breathing prevents me from completing the full mile."	"I feel great that I can finally cut my lawn without taking a break."	"My fitness club membership is too expensive, so I decided to invest in a home gym so I can continue my current routine."	"Over the holiday break, I just stopped taking my walks in the park."
Intervention	Begin dialogue regarding health risks with inactivity. Discuss the benefits of exercise for risk reduction. Evaluate environmental and social determinants of physical inactivity.	Counsel on patient-specific health risks. Link pros and cons of physical activity to personal goals.	Assist with strategic planning for exercise. Make referrals to an exercise specialist, dietitian, etc. Set a start date for the action plan. Delineate health and exercise goals.	Implement an exercise routine. Identify health team resources. Establish social support. Schedule follow-up visits and reminders. Discuss problem-solving strategies.	Schedule regular follow-up visits and reminders. Reevaluate goals and adjust accordingly. Develop a reward system to affirm goal attainment.	Provide resources for support and self-directed activities.	See precontemplation and contemplation.

| Strategies | Assist patient to consider advantages of behavior change. Discuss medical conditions and implications of nonaction. Motivational interviewing. | Facilitate reduction in ambivalence about changing. Discuss potential barriers to change. Determine available resources to support behavior change. | Initiate action-oriented measures. Write an exercise prescription. | Reinforce and encourage changed behavior. Review barriers and facilitators of change. Revise action plan as needed. | Reinforce and encourage changed behavior. Review barriers and facilitators of change. Revise action plan as needed. Develop coping strategies. | Reinforce and encourage changed behavior. Maintain coping strategies. | See precontemplation and contemplation. |

Data from Rippe, J. M. (2019). *Lifestyle medicine* (3rd ed.). CRC Press.

approach to promoting physical activity based on the patients' values, needs, physical limitations, personal resources, and preferred activities. Additionally, the model identifies 10 processes of change that change agents can use to facilitate change. It is important to note that progression through the stages of change does not constitute achievement of the goal behavior but instead represents movement toward the targeted goal.

Precontemplation

In the precontemplation stage, patients are not motivated to increase physical activity due to a lack of awareness or misinformation regarding the need for change. Statements such as *I feel fine; why do I need to increase my physical activity?* serve as an opportunity for the APP to share information about the patients' condition that puts them at increased risk for poor health and to describe the potential benefits of physical activity. Some individuals may have even attempted to increase their physical activity in the past and were either defeated by perceived failure to achieve their goal or perhaps challenges greatly outweighed resources to make the change. The APP may hear statements from the patient such as *I am not interested in exercising because I cannot fit it into my schedule right now.*

Practical interventions for this stage include consciousness-raising, dramatic relief, and environmental reevaluation with the expected outcome of patient acknowledgment of potential behavior change benefits. The purpose of *consciousness-raising* is to increase patient acceptance of the health benefits associated with increased physical activity. The APP can share relevant information with patients, including potential outcomes associated with their health issue, while allowing for questions and clarification. *Dramatic relief* involves evoking the patients' emotions, such as fear, excitement, anger, grief, or guilt, and relating them to their unhealthy behavior. Personal testimony or sharing

other patient stories can provide a narrative for patients to visualize the experience of being physically fit. The purpose is not to shame the patients into action but rather to allow for expression and resolution of emotions to elicit motivation to change. An example of *environmental reevaluation* can be discerned in the statement *I don't know what my family will do if I die of a heart attack.* This technique reflects the patients' ability to notice how their behavior will affect others or their environment and may influence them to make healthier choices based on their desire to preserve the integrity of their family or surroundings.

Contemplation

Often, patients are aware of the need for change but may be experiencing a conflict in whether they are ready to make the necessary changes. This ambivalence is characteristic of the contemplation stage. APPs can assist patients in resolving ambivalence by exploring the pros and cons of the changed behavior. In some cases, the ambivalence may be related to perceived barriers to recommended activity. Consequently, exploring resources to overcome the obstacles can be a helpful strategy. Additionally, *self-reevaluation* can help contemplators imagine living without their health condition. Through self-reflection and futuristic planning, patients can reinvent themselves by comparing their present life experience with illness to the imagined self enjoying an active life.

Preparation

Entrance into the preparation stage of behavior change is evidenced by planned measures by the patients to increase physical activity, such as participation in social groups with a focus on exercise, meeting with an exercise specialist for guidance, or reading a book on exercise. This stage is characterized by patients' readiness to enact needed behavior change despite challenges or barriers. It also marks a pivotal moment when patients are amenable to a more tangible action-oriented intervention plan instead of the cognitive measures taken in the precontemplation and contemplation stages. Although the patients have not yet started to engage in the prescribed activity, they are motivated to *prepare* to be more physically active. The preparation stage is often called the commitment stage because the patients become more decisive about increasing physical activity. Their commitment builds on the growing belief that they can accomplish the stated health goal. This self-efficacy will ensure patient success along the behavior change continuum and progression to the next stages.

Action

During the action stage, the patients begin to engage in the prescribed activity and appreciate the mental and physical health benefits conceptualized in earlier stages. These benefits may nurture continued motivation and adherence to the prescribed physical activity, though it is not expected that the patients will reach the final goal until the maintenance stage. The APP should offer *reinforcement* through verbal affirmation and noting improvement in outcomes measures (e.g., decreased blood pressure). Encouraging the patients to use *contingency management*, such as identifying rewards for physical activity and decreasing rewards of sedentary behavior, provides additional reinforcement. *Helping relationships* can be formed between the APP and the patients or with a social group that fosters support through trust, connection, and accountability. Two additional techniques in the action stage are *counterconditioning* (substituting active behaviors for sedentary behaviors) and *stimulus control* (restructuring the environment to encourage increased activity). These measures may ward against relapse and offer emotional and motivational incentives to continue the new behavior until goal attainment.

Maintenance

Individuals who have reached the targeted goal behavior characterized by consistent engagement in the prescribed activity for at least 6 months or more are in the maintenance stage. Rippe (2019) notes that individuals are at risk of relapsing into old behaviors for up to five years after the behavior change. Therefore, APPs must continue to utilize reinforcement, counterconditioning, and stimulus control as needed while consistently addressing barriers to change. At times, the action plan may need revision due to changes in motivational or situational factors. APPs should also encourage the development of coping strategies to prevent relapse associated with emotional distress, boredom, or situational stress.

Termination

The termination stage is the complete remission of unhealthy habits and acceptance of newly acquired behaviors as a permanent lifestyle. The temptation to return to old habits and sedentary behavior is absent, so the risk of relapse is low. Nevertheless, relapse is always possible, so techniques such as reinforcement management, counterconditioning, and stimulus control are still relevant for this stage. Patients in the termination stage still require regular follow-up visits to monitor continued maintenance of targeted behaviors.

Relapse

Although the ultimate goal in behavior change is to avoid relapse, defined as cessation of goal behavior, it is common for patients to experience setbacks. However, success is still obtainable by using the strategies just mentioned in the context of the TTM. Many patients may recycle back through the various stages several times before reaching the targeted behavior goal. Even though the desire is to reach goal behavior, emphasis should be made on progression through the stages of change to reduce undue pressure and negative repercussions of unsuccessful attempts at increasing physical activity.

Exercise Assessment

Exercise Vital Sign

The exercise vital sign, a self-reported exercise assessment, is a valid measurement for adults and children that can be incorporated into the electronic medical record and used to initiate the conversation about exercise habits with each patient (Coleman et al., 2012; Young et al., 2022). The exercise vital sign consists of the following two questions:

1. On average, how many days per week do you engage in moderate to strenuous exercise (like a brisk walk)?
2. On average, how many minutes do you engage in exercise at this level?

Response choices for days are categorical from 0 to 7, and minutes are recorded in blocks of 10: 0, 10, 20, 30, 40, 50, 60, 90, 120, and 150 or greater. An additional question that APPs should consider asking is *How many days per week do you perform muscle-strengthening exercises, such as bodyweight exercises or resistance training?* All patients should be asked the exercise vital sign questions at each visit and screened according to the current ACSM preparticipation screening recommendation.

Exercise Preparticipation Screening

In 2016, the ACSM updated and simplified its exercise preparticipation screening guidelines. The rationale for the update was that exercise, especially light- to moderate-intensity exercise, is safe for most people (Riebe et al., 2015). Before the changes, recommendations included health screening for known diseases, signs and symptoms suggestive of disease, and cardiovascular risk factors. This information was used to classify individuals into low-risk,

moderate-risk, and high-risk categories. These classifications led to recommendations on medical clearance or evaluation and/or exercise testing before clearing the individual for exercise. This led to excessive physician referrals and created a burden on the medical system as well as potential barriers to exercise, resulting in the new screening recommendations. Other factors rationalizing the updated screening guidance include the fact that transient risk of exercise-related sudden cardiac death and acute myocardial infarction are much lower during light to moderate exercise than vigorous exercise and that cardiovascular disease risk factors do not predict adverse cardiovascular events.

The new preparticipation health screening process no longer includes risk factor analysis or risk-level classifications. Instead, recommendations for clearance by the healthcare provider have replaced specific recommendations for medical clearance or exercise testing. This clearance is based on the following:

- The individual's current level of structured exercise
- The presence of major signs and symptoms suggestive of cardiovascular, metabolic, or renal disease
- The desired intensity of exercise

The first step in this screening process is to determine whether the individual currently engages in structured exercise and, if so, to what level of intensity. The next step is to determine the recognition of cardiovascular, metabolic, or renal disease and the presence of major signs and symptoms suggestive of these diseases. Finally, medical clearance is determined based on the ACSM algorithm (see Table 13.12 at the end of this chapter).

Physical Activity Readiness Questionnaire

Before starting an exercise program, patients should fill out a physical activity readiness questionnaire (PAR-Q+). The PAR-Q+ is a screening tool to uncover potential health and lifestyle issues. It consists of seven questions that may reveal heart, circulatory, balance, medical, emotional, or joint problems that could make exercise difficult or dangerous. The exercise specialist typically administers the PAR-Q+ during the initial exercise consultation. A link to a sample PAR-Q+ form can be found in Table 13.12 at the end of this chapter.

Physical Activity Assessment

The physical activity assessment is a critical component in designing a safe, efficient, and effective exercise program. The rationale for performing an initial physical activity assessment includes the following:

- Identify current fitness level.
- Establish a baseline for future comparison of improvement or rate of progress.
- Identify needs and limitations.
- Develop a safe and an effective exercise program.
- Develop short-, medium-, and long-term goals.

An exercise specialist usually conducts physical activity assessments. These assessments fall into six general categories:

- Body composition
- Cardiovascular endurance
- Muscular strength
- Local muscular endurance
- Flexibility
- Neuromotor training

Body Composition

Body fat is associated with many chronic conditions, including hypertension, metabolic syndrome, type 2 diabetes mellitus, cardiovascular disease, and dyslipidemia. Therefore, it is important to monitor changes in body composition over time. Body composition testing estimates the relative amount of body fat in proportion to lean tissue mass, and some tests can also estimate body fat distribution. Body composition may be conveniently assessed and monitored by measuring waist circumference, skinfold measurements, or bioelectrical impedance. Other, less accessible methods used to measure body composition include air displacement plethysmography (BOD POD), underwater weighing, and dual-energy X-ray absorptiometry (DEXA). While underwater weighing, BOD POD, and DEXA are considered gold standard methods for assessing body composition, all methods include a window of error. Standard field tests such as body mass index (BMI), waist circumference, skinfold measurement, and bioelectrical impedance include windows of error of approximately ± 4% to 6% (Kuriyan, 2018).

Cardiovascular Endurance

Cardiovascular (also referred to as cardiorespiratory) endurance is the ability to perform large-muscle, dynamic, moderate- to high-intensity exercise for prolonged periods. An individual's cardiovascular fitness level (i.e., aerobic capacity, or VO_2 max) is the number one predictor of all-cause mortality (Kodama, 2009). Cardiovascular fitness is often expressed as metabolic equivalent of task (MET), where one MET is roughly the metabolic cost or amount of oxygen consumed while sitting quietly (Jetté et al., 1990). This is equivalent to 3.5 milliliters per kilogram per minute. Above a resting state, METs are expressed as the ratio of the working metabolic rate to the resting metabolic rate. APPs should be aware that METs describe absolute intensity, but they may not describe accurate intensity relative to the patient (Strath et al., 2013). For example, walking is considered moderate-intensity physical activity; however, the intensity for each individual may vary. In absolute terms, walking at a speed of 3 mph is equivalent to ~3 METs. Compare person A, with an aerobic capacity of 5 METs, with person B with an aerobic capacity of 12 METs. When walking at the same speed and absolute intensity of

Table 13.3 Rating of Perceived Exertion (RPE) OMNI-RES Scale

1	2	3 to 4	5 to 6	7 to 8	9 to 10
Very easy	Easy	Somewhat easy	Somewhat hard	Hard	Extremely hard

Data from Naclerio, F., Rodríguez-Romo, G., Barriopedro-Moro, M. I., Jiménez, A., Alvar, B. A., & Triplett, N. T. (2011). Control of resistance training intensity by the Omni Perceived Exertion Scale. *Journal of Strength and Conditioning Research, 25*(7), 1879–1888. https://doi.org/10.1519/jsc.0b013e3181e501e9

3 METs, person A performs hard-intensity activity (60% of their aerobic capacity), and person B performs light-intensity activity (25% of their aerobic capacity). This underscores the need to assess each patient's cardiovascular endurance level and place them on an appropriate aerobic exercise program.

Field tests for cardiovascular endurance include treadmill tests, various walk/run tests (e.g., Rockport walking test and 12-minute walk/run), step testing, and ergometer testing (Liguori et al., 2021). Nonexercise methods of assessing cardiovascular fitness have also been developed when traditional exercise testing is not feasible. Nonexercise methods are prediction equations that commonly include age, gender, percent body fat, BMI, weight, height, and physical activity status (measured either objectively or subjectively) to estimate cardiorespiratory fitness (Wang et al., 2019).

Muscular Strength

Muscular strength is the maximum force a muscle group can produce at a specified velocity (Kell et al., 2001). It is expressed as an individual's one-repetition maximum, or the maximum load an individual can lift while maintaining proper form. Because of the equipment and expertise needed for these assessments, they are best utilized by a qualified exercise specialist. Common methods to assess muscular strength include the following:

- Bench press and overhead press (upper body)
- Smith machine squat, leg press, and knee extension (lower body)

Rating of perceived exertion (RPE) scales, such as the OMNI (see **Table 13.3**) and repetitions in reserve (RIR) scales, are also valid and reliable methods to provide a baseline strength measurement and track changes over time. The RPE and RIR scales measure the individual's subjective (perceived) level of effort. Specifically, they measure the set's proximity to momentary muscular failure. Older adults and special populations may find this type of testing more practical than repetition maximum testing because it negates the need to perform a set to momentary muscular failure.

Local Muscular Endurance

Muscular endurance is the ability of a muscle group to execute repeated contractions over time sufficient to cause muscular fatigue or maintain a specific percentage of maximum voluntary contraction for a prolonged time. Absolute muscular endurance refers to the total number of repetitions at a given amount of resistance. Relative muscular endurance refers to the number of repetitions performed at a percentage of the one-repetition maximum (e.g., 70%). Similar to the muscular strength assessment, depending on the time and resources available to the APP, the local muscular endurance assessment may also need to be performed by an exercise specialist. Common methods to assess muscular endurance include curl-ups (crunches) and push-ups.

The exercise specialist can make modifications based on musculoskeletal conditions. Similar to their usefulness with muscular strength assessments, RPE scales are a valid and reliable way to assess muscular endurance and can be used by an exercise specialist under appropriate conditions (e.g., joint pain). While the exercise specialist will perform the assessment and potentially modify the exercise prescription based on the results of the tests, this information is important for APPs to understand. It can be used as a method of vetting the skill set of exercise specialists and as communication between the APP and the patient or between the APP and the trainer. Trainers should provide data to the APP in the form of progress reports or updates regarding the assessment and outcomes of the exercise prescription.

Flexibility

Flexibility is the ability to move a joint through its complete range of motion. Common methods to assess flexibility include joint range of motion assessment and sit-and-reach (or modified/unilateral sit-and-reach). While time constraints and the knowledge and skill of an exercise specialist may limit the thoroughness of a flexibility assessment, comprehensive joint range of motion assessments are preferable whenever possible since movement restrictions or hypermobility may predispose an individual to injury.

Neuromotor Training

Neuromotor training includes exercises involving balance, agility, coordination, proprioception, and gait. Common clinical assessments include the following:

- Single-leg balance test
- Y-balance test
- Timed up-and-go
- Backward walk test
- Step-down test

Neuromotor assessments and training are important with older adults, especially those diagnosed with sarcopenia or otherwise at moderate to high risk for falling.

Starting the Conversation

APPs should discuss physical activity and exercise with all patients, regardless of age, health conditions, or other factors. It is essential to meet patients where they are and then provide inspiration and support to optimize physical activity and exercise as they are willing to do so. Just telling people to *move often* is unlikely to be enough. This conversation should be two way, with APPs listening at least as much as they speak.

Besides knowing the answers to the exercise vital sign questions, asking for permission to discuss the topic of exercise as it specifically relates to patients' health is a great way to start the conversation. Most people are interested in learning how something could directly affect their health conditions, especially if one behavior change could improve several issues or prevent undesired outcomes. For patients open to further discussion, open-ended questions can begin the conversation. The answers to these questions will then serve as the basis for personalized patient education and counseling. Based on patient responses, some follow-up closed-ended questions may also be important in the initial conversation. For example, discomfort or injuries from trying to exercise in improper shoes could be prevented by asking if the patients have appropriate footwear for exercise. **Table 13.4** provides questions and tips for starting the conversation.

Exercise Prescription

As previously stated, the exercise prescription must match the patients' needs, goals, and abilities. A simple acronym known as the FITT-P principle, where *F* stands for *frequency*, *I* for *intensity*, the first *T* for *time* (duration), the second *T* for *type*, and *P* for *progression*, can be used to design both flexibility and cardiovascular exercise prescriptions.

Table 13.4 Starting the Conversation

Question	APP Tips
Tell me about your current exercise.	Start with an open-ended question. Elicit information about aerobic, strength, flexibility, and neuromuscular activities. Meet patients where they are. Once a baseline of physical activity and exercise habits is established, suggestions can be offered for adjustments or improvements using the physical activity guidelines.
What types of exercise do you most enjoy or have you enjoyed in the past?	Discuss how starting with activities that have something in common with previous favorites may make exercise more enjoyable and easier to establish as a habit.
How do you feel about exercising on your own? Is there any type of exercise you would like to do but currently cannot?	Determine whether the patient might benefit from referral to a physical therapist, personal trainer, or other exercise specialist. Referrals are recommended if the patient has any injuries or was injured in the past during exercise.
Do you like to exercise with others, by yourself, or with a combination of both?	Help the patient match desired interaction to potential activities.
Does daily exercise seem hard or unrealistic? Do you have any limitations that could hold you back from optimizing your physical activity?	Identify whether there are barriers, and brainstorm solutions together.
What types of exercises can you do at home? What exercise equipment or facilities can you access outside your home?	Help the patient start thinking about options (e.g., gym, community center, parks/trails, local school track or field, or pool).
How could exercise best fit into your schedule?	Help the patient determine whether scheduling exercise like other appointments might be beneficial.
What benefits would you like to get from increasing exercise?	Have the patient state desired benefits for increasing exercise. These benefits (e.g., improved A1C) can then be regularly monitored and reported to the patient to help measure success.
How motivated are you about moving more daily and increasing regular exercise each week?	The patient's level of motivation should guide the discussion. Motivational interviewing is particularly effective for patients in the precontemplation or contemplation stages of change.
What can I do to best support you in safely increasing your exercise?	Decide together if a quick phone call by the APP or medical staff, a short-term follow-up office visit, or other communication might be helpful.

Flexibility Exercise Prescription

Flexibility and mobility tend to decrease over the life span, which may in part be attributed to a decrease in physical activity (McKay et al., 2017; Medieros et al., 2013; Stathokostas & Vandervoort, 2016). Maintaining adequate flexibility is important for ease of movement and the ability to perform activities of daily living (ADLs), such as tying shoes and safely picking up an object from the floor. Soft tissue injuries usually occur when tissue is maximally stretched (Verrall, 2016). Restricted joint range of motion would increase the risk of injury, underscoring the need for a proper flexibility program. Ideally, assessment of joint range of motion would precede the design of a flexibility or stretching program. A joint range of motion assessment performed at each major joint can determine areas that are normal, restricted (tight), or hypermobile (loose). This allows for the program design to create flexibility balance around each joint. Refer to the description of each component of the FITT-P principle in **Table 13.5** regarding the flexibility exercise prescription.

Cardiovascular Exercise Prescription

Since cardiovascular fitness is the number one predictor of all-cause mortality, APPs need to advise patients to engage in a progressive cardiovascular exercise program, preferably with a minimum goal of training in the middle of their aerobic training zone.

The following are the four most common forms of cardiovascular exercise:

1. *Long, slow duration* (LSD): Exercising in the low to moderate aerobic intensity domain (e.g., walking briskly on a treadmill).

Table 13.5 FITT-P Principle for Flexibility Program Design

Component	Description
Frequency	Frequency can range from 2 to 7 days per week. Restricted (tighter) areas may require higher frequency to create greater weekly stretching volume. Volume can also be increased via additional sets.
Intensity	The intensity of a stretch may vary based on an individual's tolerance of discomfort. The general recommendation is to stretch to the point of mild or moderate discomfort, equivalent to 4–6 on a 1–10 discomfort scale, and to avoid bouncing a stretch.
Time (duration)	The time, or duration, of a stretch can range from 20 seconds to greater than a minute and depends on the goal (i.e., maintain or improve joint range of motion) or type of stretch.
Type	Common types of stretching include passive, active, proprioceptive neuromuscular facilitation (PNF), and dynamic. While all types of stretching improve joint range of motion when performed properly, PNF stretching has been shown to be the most effective primarily because progression is built into this type of stretch (Page, 2012).
Progression	Progress is indicated only in areas where movement restriction exists. To progress, or increase joint range of motion, the individual should be instructed to stretch to their first *end range* of motion, hold for 10–20 seconds and relax, followed by stretching slightly further to find a new end range (i.e., move further into the stretch).

Based on Liguori, G., Feito, Y., Fountaine, C., Roy, B., & American College of Sports Medicine. (2021). *ACSM's guidelines for exercise testing and prescription.* Wolters Kluwer.

2. *Tempo training*: Exercising near the lactate or anaerobic threshold, which can usually be sustained for only 15 to 25 minutes (e.g., running at the highest level possible within the aerobic training zone).

3. *High-intensity interval training* (HIIT): Exercise that includes a *work* portion, usually above the anaerobic threshold (i.e., the work rate at which exercise is no longer aerobic) but shy of an all-out sprint, and a *recovery* portion, usually at light intensity (e.g., doing a 5-minute warm-up on the elliptical machine, then increasing speed to a *near sprint* for 2 minutes, followed by reducing to just above the warm-up speed for 2 minutes, then cycling through the work and recovery periods 3 to 5 times, and finishing with a 5-minute cooldown).

4. *Sprint interval training* (SIT): Exercise that includes a *work* portion at or near an all-out sprint and a *recovery* portion, usually at a light intensity (e.g., doing a 5-minute warm-up on a stationary bicycle, then increasing speed to an *all-out sprint* for 15 seconds, followed by reducing to just above the warm-up speed for 75 seconds, then cycling through the work and recovery periods 3 to 5 times, and finishing with a 5-minute cooldown).

As noted in **Table 13.6**, the FITT-P principle may also be used to design cardiovascular training programs.

Strength Exercise Prescription

Mounting evidence indicates that resistance (strength) training is as beneficial as cardiovascular exercise at mitigating chronic disease (Tavoian et al., 2020). Regular strength training prevents or reverses sarcopenia, osteopenia, and osteoporosis; prevents injury; improves functional capacity and ease of ADLs; improves balance; and provides a variety of other benefits. Because of loss of muscle and strength with aging, which in the absence of strength training occurs at a rate of ~10% per decade from age 30 to 50 and ~15% per decade thereafter (Keller & Engelhardt, 2014), routine ADLs may become the equivalent of heavy lifting or high-intensity tasks for older adults (Hortobágyi et al., 2003). Therefore, the older one gets, the more important it becomes to engage in regular strength training.

Unlike flexibility and cardiovascular program design, where the prescription can follow the FITT-P principle, designing a strength training program is more complex and usually requires referral to a qualified exercise specialist. While the strength exercise prescription will typically be designed and coached by an exercise specialist, the information in this section is important for APPs to understand. Progressive resistance training is underutilized (and often underappreciated) in many areas of medicine, including geriatrics, oncology, cardiac rehab, obesity, and diabetes management, to name a few (Kennedy et al., 2021; Mandic et al., 2011; Sundell, 2011). APPs should become familiar with the language and process to better discuss and disseminate this information with their patients and qualified exercise specialists.

Examples of the variables involved in designing a strength training program include the following:

- Frequency
- Sets per muscle group
- Repetitions per set
- Objective (load) and subjective (relative effort) intensity
- Choice of exercise
- Order of exercise
- Rest between sets and exercise sessions
- Repetition tempo

Individuals new to strength training will have a learning curve for developing proper form, mind–muscle connections, determining initial loads and available range of motion, and understanding the general flow of a strength workout. This initial phase, known as the familiarization phase, may take several weeks

Table 13.6 FITT-P Principle for Aerobic Program Design

Component	Description
Frequency	Frequency can range from 1–7 days per week. When the goals pertain to weight loss or improvement in aerobic capacity, increasing frequency is indicated.
Intensity	Intensity of cardiovascular exercise can be measured objectively by measuring heart rate in beats per minute and subjectively by measuring RPE scales. The most convenient way to measure heart rate is using a heart rate monitor. RPE scales are most accurate when combined with another method of assessing subjective intensity known as the talk test. When using the talk test, the APP or exercise specialist asks the patient (or client) to say a few sentences while performing aerobic exercise and simultaneously shows the patient a chart (see **Table 13.7**) that equates the rate of ventilation with the rate of perceived effort.
Time (duration)	The duration of cardiovascular exercise can vary from very short bouts (e.g., 5 minutes for the very deconditioned) to 60 minutes or greater. Fitness level, individual goals, motivation, and the type of cardiovascular exercise determine duration. Individuals with weight loss as a goal should strive to maximize weekly duration (e.g., 150–250 minutes per week).
Type	The type of cardiovascular exercise includes the following: 1. Impact (e.g., running) 2. Nonimpact (e.g., elliptical machine, swimming, and cycling) The general recommendation is to alternate between impact and nonimpact from session to session. The ratio is at the discretion of the individual.
Progression	Progression can occur by increasing frequency, duration, or intensity of exercise and is at the clinician's, trainer's, or individual's discretion. For safety reasons, HIIT and SIT should not be programmed until the person can comfortably sustain at least 15–20 minutes of continuous aerobic exercise at moderate intensity.

Based on information from Liguori et al. (2021); Ribeiro et al. (2017); Woltmann et al. (2015).

before the individual is ready to progress. This underscores the need for professional guidance, at least initially.

Frequency

Current ACSM guidelines suggest strengthening exercises for each major muscle group two to three times per week (Liguori et al., 2021). Individuals who have the time or desire to train only two or three times per week should engage in total-body training sessions (Liguori et al., 2021). Those who have the time or desire to train four or more times per week should train in a split-routine format (ACSM, 2009). Examples of a split-routine format would include two lower-body and two upper-body training sessions or two push-dominant (e.g., squat and chest press) and two pull-dominant (e.g., deadlift and back row) training sessions within one week.

Sets per Muscle Group

Sets per muscle group can be viewed by session and by training week. Current guidelines recommend 10 to 15 sets per major muscle group per week to optimize the adaptations and associated benefits of strength training (Morton et al., 2019). Novices should begin with less weekly volume, such as 4 to 6 sets per muscle group per week (i.e., 2 to 3 sets

Table 13.7 Rating of Perceived Exertion Combined with Talk Test

RPE	Perceived Exertion/Talk Test
17–19	Very vigorous/hard activity Speech is very difficult.
14–16	Vigorous/hard activity Speech is limited to short phrases.
12–13	Moderate activity Speech is possible with some difficulty.
10–11	Light activity Comfortable speech is possible.
<10	Very light activity Speech is unaffected from rest.

Data from Webster, A. L., & Aznar-Laín, S. (2008). Intensity of physical activity and the "Talk Test." *ACSM's Health & Fitness Journal, 12*(3), 13–17. https://doi.org/10.1249/fit.0b013e31817047b4

Woltmann, M. L., Foster, C., Porcari, J. P., Camic, C. L., Dodge, C., Haible, S., & Mikat, R. P. (2015). Evidence that the talk test can be used to regulate exercise intensity. *Journal of Strength and Conditioning Research, 29*(5), 1248–1254. https://doi.org/10.1519/jsc.0000000000000811

per muscle group per session), and progress with the previously stated goal in mind (Liguori et al., 2021).

Repetitions per Set

The ACSM (2009) defines the 6- to 15-repetition range as the primary repetition range for general strength fitness. As strength fitness increases, there is a corresponding need to decrease the repetitions performed and increase the loads being lifted accordingly. Therefore, it is recommended that intermediate and advanced lifters spend most of their time training in the 4- to 12-repetition range, using heavier weights when doing fewer lifts (ACSM, 2009; Garber et al., 2011; Loveless & Ihm, 2015). While there are numerous ways to train across this spectrum, a common method is via a linear periodized approach. Refer to **Table 13.8** for an example.

Objective Intensity

Objective intensity refers to the load lifted, assuming that the lifters choose the maximal or near-maximal weight they can lift with good form for that number of repetitions (i.e., repetition maximum). If the load is such that the lifters can lift it only one to four times, the objective load is considered *very heavy*, and so on (see **Table 13.9**).

Subjective Intensity

Subjective intensity refers to the lifter's perceived effort. More specifically, it refers to proximity to muscle failure, where muscle failure is defined as the maximum number of repetitions the individual could have performed with proper form (Steele et al., 2017), with neuromuscular fatigue being the limiter to performing additional repetitions. Subjective intensity is defined by RPE scales. Intensity can be broken down further into two domains, a warm-up set and a working set.

Choice of Exercise

Strength exercises are virtually unlimited in number, but all exercises can be distributed into two categories, primary and assistance.

Table 13.8 Linear Periodization

Repeat Range (per Set)	Phase Length	Primary Purpose
12–15	3–4 weeks	Increase strength within this repetition range by the end of the phase.
10–12	3–4 weeks	Increase strength within this repetition range by the end of the phase.
8–10	3–4 weeks	Increase strength within this repetition range by the end of the phase.
6–8	3–4 weeks	Increase strength within this repetition range by the end of the phase.

Other considerations:

- Vary session intensities (i.e., light to moderate sessions or hard sessions).
- Vary exercise selection.
- Weekly set volume = ~10–15 sets per major muscle group.

Data from Liguori, G., Feito, Y., Fountaine, C., Roy, B., & American College of Sports Medicine. (2021). *ACSM's guidelines for exercise testing and prescription.* Wolters Kluwer.
Morton, R. W., Colenso-Semple, L., & Phillips, S. M. (2019). Training for strength and hypertrophy: An evidence-based approach. *Current Opinion in Physiology,* *10*, 90–95. https://doi.org/10.1016/j.cophys.2019.04.006

Table 13.9 Strength Continuum

Repetition Range (RM)*	Objective Intensity
1–4	Very heavy
4–7	Heavy
8–12	Moderate
12–15	Light
15–20	Very light

*RM is repetition maximum, or the maximum weight a person can lift for a defined number of exercise movements.

Traditional primary lower-body strengthening exercises include squats, deadlifts, and multidirectional lunges; upper-body exercises include presses (e.g., chest and shoulder) and rows. All other exercises are defined as assistance exercises. Historically, assistance exercises are implemented into a program to increase strength in primary exercises, create strength balance around joints, and strengthen intrinsic musculature (e.g., multifidi, serratus anterior, and rotator cuff).

Order of Exercises

Generally, the order of exercises is in accordance with the following:

- Most important muscle group or movement (e.g., muscle group to rehabilitate or movement to improve performance) to least important muscle group or movement (e.g., smaller muscle groups)
- Explosive movements (e.g., Olympic lifts or hops, bounds, and jumps) to nonexplosive movements (e.g., squats, deadlifts, and lunges)
- Large-muscle group (e.g., legs, back, and chest) to small-muscle group (e.g., hips and calves)

- Multijoint movement (e.g., squat, dead-lift, lunge, pull, and press) to single-joint movement (e.g., knee extension, knee curl, calf raise, and chest flye)
- Complex exercise to simple exercise (same as above)

Following a warm-up, in a total-body training session, this commonly equates to performing multijoint lower-body exercises (e.g., squats and deadlifts) early in a training session, followed by multijoint back row (e.g., lat pulldown), multijoint chest press (e.g., bench press), and multijoint shoulder press (e.g., military press). Assistance exercises such as knee extension, knee curl, and calf raise are typically performed at the end of a session. Core strengthening exercises, such as abdominal exercises, can be inserted in the middle of a training session, after the multijoint exercises have been completed, at the end of a training session, or on separate days.

Rest Between Sets

If the goal is to improve metabolic conditioning or local muscle endurance, rest between working sets should be 30 seconds (for smaller-muscle groups) to 90 seconds (for larger-muscle groups). Otherwise, lifters should rest 2 to 5 minutes prior to performing a set for the same muscle group.

Rest Between Training Sessions

It normally takes 24 to 72 hours for a muscle group to recover from a strength training session—most commonly 24 to 48 hours. Therefore, muscle groups should be trained on nonconsecutive days. For general fitness, adequate recovery is determined by little to no soreness in the muscle groups and the individual feels mentally ready to train those muscle groups again.

Repetition Tempo

During the initial familiarization phase, where the individual is developing mind–muscle connections and learning proper form, names of exercises, and flow of a session, it is suggested that lifters control the tempo during both the lifting (concentric) and the lowering (eccentric) portion of the movement at their desired pace. Following the initial phase, the same suggestion applies when the goal is to improve local muscle endurance. Otherwise, in most situations, it is preferable to lift with the intent of velocity and to lower with control. Lifting with the goal of velocity increases neural drive and intramuscular coordination, allowing greater loads to be lifted. It also improves the rate of force development, a neuromuscular function that decreases during the aging process and may play a role in an increased risk of falling (Maffiuletti et al., 2016).

Neuromotor Training Exercise Prescription

Unlike program design recommendations for flexibility, cardiovascular, and strength exercise, less is known about recommended dosing for improving neuromotor skills. Nevertheless, APPs should be aware that increases in baseline strength will often transfer to improvements in neuromotor skills (Izquierdo et al., 2021). This follows an exercise principle called the principle of initial value, which states that individuals with lower fitness levels have the greatest capacity for improvement and commonly have a greater transfer effect from general strength and conditioning to specific tasks. Therefore, while neuromotor training should be included in a comprehensive exercise program, a critical part of the exercise prescription is addressed via the progressive strength training program. **Table 13.10** summarizes FITT-P recommendations for neuromotor training exercise.

Exercise Progression

Fitness improvement is dependent on intensity. While frequency and volume/duration are critical variables in the development of an

Table 13.10 FITT-P Recommendations for Neuromotor Training Exercise

Component	Description
Frequency	A frequency of 2–3 days per week is recommended.
Intensity	There is no recommendation regarding intensity for neuromotor training.
Time (duration)	The ACSM recommends 20–30 minutes per day (Liguori et al., 2021).
Type	A wide spectrum of exercises can be used to improve motor control, including the following: ■ Static and transitional balance exercises (e.g., single-leg balance, single-leg balance with forward lean) ■ Dynamic balance exercises (e.g., Y-balance, tandem walk, backward walk) ■ Traditional lower-body resistance training exercises (e.g., step-ups, step-downs, multidirectional lunges) ■ Yoga and tai chi ■ Competitive or recreational sports (e.g., tennis and basketball) The general recommendation is to alternate between impact and nonimpact from session to session. The ratio is at the discretion of the individual.
Progression	Progressively difficult postures, dynamic movements that perturb the center of gravity, and exercises that progressively challenge sensory input should be appropriately utilized.

effective exercise program, it is theoretically possible to meet physical activity guidelines but remain unfit. Since cardiorespiratory and strength fitness are predictors of all-cause mortality in men and women, with no upper limit of benefit, the importance of progression cannot be overstated (Lee et al., 2010; Mandsager et al., 2018). APPs should encourage patients to increase fitness beyond beginner level and encourage continuous gradual increases in the challenge in flexibility, cardiovascular exercise, and strength training.

Exercise Considerations

In almost all cases, the benefits of exercise outweigh potential risks. However, commonsense precautions, modifications, or monitoring might be needed for patients with specific issues. These include but are not limited to those with pain or swelling that reduces the joint range of motion, insulin-dependent diabetes, pregnancy, arrhythmias, asthma, or chronic obstructive pulmonary disease (Moore et al., 2016). Before each exercise session, a patient's readiness to exercise should be assessed. Exercise may begin if the person feels good, has taken regular daily medications, is hydrated, and has blood sugar and blood pressure levels in acceptable ranges. A graded warm-up should gradually increase heart rate and breathing rate. After exercise, a cooldown period should be performed to allow both rates to return to the normal range.

One additional consideration concerning exercise is setting. Regular outdoor exercise can be beneficial, especially if done in nature. Spending time outdoors in green space is associated with increased physical activity, improved BMI, better mood, lower blood pressure, and reduced stress (Gladwell et al., 2013). For a platform APPs can use to prescribe exercise in parks, see Table 13.12.

Health Promotion Case Study Exercise Prescription for Female College Student

---

Case Description: A 19-year-old Caucasian female college student presented to her APP frustrated by fatigue, chronic joint pain, ribs that dislocated with coughing or sneezing, and history of multiple joint injuries (foot stress fracture, tibial plateau fracture, shoulder labral tear, dislocations, wrist fracture, and ankle sprain), all within the past few years.

- Allergies: Dairy products (since infancy).

- Medications: Daily multivitamin; no prescription or over-the-counter meds.

- Medical history: High cholesterol (diagnosed at 13 years old); irritable bowel syndrome (colonoscopy done at age 18 to rule out other possibilities).

- Surgical history: Supra-umbilical hernia repair (at 6 months old); wisdom teeth removal (at age 18); laparoscopic R shoulder labrum repair (at age 19).

- Family history: Mother alive and well; father high cholesterol; paternal grandmother high cholesterol; maternal grandfather high cholesterol; younger sister and older brother alive and well.

- Social history: Never smoker, no alcohol, no drugs, 1 cup caffeine daily. Recreational figure skater; undergraduate student living on campus. Drinks 2 liters of water daily, no sodas. Eats three meals and two snacks daily, following the Plate Method with fruit and vegetables, lean proteins, and a mix of whole grains and refined grains.

- Vitals: 5'3", 145 lb, blood pressure 100/60 mmHg, heart rate 58 bpm.

- Physical exam: Remarkable only for hypermobile joints and multiple old scars.

- Labs: Complete blood count, complete metabolic panel, thyroid stimulating hormone, c-reactive protein, autoimmune (lupus, rheumatoid arthritis, etc.) panel within normal limits; total cholesterol 260 (high), LDL 165 (high), triglycerides 180 (high), HDL 40 (low).

The patient was given the following exercise prescription.

EXERCISE $\mathbf{R_x}$

APP LifeStyle Medicine Center
1 (800) 000-0000

Date: _ _ _ _ _ _ _ _ _ _
Expires: 60 days from today

Exercise:

- **Aerobic:** Combination of swimming, jogging, cycling, and team sports for a combination of moderate and vigorous intensity for 30-60 minutes 5x per week

- **Strength:** See exercise specialist to develop personalized progressive resistance training program

- **Flexibility/mobility:** Foam roll, assisted yoga, Pilates, and/or myofascial release 10-15 minutes daily

- **Balance:** Tai chi and balance techniques for 20 minutes 2x per week

Patient objectives:

- Increase joint stability
- Increase total body strength
- Maintain aerobic conditioning
- Improve muscle relaxation capabilities without straining supporting structures
- Incorporate mind-body movements to improve mental and physical stamina

Patient info:

Jane Doe

01/01/2003

Clinician info:

Provider S, APP

Print   *Provider S, APP*

Sign

Medical considerations:

- **Current conditions:** Fatigue, generalized joint pain, generalized hypermobility

- **History:** Several previous orthopedic injuries, no current exercise restrictions

- **Current medications:** Multivitamin daily

- **Medical restrictions:** None currently

Exercise Outcome: The patient began a progressive strength training program designed using exercise science principles and guidelines, adding this to her regular 5 days a week of cardiovascular exercise. She also began to shift more toward a whole-food plant-based diet. Initially, she planned to try this combination of changes for one month; however, she was so impressed by improvement in symptoms that she continued this exercise and eating plan long term. Several months into the change, she was finally diagnosed by a rheumatologist with Ehlers-Danlos syndrome (connective tissue disorder), which explained the symptoms she had been having for years as well as her predisposition to joint injuries. Her rheumatologist said that she should continue her robust exercise plan, which now included regular strength training, and her healthy anti-inflammatory diet since those were the best things she could do for her health.

Over the next 2 years, she lost over 20 pounds of fat mass and over 10% body fat while maintaining her lean muscle mass within 1–5 pounds of baseline measurements (validated via InBody bioelectrical impedance analysis measurements). Total cholesterol, LDL, and triglycerides normalized while HDL increased. Chronic joint pain improved. Energy and recovery somewhat improved; however, she still needs extra rest after high-intensity exercise, and she rarely trains above 85% of one-repetition maximum to avoid the strain that level of intensity of resistance training would produce on her muscles and joints even when maintaining proper form. She remained cautious about maintaining proper form and taking extra rest as necessary to prevent further injuries from the hypermobility and hyperlaxity in her joints. Another two years later, weight and biomarkers were stable. She continued regular daily exercise, focusing on functional fitness and circuit training, which included mind–body exercises of yoga, tai chi, and Pilates as well as cardiovascular training and free weight resistance training. She believes that her well-rounded exercise program has played a primary role in improving her quality of life, and her healthcare providers agree based on objective labs and exams.

Critical Thinking Questions

1. Explain specific mechanisms for how strength training benefited this patient's chronic joint pain, cholesterol panel, and body composition.

2. Considering exercise guidelines, how should this patient's exercise program change over time so that overall health continues to be optimized?

Translating the Physical Activity Prescription Into an Action Plan

5As Framework

The APP can assist the patient in developing an exercise program and physical activity objectives using the 5As framework: assess, advise, agree, assist, and arrange (see **Table 13.11**). This framework originated with the U.S. Department of Health and Human Services for tobacco cessation and is commonly used for therapeutic behavior change (Tobacco Use and Dependence Guideline Panel, 2008).

SMART Goals

Increasing physical activity can be challenging, especially for those engaging in such activity for the first time. The journey from a sedentary lifestyle to one characterized by consistent energy-expending daily activity takes time and careful planning. For many, change can take up to 60 days to actualize their physical activity goals (Rippe, 2019). Various factors that can challenge the best intentions include the patient's fitness level, physical disabilities, ambient support, and access to the resources needed to achieve targeted goals.

SMART is an acronym that stands for specific, measurable, achievable, relevant, and time-bound. A SMART goal incorporates these

Table 13.11 Using the 5As Framework for Physical Activity Counseling

5A Component	Approach
Assess	What stage of change is the patient in? Measure the patient's exercise vital signs at every visit. Determine the patient's physical activity readiness. Conduct a preparticipation screen and exercise assessments.
Advise	Discuss disease risk profile. Relate the patient's symptoms and laboratory results to physical inactivity. Review health benefits of exercise/physical activity, and correlate to specific patient medical history. Share success stories of individuals similar to the patient.
Agree	Based on the stage of change, collaborate with the patient to set SMART (specific, measurable, achievable, relevant, time-bound) physical activity goals. Provide detailed FITT-P plan for cardiovascular, flexibility, and neuromotor training exercises.
Assist	Identify barriers to engaging in exercise. Outline strategies to incorporate physical activity into daily living. Establish social support that will augment exercise goals. Devise an accountability plan for compliance with physical activity targets.
Arrange	Outline follow-up plan (e.g., telephone, email, or remote patient monitoring). Schedule necessary referrals (e.g., exercise specialist for strength exercise prescription, physical therapy, occupational therapy, or health coach).

criteria to help focus the patients' efforts and increase their chance of achieving their physical activity and exercise goals. However, setting SMART goals will be effective only if the goals result from collaboration between the APP and the patient once the patient's readiness and motivation are determined. These are generally determined during the preparation stage of change.

SMART goals should articulate the particular activity to perform, such as brisk walking (specific), how many days per week and how long it should be performed in minutes or hours (measurable), and the time frame in which it needs to be completed (time-bound). SMART goals also must be matched with the patient's desired outcome, motivation, ability, and willingness to perform the physical activity (relevant). The patients should also be confident that they can navigate the required logistics to engage

in the action as prescribed (achievable). If goals are well planned and meaningful to the patients, they are more likely to be achieved and lead to the overall objective of moving often. Once SMART goals are agreed upon, then an exercise prescription can be created by the APP for accountability and to measure progress toward the stated goals. **Figure 13.1** provides examples of SMART exercise goals.

Interprofessional Approach to Improving Physical Fitness

Clinicians, allied health professionals, and other specialists should collaborate to help patients achieve the goals of moving often, meeting exercise guidelines, and increasing fitness levels.

SMART Goals
- I will do total body progressive resistance training 3 days a week for the next 3 months.
- I will increase weekly cardio activity by walking 10 minutes after dinner at least 5 days a week for the next month.

Figure 13.1 Examples of SMART exercise goals.

The following professionals are commonly involved in this interprofessional approach (U.S. Bureau of Labor Statistics, 2018):

- Primary care provider (medical doctor (MD)/doctor of osteopathic medicine (DO), APP): Clinician responsible for the coordination of the patient's health, handling minor acute concerns, and managing chronic conditions.
- Specialist (MD/DO, APP): Clinician whose scope focuses on a particular branch of medicine rather than primary care, often due to advanced training in a specific area.
  - Physiatrist: Specializes in restoring functional ability and quality of life.
  - Orthopedist: Specializes in the correction of disorders of the musculoskeletal system.
  - Cardiologist: Specializes in the heart and blood vessels and can provide cardiac testing to clear patients for exercise.
- Chiropractor: Allied health professional who treats problems with the neuromusculoskeletal system.
- Physical therapist (PT): Allied health professional who prescribes therapeutic exercise, provides hands-on care, and delivers patient education regarding rehabilitation and injury prevention.
- Occupational therapist (OT): Allied health professional who helps people across the life span do the things they want and need to do through the therapeutic use of daily activities.

- Athletic trainer (AT): Allied health professional who collaborates with sports medicine specialists to provide services such as prevention, therapeutic intervention, and rehabilitation of injuries and medical conditions.
- Health coach: Specialist in utilizing strategies to encourage health behavior change.
- Exercise specialist: Umbrella term that includes kinesiologists, personal trainers, and exercise physiologists, all of whom can develop fitness and exercise programs.

The Medicine - Rehab - Fitness Institute is a helpful resource for interprofessional collaboration (see **Table 13.12**). The institute provides current, evidence-informed content on bridging the gap to connect medicine, rehabilitation, and fitness.

Referral to an Exercise Specialist

Regarding the continuum of care in lifestyle medicine, clinicians and allied health professionals should be regularly referring patients to exercise specialists. Unfortunately, the fitness industry is unregulated, which presents a challenge for the APP in making effective referrals. The following are factors to consider.

Qualifications

Ideally, APPs should refer patients to exercise specialists who

- hold a degree in exercise physiology, kinesiology, athletic training, or a related field;

TABLE 13.12	Evidence-Based Resources for Exercise

Resource	URL
American College of Lifestyle Medicine (ACLM)	https://lifestylemedicine.org
American College of Sports Medicine (ACSM)	https://www.acsm.org
ACSM preparticipation health screening tool	http://links.lww.com/FIT/A31
ACSM Exercise Is Medicine	https://www.exerciseismedicine.org
Medicine - Rehab - Fitness Institute	http://www.MRFInstitute.org
Institute for Credentialing Excellence	https://ice.learningbuilder.com/Public/MemberSearch/Program Verification
Park Rx America	https://parkrxamerica.org
PAR-Q+ form	http://eparmedx.com/wp-content/uploads/2013/03/January2020 PARQPlusFillable.pdf
Readiness Ruler	https://iprc.iu.edu/sbirtapp/mi/ruler.php
Walk with a Doc	https://walkwithadoc.org

- hold at least one NCCA-accredited certification; and
- have at least 2 years of experience training clients similar to the APP's patient population.

The National Commission for Certifying Agencies (NCCA) is the body that accredits fitness certifying organizations. The phrase *nationally recognized certification* implies that an organization is accredited through the NCCA. Countless fitness organizations offer various certifications, but only 18 are currently accredited through the NCCA. The most highly recognized are the two governing bodies in exercise science: (1) the American College of Sports Medicine (ACSM) and (2) the National Strength and Conditioning Association (NSCA). Others include the American Council on Exercise (ACE) and the National Academy of Sports Medicine (NASM). These organizations also offer certifications that cover pathophysiology and program design for special populations.

Setting

Patients can be referred to exercise specialists in hospitals, independent clinics (e.g., rehabilitation or wellness), or commercial settings. Hospitals and independent clinics may provide an additional layer of safety since the patient is being trained within a clinical environment under the watchful eye of other healthcare providers.

Cost

A question commonly asked is *Does insurance cover fitness training sessions?* The

Personal Health Investment Today (PHIT) Act is proposed legislation in Congress to allow all Americans to use pretax dollars to pay for physical activity expenses just like other qualified medical expenses reimbursed from a health savings account (HSA). The Physical Activity Alliance (a merging of the National Physical Activity Plan Alliance, National Physical Activity Society, and National Coalition for Promoting Physical Activity) is working to ultimately provide reduced costs for patients through insurance reimbursements and the promise of exercise billing codes. Until these efforts are finalized, fitness training sessions are an out-of-pocket expense. Several payers offer reimbursement, but it depends on the insurance company and the individual policy. Therefore, patients would need to determine whether their current policy includes fitness reimbursement or if it can be added to the policy. Some employers provide fitness incentives to their employees, so patients should check with their employer about this benefit.

Collaboration

Another opportunity for APPs to partner with exercise specialists is to collaborate directly to provide exercise counseling to patients in the office or via telemedicine. By offering this counseling during the regular office visit, the APP can utilize the expertise of the exercise professional to determine starting points for flexibility, cardiovascular, and strength training exercise as well as to write a detailed exercise prescription. An internationally recognized diagnosis code for physical inactivity exists: Z72.3 is the ICD-10 code (World Health Organization, 2019). The APP can document the need for increased exercise in the subjective and assessment parts of the visit note, and the exercise specialist's prescription and counseling notes can be added to the plan. Exercise counseling can be part of a routine visit that is billable to many commercial insurance providers. APPs should check with the particular insurance provider to determine whether the Z71.82 ICD-10 code for exercise counseling (ICD10data.com, 2021) is billable. Exercise counseling can be considered preventive counseling, so patients may not have to pay a copay if this is billed as a preventive counseling visit (e.g., using the 99403 CPT code with the appropriate Z code).

Summary

In conclusion, making practical the advice to *move often* is vital for improving both patient

---

Health Promotion Activity: Develop an Exercise Plan

Using the principles described in this chapter, develop a realistic 7-day plan for yourself that follows the guideline-recommended amount of time for aerobic, strength, and flexibility training. You may use input from a qualified exercise specialist if desired.
   Try out your plan. Then reflect on the following:

1. How difficult was it to incorporate your 7-day plan into your life?
2. What barriers did you have to overcome to complete this?
3. What would it take for you to sustain this amount of activity long term?
4. Looking back, would there have been anything you could have done differently to make your exercise more enjoyable?
5. How did doing this for 7 days change how you feel about any aspect of exercise or your health?
6. What benefits to your overall health or lifestyle did you notice (e.g., better sleep, mood, food choices, and hydration)?

   Based on your experience with your 7-day exercise plan, how would you recommend patients develop and implement exercise plans?

and population health. Regular physical activity throughout the day plus regular exercise throughout the week is ideal and beneficial for everyone of any ability or age. APPs should understand physical activity guidelines and stages of change, discuss exercise with every patient, and collaborate with other professionals to optimize each patient's fitness level. Exercise assessment, prescriptions, and counseling can be done in the clinic during regular office visits. For progressive strength training or for patients who would benefit from supervised exercise, APPs should provide a referral to a qualified exercise specialist. Optimizing physical fitness will not only improve patients' mental and physical health but also can prevent or reverse chronic disease and improve quality and length of life. This should be a win-win-win situation for patients, APPs, and exercise professionals. Refer to Table 13.12 for evidence-based resources for exercise. For additional application, see the bonus case study on the previous page and the case study workouts in Table 13.13, Table 13.14, Table 13.15, and Table 13.16.

Acronyms

ACE: American Council on Exercise
ACSM: American College of Sports Medicine
ADLs: activities of daily living
APP: advanced practice provider
AT: athletic trainer
BMI: body mass index
FITT-P: frequency, intensity, time, type, progression
HIIT: high-intensity interval training
LSD: long, slow duration
MD/DO: medical doctor/doctor of osteopathic medicine
MET: metabolic equivalent of task
NASM: National Academy of Sports Medicine
NCCA: National Commission for Certifying Agencies

NSCA: National Strength and Conditioning Association
OT: occupational therapist
PAGC: Physical Activity Guidelines Committee
PAR-Q+: Physical Activity Readiness Questionnaire
PNF: proprioceptive neuromuscular facilitation
PT: physical therapist
RPE: rating of perceived exertion
SIT: sprint interval training
SMART: specific, measurable, achievable, relevant, and time-bound
TTM: transtheoretical model

References

American College of Obstetricians and Gynecologists. (2022). *Exercise after pregnancy*. https://www.acog.org/womens-health/faqs/exercise-after-pregnancy

American College of Sports Medicine. (2009). Progression models in resistance training for healthy adults. *Medicine & Science in Sports & Exercise, 41*(3), 687–708. https://doi.org/10.1249/mss.0b013e3181915670

Buresh, R., & Berg, K. (2014). Role of exercise on inflammation and chronic disease. *Strength and Conditioning Journal, 36*(4), 87–93. https://doi.org/10.1519/ssc.0000000000000071

Carlson, S. A., Adams, E. K., Yang, Z., & Fulton, J. E. (2018). Percentage of deaths associated with inadequate physical activity in the United States. *Preventing Chronic Disease, 15*. https://doi.org/10.5888/pcd18.170354

Centers for Disease Control and Prevention. (2019). *Trends in meeting the 2008 Physical Activity Guidelines, 2008–2018*. https://www.cdc.gov/physicalactivity/downloads/trends-in-the-prevalence-of-physical-activity-508.pdf

Coleman, K. J., Ngor, E., Reynolds, K., Quinn, V. P., Koebnick, C., Young, D. R., Sternfeld, B., & Sallis, R. E. (2012). Initial validation of an exercise "vital sign" in electronic medical records. *Medicine & Science in Sports & Exercise*, *44*(11), 2071–2076. https://doi.org/10.1249/mss.0b013e3182630ec1

Collado-Mateo, D., Lavín-Pérez, A. M., Peñacoba, C., Del Coso, J., Leyton-Román, M., Luque-Casado, A., Gasque, P., Fernández-del-Olmo, M. Á., & Amado-Alonso, D. (2021). Key factors associated with adherence to physical exercise in patients with chronic diseases and older adults: An umbrella review. *International Journal of Environmental Research and Public Health*, *18*(4), 2023. https://doi.org/10.3390/ijerph18042023

Fiatarone, M. A. (1990). High-intensity strength training in nonagenarians. *JAMA*, *263*(22), 3029. https://doi.org/10.1001/jama.1990.03440220053029

Fragala, M. S., Cadore, E. L., Dorgo, S., Izquierdo, M., Kraemer, W. J., Peterson, M. D., & Ryan, E. D. (2019). Resistance training for older adults. *Journal of Strength and Conditioning Research*, *33*(8), 2019–2052. https://doi.org/10.1519/jsc.0000000000003230

Freitas, P. P., Menezes, M. C., Santos, L. C., Pimenta, A. M., Ferreira, A. V. M., & Lopes, A. C. S. (2020). The transtheoretical model is an effective weight management intervention: A randomized controlled trial. *BMC Public Health*, *20*(652). https://doi.org/10.1186/s12889-020-08796-1

Garber, C. E., Blissmer, B., Deschenes, M. R., Franklin, B. A., Lamonte, M. J., Lee, I-Min., Nieman, D. C., & Swain, D. P. (2011). Quantity and quality of exercise for developing and maintaining cardiorespiratory, musculoskeletal, and neuromotor fitness in apparently healthy adults. *Medicine & Science in Sports & Exercise*, *43*(7), 1334–1359. https://doi.org/10.1249/mss.0b013e318213fefb

Gladwell, V. F., Brown, D. K., Wood, C., Sandercock, G. R., & Barton, J. L. (2013). The great outdoors: How a green exercise environment can benefit all. *Extreme Physiology & Medicine*, *2*(3). https://doi.org/10.1186/2046-7648-2-3

Hortobágyi, T., Mizelle, C., Beam, S., & DeVita, P. (2003). Old adults perform activities of daily living near their maximal capabilities. *The Journals of Gerontology: Series A*, *58*(5), M453–M460. https://doi.org/10.1093/gerona/58.5.m453

ICD10data.com. (2021). *2023 ICD-10-CM diagnosis code Z71.82.* https://www.icd10data.com/ICD10CM/Codes/Z00-Z99/Z69-Z76/Z71-/Z71.82

Izquierdo, M., Merchant, R. A., Morley, J. E., Anker, S. D., Aprahamian, I., Arai, H., Aubertin-Leheudre, M., Bernabei, R., Cadore, E. L., Cesari, M., Chen, L.-K., de Souto Barreto, P., Duque, G., Ferrucci, L., Fielding, R. A., García-Hermoso, A., Gutiérrez-Robledo, L. M., Harridge, S. D. R., Kirk, B., &

Kritchevsky, S. (2021). International exercise recommendations in older adults (ICFSR): Expert consensus guidelines. *Journal of Nutrition, Health & Aging*, *25*(7), 824–853. https://doi.org/10.1007/s12603-021-1665-8

Jetté, M., Sidney, K., & Blümchen, G. (1990). Metabolic equivalents (METS) in exercise testing, exercise prescription, and evaluation of functional capacity. *Clinical Cardiology*, *13*(8), 555–565. https://doi.org/10.1002/clc.4960130809

Kell, R. T., Bell, G., & Quinney, A. (2001). Musculoskeletal fitness, health outcomes and quality of life. *Sports Medicine*, *31*(12), 863–873. https://doi.org/10.2165/00007256-200131120-00003

Keller, K., & Engelhardt, M. (2014). Strength and muscle mass loss with aging process: Age and strength loss. *Muscles, Ligaments and Tendons Journal*, *3*(4), 346–350.

Kennedy, M. A., Bayes, S., Newton, R. U., Zissiadis, Y., Spry, N. A., Taaffe, D. R., Hart, N. H., & Galvão, D. A. (2021). Implementation barriers to integrating exercise as medicine in oncology: An ecological scoping review. *Journal of Cancer Survivorship*. https://doi.org/10.1007/s11764-021-01080-0

Kirk, A., MacMillan, F., & Webster, N. (2010). Application of the transtheoretical model to physical activity in older adults with type 2 diabetes and/or cardiovascular disease. *Psychology of Sport and Exercise*, *11*, 320–324. https://doi.org/10.1016/j.psychsport.2010.03.001

Kodama, S. (2009). Cardiorespiratory fitness as a quantitative predictor of all-cause mortality and cardiovascular events in healthy men and women. *JAMA*, *301*(19), 2024. https://doi.org/10.1001/jama.2009.681

Kuriyan, R. (2018). Body composition techniques. *Indian Journal of Medical Research*, *148*(5), 648. https://doi.org/10.4103/ijmr.ijmr_1777_18

Lee, D-C., Sui, X., Ortega, F. B., Kim, Y-S., Church, T. S., Winett, R. A., Ekelund, U., Katzmarzyk, P. T., & Blair, S. N. (2010). Comparisons of leisure-time physical activity and cardiorespiratory fitness as predictors of all-cause mortality in men and women. *British Journal of Sports Medicine*, *45*(6), 504–510. https://doi.org/10.1136/bjsm.2009.066209

Liguori, G., Feito, Y., Fountaine, C., Roy, B., & American College of Sports Medicine. (2021). *ACSM's guidelines for exercise testing and prescription.* Wolters Kluwer.

Loveless, M. S., & Ihm, J. M. (2015). Resistance exercise. *Current Sports Medicine Reports*, *14*(3), 221–226. https://doi.org/10.1249/jsr.0000000000000149

Maffiuletti, N. A., Aagaard, P., Blazevich, A. J., Folland, J., Tillin, N., & Duchateau, J. (2016). Rate of force development: Physiological and methodological considerations. *European Journal of Applied Physiology*, *116*(6), 1091–1116. https://doi.org/10.1007/s00421-016-3346-6

Mandic, S., Myers, J., Selig, S. E., & Levinger, I. (2011). Resistance versus aerobic exercise training in chronic heart failure. *Current Heart Failure Reports*, 9(1), 57–64. https://doi.org/10.1007/s11897-011-0078-0

Mandsager, K., Harb, S., Cremer, P., Phelan, D., Nissen, S. E., & Jaber, W. (2018). Association of cardiorespiratory fitness with long-term mortality among adults undergoing exercise treadmill testing. *JAMA Network Open*, 1(6), e183605. https://doi.org/10.1001/jamanetworkopen.2018.3605

McKay, M. J., Baldwin, J. N., Ferreira, P., Simic, M., Vanicek, N., & Burns, J. (2017). Normative reference values for strength and flexibility of 1,000 children and adults. *Neurology*, 88(1), 36–43. https://doi.org/10.1212/WNL.0000000000003466

Medeiros, H. B. O., de Araújo, D. S. M. S., & Araújo, C. G. S. (2013). Age-related mobility loss is joint-specific: An analysis from 6,000 Flexitest results. *AGE*, 35(6), 2399–2407. https://doi.org/10.1007/s11357-013-9525-z

Menezes, M. C., Bedeschi, L. B., Santos, L. C., & Lopes, A. C. S. (2016). Interventions directed at eating habits and physical activity using the transtheoretical model: A systematic review. *Nutricion Hospitalaria*, 33(5), 1194–1204. https://doi.org/10.20960/nh.58

Moore, G. E., Durstine, J. L., & Painter, P. L. (Eds.). (2016). *ACSM's exercise management for persons with chronic diseases and disabilities*. Human Kinetics.

Morton, R. W., Colenso-Semple, L., & Phillips, S. M. (2019). Training for strength and hypertrophy: An evidence-based approach. *Current Opinion in Physiology*, 10, 90–95. https://doi.org/10.1016/j.cophys.2019.04.006

Mostafavi, F., Ghofranipour, F., Feizi, A., & Pirzadeh, A. (2015). Improving physical activity and metabolic syndrome indicators in women: A transtheoretical model-based intervention. *International Journal of Preventative Medicine*, 6(28). https://doi.org/10.4103/2008-7802.154382

Naclerio, F., Rodríguez-Romo, G., Barriopedro-Moro, M. I., Jiménez, A., Alvar, B. A., & Triplett, N. T. (2011). Control of resistance training intensity by the Omni Perceived Exertion Scale. *Journal of Strength and Conditioning Research*, 25(7), 1879–1888. https://doi.org/10.1519/jsc.0b013e3181e501e9

National Center for Health Statistics. (2019). *National health interview survey: Glossary*. Centers for Disease Control and Prevention. https://www.cdc.gov/nchs/nhis/physical_activity/pa_glossary.htm

Nay, K., Smiles, W. J., Kaiser, J., McAloon, L. M., Loh, K., Galic, S., Oakhill, J. S., Gundlach, A. L., & Scott, J. W. (2021). Molecular mechanisms underlying the beneficial effects of exercise on brain function and neurological disorders. *International Journal of Molecular Sciences*, 22(8), 4052. https://doi.org/10.3390/ijms22084052

Page, P. (2012). Current concepts in muscle stretching for exercise and rehabilitation. *International Journal of Sports Physical Therapy*, 7(1), 109–119.

Pedersen, B. K., & Saltin, B. (2006). Evidence for prescribing exercise as therapy in chronic disease. *Scandinavian Journal of Medicine & Science in Sports*, 16(S1), 3–63. https://doi.org/10.1111/j.1600-0838.2006.00520.x

Piercy, K. L., Troiano, R. P., Ballard, R. M., Carlson, S. A., Fulton, J. E., Galuska, D. A., George, S. M., & Olson, R. D. (2018). The Physical Activity Guidelines for Americans. *JAMA*, 320(19), 2020–2028. https://doi.org/10.1001/jama.2018.14854

Raghupathi, V., & Raghupathi, W. (2020). Healthcare expenditure and economic performance: Insights from the United States data. *Frontiers in Public Health*, 8(156). https://doi.org/10.3389/fpubh.2020.00156

Riebe, D., Franklin, B. A., Thompson, P. D., Garber, C. E., Whitfield, G. P., Magal, M., & Pescatello, L. S. (2015). Updating ACSM's recommendations for exercise preparticipation health screening. *Medicine & Science in Sports & Exercise*, 47(11), 2473–2479. https://doi.org/10.1249/mss.0000000000000664

Rippe, J. M. (2019). *Lifestyle medicine* (3rd ed.). CRC Press.

Schuch, F. B., Vancampfort, D., Firth, J., Rosenbaum, S., Ward, P. B., Silva, E. S., Hallgren, M., Ponce De Leon, A., Dunn, A. L., Deslandes, A. C., Fleck, M. P., Carvalho, A. F., & Stubbs, B. (2018). Physical activity and incident depression: A meta-analysis of prospective cohort studies. *American Journal of Psychiatry*, 175(7), 631–648. https://doi.org/10.1176/appi.ajp.2018.17111194

Stathokostas, L., & Vandervoort, A. A. (2016). The flexibility debate: Implications for health and function as we age. *Annual Review of Gerontology and Geriatrics*, 36(1), 169–192. https://doi.org/10.1891/0198-8794.36.169

Steele, J., Fisher, J., Giessing, J., & Gentil, P. (2017). Clarity in reporting terminology and definitions of set endpoints in resistance training. *Muscle & Nerve*, 56(3), 368–374. https://doi.org/10.1002/mus.25557

Strath, S. J., Kaminsky, L. A., Ainsworth, B. E., Ekelund, U., Freedson, P. S., Gary, R. A., Richardson, C. R., Smith, D. T., & Swartz, A. M. (2013). Guide to the assessment of physical activity: Clinical and research applications: A scientific statement from the American Heart Association. *Circulation*, 128(20), 2259–2279. https://doi.org/10.1161/01.cir.0000435708.67487.da

Sundell, J. (2011). Lihasvoimaharjoittelu on liian vähän käytetty täsmälääke lihavuudessa ja vanhuudessa [Resistance training is an underutilized therapy in obesity and advanced age]. *Duodecim*, 127(4), 335–341. https://pubmed.ncbi.nlm.nih.gov/21442853/

Tavoian, D., Russ, D. W., Consitt, L. A., & Clark, B. C. (2020). Perspective: Pragmatic exercise recommendations for older adults: The case for emphasizing resistance training. *Frontiers in Physiology, 11.* https://doi.org/10.3389/fphys.2020.00799

Tobacco Use and Dependence Guideline Panel. (2008). *Treating tobacco use and dependence: 2008 update.* U.S. Department of Health and Human Services. https://www.ncbi.nlm.nih.gov/books/NBK63952

U.S. Bureau of Labor Statistics. (2018, April 13). *Healthcare occupations.* https://www.bls.gov/ooh/healthcare/home.htm

Verrall, G. (2016). Deducing a mechanism of all musculoskeletal injuries. *Muscles, Ligaments and Tendons Journal, 6*(2), 174–182. https://doi.org/10.11138/mltj/2016.6.2.174

Wang, Y., Chen, S., Lavie, C. J., Zhang, J., & Sui, X. (2019). An overview of non-exercise estimated cardiorespiratory fitness: Estimation equations, cross-validation and application. *Journal of Science in Sport and Exercise, 1*(1), 38–53. https://doi.org/10.1007/s42978-019-0003-x

Webster, A. L., & Aznar-Laín, S. (2008). Intensity of physical activity and the "Talk Test." *ACSM's Health & Fitness Journal, 12*(3), 13–17. https://doi.org/10.1249/fit.0b013e31817047b4

Woltmann, M. L., Foster, C., Porcari, J. P., Camic, C. L., Dodge, C., Haible, S., & Mikat, R. P. (2015). Evidence that the talk test can be used to regulate exercise intensity. *Journal of Strength and Conditioning Research, 29*(5), 1248–1254. https://doi.org/10.1519/jsc.0000000000000811

World Health Organization. (2019). Z72.3 Lack of physical exercise. In *International statistical classification of diseases and related health problems* (10th ed.). https://icd.who.int/browse10/2019/en#/Z72.3

World Health Organization. (2020, November 26). *Physical activity.* https://www.who.int/news-room/fact-sheets/detail/physical-activity

Young, J. A., Hand, B. N., Onate, J. A., & Valasek, A. E. (2022). Clinical utility and validity of exercise vital signs in children. *Current Sports Medicine Reports, 21*(1), 28–33. https://doi.org/10.1249/JSR.0000000000000928

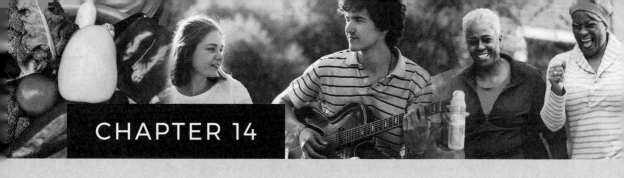

CHAPTER 14

Avoid Alcohol

Sara B. Adams, PhD, RN, CNE
Carol Essenmacher, DNP, PMHCNS-BC

We are socialized to think that unless a person drinks excessive alcohol, there is no harm; however, alcohol is toxic, and even a small amount can lead to health problems.

Dr. Loureen Downes

OBJECTIVES

This chapter will enable the reader to:

1. Integrate knowledge of the biological and health effects of alcohol into effective healthy lifestyle strategies.
2. Describe and discuss evidence-informed clinical practice recommendations for alcohol use and assessment.
3. Utilize the screening, brief intervention, and referral to treatment (SBIRT) approach for early identification and intervention for risky alcohol use.
4. Design lifestyle prescriptions for avoiding, reducing, or eliminating alcohol use.
5. Engage with other healthcare professionals to ensure a comprehensive and interprofessional approach for treating risky alcohol use.

Overview

Alcohol use affects health. As an advanced practice provider (APP), implications for assessing, preventing, and providing treatment options for alcohol use are an important part of professional practice. In this chapter, the reader will gain a basic understanding of alcohol use, its effect on body systems, and its contribution to chronic disease. Strategies for assessing alcohol use and lifestyle modifications for decreasing and preventing alcohol use will be examined. Information related to excessive use of alcohol is readily available. However, when exploring the health effects of low to moderate use of alcohol, information on the benefits and harms remains unclear. There is a significant need for objective, evidence-based information on the consequences of alcohol use to support patients striving for healthy lifestyles effectively. Strategies to incorporate evidence-informed, healthy lifestyle practices to reduce or eliminate alcohol consumption and pearls about

© Kathleen Gail/Shutterstock; © StoryTime Studio/Shutterstock; © kali9/Getty Images

how to start these conversations with patients will also be offered.

Up-to-date, high-quality evidence-based information is a critical component of advanced practice. Yet information alone is inadequate to assist providers in developing therapeutic strategies with patients related to the use of alcohol. APPs should combine the available evidence with reflective practices to develop a treatment philosophy and skill set to address alcohol use and apply these as an important component of interprofessional care.

Prevalence of Alcohol Use

To gain a foundational understanding of the health implications of alcohol use, it is beneficial to review the populations most affected by alcohol use and other demographic information. According to the Centers for Disease Control and Prevention (CDC), the death toll due to excessive alcohol intake is about 1 in 10 adults ages 20 to 64 years old (National Center for Chronic Disease Prevention and Health Promotion [NCCDPHP], 2021). The Behavior Risk Factor Surveillance System (BRFSS) survey showed that over half of U.S. adult citizens drank alcohol within the previous 30 days, with 16% attributed to binge drinking and 7% engaging in heavy drinking (CDC, 2022a). The National Institute on Alcohol Abuse and Alcoholism (NIAAA, 2022a) reports an emerging trend of *high-intensity* drinking, which is defined as consuming twice as much as the binge drinking threshold. This phenomenon is more likely to result in medical emergencies related to alcohol (NIAAA, 2022). These data are not limited to adult alcohol use. In fact, 14.5 million people over the age of 12 in the United States have alcohol use disorder (AUD), and 414,000 are between the ages of 12 and 17 years (Substance Abuse and Mental Health Services Administration [SAMHSA], 2021).

These demographic data provide necessary information outlining the pervasive nature of alcohol use in the United States and the vastness of the problems associated with alcohol, including addiction. Understanding how the body interacts with alcohol on a cellular level and the multiple body systems associated with these dynamic processes is important as APPs work to plan care.

Biological Effects of Alcohol

Through a deeper understanding of the biological effects of alcohol, APPs can help individuals sustain healthy lifestyles. A brief discussion of the pharmacology of alcohol is helpful for understanding the effect of alcohol on the body. The discussion can be broken down into three noteworthy areas for understanding the implications of alcohol use. These include pharmacokinetics (what the body does to the drug), pharmacodynamics (what the drug does to the body), and pharmacogenomics (the effects of gene expression influences) (Herron & Brennan, 2019). Most APPs have studied these effects; therefore, only a brief overview of treatment strategies is provided here for context.

The most compelling piece of pharmacokinetic information about alcohol is that the body distributes this tiny, water-soluble molecule very swiftly and efficiently throughout the body. This includes all tissues and includes rapid absorption of alcohol to the fetus of pregnant women. Alcohol is metabolized (broken down) into alcohol dehydrogenase (ADH) by the liver. Men and women metabolize alcohol differently, with women having 20% to 25% higher blood alcohol levels than men who have consumed the same amount of alcohol (Woodward, 2019).

A significant pharmacodynamic effect of alcohol stems from the chemical's effect on the central nervous system. At low levels of alcohol use, people experience less anxiety, increased feelings of well-being and euphoria, and a rise in impaired judgment (Woodward, 2019). Alcohol acts as a central nervous system depressant, and acute intoxication can result in disorientation, confusion, hallucinations, reduced gag reflex, bradycardia, and depressed respirations (Marshall & Spencer, 2019; Stahl, 2021). These symptoms can progress to seizures and death.

Zajicek and Karan (2019) describe pharmacogenomics as the "study of the relationship between genetic variations and drug disposition and response" (p. 41). This is important to know, as one's genetic makeup may influence the metabolism of alcohol and the risk of addiction. Information about genetic vulnerability to alcohol has the potential to inform prevention strategies.

Pharmacokinetics, pharmacodynamics, and pharmacogenomics of alcohol can inform clinical practice. This is undoubtedly the case when applied to different populations who are the most highly affected by alcohol use and AUD. The foundational knowledge this provides plays a role in how the health effects of alcohol use are understood.

Health Effects of Alcohol

It is widely understood that excessive alcohol use contributes to numerous adverse health outcomes, including liver disease, high blood pressure, heart disease, stroke, cognitive function disorders, and multiple types of cancer (NCCDPHP, 2021; Stahl, 2021). Since most studies related to alcohol use and chronic disease are based on moderate to heavy alcohol use, it is necessary to explore the link between low and moderate use of alcohol. Low to moderate alcohol use is implicated in several chronic diseases. For example, studies are available that link as little as one drink per day to significant increases in the risk of female breast cancer as well as a variety of other cancers (Bagnardi et al., 2015; Ko et al., 2021). Alcohol is also directly linked to overall cancer mortality, specifically when compared to lifetime abstinence (Ko et al., 2021).

In addition to physical health risks, alcohol is a significant contributor to poor mental health outcomes. About 17 million adults have an overlapping mental illness alongside substance use disorder (SAMHSA, 2021). Of those with serious mental illness, 5.7 million have a substance use disorder. Alcohol contributes to poor outcomes among people with mental diagnoses, and since it is a central nervous system depressant, it can lead to depression and increased risk of suicidal ideation (Lynch et al., 2020).

Vistonay et al. (2022) discovered, in a systematic review of the evidence related to alcohol use and health, that there were several incidences where alcohol use had an effect on health outcomes, including cardiovascular lipid profile, cardiovascular events, mental health, diabetes, dementia, HIV seroconversion, and musculoskeletal health. However, given the nature of studies related to alcohol use, it is often difficult to link causal inference to alcohol alone in these cases, as there is little to no researcher control over the variable of interest (Vistonay et al., 2022).

The pharmacology and health effects of alcohol are clear that even small amounts of alcohol have an effect on body systems and disease risk. Although one cannot determine causality when exploring the effects of alcohol use on health, the effect at the cellular level on body systems is evident. Therefore, based on this data, the APP can create educational interventions that any amount of alcohol affects body processes. According to Burton and Sheron (2018), no amount of alcohol is beneficial, and even small amounts can be dangerous given the evidence explored (Ko et al., 2021; Lynch et al., 2020). It is necessary to understand the amount of alcohol consumed by patients, and therefore defining alcohol consumption becomes an important factor in the discussion of alcohol use with a patient. It is imperative to understand the prevailing definitions of low to moderate drinking as well as definitions of excessive and binge drinking.

Evidence-Informed Clinical Practice Recommendations

The *Dietary Guidelines for Americans, 2020–2025* recommends that the consumption of alcohol be limited to one drink or less per day for women and two drinks or less per day for men, to reduce health risks, or abstinence from drinking entirely (U.S. Department of Agriculture and U.S. Department of Health and Human Services, 2020) (see **Figure 14.1**). Several groups should completely abstain from alcohol, including pregnant women, people under the age of 21, those recovering from AUD, and anyone taking medications or having a diagnosis that is contraindicated in combination with alcohol use.

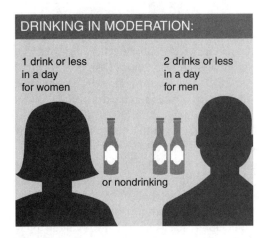

Figure 14.1 Dietary guidelines for alcohol.

Centers for Disease Control and Prevention. (2022, April 19). *Facts about moderate drinking.* https://www.cdc.gov/alcohol/fact-sheets/moderate-drinking.htm

Health Promotion Research Study

Excessive Alcohol Use and Parenting Status

Background: Excessive alcohol use, a leading cause of death and disability, has been increasing in the United States. Although recent attention has focused on the drinking status of child-rearing women, it remains unclear whether binge and heavy drinking vary by parenting status and sex. This descriptive study aimed to discover trends in binge and heavy drinking among men and women according to parenting status and age.

Methodology: Secondary data analysis was conducted on survey information from respondents to the National Health Interview Survey (n = 239,944 of the original sample, which was 477,409 [cohort number from 2006 to 2018]). Study subjects were categorized by various combinations based on marital status, age groups, race, socioeconomic status, and year (2008–2014). Terms such as *heavy drinking* and *binge drinking* were described.

Results: The study found that binge drinking increased and alcohol abstention decreased for all groups except for young men (ages 18–29) with children. Heavy drinking decreased for all ages except women ages 44–55 years old.

Implication for Advanced Practice: APPs should be made aware of trends and be advised to conduct thorough assessments and screenings for alcohol use in all adults—not just select groups of men and women. Everyone should be considered at risk and receive screening and treatment when appropriate.

Reference: Data from McKetta, S., & Keyes, K. M. (2019). Heavy and binge drinking and parenting status in the United States from 2006 to 2018: An analysis of nationally representative cross-sectional surveys. *PLoS Medicine, 16*(11), e1002954. https://doi.org/10.1371/journal.pmed.1002954

Because of the many adverse health effects of alcohol, the U.S. Preventive Services Task Force (2018) and other professional organizations (Committee on Health Care for Underserved Women, 2011; Salisbury-Afshar & Fleming, 2019) have recommended that alcohol screening be implemented in primary care settings for all adults 18 years and older and that brief behavioral counseling interventions be provided to persons engaged in risky or hazardous drinking to reduce unhealthy alcohol use. The American Academy of Pediatrics supports similar recommendations for focused screening and education in adolescents due to the potential adverse effect of alcohol on the developing brain (Quigley et al., 2019).

Understanding Risky Alcohol Use

Risky alcohol use is defined as "any level of alcohol consumption that increases the risk of harm to a person's health or well-being or that of others" (National Center on Birth Defects and Developmental Disabilities [NCBDDD], 2014, p. 7). Several sources describe risky drinking, or excessive alcohol use, for men as binge drinking five or more drinks at any one time or 15 or more drinks per week. For women, excessive drinking is defined as four or more drinks on one occasion or eight or more drinks per week (CDC, 2022b; Herron & Brennan, 2019; National Institute on Drug Abuse, 2021). For some individuals, a lower level than just described or even any drinking is considered risky due to health conditions and activities (NCBDDD, 2014).

"*Alcohol use disorder* is defined as a cluster of behavioral and physical symptoms, such as withdrawal, tolerance, and craving" (American Psychiatric Association, 2022, p. 555). **Table 14.1** lists the criteria and sample

assessment questions that the APP can use when evaluating alcohol use. Depending on how many of the diagnostic criteria are met, AUD is classified as either mild (2–3), moderate (3–5), or severe (≥6).

Misunderstandings About Alcohol Use

Clarifying the type and amount of alcohol consumed is an essential component of the patient assessment. An important part of understanding the effects of alcohol stems from typical formulations of it into a variety of enticing drinks. In the United States, a standard drink of alcohol is the amount contained in 12 ounces of beer, 5 ounces of wine, or 1.5 ounces of distilled hard liquor (see **Figure 14.2**). This is a source of confusion for people when they report the amount of alcohol they typically ingest since many wine glasses hold 6 to 8 ounces and servings of beer often come in 20-ounce containers. This leads to reported and perceptual differences between actual and perceived amounts ingested.

Hunter et al. (2017) remind providers that erroneous assumptions about alcohol use confound reporting of amounts and types of alcohol ingested and exacerbate access to care. For example, people who use alcohol may misperceive one type of alcohol as *worse* than another when there are no differences in effects between different types of alcohol (Hunter et al., 2017). Inconsistent and inaccurate reporting of alcohol use in the patient assessment can lead to ineffective treatment. Additionally, most people who use alcohol do not drink every day. Therefore, it is essential to focus on the alcohol consumed on the days that they do drink.

People tend to equate drinking too much with alcoholism, further affecting conversations about the amount of alcohol consumed (NCBDDD, 2014). People may believe that they are not at risk because they can "handle"

Table 14.1 DSM-5 Alcohol Use Disorder Diagnosis Criteria and Assessment Questions

Diagnosis Criteria	Assessment Question
1. Alcohol is often taken in larger amounts or over a longer period than was intended.	Do you drink more than you mean to?
2. There is a persistent desire or unsuccessful efforts to cut down or control alcohol use.	Do you want to stop but can't?
3. A great deal of time is spent in activities necessary to obtain alcohol, use alcohol, or recover from its effects.	Is drinking taking over your life?
4. Craving, or a strong desire or urge to use alcohol.	If you can't drink, are you thinking about drinking?
5. Recurrent alcohol use resulting in a failure to fulfill major role obligations at work, school, or home.	Is your drinking getting in the way of day-to-day activities?
6. Continued alcohol use despite having persistent or recurrent social or interpersonal problems caused or exacerbated by the effects of alcohol.	Is drinking getting in the way of your relationships?
7. Important social, occupational, or recreational activities are given up or reduced because of alcohol use.	Are you sitting things out because of alcohol?
8. Recurrent alcohol use in situations in which it is physically hazardous.	Are you drinking in risky settings or doing risky things while drinking?
9. Alcohol use is continued despite knowledge of having a persistent or recurrent physical or psychological problem that is likely to have been caused or exacerbated by alcohol.	Do you know drinking isn't good for you, but you do it anyway?
10. Tolerance, as defined by either of the following: a need for markedly increased amounts of alcohol to achieve intoxication or desired effect, or a markedly diminished effect with continued use of the same amount of alcohol.	Do you need to drink more than you used to?
11. Withdrawal, as manifested by either of the following: the characteristic withdrawal syndrome for alcohol, or alcohol (or a closely related substance, such as a benzodiazepine) is taken to relieve or avoid alcohol withdrawal symptoms.	Do you feel it when you stop drinking?

Data from Gasser, M. (2022, March 28). *The truth about alcohol and why it is so dangerous.* Transcendence Treatment Center. https://ttreatment.org/the-truth-about-alcohol-and-why-it-is-so-dangerous

their alcohol intake. The APP should recognize that screening aims to identify both patients with AUD and those who drink too much but are not dependent on alcohol. The APP's goal is to motivate the former to seek help while the goal for the latter is to motivate them to cut down or stop drinking (NCBDDD, 2014).

Screening, Brief Intervention, and Referral to Treatment

Screening, brief intervention, and referral to treatment (SBIRT) is a comprehensive and integrated approach for early identification

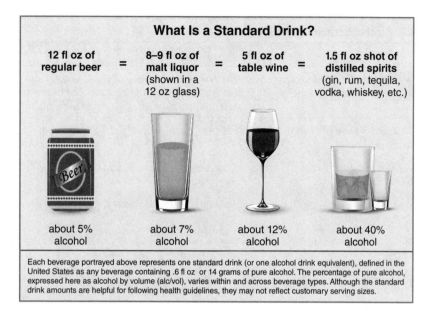

Figure 14.2 Alcohol drink equivalents.

National Institute on Alcohol Abuse and Alcoholism. (2022b). *What is a standard drink?* https://www.niaaa.nih.gov/alcohols-effects-health/overview-alcohol-consumption
/what-standard-drink

and intervention with patients whose patterns of alcohol drinking put their health at risk (SAMHSA, 2022). SBIRT targets patients who use alcohol at risky or harmful levels. Its components include the following:

- The use of standardized screening tools to quickly assess the risk level of alcohol use and identify the appropriate intervention or treatment.
- A brief intervention to increase patients' awareness and insight about their use of alcohol, relate patient-specific health effects of drinking, and enhance motivation for behavior change.
- Referral to treatment for patients showing signs of AUD to access specialty care.

Starting the Conversation

The relationship between the APP and the patient is foundational to assessing alcohol use and addressing any lifestyle or behavioral intervention. The APP is responsible for beginning an honest conversation about alcohol use, providing education on the effect of alcohol on multiple body systems, and establishing enough rapport with patients to gather an accurate assessment of alcohol use.

Screening for Risky or Harmful Alcohol Use

When APPs use objective screening tools, disease and risk can be detected much earlier than when the disease has progressed enough to reveal physical symptoms (Iragorri & Spackman, 2018). According to O'Connor et al. (2018), screening and brief interventions for alcohol use are helpful across disciplines and settings and appropriate in community, primary care, and inpatient settings. These assessments and interventions help identify unhealthy levels of alcohol use and can contribute to the initiation of effective treatment (O'Connor et al., 2018).

Using valid and reliable assessment and screening tools can augment the initial conversation about alcohol use. The NIAAA

Table 14.2 Alcohol Screening Tools

Tool	URL
Alcohol Screening and Brief Intervention for Youth: A Practitioner's Guide*	https://www.niaaa.nih.gov/alcohols-effects-health /professional-education-materials/alcohol-screening -and-brief-intervention-youth-practitioners-guide
Alcohol Use Disorders Identification Test (AUDIT)	https://nida.nih.gov/sites/default/files/audit.pdf
Alcohol Use Disorders Identification Test-Concise (AUDIT-C)	https://cde.drugabuse.gov/sites/nida_cde/files/Audit -C_2014Mar24.pdf
Brief Screener for Tobacco, Alcohol, and Other Drugs (BSTAD)*	https://nida.nih.gov/ast/bstad/#
CAGE (cut down, annoyed, guilty, eye-opener) Questionnaire	https://www.mirecc.va.gov/cih-visn2/Documents/Provider _Education_Handouts/CAGE_Version_3.pdf
The CRAFFT* Interview	https://crafft.org/wp-content/uploads/2019/02/CRAFFT-2.0 _Clinician-Interview.pdf
Planning and Implementing Screening and Brief Intervention for Risky Alcohol Use (SBI)	https://www.cdc.gov/ncbddd/fasd/documents /AlcoholSBIImplementationGuide-P.pdf
Screening to Brief Intervention (S2BI)*	https://nida.nih.gov/ast/s2bi/#
T-ACE (tolerance, annoyance, cut down, eye-opener) Screening Tool	https://www.mirecc.va.gov/visn22/T-ACE_alcohol_screen.pdf
Tobacco, Alcohol, Prescription Medication, and Other Substance Use Tool (TAPS)	https://nida.nih.gov/taps/#
TWEAK (tolerance, worried, eye-opener, amnesia, k/cut down)**	https://pubs.niaaa.nih.gov/publications/assessingalcohol /instrumentpdfs/74_tweak.pdf

*Appropriate for use with youth and adolescent populations.
**Assessment for pregnancy-related risk of alcohol use.

recommends asking, *How many times in the past year have you had five (four for women) or more drinks in a day?* This single screening question has 73% to 88% sensitivity and 74% to 100% specificity for detecting unhealthy alcohol use in U.S. primary care settings (O'Connor et al., 2018). It is helpful as a universal prescreening for all patients during each visit to rule out patients at low or no risk. More detailed screening instruments are recommended if the patient's response to the single screening question is one or more. Multiple screening tools for different patient populations, including adults, pregnant women, children, and adolescents can be found in **Table 14.2**.

Brief Interventions to Address Alcohol Use

After APPs have surmised that alcohol use might be an issue for patients, the next step involves enhancing their motivation to change their behavior (or to motivate patients with more severe risk to seek treatment). Motivational interviewing (MI) is one evidence-informed strategy to engage patients in a conversation about behavior change. Using MI, the APP can initiate a discussion related to alcohol use. According to Levounis et al. (2017), MI does not honor the tradition of confrontation in addiction treatment. Instead, MI uses the principles of collaboration, evocation, and autonomy to engage in a conversation between patients and providers. Collaboration is a concept that breaks from the authoritative and prescriptive approach of providers making decisions on the patient's behalf. In MI, providers and patients work together to make decisions about care. The provider seeks to discover what values the patients hold as important and then helps the patients notice any discrepancies between their behavior and their values. MI recognizes that the patients are in charge of

their own health, care, and life and are able to make choices to support their values (Levounis et al., 2017). The steps for a brief intervention are summarized in **Table 14.3**.

In a Cochrane Review of Evidence, Kaner et al. (2018) describe brief interventions to reduce alcohol consumption, specifically in harmful- or hazardous-level consumers of alcohol, compared to no intervention. A brief intervention was defined as "a conversation comprising five or fewer sessions of brief advice or brief lifestyle counseling and a total duration of less than 60 minutes" (Kaner et al., 2018, p. 1). The interventions typically included a discussion of the patient's risk compared with national norms, patient-specific adverse alcohol effects, tips for decreasing drinking, MI strategies, or the development of an action plan. The researchers found

Table 14.3 Brief Intervention Steps

Step	Description	Sample
Raise the subject	■ Explain your role; ask permission to discuss the alcohol use screening form.	■ "Hi, my name is _____. I'm one of the advanced practice providers here at the clinic. Would it be OK if we talked about the annual screening forms you filled out today?"
	■ Ask about alcohol use patterns, using the patient's own words. Listen carefully; use reflections to demonstrate understanding.	■ "What does your alcohol use look like in a typical week?"
Provide feedback	■ Share alcohol use screening results; explore the patient's reaction.	■ "Your score puts you in the _____ zone, which means _____. The low-risk limits are _____. What do you think about that?"
	■ Provide patient education materials, and highlight a few health/social/work issues related to risky alcohol use. ■ Explore the patient's reaction to the information. Listen closely and reflect.	■ "What connection might there be between your alcohol use and why you came in today?"

(continues)

Table 14.3 Brief Intervention Steps   (continued)

Step	Description	Sample
Enhance motivation	■ Ask about the pros and cons for changing their behavior.	■ "What do you like most about drinking? What don't you like?"
	■ Explore their readiness to change.	■ "On a scale of 0–10, how ready are you to make a change in your drinking?"
	■ Ask about their response to elicit change talk.	■ If readiness is >2: "Why that number and not a _____ (lower one)?" ■ If 0–2: "How would your drinking have to affect your life for you to start thinking about cutting back?"
Negotiate plan	■ Summarize the conversation (risk, pros/cons, readiness), including reasons for change identified by the patient.	■ "We talked about your risk score and how your drinking may be affecting your blood pressure and insomnia. Although you enjoy the way alcohol helps you relax, you are noticing some unwanted weight gain. You rated your readiness to cut back as a 6/10 because you've already cut out wine at dinner."
	■ Ask a key open-ended question. ■ If not ready to plan, stop the intervention, thank the patient, and offer patient education materials. ■ If needed, offer options for change (can use patient education materials). Write down agreed-to steps and give them to the patient.	■ "What do you think you will do? What steps are you willing to take to cut back?"
	■ Assess the patient's confidence in achieving the steps.	■ "On a scale of 0–10, how confident are you to make these changes?"
	■ Negotiate a follow-up visit and thank the patient.	

Data from Gotham, H. (n.d.). Screening and brief intervention for substance use: A health imperative [PowerPoint slides]. Retrieved May 12, 2023, from https://umkc.app.box.com/s/mvwt992izkokxeswhso6iss2w9azbt6p

moderate-quality evidence of the effectiveness of brief interventions for reducing alcohol consumption compared to minimal or no intervention. APPs in primary care are well positioned for such brief interventions, as they have in-depth knowledge of the patient and the opportunity for regular one-to-one conversations. Studies reviewed on brief interventions that included counseling and lifestyle interventions had few to no associated adverse problems, making these interventions low cost and effective (O'Connor et al., 2018).

Lifestyle Prescriptions for Avoiding Alcohol

Once collaboration and motivation to change behavior are established, the APP might consider writing a lifestyle prescription for avoiding alcohol. Due to the reciprocal relationship between the A-SMART components (adopt healthy eating, stress less, move often, avoid alcohol, rest more, treat tobacco use), a multifaceted plan of care offers a holistic approach to reducing or eliminating alcohol use.

Adopt Healthy Eating

Nutrition can be negatively affected by alcohol use, as alcohol consumption can replace calories that would otherwise be gained through eating nutrient-dense calories. Alcohol is often consumed with or in addition to regular meals, leading to excess caloric intake. Additionally, people with sustained heavy alcohol use often suffer from inadequate nutrient absorption, even if enough calories are consumed (Gramlich et al., 2021). According to Gramlich et al., it is necessary to assess for alcohol-related malnutrition and include strategies for improving nutritional status as part of the plan of care for the patient with AUD.

Stress Less

Reduction of stress and improvement in social connections are important to improving health. For those who use alcohol, according to Kelly et al. (2020), Alcoholics Anonymous (AA) and other 12-step facilitated programs are among the best interventions for improving abstinence and reducing drinking intensity, alcohol addiction severity, and alcohol-related consequences.

This is likely related to the social nature and the one-to-one support for reducing and eliminating alcohol from a person's lifestyle (Kelly et al., 2020). Social media may also provide a source of exploration and support for cutting down on drinking, with examples such as the sober curious movement and Dry January, a month of voluntary sobriety. More evidence is necessary to determine how social support, particularly in social media, can affect alcohol use.

Move Often

Physical activity is essential to effective treatment for alcohol recovery (Manthou et al., 2016). When introduced into alcohol recovery programs, physical activity reduces binge drinking and drinking days in people who use alcohol. Additionally, physical activity elevates serotonin levels and brain-derived neurotrophic factor (BDN), which has been shown to improve mood and cognitive functioning (Pitrelli et al., 2018). Low mood and alcohol use are often correlated. However, it is not well understood whether people use alcohol because of low mood or have a depressed mood related to alcohol use. Both are evident in the literature.

Avoid Alcohol

SAMHSA (n.d.) provides tips for cutting down on alcohol intake. These include monitoring alcohol use to prevent risky drinking, setting a daily and weekly drinking limit, pacing drinking to no more than one standard drink per hour, recording how much alcohol is consumed each day, avoiding situations and triggers that lead to drinking, asking a friend who does not drink for help in staying within limits, and seeking professional help and treatment. A handout can be presented to the patient with a list of tips from which they can choose the one(s) that resonate or seem most actionable.

Rest More

Adequate sleep protects mental well-being and functioning and is a part of a lifestyle treatment plan for alcohol use. According to Scott et al. (2021), improved sleep quality is directly linked to improved mental health. People with insomnia have a 10% greater risk of depression and a 17% greater risk of depression (Scott et al., 2021). Both anxiety and depression are linked to increases in alcohol and substance use (SAMHSA, 2021). When

---

Health Promotion Case Study Addressing Alcohol Use in an Adult Female

Case Description: S.T. is a 61-year-old female of mixed-race ethnicity who has generally been healthy. At her initial visit 3 months ago, her APP noted that her weight has slowly crept up over the years and her BMI indicated that she falls within the parameters for obesity. Additionally, her laboratory studies showed a steady increase in her FBS readings, and her HgbA1c indicated she was prediabetic. In the 3 months since her initial visit, she has made some lifestyle changes toward the goal of losing 20 pounds and reversing her progression toward a diagnosis of type 2 diabetes. When the APP sees her today, S.T. has lost only 3 pounds, and while there is a slight improvement in her lab values, she remains at risk for type 2 diabetes. In reviewing her efforts in changing her behaviors, the APP learns that she is drinking more water, walking 1–2 miles every other day, and has started attending a yoga class at a local facility. However, when queried, she admits that she "enjoys a nightcap every evening." Upon further questioning, she reveals that she has 1–2 glasses of wine about 5–7 days per week. She estimates that the glasses that she uses are 6 to 8 ounces. She is very ambivalent and skeptical about giving up this ritual. She tells you, "Well, everyone will die of something. I don't think my drinking is that bad."

- Family history: Positive for cancer, with several members succumbing to colon cancer.
- Vital signs: Blood pressure 138/86 mmHg, heart rate 80 bpm, respiratory rate 18 bpm, temp 98.9°F.

Lifestyle Vital Signs
- Adopt healthy eating: States drinking more water in place of sweetened beverages.
- Stress less: Denies new stressors. States that stress levels are manageable.
- Move often: Walks 1–2 miles every other day. She has started attending a yoga class at a local facility.
- Avoid alcohol: Admits 1–2 glasses of wine about 5–7 days per week.
- Rest more: Not assessed.
- Treat tobacco use: Denies.
- BMI: 32 kg/m^2 (down 3 pounds from last visit).

Critical Thinking Questions
1. How do you establish effective therapeutic communication with a patient who does not perceive that their lifestyle choices need changing?
2. Describe how you might use SBIRT at this visit.
3. How would you help motivate S.T., at minimum, to begin thinking about changing her nightcap ritual?
4. What lifestyle strategies would you recommend for S.T. at the present time?
5. How would you motivate someone to change a behavior that you also engage in or feel is not that harmful?

making decisions about drinking alcohol, whether it is reducing alcohol from heavy to light use or eliminating alcohol, mental health matters. Lifestyle change takes determination and strategy. Therefore, getting adequate rest can be essential to support mental health.

Treat Tobacco Use Disorder

If a person uses tobacco alongside alcohol, it is recommended that the person try to quit all substances simultaneously. Treating tobacco use disorder can improve outcomes for alcohol treatment. The rationale is that if a person continues one addictive substance, the cycle continues in the neuropathways and makes it more difficult for the patient to abstain from the other substance and can drive cravings (Essenmacher et al., 2021).

Implications for APPs

Evidence-informed practice is the cornerstone of advanced practice. A continual review of the available literature creates the opportunity to enhance assessment measures and interventions that improve patient outcomes. Research must be evaluated for its level on the evidence hierarchy and what the research is intended to provide. Descriptive, nonexperimental studies are designed to inform while experimental studies are intended to describe the effect of interventions on outcome measures. McKetta and Keyes (2019) completed a secondary data analysis of national-level data to describe the patterns of alcohol use and parenting status broken down by demographics. Since these data are informative only, it is impossible to draw causal inferences. However, these data can inform how risk is assessed and among which groups risk tends to be greater.

Continuing to evaluate the most recent and highest level of evidence is one way for APPs to stay up to date with best practices and emerging evidence for alcohol use. Another strategy is to use health promotion practices related to alcohol use with every patient, at every visit, and in every setting. Since the risks associated with alcohol use are well defined, beginning a conversation about alcohol is appropriate with children over 12 through the aging adult. Primary prevention strategies are the most effective; however, secondary prevention (e.g., screening) and tertiary prevention (e.g., treatment and referral for rehabilitation and support systems) are also useful.

As discussed, lifestyle changes and interventions are best addressed in a multifaceted manner. This includes the use of an interprofessional care model that involves psychiatrists and addiction treatment specialists who can prescribe medication if necessary; social workers, psychologists, and therapists who can provide one-to-one counseling; dietitians who can assess and address nutritional deficiencies; exercise specialists who can assist the patient in meeting physical activity guidelines; community health workers who know and understand community resources; and physicians or APPs who can manage chronic health issues resulting from or affected by alcohol use. Outpatient and residential alcohol treatment programs are also available.

Health Promotion Activity: Describing a Healthy Use of Alcohol

After reading this chapter, if you were to engage in conversations with colleagues about the role of alcohol use in terms of a healthy lifestyle, how would you describe a healthy use of alcohol? Would your perspective be that one should not use alcohol at all, or is it OK to use small amounts regularly? Describe your rationale for your position.

Summary

Although some existing data support low levels of drinking and improvement in cognitive function (Zhang et al., 2020), the evidence is far from conclusive. APPs must use extreme caution advising practices (i.e., low to moderate alcohol use) that have known negative physical and psychological consequences. Most of the evidence that supports alcohol use is inconclusive. Additionally, all the potential benefits of alcohol use can be mimicked through other means without the potential for toxic effects on multiple body systems. This chapter has provided foundational information; however, a thorough and continual review of the evidence and current recommendations is essential.

Prescriptions for healthy lifestyles should include avoiding alcohol due to a lack of consistent evidence that alcohol use is the only mechanism for improving purported health outcomes, whereas the potential risks to morbidity and mortality are well established (CDC, 2022b; SAMHSA, 2021). When assessing alcohol consumption, APPs should be aware of the misunderstandings around the type and amount of alcohol used. The SBIRT approach is helpful for early identification and intervention with patients at risk for harmful alcohol use. A-SMART prescriptions and an interprofessional care team are among the best strategies for addressing risky alcohol use and have the potential to act as a care bundle of evidence-informed practices that can help reduce or eliminate alcohol consumption.

TABLE 14.4	Evidence-Based Resources for Avoiding Alcohol	
Organization	**Resource**	**URL**
Alcoholics Anonymous	International mutual aid fellowship dedicated to abstinence-based recovery from alcoholism through its 12-step program	https://www.aa.org
American Addiction Centers	Research-based information on the nature of alcohol abuse and addiction; helpline/chat	https://www.alcohol.org
American Family Physician (*AFP*, journal of the American Academy of Family Physicians)	Collection of *AFP* content on alcohol use disorders and related issues	https://www.aafp.org/afp/topicModules/viewTopicModule.htm?topicModuleId=1
American Society of Addiction Medicine (ASAM)	*The ASAM Essentials of Addiction Medicine* and other clinician guidelines and resources	https://www.asam.org
Healthy People 2030	Objectives and resources related to drug and alcohol use	https://health.gov/healthypeople/objectives-and-data/browse-objectives/drug-and-alcohol-use

Organization	Resource	URL
National Institute on Alcohol Abuse and Alcoholism	Alcohol Treatment Navigator	https://alcoholtreatment.niaaa.nih.gov
National Institute on Alcohol Abuse and Alcoholism	Alcohol Screening and Brief Intervention for Youth: A Practitioner's Guide	https://www.niaaa.nih.gov/alcohols-effects-health/professional-education-materials/alcohol-screening-and-brief-intervention-youth-practitioners-guide
National Institute on Alcohol Abuse and Alcoholism	Health Professional's Core Resource on Alcohol	https://www.niaaa.nih.gov/health-professionals-communities/core-resource-on-alcohol
Substance Abuse and Mental Health Services Administration	2020 Report: Key Substance Use and Mental Health Indicators	https://www.samhsa.gov/data/sites/default/files/reports/rpt35325/NSDUHFFRPDFWHTMLFiles2020/2020NSDUHFFR1PDFW102121.pdf
Substance Abuse and Mental Health Services Administration	Alcohol Use Facts and Resources (patient handout)	https://www.samhsa.gov/sites/default/files/alcohol-use-facts-resources-fact-sheet.pdf
University of Missouri–Kansas City School of Nursing and Health Studies	SBIRT clinician tools and training videos	https://www.sbirt.care/tools.aspx

Acronyms

AA: Alcoholics Anonymous
ADH: alcohol dehydrogenase
APP: advanced practice provider
A-SMART: adopt healthy eating, stress less, move often, avoid alcohol, rest more, treat tobacco use
AUD: alcohol use disorder
BRFSS: Behavior Risk Factor Surveillance System

MI: motivational interviewing
NCBDDD: National Center on Birth Defects and Developmental Disabilities
NIAAA: National Institute on Alcohol Abuse and Alcoholism
SAMHSA: Substance Abuse and Mental Health Services Administration
SBIRT: screening, behavioral intervention, and referral to treatment

References

American Psychiatric Association. (2022). Alcohol-related disorders. In *Diagnostic and statistical manual of mental disorders text revision* (5th ed., pp. 553-568). Author.

Bagnardi, V., Rota, M., Botteri, E., Tramacere, I., Islami, F., Fedirko, V., Scotti, L., Jenab, M., Turati, F., Pasquali, E., Pelucchi, C., Galeone, C., Bellocco, R., Negri, E.,

Corrao, G., Boffetta, P., & La Vecchia, C. (2015). Alcohol consumption and site-specific cancer risk: A comprehensive dose-response meta-analysis. *British Journal of Cancer, 112*(3), 580–593. https://doi.org/10.1038/bjc.2014.579

Burton, R., & Sheron, N. (2018). No level of alcohol consumption improves health. *The Lancet, 392*(10152), 987–988. http://doi.org/10.1016/S0140-6736(18)31571-X

Centers for Disease Control and Prevention. (2022a). *Alcohol and public health: Data on excessive drinking.* https://www.cdc.gov/alcohol/data-stats.htm

Centers for Disease Control and Prevention. (2022b). *Alcohol and public health: Dietary guidelines for alcohol.* https://www.cdc.gov/alcohol/fact-sheets/moderate-drinking.htm

Committee on Health Care for Underserved Women. (2011). Committee opinion no. 496: At-risk drinking and alcohol dependence: Obstetric and gynecologic implications. *Obstetrics & Gynecology, 118*(2), 383–388. https://doi.org/10.1097/AOG.0b013e31822c9906

Essenmacher, C., Baird, C., Houfek, J., Spielman, M. R., & Adams, S. (2021). Nursing competencies for treating tobacco use and dependence: A systems-level change invitation to improve healthcare. *Journal of the American Psychiatric Nurses Association, 28*(1), 23–36. https://doi.org/10.1177/10783903211058785

Gasser, M. (2022, March 28). *The truth about alcohol and why it is so dangerous.* Transcendence Treatment Center. https://ttreatment.org/the-truth-about-alcohol-and-why-it-is-so-dangerous

Gotham, H. (n.d.). Screening and brief intervention for substance use: A health imperative [PowerPoint slides]. Retrieved May 12, 2023, from https://umkc.app.box.com/s/mvwt992izkokxeswhso6iss2w9azbt6p

Gramlich, L., Tandon, P., & Rahman, A. (2021). Nutritional status in patients with sustained heavy alcohol use. *UpToDate.* https://www.uptodate.com/contents/nutritional-status-in-patients-with-sustained-heavy-alcohol-use

Herron, A. J., & Brennan, T. K. (2019). *The ASAM essentials of addiction medicine* (3rd ed.). Wolters Kluwer and the American Society of Addiction Medicine.

Hunter, C. L., Goodie, J. L., Oordt, M. S., & Dobmeyer, A. C. (2017). *Integrated behavior health in primary care: Step-by-step guidance for assessment and intervention* (2nd ed.). American Psychological Association.

Iragorri, N., & Spackman, E. (2018). Assessing the value of screening tools: Reviewing the challenges and opportunities of cost-effective analysis. *Public Health Reviews, 39*(17). https://doi.org/10.1186/s40985-018-0093-8

Kaner, E. F. S., Beyer, F. R., Muirhead, C., Campbell, F., Pienaar, E. D., Bertholet, N., Daeppen, J. B., Saunders, J. B., & Burnand, B. (2018). Effectiveness of brief alcohol interventions in primary care populations. *Cochrane Database of Systematic Reviews 2018, 2*(CD004148). https://doi.org/10.1002/14651858.CD004148.pub4

Kelly, J. F., Humphreys, K., & Ferri, M. (2020). Alcoholics Anonymous and other 12-step programs for alcohol use disorder. *Cochrane Database of Systematic Reviews 2020, 3*(CD012880). https://doi.org/10.1002/14651858.CD012880.pub2

Ko, H., Chang, Y., Kim, H-N., Kang, J-H., Shin, H., Sung, E., & Ryu, S. (2021). Low-level alcohol consumption and cancer mortality. *Scientific Reports, 11*, 4585. https://doi.org/10.1038/s41598-021-84181-1

Levounis, P., Atnaout, B., & Marienfeld, C. (2017). *Motivational interviewing for clinical practice.* American Psychiatric Association.

Lynch, F. L., Peterson, E. L., Lu, C. Y., Rossom, R. C., Waitzfalder, B. E., Owen-Smith, A. A., Hubley, S., Prabhakar, D., Williams, L. K., Beck, A., Simon, G. E., & Ahmendani, B. K. (2020). Substance use disorders and risk of suicide in a general U.S. population: A case control study. *Addiction Science and Clinical Practice, 15*(14). https://doi.org/10.1186/s13722-020-0181-1

Manthou, E., Georgakouli, K., Fatouros, I. G., Gianoulakis, C., Theodorakis, Y., & Jamurtas, A. Z. (2016). Role of exercise in the treatment of alcohol use disorders: Review. *Biomedical Reports, 4*, 535–545. https://doi.org/10.3892/br.2016.626

Marshall, B., & Spencer, J. (2019). *Fast facts about substance use disorders: What every nurse, APRN, and PA needs to know.* Springer.

McKetta, S., & Keyes, K. M. (2019). Heavy and binge alcohol drinking and parenting status in the United States from 2006 to 2018: An analysis of nationally representative cross-sectional surveys. *PLoS Medicine, 16*(11), e1002954. https://doi.org/10.1371/journal.pmed.1002954

National Center for Chronic Disease Prevention and Health Promotion. (2021). *Excessive alcohol use.* Centers for Disease Control and Prevention. https://www.cdc.gov/chronicdisease/resources/publications/factsheets/alcohol.htm

National Center on Birth Defects and Developmental Disabilities. (2014). *Planning and implementing screening and brief intervention for risky alcohol use: A step-by-step guide for primary care practices.* Centers for Disease Control and Prevention. https://www.cdc.gov/ncbddd/fasd/documents/AlcoholSBIImplementationGuide-P.pdf

National Institute on Alcohol Abuse and Alcoholism. (2022a). *Alcohol facts and statistics.* https://www.niaaa.nih.gov/publications/brochures-and-fact-sheets/alcohol-facts-and-statistics

National Institute on Alcohol Abuse and Alcoholism. (2022b). *What is a standard drink?* https://www.niaaa

.nih.gov/alcohols-effects-health/overview-alcohol
-consumption/what-standard-drink

National Institute on Drug Abuse. (2021). *Alcohol: Key takeaways*. U.S. Department of Health and Human Services, National Institutes of Health. https://www .drugabuse.gov/drug-topics/alcohol

O'Connor, E., Perdue, L. A., Senger, C. A., Rushkin, M., Patnode, C. D., Bean, S. L., & Jonas, D. E. (2018). Screening and behavioral counseling interventions to reduce unhealthy alcohol use in adolescents and adults: Updated evidence report and systematic review for the U.S. Preventive Services Task Force Services. *JAMA*, *320*(18), 1910–1928. https://doi.org /doi:10.1001/jama.2018.12086

Pitrelli, A., Matkovic, L., Vacotto, M., Lopez-Costa, J. J., Basso, N., & Bruysco, A. (2018). Aerobic exercise upregulated the BDNF-serotonin systems and improves cognitive functioning in rats. *Neurobiology of Learning and Memory*, *155*, 528–542. https://doi .org/10.1016/j.nlm.2018.05.007

Quigley, J., Committee on Substance Use and Prevention, Ryan, S. A., Camenga, D. R., Patrick, S. W., Plumb, J., & Walker-Harding, L. (2019). Policy statement: Alcohol use by youth. *Pediatrics*, *144*(1), e20191356. https:// doi.org/10.1542/peds.2019-1356

Salisbury-Afshar, E., & Fleming, M. (2019). Identification of and treatment for unhealthy alcohol use in primary care settings. *American Family Physician*, *99*(12), 733–734.

Scott, A. J., Webb, T. L., St. James, M. M., Rowse, G., & Weich, S. (2021). Improving sleep quality leads to better mental health: A meta-analysis of randomized controlled trials. *Sleep Medicine Reviews*, *60*, 101556. https://doi.org/10.1016/j.smrv.2021.101556

Stahl, S. (2021). *Stahl's essential psychopharmacology* (5th ed.). Cambridge.

Substance Abuse and Mental Health Services Administration. (n.d.). *Alcohol use facts and resources*. Retrieved May 22, 2023, from https://www.samhsa.gov/sites /default/files/alcohol-use-facts-resources-fact-sheet.pdf

Substance Abuse and Mental Health Services Administration. (2021). *Key substance use and mental health indicators in the United States: Results from the 2020 National Survey on Drug Use and Health* (Publication No. PEP21-07-01-003). U.S. Department of Health and Human Services. https://www.samhsa .gov/data/sites/default/files/reports/rpt35325 /NSDUHFFRPDFWHTMLFiles2020/2020NSDUHFFR1 PDFW102121.pdf

Substance Abuse and Mental Health Services Administration. (2022). *Screening, brief intervention, and referral to treatment (SBIRT)*. https://www.samhsa .gov/sbirt

U.S. Department of Agriculture and U.S. Department of Health and Human Services. (2020). *Dietary guidelines for Americans, 2020-2025* (9th ed.). www .dietaryguidelines.gov

U.S. Preventive Services Task Force. (2018). *Final recommendation statement: Unhealthy alcohol use in adolescents and adults: Screening and behavioral counseling recommendations*. https://www.uspreventiveservicestaskforce.org /uspstf/recommendation/unhealthy-alcohol-use -in-adolescents-and-adults-screening-and-behavioral -counseling-interventions#fullrecommendationstart

Vistonay, R., Sunderland, M., Slade, T., Wilson, J., & Mewton, L. (2022). Are there non-linear relationships between alcohol consumption and long-term health? A systematic review of observational studies employing approaches to improve causal inference. *BMC Medical Research Methodology*, *22*(16). https:// doi.org/10.1186/s12874-021-01486-5

Woodward, J. J. (2019). The pharmacology of alcohol. In A. J. Herron & T. K. Brennan (Eds.), *The ASAM essentials of addiction medicine* (3rd ed.). Wolters Kluwer.

Zajicek, A., & Karan, L. D. (2019). Pharmacokinetic, pharmacodynamic, and pharmacogenomic principles. In A. J. Herron & T. K. Brennan (Eds.), *The ASAM essentials of addiction medicine* (3rd ed.). Wolters Kluwer.

Zhang, R., Shen, L., Miles, T., Shen, Y., Cordero, J., Qi, Y., Liang, L., & Li, C. (2020). Association of low to moderate alcohol drinking with cognitive functions from middle to older age among US adults. *JAMA Network Open*, *3*(6), e207922. https://doi.org/10.1001 /jamanetworkopen.2020.7922

CHAPTER 15

Rest More

Josie H. Bidwell, DNP, RN, FNP-C, DipACLM
Cindy Secrist Rima, DNP, APRN, ANP-BC, DipACLM
Lawrence Chan, DO

Sleep is medicine with many health benefits, as recommended, and can be taken every 24 hours without side effects.

Dr. Loureen Downes

OBJECTIVES

This chapter will enable the reader to:

1. Describe concepts of sleep–wakefulness regulation and sleep stages in sleep physiology.
2. Discuss the effect of sleep on select health conditions.
3. Describe appropriate sleep assessment strategies.
4. Discuss select sleep disorders.
5. Explain basic sleep hygiene principles.
6. Discuss the importance of an interprofessional approach to sleep health.
7. Examine the use of goal setting in optimizing sleep habits.
8. Formulate a lifestyle management prescription to address selected sleep-related issues.

Overview

This chapter will introduce the advanced practice provider (APP) to the role of restful sleep in overall health promotion and disease prevention. Sleep is essential to sustain human life (Sullivan et al., 2022). By understanding the basic physiology of sleep and its effect on select body systems, the APP will be prepared to provide sleep assessments, sleep hygiene counseling, and lifestyle-based sleep prescriptions.

Sleep Physiology

Sleep can be described as "a reversible behavioral state of perceptual disengagement from and unresponsiveness to the environment" (Sullivan et al., 2022, p. 16). While sleep is not fully understood, multiple physiological effects have been theorized, including restoration, clearance function, neural plasticity, memory consolidation, and energy conservation. Ideally, periods of sleep and wakefulness

© Kathleen Gail/Shutterstock; © StoryTime Studio/Shutterstock; © kali9/Getty Images

exist in a pattern that supports optimal mental and physical homeostasis and health.

Regulation of Sleep and Wakefulness

Historically, the process of sleep was thought of as a passive activity. However, it is now recognized as an active process primarily controlled by sleep-promoting and wakefulness-promoting neurotransmitter systems and the individual's circadian rhythm. Circadian rhythms are heavily influenced by the suprachiasmatic nucleus, also known as the master clock.

Critical factors in the sleep–wakefulness regulation processes include exposure to daylight or a similar light spectrum and the accumulation of adenosine, which occurs at a higher rate throughout the wakefulness cycle. The presence or absence of light is perceived by specialized sensory cells in the retina—the intrinsic photosensitive retinal ganglion cells (ipRGCs). Although ipRGCs do not transmit visual images, their ability to perceive light facilitates the pupillary constriction response to light stimulus. More importantly, ipRGCs provide the input for the retino-hypothalamo-pineal pathway, which synchronizes the sleep–wake cycle with the light–dark cycle. The ipRGCs signal the suprachiasmatic nucleus in the hypothalamus when the presence of light is of a wavelength associated with the natural light spectrum. The pathway then signals the pineal gland to either increase the production and release of melatonin, a hormone long associated with controlling the sleep–wake cycle, as darkness approaches or to block melatonin production in the presence of natural light (Mure, 2021; Wyatt, 2020). See **Figure 15.1**.

Additional mechanisms are in place to support arousal. The thalamocortical network, arousal centers located in the brain stem and hypothalamus, supports wakefulness (Luppi & Fort, 2019). One family of primarily excitatory neuropeptides produced by the hypothalamus are the orexins. It is thought that orexins regulate behavior during times of threat exposure, physiological need, and opportunities for reward by stimulating the release of additional alertness-promoting neurotransmitters such as norepinephrine, serotonin, and dopamine and affecting multiple structures across the central nervous system. Of note, two groups of researchers discovered these neuropeptides near the same time; therefore, these neuropeptides are known in the scientific community by the interchangeable names of orexin or hypocretin (de Lecea et al., 1998).

A powerful driver for sleep in the sleep–wake cycle is adenosine. Adenosine is released when adenosine triphosphate (ATP) is broken down to release energy for physiological functions such as active transport, the synthesis of protein and other chemical compounds, and muscle contraction (Barrett et al., 2019). As energy is needed and produced throughout the day, adenosine accumulates. This progressive accumulation of adenosine is sensed by specialized cells and is the predominant factor contributing to increasing sleep pressure and the homeostatic sleep drive (Lazarus et al., 2019). Interestingly, caffeine enhances wakefulness due to its ability to block the action of adenosine.

As one engages in restful slumber, the benefits include many restorative processes: the clearance of metabolic waste, support of neural plasticity and memory consolidation, and energy conservation. However, if one chooses to disregard these signals and remain in the wakefulness phase for extended periods, adenosine levels continue to rise, progressively increasing the drive for sleep, especially if wakefulness continues into the early-morning hours. Eventually, the sleep drive reaches undeniable levels, which may no longer be willfully deferred (Wyatt, 2020).

As night and darkness fade, the arousing effect of sunlight and the light phase again initiate wakefulness. This stimulation can also occur with artificial light sources, especially within the sunlight spectrum, and may influence the overall timing of the sleep–wake cycle.

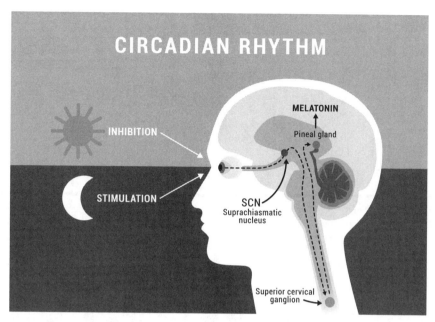

Figure 15.1 Circadian rhythm.

© elenabsl/Shutterstock

Light exposure near the end of a sleep event or early in wakefulness can aid in advancing sleep cycles to earlier in the day (phase advance). Conversely, light exposure in the evening or first half of one's typical period causes a later circadian rhythm (phase delay) (Wyatt, 2020).

Stages of Sleep

The stages of sleep can be loosely grouped into nonrapid eye movement (NREM) and rapid eye movement (REM) states. Sleep staging is determined through the use of electroencephalogram (EEG) evaluation. NREM is comprised of several individual stages. Historically, four phases (stages 1, 2, 3, and 4) were delineated in the NREM state. However, a newer classification consolidates the two later NREM sleep stages into one stage. Therefore, the most current nomenclature utilized to describe NREM sleep is N1, N2, and N3 (Berry et al., 2020). See sleep stages in **Table 15.1**.

Stage N1 is described as the lightest phase of sleep and is characterized by easy arousability. Healthy young adults spend approximately 5% to 10% of a sleep episode in this stage. Stage N2 is characterized by the appearance of sleep spindles and K complexes, which are associated with memory consolidation. Stage N2 comprises the largest total amount of sleep (45–55%) during a sleep event. The final stage of NREM sleep, N3, is also known as slow-wave sleep (SWS), or deep sleep. Adults spend approximately 10% to 20% of a sleep episode in this stage of sleep. Arousability during NREM sleep is most difficult during this stage (Kirsch, 2021).

REM sleep is characterized by rapid eye movements and dreaming. Approximately 18% to 23% of total sleep time is spent in REM sleep (Kirsch, 2021). REM sleep is distinctive for irregular respiratory rate, heart rate, ventilation, and blood pressure as well as atonia on electromyogram (EMG) due to direct alpha motor neuron inhibition occurring. Atonia results from direct blocking of alpha motor neurons resulting in the inactivity of all voluntary muscles except the diaphragm and extraocular muscles. It has the net benefit of minimizing the risk of injury during REM's active dream state (Luppi & Fort, 2019).

Table 15.1 Sleep Stages

Category	Stage	Characteristic	Percentage of Sleep Episode
NREM	N1	Lightest phase; easy arousability	5–10%
NREM	N2	Sleep spindles and K complexes; memory consolidation	45–55%
NREM	N3	Slow-wave, or deep, sleep; arousability difficult	10–20%
REM		Rapid eye movements; dreaming	18–23%

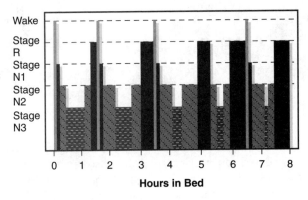

Figure 15.2 Sleep hypnogram.

Data from Roehrs, T. & Roth, T. (2020). The effects of medications on sleep quality and sleep architecture. UpToDate. Retrieved January 6, 2022, from https://www.uptodate.com/contents/the-effects-of-medications-on-sleep-quality-and-sleep-architecture.

Sleep Architecture

An individual's sleep event does not progress linearly from wakefulness to N1, N2, N3, and REM sleep. Instead, sleep events are categorized by cycles of both NREM and REM states that change in duration and frequency during the sleep episode (McGinty & Szymusiak, 2022). The cyclical progression of sleep staging is depicted in the sleep hypnogram in **Figure 15.2**. In this example, the individual progresses from wakefulness to N1, followed by progression to N2 and then N3 but returns to N2 before proceeding to REM sleep (Miller et al., 2015). The duration of time spent in each stage changes as the sleep episode progresses with increases in REM duration and decreases in N3. In general, REM sleep occurs every 90 to 120 minutes. Brief periods of wakefulness that the individual often does not appreciate are also part of normal sleep architecture (Kirsch, 2021).

Sleep architecture is influenced by intrinsic and extrinsic factors. One of the most important intrinsic factors is age. Sleep architecture changes across the life span. In early infancy, sleep onset is characterized by REM sleep (Wise & Glaze, 2021). This changes over to NREM entry into sleep at approximately 3 months (Kirsch, 2021). Babies also spend much longer in REM sleep, and sleep cycles are shorter in duration than in other age categories. Children and adolescents begin a sleep event in NREM and spend about 75% of a sleep episode in this phase. Sleep cycles occur approximately every 90 to 100 minutes. Additionally, the amount of time spent in stage N3 begins to decrease during puberty and extends into adulthood (Wise & Glaze, 2021). Middle-aged and older adults spend less time in N3 and have more periods of awakenings and N1 sleep (Kirsch, 2021).

Medications are a common extrinsic factor that can disrupt sleep architecture. Any medication or substance that crosses the blood–brain barrier can affect sleep quality and staging. Common medications and their effect on sleep are presented in **Table 15.2**.

Table 15.2 Effect of Select Medications on Sleep Quality and Architecture

Medication Class	Effect on Sleep
Benzodiazepines	Reduce time to sleep onset Reduce N1 sleep time Increase N2 sleep time Rebound insomnia upon cessation
Anti-seizure	Reduce time to sleep onset Increase total sleep time Reduce REM sleep
Tricyclic antidepressants (tertiary)	Reduce time to sleep onset Reduce wakefulness after sleep initiation Reduce REM sleep
Selective serotonin reuptake inhibitors (SSRIs)	Reduce total sleep time Increase wakefulness after sleep initiation Reduce REM sleep
Lithium	Increase total sleep time Reduce REM sleep Increase N3 sleep time
Opioids	Reduce N3 sleep time May reduce REM sleep
Central nervous system (CNS) stimulants	Increase time to sleep onset Increase wakefulness after sleep initiation Increase N1 sleep time Reduce N3 sleep time Reduce REM sleep time
Atypical antipsychotics	Reduce time to sleep onset Increase total sleep time Increase N3 sleep time Reduce REM sleep time
Beta blockers	Increase wakefulness following sleep initiation Reduce REM sleep time

Data from Roehrs, T., & Roth, T. (2020). The effects of medications on sleep quality and sleep architecture. *UpToDate*. https://www.uptodate.com/contents/the-effects-of-medications-on-sleep-quality-and-sleep-architecture

Sleep Effect on Health

Sleep is believed to play an important physiological role in health, as evidenced by the negative effects of decreased sleep duration. Liew and Aung (2021) reviewed 135 original English articles on sleep deprivation and diseases published between January 2014 and March 2020. While some findings were inconclusive, the preponderance of data concluded that sleep deprivation is associated with a vast array of pathophysiological sequelae and diseases.

The link between sleep and cardiovascular outcomes has become increasingly apparent. Sleep deprivation increases the risk of hypertension, stroke, and coronary heart disease (Cappuccio et al., 2011; Khani et al., 2018; Matthews et al., 2018; Patyar & Patyar, 2015). Obstructive sleep apnea has also been identified as an independent risk factor for several cardiovascular diseases, including hypertension, pulmonary hypertension, heart failure, arrhythmias, coronary artery disease, and stroke (Javaheri et al., 2017). Due to destabilizing normal sleep patterns, shift work and subsequent insufficient sleep have

Effect of Impaired Sleep and Sleep Deprivation

- Impaired memory and attention control
- Emotional lability
- Aggressive behavior and socialization problems
- Cognitive instability and structural brain function lapses
- Accumulation of CNS waste products due to glymphatic pathway dysfunction
- Impaired protein synthesis, myelination, synapse formation, and cellular detoxification
- Altered amyloid-beta precursor processing
- Increased tau accumulation, plaque deposits, and amyloid-beta accumulation
- Higher sympathetic nervous system activation
- Dysfunction of nitric oxide–mediated vasodilation
- Endothelial dysfunction–associated reduction in REM sleep
- Blood pressure remains higher during sleep
- Impaired heart rate recovery after exercise
- Higher risk for hypertension, stroke, and diabetes
- Increased metabolic syndrome and central obesity
- Hepatic inflammation and apoptosis of hepatocytes
- Non-alcoholic fatty liver disease (NAFLD) associated with repetitive sleep reductions
- Glucose and lipid metabolism dysfunction
- Loss of bone density (sarcopenia and osteopenia)
- Impaired wound healing
- Exacerbation of early-stage psoriasis
- Increased wrinkles
- Immune system dysfunction
- Increased inflammatory mediator biomarkers, negatively affecting clotting and inducing blood–brain barrier leakage
- Augmented neutrophil response
- Induction of pro-inflammatory cytokines
- Reduced mast cell regulation
- Blunted responses of the autonomic nervous system to environmental cues

Data from Liew, S. C., & Aung, T. (2021). Sleep deprivation and its association with diseases: A review. *Sleep Medicine, 77*, 192–204. https://doi.org/10.1016/j.sleep.2020.07.048

been associated with accidents, coronary heart disease, stroke, and cancer (Kecklund & Axelsson, 2016). Chronic sleep disruption has been linked to abnormal glucose metabolism through its effects on leptin, ghrelin, and appetite regulation as well as the increased risk of obesity. Decreased sleep is also associated with breast, colorectal, and prostate cancer (Gapstur et al., 2014; Lehrer et al., 2013; Luyster et al., 2012). These risks make assessing sleep an important part of the APP's tool kit.

Sleep Disorders

Sleep disorders are broadly categorized into insomnias, sleep-related breathing disorders, central disorders of hypersomnolence, circadian rhythm sleep–wake disorders, parasomnias, and sleep-related movement disorders (American Academy of Sleep Medicine [AASM], 2014; Sateia & Thorpy, 2022). Awareness of these disorders will help identify patients who may need a sleep specialist referral.

Insomnia is persistent difficulty falling asleep or staying asleep with associated daytime symptoms such as fatigue, irritability, inattention, and impaired school or work performance. It is separated into short-term versus chronic insomnia by a time frame of 3 months (AASM, 2014). Insomnia is a common complaint in clinical practice. Still, it is essential to consider other sleep disorders as potential causes as well as chronic medical conditions and medications that may be contributing factors.

Sleep-related breathing disorders include various forms of sleep apnea and sleep-related hypoventilation (Sateia & Thorpy, 2022). Patients will typically present with sleep disturbance; daytime sleepiness; and symptoms suggestive of breathing difficulty, including snoring, gasping, or choking. Bed partners may be the ones to identify symptoms instead of patients themselves. Individuals with sleep-related breathing disorders tend to have a higher body mass index, enlarged neck circumference, and crowded upper airways and may have comorbid medical issues like hypertension and diabetes (AASM, 2014).

Central disorders of hypersomnolence include diagnoses of narcolepsy and idiopathic hypersomnia and are characterized by persistent daytime sleepiness despite obtaining adequate sleep at night. Narcolepsy can include symptoms of sleep paralysis and hallucinations while transitioning between sleep and wake. Cataplexy, a symptom specific to narcolepsy, is sudden muscle weakness triggered by sudden strong emotions such as laughter, anger, stress, and excitement. Patients do not lose consciousness during cataplexy (AASM, 2014; Sateia & Thorpy, 2022).

Circadian rhythm sleep–wake disorders describe a misalignment between a patient's sleep–wake cycle and a conventional or patient-specific environmental schedule. Most encountered are delayed sleep–wake phase disorders, which result in difficulty falling asleep and problems waking up in the morning. In contrast, advanced sleep–wake phase disorders manifest as falling asleep and waking up too early (AASM, 2014; Sateia & Thorpy, 2022).

Parasomnias describe several sleep-related phenomena, including sleepwalking, sleep terrors, and nightmares. Although most are benign, one specific parasomnia, REM behavior disorder, is associated with neurodegenerative disorders such as Parkinson's disease (AASM, 2014; Sateia & Thorpy, 2022). The primary focus in the management of parasomnias is maintaining the safety of the patient and others.

Sleep-related movement disorders include restless legs syndrome, periodic limb movement disorder, and bruxism. Symptoms are typically managed only if they cause sleep disruption. Restless legs syndrome is the most common of these disorders and is described as an urge to move one's legs, which is worse in the evening and at rest and is improved with movement (AASM, 2014; Sateia & Thorpy, 2022).

Health Promotion Research Study

Effects of Diet on Sleep

Background: Cardiometabolic diseases, including obesity, diabetes, and hypertension, have been associated with poor sleep quantity and quality. Because diet plays a foundational role in the prevention, treatment, and reversal of chronic disease, this study aimed to review the available evidence related to sleep-promoting foods.

Methodology: A systematic review strategy was employed to search multiple databases for study review. Review authors searched PubMed (MEDLINE), Cumulative Index of Nursing and Allied Health Literature (CINAHL), and Cochrane for studies examining diet and sleep in healthy adults between 1990 and 2019. Studies were excluded if they included any other sleep-promoting interventions or if participants had acute or chronic health conditions. Studies were also excluded from the review if full-text English versions were not available. In the initial literature search, 3,545 studies were identified. However, following the removal of duplicates and application of exclusion criteria, 32 studies were appropriate for inclusion in the full review.

Results: Tryptophan-rich foods led to improvements in sleep quality and quantity when compared to controls while tryptophan-depleted foods were associated with less overall sleep time and sleep efficiency. There was variable, low-quality evidence on the use of certain supplements for sleep improvement. However, when consumed as part of a whole food, the evidence for the addition of cherries, which are a source of melatonin, was more consistent. Cherries (Jerte Valley or Montgomery tart) were associated with improved sleep time and efficiency. This finding was most significant for those middle-aged or older. Adjusting the ratio of macronutrient groups also produced changes in sleep quality and quantity. High carbohydrate meals when eaten 4 hours before bedtime did produce a shortened sleep onset latency. Of note, the quality of the carbohydrate was important because refined sugar led to increased arousal. Furthermore, fiber-rich meals were associated with less time in N1 and more time in N3. While these results are promising, further research is needed to fully understand the effect of macronutrients, supplements, and specific whole foods on sleep.

Implications for Advanced Practice: Understanding the role of nutrition in healthy, restful, sleep is an important skill for the APP. The APP should be able to not only draw the correlation between diet and chronic disease but also how to add or remove foods to improve the condition.

Reference: Data from Binks, H., Vincent, G. E., Gupta, C., Irwin, C., & Khalesi, S. (2020). Effects of diet on sleep: A narrative review. *Nutrients*, *12*, 936. https://doi.org/ doi:10.3390/nu12040936

Sleep Assessment

A thorough sleep assessment will attempt to identify a patient's concerns, sleep–wake pattern, bedtime environment, and behaviors while also identifying any potential disorders that might affect their sleep (Berry & Wagner, 2014; Goldstein & Chervin, 2022). These findings will allow the APP to take appropriate action and provide suitable prescriptions. The sleep assessment typically begins with an open-ended question regarding sleep concerns, obtaining broad categories that are later explored in greater detail. Any recent changes, stressors, or triggers should be explored.

The patient's general sleep schedule is obtained by asking when they go to bed and how long it takes to fall asleep. Sleep duration varies by age, with more sleep required in infancy, childhood, and adolescence. Most adults need between 7 and 9 hours of sleep daily (Hirshkowitz et al., 2015). Age-specific guidelines are presented in **Table 15.3**.

The number and duration of nocturnal awakenings help determine the level of fragmentation. Asking what causes the awakenings

Table 15.3 National Sleep Foundation–Recommended Sleep Duration

Age	Number of Hours
Newborns	14–17 hours
Infants	12–15 hours
Toddlers	11–14 hours
Preschoolers	10–13 hours
School-aged children	9–11 hours
Teenagers	8–10 hours
Young adults/adults	7–9 hours
Older adults	7–8 hours

Data from Hirshkowitz, M., Whiton, K., Albert, S. M., Alessi, C., Bruni, O., DonCarlos, L., Hazen, N., Herman, J., Katz, E. S., Kheirandish-Gozal, L., Neubauer, D. N., O'Donnell, A. E., Ohayon, M., Peever, J., Rawding, R., Sachdeva, R. C., Setters, B., Vitiello, M. V., Ware, J. C., & Adams Hillard, P. J. (2015). National Sleep Foundation's sleep time duration recommendations: Methodology and results summary. *Sleep Health, 1*(1), 40–43. https://doi.org/10.1016/j.sleh.2014.12.010

(e.g., sound, pain, urination) provides clues to possible sleep disturbance causes. The final wake-up time and overall subjective sleep time help determine whether the patient is getting adequate amounts. Comparing weekday (workday) and weekend (off-day) schedules shows the effects of work and other responsibilities on sleep and may reveal patterns of sleep deprivation and attempts to catch up. For a more thorough assessment, ask the patient to complete a two-week sleep diary, which helps both the patient and the APP visualize irregular sleep schedules and circadian rhythm disorders (see Table 15.5).

The patient's nighttime routine may identify behaviors or environmental factors that affect their sleep quality (Berry & Wagner, 2014; Goldstein & Chervin, 2022). Review the patient's sleep environment, including noise levels, extraneous light, bed mattress comfort, temperature, and screen time around bedtime. Explore whether they have children, pets, or bed partners that contribute to awakenings. Behaviors such as clock watching, completing work tasks, and watching television increase wakefulness and weaken the association

between the bed and sleep. The light produced by screens tends to fall in the blue wavelength, which potently and quickly suppresses melatonin. Caffeine, alcohol, and nicotine all have negative effects on sleep as well.

Daytime activities also are key, as decreased exercise and daytime light exposure may worsen sleep quality. Inquire about anxiety and worries that lead to ruminations that commonly impede sleep onset. Frequent and long naps are also known to disrupt sleep (Berry & Wagner, 2014; Goldstein & Chervin, 2022).

Broadly screen for common sleep disorders. Ask about snoring or episodes of gasping or observed apneic episodes. Review morning symptoms such as unrefreshing sleep, dry mouth, or morning headaches. Inquire about bothersome movements when trying to fall asleep or after falling asleep. Review symptoms of daytime sleepiness, particularly when the patient is driving or operating heavy machinery (Berry & Wagner, 2014; Goldstein & Chervin, 2022). Collateral information from close friends, spouses, or family members is often helpful.

Consider using questionnaires like the Pittsburgh Sleep Quality Index to assess general sleep quality. The Functional Outcomes of Sleep Questionnaire measures the effect of sleepiness on daily activities. Other scales, such as the STOP-BANG, Insomnia Severity Index, Epworth Sleepiness Scale, and International Restless Legs Scale, can be used when specific disorders are suspected (Berry & Wagner, 2014; Goldstein & Chervin, 2022).

An actigraph is a device that is typically worn on the wrist and estimates sleep primarily based on movement. Manufacturer algorithms score sleep during periods when activity is significantly reduced while periods with more activity are scored as awake. Some devices will capture noise and light levels as well. Actigraphy is attractive because it is noninvasive, can be utilized in one's home, and can help assess circadian rhythm disorders and sleep patterns (Berry & Wagner, 2014;

Goldstein & Chervin, 2022). However, given the lack of additional parameters such as EEG, sleep staging is unavailable, and the total sleep time is considered an estimation.

Polysomnography (PSG) performed in a sleep laboratory is currently the most complete sleep assessment. During PSG, information is obtained by monitoring EEG, EMG, electrooculogram (EOG), electrocardiogram (ECG), snoring, airflow, nasal pressure, breathing effort, pulse oximetry, and body position. PSG is primarily used to diagnose sleep-related breathing and movement disorders, central disorders of hypersomnolence, and specific parasomnias (Berry & Wagner, 2014; Goldstein & Chervin, 2022).

Health Promotion

Interprofessional Team

APPs should initiate a discussion with patients about the importance of sleep in preventing, treating, and reversing chronic disease. The APP can also play an essential role in determining the current state of a patient's rest and the effect on overall health. However, an interprofessional approach should be utilized in suspected sleep disorders or comorbid psychiatric conditions. Additional team members may include a sleep medicine specialist and a mental health professional.

A sleep medicine specialist is a physician specially trained in the assessment, diagnosis, and treatment of sleep disorders, including but not limited to insomnia, obstructive sleep apnea, and periodic limb movement disorders. Treatment may include both pharmacological and nonpharmacological therapy. When the underlying cause of the sleep disturbance is not readily apparent, it is appropriate to consult a sleep medicine specialist (AASM, 2022).

Mental health professionals addressing sleep health may be psychiatrists, psychiatric–mental health nurse practitioners, clinical psychologists, or licensed professional counselors. Treatment of comorbid psychiatric disorders

such as depression and anxiety can often be beneficial in treating insomnia and other sleep disorders (Alvaro et al., 2013). Cognitive behavioral therapy for insomnia (CBT-I) is a powerful tool in treating insomnia, improving the amount of time spent in restful sleep for 70% to 80% of patients (Trauer et al., 2015).

Starting the Conversation

As with most health behavior changes, motivational interviewing techniques should be employed to start the conversation and gauge individual interest in the anticipated change. One of the quickest and easiest to implement tools is the Sleep Readiness-to-Change Ruler (see **Figure 15.3**). By discerning the importance and confidence around health behavior change related to sleep, the APP can gauge interest in change and any barriers in enacting that change.

For optimal likelihood of behavior change adoption, the patient should choose a rating of 7 or higher for importance and confidence (Boudreaux et al., 2012; Hesse, 2006). The APP can address a low importance rating by sharing information about the effect of sleep health on other chronic conditions (e.g., heart disease, diabetes, weight management) to increase relevance to the patient. Additionally, interventions matched with the patient's stage of change should be employed for any stage (Prochaska & DiClemente, 2005).

Sleep Hygiene and Counseling

Consistent restorative sleep requires planning and adjustments to daily habits and routines. Sleep hygiene counseling should focus on sleep preparation, maximization of positive daily habits, and a restful sleep environment.

Consistency is fundamental to establishing and maintaining a healthy sleep pattern. It is crucial to maintain a schedule and routine for sleep that is consistent from day to day to support a well-functioning circadian rhythm.

Sleep Readiness-to-Change Ruler

How important is it to you to make changes to your sleep habits? (Circle the number)

0	1	2	3	4	5	6	7	8	9	10
Not important										Very important

How confident are you that you can make changes to your sleep habits? (Circle the number)

0	1	2	3	4	5	6	7	8	9	10
Not important										Very important

Figure 15.3 Sleep Readiness-to-Change Ruler.

If adjustments to bedtime and wake time are required, it is best to make these changes gradually in 1- to 2-hour increments each day (National Heart, Lung, and Blood Institute [NHLBI], 2011).

In addition to maintaining a consistent sleep and wake schedule, a well-established routine can support initiating and maintaining a healthy sleep episode. A warm shower or bath can generate feelings of relaxation and sleepiness due to a drop in core body temperature following this activity. Quiet activities such as reading or listening to calming music can also benefit a daily sleep routine. Furthermore, late afternoon napping can lead to delayed sleep onset and should be avoided (NHLBI, 2011).

Food and beverage choices can have a detrimental effect on achieving and maintaining quality sleep. A large meal close to bedtime can cause dyspepsia and impaired sleep onset. Additionally, the increased consumption of fluids at night may lead to interrupted sleep due to nocturia. Alcohol is often used in the evening for relaxation and sleep induction. However, alcohol consumption contributes to lighter stages of sleep and nighttime awakenings. Even light alcohol consumption, defined as one serving per day for women and two servings per day for men, is associated with a 9.3% reduction in sleep quality (Pietila et al., 2018). Therefore, alcohol should be avoided within 4 hours of bedtime to support restful sleep (Stein & Friedman, 2006). Furthermore,

caffeine has a relatively long half-life (4–6 hours) that can delay sleep onset if consumed in the afternoon and evening (NHLBI, 2011). Caffeine should be discontinued at least 6 hours before the desired bedtime (Drake et al., 2013).

Physical activity can help support a healthy sleep pattern. However, the sleep onset may be adversely affected when exercise occurs within 2 to 3 hours of the desired bedtime. Exposure to daylight is also beneficial in establishing regular sleep–wake cycles. Acquiring 30 minutes of daily sunlight is sufficient to reinforce this benefit (NHLBI, 2011).

Maximization of a restful sleep environment should focus on light, noise, and room temperature. Most importantly, the bedroom should be used only for sleep and sexual encounters. Other leisure activities should be conducted in a separate location to reinforce the likelihood of successful sleep onset and maintenance. A decrease in core body temperature is associated with a release of melatonin. Therefore, a cool room temperature is also beneficial. A room temperature of 60 to 67 degrees Fahrenheit is considered appropriate for promoting a healthy sleep pattern in adults (Pacheco, 2021).

Exposure to excessive light can inhibit the natural release of melatonin. The use of light dimmer switches during the evening hours can begin to signal the body that bedtime is approaching. Additionally, the blue wavelength light emitted by electronics such as televisions, tablets, cellular phones, and computers can impair melatonin's natural release, leading to delayed sleep onset. Therefore, the use of electronic devices should cease at least 60 minutes before anticipated bedtime. As much as feasible, the bedroom should be technology-free. If an electronic device is required, the lowest brightness setting and any modes to assist with sleep should be employed (Suni, 2020).

Health Promotion Case Study Addressing Sleep Health in an Adult Female

Case Description: V.S. is a 45-year-old Hispanic female who presents for a follow-up visit for uncontrolled hypertension. She endorses taking her antihypertensive medication as prescribed. She has previously tried diuretic therapy and was unable to tolerate it.

- Past medical history: Hypertension, obesity (class 3), asthma.
- Medications: Amlodipine 10 mg daily; lisinopril 40 mg daily.
- Past surgical history: Hysterectomy.
- Family history: Type 2 diabetes (paternal grandfather), mitral valve prolapse (mother).
- Social history: Elementary school teacher; married for 20 years; one child, 15-year-old son.
- Review of systems: Remarkable only for daytime fatigue, snoring, and waking at least once during the night to urinate.
- Vital signs: Blood pressure 142/82 mmHg, heart rate 84 bpm, respiratory rate 16 bpm, temp 98°F, oxygen saturation 99% on room air.
- Physical exam: Unremarkable.

Lifestyle Vital Signs

- Adopt healthy eating: 24-hour diet recall includes breakfast of large coffee with three Splenda packets; no morning snack; often skips lunch; afternoon snack of chips and peanuts from a vending machine; dinner of spaghetti with garlic bread and wine.
- Stress less: Denies new stressors. States that stress levels are manageable.
- Move often: 2 days per week of walking the dog for 15 minutes; no resistance or flexibility exercises.
- Avoid alcohol: Drinks 1–2 glasses of white wine (5 oz each) daily. Denies substance use.
- Rest more: 10 p.m. bedtime; 1–2 hours to fall asleep (watching television); 1–2 awakenings during the night (to urinate); 30 minutes to fall back asleep; awakens at 5:30 a.m.; gets out of bed at 6:15 a.m. (hits snooze multiple times); 4/10 refreshed, states she feels sluggish and foggy; snores.
- Treat tobacco use: Never smoked. No smokeless tobacco.
- BMI: 36 kg/m^2.

Critical Thinking Questions

1. Does V.S. have a problem with sleep quantity, sleep quality, or both? Discuss your rationale.
2. What additional screening tests, if any, are needed to evaluate her sleep?
3. What factors in the above subjective and objective data could potentially affect V.S.'s sleep health?
4. What potential sleep-related modifications could you recommend to address V.S.'s sleep health?

Rest Prescription

A successful sleep health prescription is patient led and provider supported. After assessment and brief counseling by the APP, the patient is the expert in deciding what intervention is important and achievable in their life. The APP should clearly articulate the role of sleep in preventing, treating, or reversing the patient's medical condition. Following this, the APP may offer several potential sleep-related modifications and empower the patient to choose the modification they are most confident in incorporating into their life. For example, the APP may discuss the role of afternoon caffeine consumption and bedtime screen use in insomnia. However, if the patient enjoys watching the nighttime news in bed with their spouse, targeting afternoon caffeine consumption is more likely to be achievable and sustainable.

As with any health behavior change, a well-crafted goal is foundational to ensuring success. SMART goal methodology is a well-validated strategy in goal setting in which goals are written using specific, measurable, achievable, relevant, and time-bound language (Bodenheimer & Handley, 2009). To ensure that a goal is both achievable and relevant, the APP can utilize the change rulers. A goal that scores ≥7 on the importance and confidence scale is more likely to be achieved. In the previous example, the APP could guide the patient to set a goal to avoid caffeine consumption after lunch.

An action plan should be developed to clearly and concisely delineate the steps required to achieve the SMART goal. Additionally, acknowledging potential barriers and creating a backup plan for attaining the SMART goal are often overlooked but important steps in goal achievement. In the previous example, the patient could develop a plan to choose decaffeinated green tea instead of coffee for their afternoon beverage choice. Because the coffee is being utilized for afternoon energy, backup strategies may focus on other ways to improve energy, such as deep breathing exercises and short walk breaks. The most important factor

Table 15.4 Example of a Rest Prescription

Component	Prescription
Goal	To promote falling asleep more easily, I will avoid caffeine after lunch.
Action plan	I will choose decaffeinated green tea for my afternoon beverage.
Backup plan	If I feel tired in the afternoon, I will do some deep breathing exercises or take a 5-minute walk around my office.

Health Promotion Activity: Assessing and Addressing Sleep Health

1. Conduct a sleep screening assessment of a classmate (or as directed by your course faculty) using one of the instruments discussed in this chapter.
2. Develop two lifestyle prescriptions for rest based on the assessment findings.

in choosing the action and backup plans is that the patient designs the process. This increases the likelihood of adoption into daily living. An example of this process is depicted in the written prescription provided in **Table 15.4**.

Summary

Restful sleep is a foundational component of disease prevention, treatment, and reversal.

Alterations to quantity, quality, or both can affect many body systems and medical conditions. Sleep is not a passive process and is not merely the absence of consciousness. Through multiple physiological activities, sleep has the potential to either be beneficial or detrimental to cardiometabolic processes that involve heart disease, glycemic control, and weight management. Sleep and rest also play a fundamental role in the mental health of individuals.

The APP has a responsibility to understand the physiological implications of poor sleep, accurately assess a patient's sleep status, and facilitate the development of a person-centered treatment plan to address sleep-related issues. An accurate assessment is the basis for providing a person-centered treatment plan. At the most basic, the APP should collect information related to both sleep quality and quantity. A comprehensive sleep assessment is supported by validated screening tools (see **Table 15.5**). Not only should the APP evaluate for diagnosable sleep disorders but also environmental, behavioral, and psychological factors, which may influence rest and sleep. In particular, the APP should be familiar with the role of sleep hygiene, including but not limited to light exposure, caffeine, alcohol, and temperature, in the achievement and maintenance of quality sleep.

Through motivational interviewing techniques, SMART goal development, and action planning, the APP can design a therapeutic lifestyle prescription to promote rest and sleep. Utilization of an interprofessional team should be encouraged when applicable to fully evaluate and manage these patients. The primary care provider or the sleep subspecialist may play a role in adjusting medications that influence sleep staging and rhythms. Additionally, referral for CBT-I is an important consideration when working on behavioral aspects affecting sleep and rest. This chapter provides the foundational information needed for the APP to provide quality assessment, diagnosis, referral, and treatment for alterations in sleep and rest.

TABLE 15.5 Evidence-Based Resources: Rest

Resource	URL
American Academy of Sleep Medicine (includes practice guidelines, clinical resources, and patient information)	https://aasm.org
Sleep Foundation	https://www.sleepfoundation.org
Single-Item Sleep Quality Scale	https://www.ncbi.nlm.nih.gov/pmc/articles /PMC6223557/pdf/jcsm.14.11.1849.pdf
AASM Two-Week Sleep Diary	https://sleepeducation.org/docs/default-document -library/sleep-diary.pdf
Pittsburgh Sleep Quality Index	https://www.sleep.pitt.edu/instruments
Epworth Sleepiness Scale	https://epworthsleepinessscale.com/about-the-ess
Functional Outcomes of Sleep Questionnaire	https://www.thoracic.org/members/assemblies /assemblies/srn/questionaires/fosq.php
STOP-BANG (sleep apnea)	https://www.mdcalc.com/stop-bang-score-obstructive -sleep-apnea
Insomnia Severity Index	https://www.ons.org/sites/default/files /InsomniaSeverityIndex_ISI.pdf
International Restless Legs Scale	https://biolincc.nhlbi.nih.gov/media/studies/masm /IRLS.pdf?link_time=2019-07-07_21:09:19.282153

Acronyms

APP: advanced practice provider
ATP: adenosine triphosphate
CBT-I: cognitive behavioral therapy for insomnia
ECG: electrocardiogram
EEG: electroencephalogram
EMG: electromyogram

EOG: electrooculogram
ipRGC: intrinsic photosensitive retinal ganglion cell
NREM: nonrapid eye movement
PSG: polysomnography
REM: rapid eye movement
SWS: slow-wave sleep

References

Alvaro, P. K., Roberts, R. M., & Harris, J. K. (2013). A systematic review assessing bidirectionality between sleep disturbances, anxiety, and depression. *Sleep*, *36*(7), 1059–1086. https://doi.org/ 10.5665/sleep .2810

American Academy of Sleep Medicine. (2014). *International classification of sleep disorders* (3rd ed.). American Academy of Sleep Medicine.

American Academy of Sleep Medicine. (2022). *The path to sleep medicine*. https://aasm.org/professional-development /choose-sleep/the-path-to-sleep-medicine

Barrett, K., Barman, S., Brooks, H., & Yuan, J. (2019). *Ganong's review of medical physiology* (26th ed.). McGraw-Hill Education.

Berry, R. B., Quan, S. F., Abreau, A. R, Bibbs, M. L., DelRosso, L., Harding, S. M., Mao, M.-M., Plante, D. T., Pressman, M. R., Troester, M. M., & Vaughn, B. V. (2020). *The AASM manual for the scoring of sleep and associated events: Rules, terminology and technical specifications*. American Academy of Sleep Medicine. https://aasm.org/clinical-resources/scoring-manual

Berry, R. B., & Wagner, M. H. (2014). *Sleep medicine pearls* (3rd ed.). Elsevier.

Binks, H., Vincent, G. E., Gupta, C., Irwin, C., & Khalesi, S. (2020). Effects of diet on sleep: A narrative review. *Nutrients, 12*, 936. https://doi.org/ doi:10.3390 /nu12040936

Bodenheimer, T., & Handley, M. A. (2009). Goal setting for behavior change in primary care: An exploration and status report. *Patient Education and Counseling*, *76*(2), 174–180. https://doi.org/ 10.1016/j.pec.2009 .06.001

Boudreaux, E. D., Sullivan, A., Abar, B., Bernstein, S. L., Ginde, A. A., & Camargo, C. A., Jr. (2012). Motivation rulers for smoking cessation: A prospective observational examination of construct and predictive validity. *Addiction Science & Clinical Practice*, *7*(1), 8. https://doi.org/ 10.1186/1940-0640-7-8

Cappuccio, F. P., Cooper, D., D'Elia, L., Strazzullo, P., & Miller, M. A. (2011). Sleep duration predicts cardiovascular outcomes: A systematic review and meta-analysis of prospective studies. *European Heart Journal*, *32*(12), 1484–1492. https://doi.org/10.1093 /eurheartj/ehr007

De Lecea, L., Kilduff, T. S., Peyron, C., Gao, X.-B., Foye, P. E., Danielson, P. E., Fukuhara, C., Battenberg, E. L. F., Gautvik, V. T., Bartlet, F. S., II, Frankel, W. N., van den Pol, A. E., Bloom, F. E., Gautvik, K. M., & Sutcliffe, J. G. (1998). The hypocretins: Hypothalamus-specific peptides with neuroexcitatory activity. *Proceedings of the National Academy of Sciences of the United States of America*, *95*(1), 322–337. https://doi.org/10.1073 /pnas.95.1.322

Drake, C. D., Roehrs, T., Shambroom, J., & Roth, T. (2013). Caffeine effects on sleep taken 0, 3, or 6 hours before going to bed. *Journal of Clinical Sleep Medicine*, *9*(11), 1195–2000. https://doi.org/10.5664 /jcsm.3170

Gapstur, S. M., Diver, W. R., Stevens, V. L., Carter, B. D., Teras, L. R., & Jacobs, E. J. (2014). Work schedule, sleep duration, insomnia, and risk of fatal prostate cancer. *American Journal of Preventive Medicine*, *46*(3 Suppl 1), S26–S33. https://doi.org/10.1016/j .amepre.2013.10.033

Goldstein, C. A., & Chervin, R. (2022). Clinical tools and tests in sleep medicine. In M. Kyrger, T. Roth, C. A. Goldstein, & W. C. Dement (Eds.), *Principles and practice of sleep medicine* (pp. 666–677). Elsevier.

Hesse, M. (2006). The readiness ruler as a measure of readiness to change poly-drug use in drug abusers. *Harm Reduction Journal*, *3*(3). https://doi .org/10.1186/1477-7517-3-3

Hirshkowitz, M., Whiton, K., Albert, S. M., Alessi, C., Bruni, O., DonCarlos, L., Hazen, N., Herman, J., Katz, E. S., Kheirandish-Gozal, L., Neubauer, D. N., O'Donnell, A. E., Ohayon, M., Peever, J., Rawding, R., Sachdeva, R. C., Setters, B., Vitiello, M. V., Ware, J. C., & Adams Hillard, P. J. (2015). National Sleep Foundation's sleep time duration recommendations: Methodology and results summary. *Sleep Health*, *1*(1), 40–43. https://doi.org/10.1016/j.sleh.2014.12.010

Javaheri, S., Barbe, F., Campos-Rodriguez, F., Dempsey, J. A., Khayat, R., Javaheri, S., Malhotra, A., Martinez-Garcia, M. A., Mehra, R., Pack, A. I., Polotsky,

V. Y., Redline, S., & Somers, V. K. (2017). Sleep apnea: Types, mechanisms, and clinical cardiovascular consequences. *Journal of the American College of Cardiology, 69*(7), 841–858. https://doi.org/ 10.1016/j.jacc.2016.11.069

Kecklund, G., & Axelsson, J. (2016). Health consequences of shift work and insufficient sleep. *British Medical Journal, 355*, i5210. https://doi.org/10.1136/bmj.i5210

Khani, M., Najafian, J., Taheri, M., Akhavan-Tabib, A., & Hosseini, S. (2018). Association between sleep duration and electrocardiographic ischemic changes in middle-aged population: Isfahan Healthy Heart Program. *ARYA Atherosclerosis, 14*(3), 115–121. https://doi.org/10.22122/arya.v14i3.1656

Kirsch, D. (2021). Stages and architecture of normal sleep. *UpToDate.* https://www.uptodate.com/contents/stages-and-architecture-of-normal-sleep

Lazarus, M., Oishi, Y., Bjorness, T. E., & Greene, R. W. (2019). Gating and the need for sleep: Dissociable effects of adenosine A1 and A2A receptors. *Frontiers in Neuroscience, 13*, 740. https://doi.org/10.3389/fnins.2019.00740

Lehrer, S., Green, S., Ramanathan, L., & Rosenzweig, K. E. (2013). Insufficient sleep associated with increased breast cancer mortality. *Sleep Medicine, 14*, 469. https://doi.org/10.1016/j.sleep.2012.10.012

Liew, S. C., & Aung, T. (2021). Sleep deprivation and its association with diseases: A review. *Sleep Medicine, 77*, 192–204. https://doi.org/10.1016/j.sleep.2020.07.048

Luppi, P., & Fort, P. (2019). Sleep–wake physiology. In H. Levin & P. Chauvel (Eds.), *Handbook of clinical neurology* (pp. 359–370). Elsevier. https://doi.org/10.1016/B978-0-444-64032-1.00023-0

Luyster, F. S., Strollo, P. J., Zee, P. C., & Walsh, J. K. (2012). Sleep: A health imperative. *Sleep, 35*(6), 727–734. https://doi.org/10.5665/sleep.1846

Matthews, E. E., Li, C., Long, C. R., Narcisse, M.-R., Martin, B. C., & McElfish, P. A. (2018). Sleep deficiency among native Hawaiian/Pacific Islander, Black, and White Americans and the association with cardiometabolic diseases: Analysis of the National Health Interview Survey Data. *Sleep Health, 4*(3), 273–283. https://doi.org/10.1016/j.sleh.2018.01.004

McGinty, D., & Szymusiak, R. (2022). Neural control of sleep in mammals. In M. Kyrger, T. Roth, C. A. Goldstein, & W. C. Dement (Eds.), *Principles and practice of sleep medicine* (pp. 54–67). Elsevier.

Miller, C. B., Kyle, S. D., Melehan, K. L., & Bartlett, D. J. (2015). Methodology for the assessment of sleep. In K. Babson & M. Felder (Eds.), *Sleep and affect: Assessment, theory and clinical implications* (pp. 65–90). Oxford. https://doi.org/10.1016/B978-0-12-417188-6.00004-9

Mure, L. S. (2021). Intrinsically photosensitive retinal ganglion cells of the human retina. *Frontiers in Neurology, 12*. https://doi.org/ 10.3389/fneur.2021.636330

National Heart, Lung, and Blood Institute. (2011). *In brief: Your guide to healthy sleep.* https://www.nhlbi.nih.gov/resources/brief-your-guide-healthy-sleep

Pacheco, D. (2021). *The best temperature for sleep.* Sleep Foundation. https://www.sleepfoundation.org/bedroom-environment/best-temperature-for-sleep

Patyar, S., & Patyar, R. R. (2015). Correlation between sleep duration and risk of stroke. *Journal of Stroke and Cerebrovascular Diseases, 24*(5), 905–911. https://doi.org/10.1016/j.jstrokecerebrovasdis.2014.12.038

Pietila, J., Helander, E., Korhonen, I., Myllymaki, T., Kujala, U. M., & Lindholm, H. (2018). Acute effect of alcohol intake on cardiovascular autonomic regulation during the first hours of sleep in a large real-world sample of Finnish employees: Observational study. *JMIR Mental Health, 5*(1), e23. https://doi.org/10.2196/mental.9519

Prochaska, J. O., & DiClemente, C. C. (2005). The transtheoretical approach. In J. C. Norcross & M. R. Goldfried (Eds.), *Handbook of psychotherapy integration* (pp. 147–171). Oxford University Press. https://doi.org/10.1093/med:psych/9780195165791.003.0007

Roehrs, T., & Roth, T. (2020). The effects of medications on sleep quality and sleep architecture. *UpToDate.* https://www.uptodate.com/contents/the-effects-of-medications-on-sleep-quality-and-sleep-architecture

Sateia, M. J., & Thorpy, M. J. (2022). Classification of sleep disorders. In M. Kyrger, T. Roth, C. A. Goldstein, & W. C. Dement (Eds.), *Principles and practice of sleep medicine* (pp. 678–688). Elsevier.

Stein, M. D., & Friedmann, P. D. (2006). Disturbed sleep and its relationship to alcohol use. *Substance Abuse, 26*(1), 1–13. https://doi.org/10.1300/J465v26n01_01

Sullivan, S. S., Carskadon, M. A., Dement, W. C., & Jackson, C. L. (2022). Normal human sleep: An overview. In M. Kyrger, T. Roth, C. A. Goldstein, & W. C. Dement (Eds.), *Principles and practice of sleep medicine* (pp. 16–26). Elsevier.

Suni, E. (2020). *What is sleep hygiene?* Sleep Foundation. https://www.sleepfoundation.org/sleep-hygiene

Trauer, J. M., Qian, M. Y., Doyle, J. S., Rajaratnam, S. M., & Cunnington, D. (2015). Cognitive behavioral therapy for chronic insomnia: A systematic review and meta-analysis. *Annals of Internal Medicine, 163*(3), 191–204. https://doi.org/ 10.7326/M14-2841

Wise, M. S., & Glaze, D. G. (2021). Sleep physiology in children. *UpToDate.* https://www.uptodate.com/contents/sleep-physiology-in-children

Wyatt, J. K. (2020). Overview of circadian sleep-wake rhythm disorders. *UpToDate.* https://www.uptodate.com/contents/overview-of-circadian-sleep-wake-rhythm-disorders

CHAPTER 16

Treat Tobacco Use

Shari Hrabovsky, DEd, MSN, FNP-BC
Linda Royer, PhD, MPH, MSN, RN

Tobacco use is the leading cause of preventable disease, disability, and death in the United States.

Centers for Disease Control and Prevention

OBJECTIVES

This chapter will enable the reader to:

1. Examine the prevalence and history of tobacco use.
2. Describe the characteristics and use of various tobacco products.
3. Explain the effect of tobacco use on health and disease.
4. Analyze the addictive characteristics and physical consequences of nicotine.
5. Incorporate recommendations from the U.S. Public Health Service Tobacco Cessation Guideline.
6. Use the 5As model as a guide for tobacco use interventions.
7. Apply pharmacotherapy, behavioral counseling, and lifestyle strategies in tobacco use treatment.

Overview

Tobacco dependence is a chronic disease with deceptive control over users. National organizations such as the National Cancer Institute (NCI) and the American Cancer Society (ACS) recognize that nicotine is powerfully addictive and that tobacco use is the greatest preventable cause of premature death in the United States, accounting for one out of five deaths, 87% of lung cancer deaths, and at least 30% of all cancer deaths each year (ACS, 2020; NCI, n.d.-b).

Steinberg et al. (2008) presented the case for treating tobacco dependence as a chronic disease. They asserted that if tobacco dependence is recognized as a chronic disease, it would be treated similarly to other chronic diseases, such as hypertension and diabetes. In other words, the clinician should consistently assess nicotine use and utilize multiple treatment methods to reach the outcome of abstinence. Likewise, the U.S. Preventive Services Task Force (2021) recommends that clinicians ask all adults about tobacco use, advise them to stop using tobacco, and provide behavioral

© Kathleen Gail/Shutterstock; © StoryTime Studio/Shutterstock; © kali9/Getty Images

interventions for cessation. Its recommendation also includes offering U.S. Food and Drug Administration (FDA)-approved medications to nonpregnant adults. This chapter provides the advanced practice provider (APP) with a foundation and strategies for understanding and treating tobacco use and dependence in health promotion.

Prevalence of Tobacco Use in the United States

The National Health Survey revealed that the percentage of adult tobacco users in the United States in 2018 was 19.7% (Creamer et al., 2019). **Figure 16.1**, taken from the National Health Survey, depicts the percentage of tobacco use among adults. There can be dual use of tobacco products, meaning that some users admit to using more than one of the products listed. The percentage of use of any combustible product is 16.5%. Cigarettes are the most popular combustible product used by 13.7% of U.S. adults. Cigars, cigarillos, and little cigars follow in prevalence at 3.9%. Electronic cigarettes are used by 3.2% of the adult population, with smokeless tobacco products making up 2.4% of tobacco use (Creamer et al., 2019).

The use of tobacco products by youth is also very sobering. The Centers for Disease Control and Prevention (CDC) regularly tracks

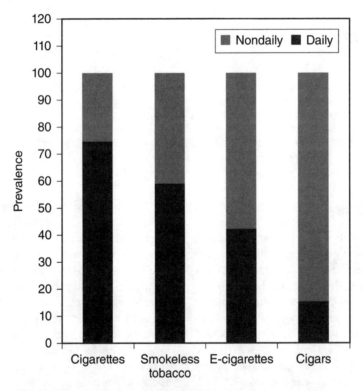

Figure 16.1 Tobacco product use among adults over the age of 18 years (2018).

Creamer, M. R., Wang, T. W., Babb, S., Cullen, K. A., Day, H., Wills, G., Jamal, A., & Neff, L. (2019). Tobacco product use and cessation indicators among adults–United States, 2018. *Morbidity and Mortality Weekly Report, 68*(45), 1013–1019. https://www.cdc.gov/mmwr/volumes/68/wr/mm6845a2.htm

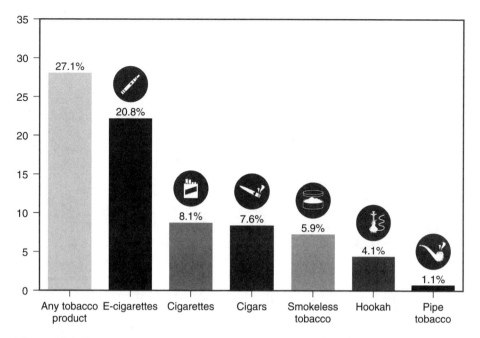

Figure 16.2 Tobacco product use among high school students (2018).

Centers for Disease Control and Prevention. (2019, February 11). *Data visualization: Tobacco product use among high school students (2018).* CDC Vital signs. https://stacks.cdc.gov/view /cdc/75893

tobacco use among high school students (see **Figure 16.2**). Ninety-nine percent of adults who have ever smoked daily report that they first smoked by the age of 26, 88% by age 18, more than one-third report by age 14, and more than one-quarter initiated tobacco use by age 12 (Campaign for Tobacco-Free Kids, 2021b; CDC, n.d.-h; Cullen et al., 2019).

Every day, about 2,000 youth under age 18 smoke their first cigarette (CDC, n.d.-a). Youth who have early exposure to tobacco are more susceptible to nicotine addiction, with symptoms appearing within weeks or even days of initiating tobacco experimentation. In addition to nicotine addiction, tobacco use can have a significant effect on health and longevity. "Overall, roughly one-third of all kids who become regular smokers before adulthood will eventually die from smoking. If current trends continue, 5.6 million of the kids under 18 who are alive today will die from tobacco-related causes" (Campaign for Tobacco-Free Kids, 2021b, p. 2).

APP Role in Promoting Tobacco Cessation

The role of health professionals is essential in facilitating health behavior change, including tobacco cessation. As such, preventive services such as screening and counseling for tobacco use are mandated by many regulatory organizations and encouraged by public health organizations. However, tobacco cessation treatment is underutilized. Geletko et al. (2022) examined tobacco cessation counseling and medications from 4,590 primary care visits by patients with current tobacco use. Of visits by current tobacco users, only 18.4% included cessation counseling.

Because 70% of smokers see a healthcare provider each year (Fiore et al., 2008), APPs have a unique opportunity to promote health by implementing tobacco use screening and counseling in primary care and many other healthcare settings. While many factors affect the availability and accessibility of tobacco use intervention, a crucial element needed to provide such services is professionals who understand the complexities of tobacco use as a chronic condition and who possess the necessary skills to apply and facilitate effective intervention.

It is imperative for APPs to know that most tobacco users want to quit. In 2015, 68% of U.S. adult smokers reported a desire to stop smoking (CDC, n.d.-a). Each year, more than half of adults who smoke try to quit. However, less than one-third use proven cessation methods (U.S. Department of Health and Human Services [HHS], n.d.). These cessation attempts could be significantly improved with the application of knowledge and skillful practice described in the remainder of this chapter.

History of Tobacco Use in the United States

Despite enormous efforts and progress in reducing smoking, tobacco use today is still the leading cause of preventable death in the United States and imposes a detrimental toll on families, businesses, the government, and the environment. Tobacco is implicated in the death of more than 480,000 people annually in the United States—more than AIDS, alcohol, car accidents, illegal drugs, murders, and suicides combined (CDC, n.d.-b). Tobacco use is the single largest preventable cause of illness and death, leading to billions of dollars spent on medical expenses and lost productivity (CDC, n.d.-f). An estimated 11.7% of U.S. annual healthcare spending was attributed to adult cigarette smoking from 2010 to 2014, translating to annual healthcare spending of more than $225 billion (Xu et al., 2021).

Cummings and Proctor (2014) provide a descriptive context of tobacco use trends in the United States. In summary, the first half of the 20th century saw an increase in tobacco use until 1964, when the U.S. surgeon general issued a report on the health risks of smoking (CDC, n.d.-d). Since that time, tobacco use has declined due to an improved understanding of the health risks of smoking,

reduced social acceptance, legal restrictions on smoking in public spaces, mass media counter-marketing campaigns, and higher taxes on cigarettes (Cummings & Proctor, 2014). Additionally, the CDC (n.d.-e) formed the Office on Smoking and Health, which has, over time, extended influence from the federal level into state and local communities for prevention and control. In addition to federal support, many organizations have come on board to provide tobacco education and intervention programs and services, including health systems, faith-based organizations, and private nonprofit organizations such as the American Lung Association. The World Health Organization (WHO, 2020) launched a yearlong campaign in 2021 to help 100 million people quit tobacco use.

Laws to Control Tobacco Use

Several methods have been used to reduce tobacco use in the United States, including taxation, the Master Settlement Agreement, the Clean Air Act, and laws related to the age of purchase. Tobacco tax is one of the most effective means of reducing use. Every 10% increase in the price of cigarettes reduces smoking in adults by 2% and in youth by about 7% (Campaign for Tobacco-Free Kids, 2021a). This action is a budget benefit because healthcare expenditures, especially Medicaid and Medicare, are reduced when tobacco use is reduced.

The Master Settlement Agreement is an agreement among 46 states, their attorney generals, four tobacco manufacturers, the public health community, the financial community, and various federal agencies. The central purpose of this 1998 agreement was to reduce smoking (particularly among youth) by placing restrictions on the advertising, marketing, and promotion of cigarettes. It also states that tobacco product manufacturers agree to pay each state a certain percentage of profit in perpetuity to compensate for the billions of dollars spent on health care (National Association of Attorneys General, n.d.).

As a result of the surgeon general's report on secondhand smoke in June 2006, 27 states and Washington, D.C., in addition to hundreds of cities, have implemented comprehensive smoke-free laws to promote clean air (Campaign for Tobacco-Free Kids, 2021b). Also, the U.S. Department of Housing and Urban Development enacted a rule that all public housing authorities must provide a completely smoke-free environment for their residents (Instituting Smoke-Free Public Housing, 2018).

As noted earlier, 88% of adult smokers begin before age 18. This early tobacco use is enhanced by the marketing practices of tobacco manufacturers to a younger population to manipulate their buying habits. In response, Congress passed a federal law in 2019 raising the age limit to *purchase* tobacco products to 21 years nationwide. However, this law does not apply to tobacco *use*, meaning it is not illegal to use tobacco under the age of 21 years. Hence, tobacco product control of use and intervention has become a societal concern leading to numerous educational, clinical, and legal efforts (Campaign for Tobacco-Free Kids, 2021b).

Tobacco Products

Although cigarette smoking is the most common form of tobacco used, a variety of tobacco products can be smoked, chewed, or sniffed. Tobacco products can generally be divided into two categories: combustible, such as cigarettes, cigars, pipes, and hookah, and noncombustible, such as chewing tobacco, snuff, dip, dissolvables, and electronic nicotine delivery systems (ENDS). **Table 16.1** and **Table 16.2** describe the characteristics and use of these products.

Table 16.1 Combustible Tobacco Products

Product	Characteristics	How Used
Cigarette	Available in tobacco or menthol flavors, cigarettes are composed of tobacco, chemical additives, filter, and paper wrapping. They are manufactured in short, regular, and long lengths and are generally sold in packs of 20 cigarettes or 10 packs per carton.	Most popular, whether store-bought or roll your own (RYO). Individuals who use RYO will purchase tubes or paper, tobacco, and sometimes a rolling machine. The open end is lit on fire with a match or lighter tool; the filter end is placed between the lips, through which air is inspired to the mouth and lungs.
Cigar	Cigars are combustible products composed of tobacco, chemical additives, and a wrapper made from a tobacco leaf instead of paper. Cigars come in a variety of sizes and many flavors. Many brands do not have a filter, but some cigars include a white filter tip.	Used similarly to a cigarette. Being larger in circumference and length, the user spends more time using it and may chew on the end. Tobacco manufacturers state that they measure the amount of nicotine to be consistent and satisfy the user in cigarettes and cigars.
Pipe	The typical pipe is of plastic construction with a hollow stem, a small mouthpiece at one end, and a bowl perched at the other end in which loose tobacco leaf is packed and lit for use.	Used similarly to the cigarette by inspiring air through the burning tobacco. The nicotine concentration is unknown because the user packs in the tobacco product.
Hookah	A waterpipe system that includes a jar, valve, hose, gasket, plate, bowl, charcoal, water, and often a wind guard.	The smoke of the tobacco passes through the water before inhalation.

Data from U.S. Food and Drug Administration. (2020, May 28). *Products, ingredients, & components.* https://www.fda.gov/tobacco-products/products-guidance-regulations/products-ingredients-components

Table 16.2 Noncombustible Tobacco Products

Product	Characteristics	How Used
Chewing tobacco	Available as loose leaf, plugs, twists, or ropes. It also comes in a variety of flavors.	Users place the product between their cheek and gum and then suck or chew on the tobacco to extract the nicotine. The saliva that accumulates in the mouth is swallowed or spit out.
Snuff/snus/dip	Snuff is different from chew, as it is finely ground tobacco. It is available in various flavors in dry, moist, or prepackaged pouches (called snus).	Users put a pinch or dip of the powder or the pouch between their cheek and gum. The juices are swallowed or spit out.
Dissolvables	Although not very popular in the United States, dissolvables are available as lozenges that resemble a pellet or tablet, orbs that look like small mints, sticks with a toothpick-like appearance, and thin strips. They contain nicotine and other potentially harmful ingredients.	These tobacco products are dissolved in the mouth.

Data from U.S. Food and Drug Administration. (2020, May 28). *Products, ingredients, & components.* https://www.fda.gov/tobacco-products/products-guidance-regulations/products-ingredients-components

ENDS, such as vaporizers and electronic cigarettes (EC), are relatively new to the tobacco product market, arriving in the United States around 2006. These noncombustible tobacco products are battery-operated devices that heat liquid into a vapor the user inhales. The device components consist of a battery, heating element, liquid with various flavors, and nicotine of varying levels. Several types of EC are available, including cigar-like devices that look like a cigarette and closed systems that disallow customization of the nicotine content or flavor of the liquid. Advanced devices can be shaped like a pen or a box in which the user adds the liquid to a tank or drips it directly onto the heating element. The advanced level of EC allows the user to vary the voltage or wattage output of the device. This changes the amount of draw resistance and level of heat to the device. Additionally, the liquid of the EC contains varying levels of propylene glycol, vegetable glycerin, flavorings, and nicotine, which affect the vapor produced and the nicotine absorbed by the body in the type of EC (CDC, n.d.-c; Yingst et al., 2015).

The pod device, known commonly as JUUL, is a closed system that uses nicotine salts to deliver nicotine to the user. These devices have become increasingly popular due to the ease of use, size, and effective delivery of nicotine (FDA, 2022a; Yingst et al., 2019). In addition, more information about harm to the body has come to light from chemicals in the vapor, such as vitamin E acetate and marijuana oils (i.e., TCH, CBD). In June 2022, the FDA ordered JUUL Labs, Inc., to stop selling and distributing these products in the United States. This order has since been stayed for additional review (FDA, 2022b).

Effect of Tobacco on Health and Disease

Nicotine is the addictive component in tobacco and plays a significant role in why tobacco product use continues. In addition to nicotine addiction, several theories for continued tobacco use have been considered. For instance, researchers recognize that there appear to be values and beliefs around tobacco use that constitute a lifestyle (Dawkins, 2013; Hrabovsky, 2018). Behaviors such as eating, drinking, drug use, and gambling often accompany tobacco use.

Although smoking rates in the United States have decreased by 50% since 1964, smoking tobacco has continued to be a primary cause of preventable disease, disability, and death in this country, claiming nearly 500,000 lives each year (CDC, 2018). More than 16 million people already have at least one disease from smoking, and at least 58 million Americans continue to be exposed to the dangerous chemicals in secondhand smoke (CDC, n.d.-e). Although nicotine is addictive, it is not what creates the most direct harm. There are over 7,000 chemicals in cigarettes, with at least 250 known to be harmful (NCI, n.d.-b). Due to the actions of several harmful constituents of tobacco products, the functions of nearly every organ and system are affected negatively, resulting in disease (HHS, 2014). The U.S. Department of Health and Human Services report on *The Health Consequences of Smoking—50 Years of Progress: A Report of the Surgeon General* lists the diseases and other adverse health effects caused by smoking and reaffirms the widespread negative consequences of smoking (HHS, 2014).

Cancers

Of the more than 7,000 chemicals in combustible products, nearly 70 are known to cause cancer (NCI, n.d.-b). In addition to being more addictive, cigarettes have become more deadly over time. Between 1959 and 2010, lung cancer risk for smokers rose dramatically (HHS, 2014). This increased risk may be due in part to a change in the design of the cigarette. For example, tiny holes in the filter increase the intake volume of smoke. Subsequently, lung cancer has become the leading cause of cancer death among both men and women, with nearly 9 out of 10 lung cancers caused by smoking (HHS, 2014). About 20% of all cancers and about 30% of all cancer deaths in the United States are caused by smoking (ACS, 2020). In addition to a causal relationship to lung, liver, colorectal, and breast cancers, there is evidence that smoking increases the risk for many other cancers and cancer-specific mortality and that quitting smoking improves the prognosis of cancer patients (ACS, 2020; HHS, 2014).

The incidence of smokeless tobacco products has increased as users naively attempt to avoid the risk of cancer and other deleterious effects of smoking. However, noncombustible products, such as chewing tobacco, increase oral cancer by causing oral lesions, changing the cell's normal function by altering the DNA and weakening the immune system (CDC, n.d.-f; Cheng et al., 2018). There is also an increased risk of gingivitis, caries, dental stains, tooth loss, and halitosis with the use of both combustible and noncombustible tobacco products.

Respiratory Diseases

Chronic bronchitis, chronic obstructive pulmonary disease, and emphysema are respiratory diseases directly related to smoking cigarettes (HHS, 2014). Smoking reduces pulmonary function by weakening and eroding respiratory tract tissues with harmful foreign chemicals, making the lungs susceptible to invading viruses and bacteria and increasing the risk for infections and chronic disease. This negative effect also affects children of smokers, who have more respiratory infections than children of nonsmokers (American Heart Association [AHA], n.d.). Another concern has been found with vaping pods or EC liquids that have been altered with substances, generally illicit, causing severe acute pulmonary distress when inhaled. This condition is called EVALI, or e-cigarette or vaping product use-associated lung injury (Blount et al., 2020; Kligerman et al., 2020).

Cardiovascular Disease

Chemicals in cigarette smoke induce a chronic inflammatory process in the circulatory system, altered lipid metabolism, endothelial damage, and a prothrombotic effect. The longer and the more cigarettes one smokes, the more serious the damage, increasing risk for hypertension, increased heart rate, narrowing of the arteries, and hardening of the arterial walls (AHA, n.d.). Cardiovascular disease, the number one cause of all deaths in the United States, claims more than 800,000 people yearly, and smoking is a significant contributing factor. Even exposure to secondhand smoke can cause a heart attack or stroke. More than 33,000 nonsmokers die every year in the United States from heart disease caused by secondhand smoke (HHS, 2014).

Carbon monoxide (CO) is a colorless, odorless, tasteless gas that is one of the most harmful substances in tobacco smoke (Rodgman & Perfetti, 2013; SRNT Subcommittee on Biochemical Verification, 2002). Once CO is taken into the lungs, it is transferred to the bloodstream, where it takes the place of oxygen attached to red blood cells, reducing the amount of oxygen available for muscle and organ use. CO also increases the amount of cholesterol deposited into the inner lining of the arteries, which can cause atherosclerosis over time and lead to cardiovascular disease and heart attack (Calafat et al., 2004). Measuring CO levels in patients with readily available tools can provide a way to start a conversation about the physical effect of smoking (AHA, n.d.; Hrabovsky et al., 2017).

Reproductive Effects

The use of tobacco before pregnancy is a major cause of reduced fertility. Smoking may also bring about ectopic pregnancy, which usually causes fetal mortality and poses a serious risk to the mother's health. Mothers who continue to smoke during pregnancy are more likely to deliver low birth weight or preterm babies—a leading cause of death, disability, and disease among newborns. There is also sufficient evidence to infer a causal relationship between smoking during pregnancy and orofacial clefts (HHS, 2014). Smoking also contributes to male infertility. Recent evidence concludes that smoking is a cause of erectile dysfunction (HHS, 2014). Furthermore, smoking damages DNA in sperm, some of which persist even after smoking cessation (Omolaoye et al., 2022).

Other Effects

Smoking interferes with proper metabolic bodily function, causing chronic diseases such as type 2 diabetes—a growing health crisis. Smokers are 30% to 40% more likely to develop type 2 diabetes than nonsmokers. Furthermore, there is a positive dose–response relationship between the number of cigarettes smoked and the risk of developing type 2 diabetes (HHS, 2014). People who smoke and have diabetes are more likely to have other serious health problems, including heart disease, blindness, kidney failure, and nerve and blood vessel damage of the feet and legs, leading to amputation. Smoking also contributes to age-related macular degeneration and rheumatoid arthritis. It can also make interventions for rheumatoid arthritis less effective. Smoking also affects immunity and autoimmunity (HHS, 2014).

Health Risks of Smokeless Tobacco

While smokeless tobacco is also dangerous to health, the death and disease from tobacco use that continues to plague the United States are overwhelmingly caused by cigarettes and other burned tobacco products (CDC, n.d.-f).

Nicotine Dependence

Nicotine dependence as a chronic disease has deceptive control over smokers (Steinberg et al., 2008). Nicotine imitates the neurotransmitter acetylcholine, which transmits a chemical message across synapses in the brain. Acetylcholine has a receptor called the nicotinic receptor. When this receptor is activated either by acetylcholine or nicotine, channels open, and ions are released, affecting the neuron and exciting the cell. The channel then closes, and the receptor becomes temporarily inactive. With continued exposure to nicotine, the inactive period of the channel becomes prolonged, thus reducing sensitivity and requiring more nicotine to create a response (Dubuc, n.d.). The severity of tobacco dependence can vary from mild to very severe.

Addiction Cycle

Neurons in the brain's ventral tegmental area have nicotine receptors that activate dopamine release in the nucleus accumbens, setting up an addiction cycle that is crucial to understanding tobacco addiction. More nicotine to this area results in more dopamine release into the brain. However, more dopamine creates dependence on that amount to feel "normal." Furthermore, continued nicotine use upregulates the number of nicotine receptors and creates a dependency. The more nicotine exposed to the receptors in the nucleus accumbens, the slower the recovery of these receptors, thus reducing the availability of active receptors. When the nicotinic receptors upregulate, more nicotine is needed to feel good or normal. Consequently, when tobacco users go for some time without using tobacco, they will experience psychological withdrawal symptoms, such as anxiety, irritability, nervousness, and restlessness (Benowitz, 2010).

Nicotine is quickly metabolized in the liver to cotinine and has a half-life of about 2 hours (Benowitz, 2010). This short half-life creates peaks and valleys of nicotine levels in the body and requires frequent doses during the day, or withdrawal symptoms return. Additionally, social and environmental cues, such as waking, work breaks, drinking coffee, or eating dinner, reinforce the use of tobacco products as people go through their day. This concurrent engagement allows users to associate feeling good and less stressed with activities where nicotine is administered (the pleasure principle), hence solidifying a dependence on the use of the nicotine product and making it their lifestyle (Dawkins, 2013).

Nicotine withdrawal can start as soon as 20 minutes after the use of a tobacco product. It generally peaks at about day 3 of abstinence, and the physical dependence can last up to 4 weeks. The psychological cravings can last much longer, however. Smokers, in particular, report cravings well past 6 months after quitting. Common nicotine withdrawal symptoms include anger, irritability, anxiety, restlessness, difficulty concentrating, sleep disturbance, depressed mood, increased appetite, and weight gain (CDC, n.d.-f).

Benefits and Concerns Related to Tobacco Use Interventions

There are many reasons to invest time, money, and social resources into tobacco use intervention, including (1) reduction of healthcare costs for care of the health consequences already described, (2) reduction of unnecessary loss of life, (3) increased productivity from addicted individuals, and (4) reduction of environmental waste and improved atmospheric air. Additionally, there are short- and long-term benefits for the individual who quits smoking and some often-ignored concerns related to quitting (FDA, 2021; NCI, n.d.-b) (**Table 16.3**).

Table 16.3 Benefits and Concerns Related to Quitting Smoking

	Short Term	Long Term

Benefits	Lowered blood pressure and improved overall blood circulation are noted within 20 minutes.
	     Carbon monoxide levels drop in 8 hours.
	     Smell and taste are improved.
	     Lung function improves with lung cilia regrowth and activation.
		After 10 years, the chance of death from lung cancer is cut in half.
		     There is a decreased risk for mouth, throat, esophagus, bladder, kidney, and pancreas cancers.
		     The risk of heart disease is that of a nonsmoker.

Concerns	There is often a perception of increased stress.
	     When a person quits smoking, caffeine intake should be reduced. It is not metabolized the same when a person quits smoking, and adverse effects like anxiety or a jittery feeling can be experienced.
		Weight gain of 10–15 pounds is not unusual. However, nutritional techniques and regular follow up can assist in managing weight during smoking cessation.
		     Depression symptoms may need additional intervention.

Health Promotion Research Study

Lifestyle Strategies to Reduce Post-Cessation Weight Gain

Background: Weight gain following smoking cessation reduces the incentive to quit, especially among women. Exercise and diet interventions may reduce post-cessation weight gain, but their long-term effect has not been estimated in randomized trials.

Methodology: The researchers estimated the long-term reduction in post-cessation weight gain among women under smoking cessation alone or combined with (1) moderate to vigorous exercise (15, 30, 45, 60 minutes/day) and (2) exercise and diet modification (≤2 servings/week of unprocessed red meat; ≥5 servings/day of fruits and vegetables; minimal sugar-sweetened beverages, sweets, and desserts; potato chips or fried potatoes; and processed red meat).

Results: Among 10,087 eligible smokers in the Nurses' Health Study and 9,271 in the Nurses' Health Study II, the estimated 10-year mean weights under smoking cessation were 75.0 kg (95% CI = 74.7, 75.5) and 79.0 kg (78.2, 79.6), respectively. Pooling both cohorts, the estimated post-cessation mean weight gain was 4.9 kg (7.3, 2.6) lower under a hypothetical strategy of exercising at least 30 minutes/day and diet modification and 5.9 kg (8.0, 3.8) lower under exercising at least 60 minutes/day and diet modification, compared with smoking cessation without exercising.

Implications for Advanced Practice: In this study, although substantial weight gain occurred in women after smoking cessation, the researchers estimated that exercise and dietary modifications could have averted most of it. APPs can include lifestyle strategies of exercise and diet modification as adjunctive interventions when counseling patients on smoking cessation, especially when post-cessation weight gain is a concern.

Reference: Jain, P., Danaei, G., Manson, J. E., Robins, J. M., & Hernán, M. A. (2020). Weight gain after smoking cessation and lifestyle strategies to reduce it. *Epidemiology, 31*(1), 7–14. https://doi.org/10.1097/EDE.0000000000001106

Clinical Interventions for Tobacco Use and Dependence

Tobacco dependence is a chronic condition and should be treated as such. The Agency for Healthcare Research and Quality (AHRQ, 2012a) advises the use of five major steps to treat tobacco use and dependence. Commonly known as the 5As, this model provides a guide for beginning the conversation at an early visit: (1) ask about tobacco use, (2) advise quitting, (3) assess readiness to quit, (4) assist in the quit attempt, and (5) arrange for follow-up. **Table 16.4** describes strategies for implementing the 5As model in the clinical setting (Fiore et al., 2008).

Throughout the process, it is essential to use a motivational interviewing approach. Motivational interviewing (MI) is an empathic, person-centered counseling approach for increasing readiness by resolving indecisiveness about behavior change (Lindson-Hawley et al., 2015). It is widely applied in tobacco use intervention (Heckman et al., 2010) and is recommended in clinical practice guidelines (Fiore et al., 2008). Miller and Rollnick (2013) based MI on person-centered counseling, a model of behavior change that provides support and guidance to patients while respecting their autonomy and limitations.

Table 16.4 The 5As Model for Tobacco Treatment

Step	Intervention	Tools
Ask about tobacco use	Ask patients at every visit about tobacco use. If patients use tobacco, verify what they are using, how often, and for how long. If they have quit, ask for how long and acknowledge their success.	▪ Fagerström Test for Nicotine Dependence ▪ Cotinine or carbon monoxide levels
Advise quitting	Advise patients to quit tobacco use. Offer the statement, "The best thing to do for your health is to quit, and I can help."	▪ Decisional balance
Assess readiness to quit	Assess readiness to quit by using the techniques outlined in this chapter. However, even if patients do not show interest in quitting, it is still the role of the APP to offer support.	▪ Transtheoretical model ▪ Importance and confidence rulers
Assist in developing a quit plan	Assist patients in quitting by collaborating with them to design an individualized quit plan, including FDA-approved tobacco treatment medications, behavioral counseling, and lifestyle strategies to support quitting.	
Arrange for follow up	Arrange for a follow-up visit by phone or in person to assess the effectiveness of medications, counseling services, and behavior change plans. If necessary, refer patients to tobacco cessation programs, counseling services, and lifestyle medicine specialists.	

Adapted from Fiore, M. C., Jaén, C. R., Baker, T. B., Bailey, W. C., Benowitz, N. L., Curry, S. J., Dorfman, S. F., Froelicher, E. S., Goldstein, M. G., Healton, C. G., Henderson, P. N., Heyman, R. B., Koh, H. K., Kottke, T. E., Lando, H. A., Mecklenberg, R. E., Mermelstein, R. J., Mullen, P. D., Orleans, C. T., . . . Wewers, M. E. (2008). *Treating tobacco use and dependence: 2008 Update*. Clinical Practice Guideline. U.S. Department of Health and Human Services. Public Health Service.

The MI process involves the exploration of the person's ambivalence (e.g., "I know smoking is not good for me, but it helps me manage my stress") in an atmosphere of acceptance, warmth, and regard. Direct persuasion and coercion are to be avoided. Instead, the objective is to enhance the discrepancy between the reasons for changing (e.g., risks to self or family health) versus reasons for staying the same (e.g., smoking helps them relax when stressed). As they explore their own arguments for change, their motivation for and movement toward a target behavior is strengthened.

Ask About Tobacco Use

During the first step of the 5As model, *ask*, the APP takes a few minutes to learn about the patients' tobacco use and habits. Questions about tobacco use should be incorporated into standard data collection at every visit. Knowing this information will allow APPs to address their patients' needs and provide relevant education.

The APP should also ask about several informative characteristics of tobacco use, such as the type of tobacco product used, the number of cigarettes or amount of tobacco product used per day, the time to first cigarette or use of tobacco product after waking, how many years patients have used tobacco products, how many times patients have quit in the past, how long since the last quit attempt, methods or medications used to quit, and carbon monoxide level (if a measurement machine is available). Cigarette smoking should be translated into pack-years, which relate to cancer risk and severity of lung disease, by multiplying the number of packs smoked per day times the number of years smoked (Al-Ibrahim & Gross, 1990). For example, a patient who has smoked one-half pack per day for 15 years would have a history of 7.5 pack-years, and a patient who has smoked two packs per day for 10 years would have a history of 20 pack-years. It may also be helpful to assess the severity of tobacco dependency. The Fagerström Test for Nicotine

Dependence is a standardized tool for assessing the intensity of nicotine addiction (see **Table 16.5**).

It is plausible that asking about tobacco use in a reflective, nonjudgmental interviewing style may increase awareness and problem recognition, processes known to promote behavior change. As patients experience a nonjudgmental attitude, respectful interest, and understanding, they feel safe to discuss their ambivalence about tobacco intervention openly. When they verbalize their ambivalence about tobacco use intervention, the APP can promote exploration of abstinence in their lives by asking open-ended questions such as "What will staying tobacco-free take from you?" or "What will you lose by staying tobacco-free?" The sooner patients address ambivalence, the sooner they can progress toward change.

Advise Quitting

During the *advise* step, the APP provides information to patients to help them understand the current and potential health risks of tobacco use and the connection with their current lab results or symptoms. Additionally, patients should be advised on the potential benefits of quitting tobacco use. Information should be tailored for each patient. For example, the dangers of secondhand smoke can be shared with parents with children at home, or the effects of smoking on fertility can be discussed with women of childbearing age. An MI approach is critical during the *advise* step to avoid creating resistance to change. Wyatt (2016) asserts that providers need a way to share information with patients "to assist them in changing harmful behaviors while respecting their autonomy to choose if, when, and how they will change. Giving advice or making suggestions is likely to elicit pushback from clients. . . . [E]ven in the absence of active resistance, client replies to well-meaning clinician-generated solutions might sound like, 'I've already tried that' or 'That won't

---

Table 16.5 Fagerström Test for Nicotine Dependence

Do you currently smoke cigarettes?
____ No ____ Yes

If yes, read each question below. For each question, enter the answer choice that best describes your response:

1. How soon after you wake up do you smoke your first cigarette?
   ____ Within 5 minutes ____ 6 to 30 minutes
   ____ 31 to 60 minutes ____ After 60 minutes

2. Do you find it difficult to refrain from smoking in places where it is forbidden (e.g., in church, at the library, in the cinema)?
   _____ No _____ Yes

3. Which cigarette would you hate most to give up?
   _____ The first one in the morning _____ Any other

4. How many cigarettes per day do you smoke?
   _____ 10 or less _____ 11 to 20 _____ 21 to 30 _____ 31 or more

5. Do you smoke more frequently during the first hours after waking than during the rest of the day?
   _____ No _____ Yes

6. Do you smoke when you are so ill that you are in bed most of the day?
   _____ No _____ Yes

The Fagerström Test for Nicotine Dependence was designed to provide an ordinal measure of nicotine dependence related to cigarette smoking. It contains six items that evaluate the quantity of cigarette consumption, the compulsion to use, and dependence. Yes/no items are scored from 0 to 1, and multiple-choice items are scored from 0 to 3. The items are summed to yield a total score between 0 and 10. The higher the total Fagerström score, the more intense the patient's physical dependence on nicotine.
Heatherton, T. F., Kozlowski, L. T., & Frecker, R. C. (1991). The Fagerström Test for Nicotine Dependence: A revision of the Fagerström Tolerance Questionnaire. *British Journal of Addiction 86*, 1119–1127. https://cde.drugabuse.gov/instrument/d7c0b0f5-b865-e4de-e040-bb89ad43202b

---

work for me' or 'Sure, I'll try that' followed with inaction" (para. 8). Instead, the APP can offer assistance in the quit attempt when patients are ready.

As noted earlier, most patients want to quit smoking. However, they are ambivalent about quitting for various reasons. The APP can use nonjudgmental, open-ended questions to help patients explore their reasons for using a tobacco product and why they might want to quit. A tool used in MI to address ambivalence is the decisional balance techniques (see **Table 16.6**). The APP starts by asking patients to share the advantages of or what they like about their tobacco use. Next, the APP asks patients about some disadvantages of, or not-so-good reasons for, continued smoking and some things they do not like about this habit. It is important to avoid labeling these reasons as "bad things" or "problems." These reasons can be explored further with additional open-ended questions, such as "How does your family feel about your use of tobacco?" "How does this affect you?" "Could you share an example of when that happened?" Next, the APP can ask about some of the patients' fears and concerns about changing by asking, "What are some of the not-so-good reasons, or concerns, about quitting smoking?" The questioning concludes

Table 16.6 Decisional Balance Technique for Smoking Intervention

Good Reasons	Not-So-Good Reasons
1. What are the advantages of, or some of the good reasons for, smoking or using tobacco products? *This question decreases resistance to change and allows people to talk in a nondefensive way, with less resistance to change.*	2. What are the not-so-good reasons to continue to smoke or use tobacco products? *This question creates ambivalence and supports change talk.*
3. What are some good reasons for, or advantages to, changing your behavior, quitting smoking, or discontinuing tobacco products? *This question elicits change talk.*	4. What are some not-so-good reasons for changing your behavior, quitting smoking, or discontinuing tobacco products? *The APP may hear some of the patients' fears about changing and short-circuit their resistance by asking this question.*

Adapted from Miller, W., & Rollnick, S. (2013). *Motivational interviewing: Helping people change* (3rd Ed.). Guilford Press.

with the APP asking about good reasons for, or advantages, of quitting. It can also be helpful to ask questions about the possible consequences of quitting, such as "If you were completely successful in quitting smoking, how would things be different?" The use of the decisional balance technique allows patients to argue for their change and gives the APP information regarding resistance to change. It can assist patients in seeing more clearly the reasons to change or to stay the same and to evaluate more objectively if this is the right time to make a change.

Assess Readiness to Quit

The next step in the 5As model is *assess*. In this step, the APP determines patients' readiness to make a quit attempt. The transtheoretical model (TTM) is a widely accepted health behavior theory that emphasizes differences among people and places their readiness to change in a sequence of six stages (Prochaska & DiClemente, 1983). Initially developed to assess readiness for smoking cessation, the TTM has been applied in various health promotion programs, including physical activity, weight loss, and HIV prevention. **Table 16.7**

describes the constructs of the TTM in the context of tobacco cessation. Intervention based on this theory has allowed health professionals to reach more people engaged in tobacco use because it recognizes that attention must be attracted before health education is offered and that health education yields self-assessment and consideration of change.

A quick MI tool for assessing patients' readiness to discontinue tobacco use is the importance and confidence rulers (Miller & Rollnick, 2013). This tool has been found to significantly improve the prediction of smoking behavior change (Boudreaux et al., 2012). When administering the importance ruler, the APP simply asks patients to rate the importance of quitting: "How important would you say it is for you to quit tobacco use? On a scale from 0 to 10, where zero is not at all important and 10 is extremely important, where would you say you are?" For the confidence ruler, the APP asks, "How confident are you that if you decided to quit using tobacco, you could do it? On a scale from 0 to 10, where zero is not at all confident and 10 is extremely confident, where would you say you are?" Both questions should be asked because they represent different components of motivation for change. The APP

Table 16.7 Transtheoretical Model Elements Adapted for Tobacco Cessation

Constructs	Description
Stages of Change	
Precontemplation	No intention to take action toward cessation within the next 6 months
Contemplation	Intention to take action in quitting tobacco use within the next 6 months
Preparation	Intention to take action in quitting tobacco use within the next 30 days and has taken some behavioral steps in this direction
Action	Gives evidence of change in behavior toward tobacco product use for less than 6 months
Maintenance	Gives evidence of cessation from tobacco product use for more than 6 months
Termination	Shows low risk of predictability toward regression or relapse
Decisional Balance	
Pros	Benefits of changing behavior
Cons	Costs of changing behavior
Self-Efficacy	
Confidence	The belief that one can engage in the healthy behavior of the quit state from tobacco products across different challenging situations
Temptation	The pull to engage in the unhealthy behavior of tobacco product use across different challenging situations
Process of change	Ten self-regulation strategies that successful changers use to move from stage to stage
Consciousness-raising	Finding and learning new facts, ideas, and tips that support healthy behavior
Dramatic relief	Experiencing the negative emotions (fear, worry, anxiety) that go along with unhealthy behavior risks but persists in positive change
Self-evaluation	Realizing that the behavior change is important to one's identity
Environmental evaluation	Realizing the effect of one's negative or positive health behavior on their social and physical environment
Self-liberation	Making a firm commitment to change
Helping relationships	Seeking and using social support
Counterconditioning	Substituting healthier alternative behaviors for unhealthy ones
Contingency management	Rewarding positive behavior; demeriting negative behavior

Data from Prochaska, J. O., & DiClemente, C. C. (1983). Stages and processes of self-change of smoking: Toward an integrative model of change. *Journal of Consulting and Clinical Psychology, 51*(3), 390–395. https://doi.org/ 10.1037//0022-006x.51.3.390

can foster change talk and build self-efficacy by asking open-ended questions that further explore motivation and confidence. "Why are you at (patient's score) and not (a lower number)?" "What would it take for you to go from (patient's score) to (a higher number)?" When the APP determines that patients are ready to proceed with a quit attempt, they can move on to the *assist* and *arrange* steps.

If patients do not think it important to quit tobacco use at this time or do not feel confident in their ability to quit, the APP can utilize the 5Rs model (AHRQ, 2012b). There are many reasons why patients may not want to quit tobacco use. This model addresses five content areas that may motivate patients to consider a quit attempt: relevance, risks, rewards, roadblocks, and repetition. The APP should ask open-ended questions to invite patients to explore these areas: "How is quitting personally *relevant* to you?" "What do you know about the *risks* to your health of using tobacco?" "How might it be *rewarding* to you if you quit using tobacco?" "What *roadblocks* would make quitting difficult for you?" *Repetition* reminds the APP to repeat the conversation at every patient visit. Tobacco users who have been unsuccessful in previous quitting experiences should be told that smokers make an average of 30 attempts before they successfully quit smoking (Chaiton et al., 2016).

Assist in Developing a Quit Plan (Treatment Approaches)

The *assist* step is where the APP helps patients to develop a quit plan. The quit plan should be collaboratively developed and tailored to patients' needs and preferences. Treatment approaches for the quit plan should be based on recognized clinical guidelines for treating tobacco use and dependence and include pharmacotherapy, behavioral counseling, and lifestyle strategies. The U.S. Public Health Service–sponsored clinical practice guideline, *Treating Tobacco Use and Dependence: 2008*

Update, contains strategies and recommendations for helping clinicians deliver effective tobacco use and dependence interventions (Fiore et al., 2008).

Harm Reduction Theory

Historically, nicotine replacement products and devices have successfully aided individuals to quit combustible tobacco products, though often not quit nicotine altogether. Although the latter is the ultimate goal, a harm reduction process has been favored in tobacco users who cannot completely adhere to a nicotine-free use intervention plan. The harm reduction theory supports that people have a lower risk of physical harm when using noncombustible nicotine products compared to cigarettes and cigars, which are lit on fire and inhaled and deliver thousands of toxins in the smoke produced (Australian Tobacco Harm Reduction Association, n.d.). Nevertheless, the perception that nicotine is the causal agent in smoking-related diseases remains constant among medical providers (Ferrara et al., 2019).

It is essential to understand the risk profile of different tobacco products, particularly when working with tobacco users who may not be able to quit but who want to switch to a less harmful nicotine product. **Figure 16.3** displays the range of harm from various tobacco product use. Smoking cigarettes causes more harm to users and others (e.g., secondhand smoke, pollution, environmental contamination) than any other product listed. Harm reduction involves switching from nicotine products at the risky left end of the x-axis to nicotine products at the less harmful right end. For those who have difficulty quitting combustible products (e.g., cigarettes, cigars, pipes), attempts to switch to noncombustible nicotine products (e.g., snus, e-cigarettes, nicotine replacement products) might be an acceptable step toward complete tobacco cessation (Nutt et al., 2014). Additionally, using a noncombustible product provides the user

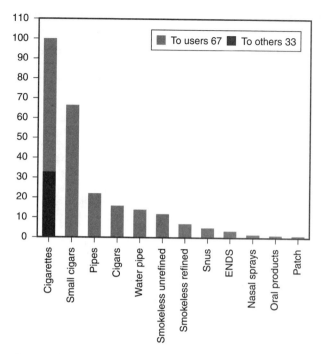

Figure 16.3 Range of harm from tobacco product use.

Nutt, D. J., Phillips, L. D., Balfour, D., Curran, H. V., Dockrell, M., Foulds, J., Fagerström, K., Letlape, K., Milton, A., Polosa, R., Ramsey, J., & Sweanor, D. (2014). Estimating the harms of nicotine-containing products using the MCDA approach. *European Addiction Research, 20,* 218–225. https://doi.org/10.1159/000360220

with additional support for lifestyle behavior changes (Australian Tobacco Harm Reduction Association, n.d.).

Pharmacotherapy

The use of medication doubles the quit rates and is suggested in every quit attempt unless contraindicated. Seven FDA-approved tobacco dependence medications are reviewed in **Table 16.8**. Nicotine replacement therapy (NRT) helps reduce symptoms and cravings to use nicotine by providing a controlled dose of the addictive chemical while a person learns to live without the tobacco product. It is safe and delivers nicotine at a reduced level, allowing a person to receive lower doses to reduce withdrawal symptoms but not support an addiction. NRT has no toxic substances such as carbon monoxide, tar, or the over 7,000 chemicals produced from burning a tobacco product. In addition, there are no dramatic

increases in nicotine levels with NRT, so dependence is significantly reduced (Fiore et al., 2008). The type of medications and doses prescribed will depend on the severity of the tobacco dependency, patient preference, comorbidities, and contraindications. Combination treatment is also an option.

Behavioral Approaches That Support Tobacco Cessation

While medication is often considered in tobacco treatment, it only acknowledges the dependent state of physical nicotine addiction. It has little effect on the social (e.g., smoking with friends) and sensory (e.g., smelling a cigarette, inhaling the smoke, seeing a plume on exhalation) experiences of a person who smokes. Therefore, the APP should offer nonpharmacotherapeutic approaches, such as patient education and cognitive-behavioral strategies, that help the patient manage triggers for

Table 16.8 FDA-Approved Tobacco Dependence Medications

Medication	Description	Additional Information

Nicotine gum	Over-the-counter (OTC) short-acting NRT product
	    May be covered by insurance if a prescription is provided
	    Dose: 2 mg or 4 mg pieces, determined by how soon the first cigarette is smoked (higher dose if the patient smokes within 30 minutes of awakening).
	    Chew one piece every 1–2 hours while awake, not to exceed 24 pieces per day.
		The chew-and-park method is recommended for optimal results. The product is chewed until a peppery taste in the mouth occurs and then it is parked between the gum and the cheek. Once the pepper taste and tingling are gone (about 10 minutes), the user repeats the chew. One piece can last about three rounds of chew and park, or about 30 minutes.
		    If chewed like a piece of regular gum, it can cause heartburn, hiccups, or jaw pain.

Nicotine patch	OTC short-acting NRT product
	    May be covered by insurance if a prescription is provided.
	    Dose: 21 mg, 14 mg, or 7 mg patch applied to the skin daily.
		The patch is placed on clean, dry skin. It is fully absorbed in about 2 hours and delivers a steady state of nicotine over 24 hours.
		    Change the location of the patch every day.
		    If the patient experiences disturbed sleep, the patch may be removed 30 minutes before bedtime.
		    If skin irritation develops, do not use the same location until all redness or irritation is resolved.

Nicotine lozenge	OTC short-acting NRT product
	    May be covered by insurance if a prescription is provided
	    Dose: 2 mg or 4 mg lozenges, determined by how soon the first cigarette is smoked (higher dose if the patient smokes within 30 minutes of awakening).
	    Use one hourly, as needed, not to exceed 20 lozenges per day.
		Available in regular or mini size and several flavors.
		    Allow the lozenge to dissolve in the mouth. Do not chew it.
		    The nicotine is absorbed in 20 minutes.

Nicotine nasal spray	A prescription is required.
	    Dose: One or two sprays in nostril per hour. Do not sniff.
	    The maximum dose is 10 sprays per hour, not to exceed 80 total sprays per day.
		The product is designed to deliver nicotine quickly via the nasal mucosa.
		    Can cause nasal irritation.

Nicotine inhaler	A prescription is required.
	    Dose: Each cartridge can deliver 4 mg of nicotine over 80 small inhalations, not to exceed 20 cartridges per day.
		The product is puffed into the oral cavity for mucosal absorption. It should not be inhaled or drawn like a cigarette, or it will cause coughing and throat irritation.
		    The nicotine inhaler is designed to combine pharmacological and behavioral support (i.e., holding a cigarette).

Medication	Description	Additional Information
Zyban (bupropion)	A prescription is required. Dose: 150 mg once daily for three days, then increase to 150 mg q12hr. Intervention should be continued for 7–12 weeks. If the patient successfully quits after 7–12 weeks, consider ongoing maintenance therapy based on individual patient risk/benefit. Zyban can also be prescribed with NRT for a personalized intervention program.	Bupropion stimulates the brain to release the feel-good hormone dopamine and reduces nicotine cravings and withdrawal symptoms. It can be prescribed as a sustained release and is not addictive. Generally, users have less weight gain. If a patient has a history of seizures, alcohol dependence, or liver disease, consider different medications.
Chantix (varenicline)	A prescription is required. Dose: 0.5 mg once a day for 3 days. Increase to 1 mg daily for 4 days, then 1 mg BID for the duration of the intervention. Doses should be spaced at least 8 hours apart. The 4-week starter pack is organized to provide correct dosing to patients.	The medication should be started 1–2 weeks before the quit date. The patient can also start the medication even if there is no interest in quitting as a possible method to reduce or quit tobacco use. Instruct the patient to always take this medication after eating with a full glass of water. The most common adverse effects are nausea and disturbed sleep. Varenicline blocks nicotine from binding to the nicotine receptors in the brain, therefore preventing the release of dopamine and reducing the rewarding aspects of smoking. Follow patients for tolerance to the medication and any new or worsening mental health symptoms.

tobacco use and cope with withdrawal symptoms. These interventions are grounded in a psychological approach.

Patient education may include information such as the immediate health benefits experienced from tobacco cessation, nicotine withdrawal symptoms, tips to manage cravings, or local tobacco cessation services (e.g., quitlines). Information on how to design a quit plan can be provided using the STAR acronym, which stands for *set* a quit date, *tell* others, *anticipate* challenges, and *remove* tobacco products from the environment (WHO, 2014). The APP should also include information and interventions to address barriers or concerns that arose during the *assess* step. **Table 16.9** lists common concerns about quitting and possible interventions.

Cognitive behavioral strategies include identifying and avoiding triggers (e.g., smoking after a meal or in the car, smoking while with friends), reducing access to cigarettes, and altering the environment to support quitting. Addressing cravings is critical. Typically, urges to use tobacco are brief, lasting only one to two minutes (WHO, 2014). The 4Ds strategy to deal with smoking cravings offers four steps for managing urges:

- Delay: Set a time limit before giving in to smoking a cigarette. Delay as long as possible.
- Deep breathing: Take 10 deep breaths to promote relaxation until the urge passes. Meditation can also be helpful during this step.

Table 16.9 Common Concerns About Tobacco Cessation

Concern	Intervention
Lack of support for cessation	▪ Schedule follow-up visits or telephone calls with patients. ▪ Urge patients to call the National Quitline Network (1-800-QUIT-NOW) or a local quitline. ▪ Help patients identify sources of support within their environment and social circles. ▪ Refer patients to an appropriate organization that offers counseling or support.
Negative mood or depression	▪ If significant, provide counseling, prescribe appropriate medication, or refer patients to a specialist.
Strong or prolonged withdrawal symptoms	▪ If patients report prolonged craving or other withdrawal symptoms, consider extending the use of an approved medication or adding/combining medications to reduce strong withdrawal symptoms.
Weight gain	▪ Recommend starting or increasing physical activity. ▪ Reassure patients that some weight gain after quitting is common and usually is self-limiting. ▪ Emphasize the health benefits of quitting relative to the health risks of modest weight gain. ▪ Emphasize the importance of a healthy diet and an active lifestyle. ▪ Suggest low-calorie substitutes such as sugarless chewing gum, vegetables, or mints. ▪ Consider medications known to delay weight gain, such as bupropion SR and NRTs (particularly 4 mg nicotine gum and lozenges). ▪ Refer patients to a registered dietitian, nutritionist, or nutritional program. Increase water intake, and use hard candies if sweets are craved (bold flavors such as peppermint or cinnamon are usually preferred).
Smoking lapses	▪ Suggest continued use of medications, reducing the likelihood that a lapse will lead to a full relapse. ▪ Encourage another quit attempt or a recommitment to total abstinence. ▪ Reassure that quitting may take multiple attempts, and use the lapse as a learning experience. ▪ Provide or refer for intensive counseling.

Adapted from Fiore, M. C., Jaén, C. R., Baker, T. B., Bailey, W. C., Benowitz, N. L., Curry, S. J., Dorfman, S. F., Froelicher, E. S., Goldstein, M. G., Healton, C. G., Henderson, P. N., Heyman, R. B., Koh, H. K., Kottke, T. E., Lando, H. A., Mecklenberg, R. E., Mermelstein, R. J., Mullen, P. D., Orleans, C. T., . . . Wewers, M. E. (2008). *Treating tobacco use and dependence: 2008 Update.* Clinical Practice Guideline. U.S. Department of Health and Human Services. Public Health Service.

- Drink water: Drinking water is a healthy alternative to putting a cigarette in the mouth and helps flush out toxins.
- Do something else: Consider activities to distract oneself from the urge, such as reading, going for a walk, listening to music, phoning a friend, watching television, or engaging in a hobby. (WHO, 2014)

While behavioral approaches are effective, these techniques may not support the sensory and motor connections that have become a way of life for the user (Dawkins, 2013). The APP should think about the ingrained ritual (e.g., lighting a cigarette first thing in the morning or as soon as one gets in the car) that is likely a subconscious behavior in a longtime daily smoker. Offering only medication and behavioral techniques (e.g., resisting urges and cravings to smoke) ignores the body's habits and way of being. Tobacco interventions should consider the strength of these habits and the relationships between smoking and the body's senses, actions, and emotions. Some patients may benefit from tobacco use interventions that include self-reflection and increased awareness of the connection to smoking through repeated actions, senses, and emotions created from years of use (Hrabovsky, 2018).

Lifestyle Strategies That Support Tobacco Cessation

Overcoming addiction to nicotine and the habits that support tobacco dependence requires a redirection of attention to establishing a different lifestyle—a health-promoting one. Lifestyle behaviors, such as those in the A-SMART (adopt a healthy diet, stress less, move often, avoid alcohol, rest more, and treat tobacco use) model, can help patients alleviate withdrawal symptoms and strengthen their immune systems (WHO, 2014). The APP can counsel patients to *adopt a healthy diet* and stay hydrated to lessen the severity of headaches, counter cravings, and prevent weight gain. Strategies to *stress less* include recruiting social support and developing relaxation and coping mechanisms to improve concentration and increase resilience. Patients who *move often* can effectively deal with restlessness and overcome insomnia. Exercise also improves cardiorespiratory fitness and lung function negatively affected by smoking. Outdoor exercise with exposure to sunlight gives the benefit of enhancing the metabolism of vitamin D, which strengthens the immune system. It is also vital to *avoid alcohol* since drinking alcohol can make quitting

smoking more difficult and increase the risk of relapse (NCI, n.d.-a). Note that reducing alcohol intake could precipitate withdrawal symptoms in alcohol-dependent persons. Finally, patients who rest more find it easier to manage the flu-like symptoms caused by nicotine withdrawal. A measured and temperate application of healthy behaviors will aid mental and emotional decision-making about one's lifestyle.

Arrange for Follow-Up

Tobacco use treatment can be time consuming and complex. It often requires multiple resources and several attempts by the tobacco user to quit. Therefore, follow-up is critical. The APP should schedule a follow-up contact via telephone, email, or personal visit during the first week and within 1 month after the quit date (WHO, 2014). The purpose of this contact is to affirm progress and efforts made, identify problems, anticipate challenges, assess medication use, and offer support. For patients who have slipped, the contact can serve to reframe the lapse as a successful learning experience, strengthen motivation and confidence, and elicit recommitment.

There are many barriers to successful tobacco use treatment. Although patients may have an attitude of well-considered decision and eagerness to engage in the tobacco cessation process, some will have motivating factors beyond the scope of APP practice. For example, patients may present out of desperation or fear because of a recent diagnosis (e.g., stroke, cancer), because their employer has mandated a tobacco-free workplace or offered a benefits package for tobacco-free workers, or because a significant person in their life is nagging or begging them to quit. Some patients may have comorbidities or stressful living conditions that make a healthy lifestyle change difficult and increase the risk of relapse. The effect of tobacco cessation on medications needs to be considered for patients with mental health disorders. Each of these factors may affect success in tobacco use intervention. Therefore, the APP should consider referral to other health professionals, such as behavioral health specialists, dietitians, exercise specialists, addiction specialists, and counselors.

Community resources, such as smoking cessation programs, healthy lifestyle classes (e.g., exercise, weight loss), support groups (e.g., Nicotine Anonymous), and telephone-based services, can provide additional support. See **Table 16.11** for evidence-based resources to treat tobacco use. In the context of community health promotion, there are opportune times to plan community-based efforts. October has been designated National Healthy Lung Month

(https://nationaltoday.com). The third Thursday in November is designated as the Great American Smokeout (www.cancer.org).

5As: Putting Them All Together

The strategies in **Table 16.10** provide guidelines for the APP when approaching, counseling, and recommending interventions to patients with tobacco use or dependence. They are taken from *Treating Tobacco Use and Dependence: 2008 Update* (Fiore et al., 2008).

Table 16.10 Strategies for Treating Tobacco Use

Step	Strategies for Implementation
Ask	Ask patients at every visit about tobacco use and document findings in the their record. If patients use tobacco: ■ Verify the tobacco products used, how often, and for how long. ■ Calculate pack-years for smoking. ■ Assess for nicotine dependence. If patients have quit, ask for how long and acknowledge their success.
Advise	In a clear, strong, and personalized manner, urge every tobacco user to quit. Advice should be: ■ Clear: "It is important that you quit smoking (or using chewing tobacco) now, and I can help you." "Cutting down while you are ill is not enough." "Occasional or light smoking is still dangerous." ■ Strong: "As your provider, I need you to know that quitting smoking is the most important thing you can do to protect your health now and in the future. The clinic staff and I will help you." ■ Personalized: Tie tobacco use to current symptoms and health concerns, social and economic costs, or the effect of tobacco use on children and others in the household. "Continuing to smoke makes your asthma worse, and quitting may dramatically improve your health." "Quitting smoking may reduce the number of ear infections your child has."
Assess	Assess patients' willingness to quit: "Are you willing to give quitting a try?" ■ If patients are willing to make a quit attempt at the time, provide assistance. ■ If patients will participate in intensive treatment, deliver such treatment or refer to intensive intervention. ■ If patients are members of a special population (e.g., adolescent, pregnant smoker, minority), consider providing additional information to address their unique needs and concerns. ■ If patients clearly state that they are unwilling to make a quit attempt at the time, use an MI approach to encourage them to identify the negative consequences of tobacco use and the positive consequences of quitting. Provide an intervention to increase future quit attempts, such as the 5Rs (relevance, risks, rewards, roadblocks, repetition), and offer to revisit at the next visit.

Step	Strategies for Implementation
Assist	Collaborate with patients to design an individualized quit plan that includes pharmacotherapy, behavioral counseling, and lifestyle strategies.
	Preparation for Quitting (STAR):
	■ Set a quit date. Ideally, the quit date should be within 2 weeks.
	■ Tell family, friends, and coworkers about quitting, and request understanding and support.
	■ Anticipate challenges to the upcoming quit attempt, particularly during the critical first few weeks. These include nicotine withdrawal symptoms.
	■ Remove tobacco products from the environment. Before quitting, avoid smoking in places where much time is spent (e.g., work, home, car). Make the home smoke-free.
	Pharmacotherapy:
	■ Recommend using an FDA-approved medication, except when contraindicated or with specific populations for which there is insufficient evidence of effectiveness (e.g., pregnant women, smokeless tobacco users, light smokers, and adolescents). Consider the use of FDA-approved medications alone or in combination.
	Behavioral Counseling:
	■ Provide practical counseling (problem-solving/skills training).
	■ Striving for total abstinence is essential. Not even a single puff after the quit date.
	■ Discuss past quit attempts. Identify what helped to build on past successes. Likewise, identify what contributed to relapses to learn from those experiences.
	■ Anticipate triggers or challenges in the upcoming attempt and how patients can successfully overcome them (e.g., avoid triggers, alter routines, employ coping mechanisms). Use decisional balance questioning to encourage tobacco users to advocate for their behavior change.
	■ Identify other smokers in the household and elicit their support or partnership. Quitting is more difficult when there is another smoker in the household. Advise patients to encourage household members to quit with them or to not smoke in their presence.
	A-SMART Lifestyle Strategies
	Encourage patients to:
	■ Adopt a healthy diet
	■ Stress less
	■ Move often
	■ Avoid alcohol
	■ Rest more
	■ Treat tobacco use
Arrange	Provide a supportive clinical environment to encourage patients in their quit attempt, and offer follow-up support. "My office staff and I are available to assist you." "I am recommending treatment that can provide ongoing support."
	Provide written materials and share about community programs and online resources that are culturally/racially/educationally/age appropriate for patients. These materials should be readily available at every clinician's workstation.
	Consider referrals to behavioral health specialists, dietitians, exercise specialists, addiction specialists, and counselors as needed.

Adapted from Fiore, M. C., Jaén, C. R., Baker, T. B., Bailey, W. C., Benowitz, N. L., Curry, S. J., Dorfman, S. F., Froelicher, E. S., Goldstein, M. G., Healton, C. G., Henderson, P. N., Heyman, R. B., Koh, H. K., Kottke, T. E., Lando, H. A., Mecklenberg, R. E., Mermelstein, R. J., Mullen, P. D., Orleans, C. T., . . . Wewers, M. E. (2008). *Treating tobacco use and dependence: 2008 Update.* Clinical Practice Guideline. U.S. Department of Health and Human Services. Public Health Service.

Health Promotion Case Study: Addressing Tobacco Dependence

Case Description: D.T. is a 46-year-old African American male who presents for his routine blood pressure follow-up. When asked about his tobacco use, he admits he is still smoking. He rates his motivation for quitting as 7/10 and his confidence for quitting as 4/10. He has tried quitting in the past via the cold turkey method (just stopping) but could not make it more than 24 hours due to irritability and feelings of anxiety. He coaches football and is worried that he may lash out at the young players if he attempts to quit again because of his nicotine withdrawal symptoms. He has considered switching from smoking cigarettes to vaping.

- Past medical history: Denies.
- Medications: Amlodipine 5 mg daily.
- Allergies: NKDA.
- Social history: Recently divorced. Drives UPS delivery truck. Lives alone.
- Vital signs: BP 140/86 mmHg left arm, heart rate 82 bpm, respirations 20 bpm, temperature 98.4°F, O_2 saturation 96% on room air, weight 225 lb, height 72 in., BMI 30.5 kg/m^2.
- Review of systems: Positive for chronic cough in the mornings that is productive at times of light-brown mucous. Denies wheezing and shortness of breath. All other systems are negative.
- Physical exam: The physical exam reveals a well-developed, well-nourished male with a positive affect. The exam is unremarkable except for a dry cough during deep inspiration and lungs with fine crackles bilaterally.
- Labs: CBC, CMP, and a lipid panel were drawn 3 months ago. All were within normal range.

Lifestyle Vital Signs
- Adopt healthy eating: Not assessed.
- Stress less: Not assessed.
- Move often: Not assessed.
- Avoid alcohol: Occasional beer in the evenings and on Sunday afternoons when watching football on television. No recreational drug use.
- Rest more: Not assessed.
- Treat tobacco use: Smokes one-half pack of cigarettes daily.

Critical Thinking Questions
- Calculate D.T.'s pack-year history.
- What additional data related to lifestyle behaviors do you want to obtain, and why?
- How might you respond to D.T.'s self-rating of motivation and confidence for quitting smoking?
- What education would you provide about the benefits and risks of switching to vaping?
- What medications would you recommend to D.T. to provide relief of nicotine withdrawal symptoms and to assist with quitting smoking?
- What behavioral counseling topics would you want to discuss?
- What lifestyle strategies would you recommend for optimizing D.T.'s quit success?
- What materials or smoking cessation resources might you share with D.T.?
- What might be your plan for follow-up? What would you want to address in future visits?
- What referrals would you consider, if any?

Reimbursement for Treatment Use Intervention

The Patient Protection and Affordable Care Act requires most health payers to cover tobacco screening, counseling, and quit attempts, including FDA-approved medications and behavior change support services (Center of Excellence for Health Systems Improvement, n.d.). Although tobacco treatment reimbursement varies by insurer and contract, clinicians can expect to be compensated for tobacco use intervention in a manner similar to compensation for other services provided. Several Current Procedural Terminology (CPT) codes are available for the provision of tobacco cessation services, depending on whether the patient is new or existing, the type of counseling (e.g., individual, group), length of counseling, and other services provided. Documentation should include time spent on counseling (i.e., patient education, guidance, and management), topics covered, the patient's stage of change, medication prescribed, support or referral provided for a quit attempt, and the follow-up plan.

When billing for tobacco use intervention, APPs can use the ICD-10 code Z72.0 to specify a diagnosis of tobacco use. Nicotine dependence codes are defined by the type of nicotine patients use (e.g., cigarettes, chewing tobacco, e-cigarettes) and whether their dependence is uncomplicated, in remission, with withdrawal symptoms, or with other nicotine-induced disorders. For example, F17.210 specifies a diagnosis of nicotine dependence, cigarette, uncomplicated. The type of product used, frequency of use, and any related complications (e.g., nicotine-induced chronic obstructive pulmonary disease [COPD]) should be documented. Some health systems incorporate automatic referrals to quitlines or community intervention centers through the electronic medical record.

Health Promotion Activity: Reflection on Trends in Tobacco Use and Quit Attempts

Review the following data. What are the implications for your practice? What knowledge, skills, and resources do you have to address tobacco use and dependence effectively?

- In 2020, an estimated 12.5% of U.S. adults were current smokers (Cornelius et al., 2020). Nearly 70% of smokers say they are "interested" in quitting (Babb et al., 2017). Less than one-third of smokers who tried to quit used proven cessation treatments, and less than 1 in 10 quit successfully in the past year (Creamer et al., 2019).
- Most quitters require multiple attempts before succeeding (WHO, 2014). Most smokers try to quit independently, but self-quitters have a success rate of 3–5% (Hughes et al., 2004).

References

Babb, S., Malarcher, A., Schauer, G., Asman, K., & Jamal, A. (2017). Quitting smoking among adults—United States, 2000–2015. *Morbidity and Mortality Weekly Report, 65*(52), 1457–1464. http://dx.doi.org/10.15585/mmwr.mm6552a1

Cornelius, M. E., Loretan, C. G., Wang, T. W., Jamal, A., & Homa, D. M. (2020). Tobacco product use among adults—United States, 2020. *Morbidity and Mortality Weekly Report, 71*(11), 397–405. http://dx.doi.org/10.15585/mmwr.mm7111a1

Creamer, M. R., Wang, T. W., Babb, S., Cullen, K. A., Day, H., Wills, G., Jamal, A., & Neff, L. (2019). Tobacco product use and cessation indicators among adults—United States, 2018. *Morbidity and Mortality Weekly Report, 68*(45), 1013–1019. https://www.cdc.gov/mmwr/volumes/68/wr/mm6845a2.htm

Hughes, J. R., Keely, J., & Naud, S. (2004). Shape of the relapse curve and long-term abstinence among untreated smokers. *Addiction, 99*(1), 29–38. https://doi.org/10.1111/j.1360-0443.2004.00540.x

World Health Organization. (2014). *A guide for tobacco users to quit.* https://apps.who.int/iris/handle/10665/112833

TABLE 16.11	Evidence-Based Resources for Treating Tobacco Use	
Organization	**Description**	**URL**
Clinician Resources		
Agency for Healthcare Research and Quality	Treatment guideline: *Treating Tobacco Use and Dependence: 2008 Update*, clinician resources	https://www.ahrq.gov/prevention/guidelines/tobacco/index.html
American Cancer Society	Extensive resources on prevention, education, and treatment of tobacco-related cancers	https://www.cancer.org/healthy/stay-away-from-tobacco.html
American College of Lifestyle Medicine	Lifestyle Medicine Core Competencies: Tobacco Cessation (continuing education course)	https://portal.lifestylemedicine.org/ACLM/Store/Education-Store/Store-Front.aspx
American Public Health Association	Fact sheets, policy statements, and reports related to advocacy on tobacco	https://apha.org/Topics-and-issues/Tobacco
Campaign for Tobacco-Free Kids	Advocacy for the protection of children and youth for 25 years	www.tobaccofreekids.org
Centers for Disease Control and Prevention	*Brief Tobacco Intervention Pocket Guide*	https://www.cdc.gov/tobacco/campaign/tips/partners/health/materials/twyd-5a-2a-tobacco-intervention-pocket-card.pdf
Center of Excellence for Health Systems Improvement	*Documenting, Coding, & Billing for Tobacco Dependence Treatment*	https://tobaccofreeny.org/images/hsi/Resources/Documenting-Coding-Billing-For-Tobacco-Dependence-Treatment.pdf
CHEST Foundation	Clinician Interactive Toolkit and downloadable *Tobacco Dependence Treatment Toolkit*	https://foundation.chestnet.org/lung-health-a-z/smoking-and-tobacco-use/?Item=For-Clinicians
Mayo Clinic	*Tobacco Dependence Treatment Medication Summary*	https://www.mayo.edu/research/documents/medication-handout-2015-02-pdf/doc-20140182

Organization	Description	URL
Merlo Lab	Motivational interviewing video examples	Bad example: https://youtu.be /80XyNE89eCs Good example: https://youtu.be /URiKA7CKtfc
National Institute on Drug Abuse	Posts the latest research facts on vaping and nicotine	https://nida.nih.gov/research -topics/tobacconicotine-vaping
New York City Health	*Smoking Cessation Medication Prescribing Chart*	https://www1.nyc.gov/assets/doh /downloads/pdf/csi/tobacco-med -brief-instructions.pdf
Centers for Disease Control and Prevention	Education, history, statistics, legislation activities against tobacco product use and tobacco cessation resources	https://www.cdc.gov/tobacco /index.htm
Substance Abuse and Mental Health Services Administration	Gives special attention to youth and young adult tobacco users. Provides training webinars. Focuses on substance and mental health.	www.samhsa.gov
Truth Initiative	Nonprofit public health organization dedicated to eliminating smoking and vaping and the resulting nicotine addiction among young people	https://truthinitiative.org /who-we-are/our-mission
U.S. Department of Health and Human Services	*E-Cigarette, or Vaping, Products Visual Dictionary*	https://www.cdc.gov/tobacco /basic_information/e-cigarettes /pdfs/ecigarette-or-vaping -products-visual-dictionary -508.pdf
World Health Organization	*Toolkit for Delivering the 5A's and 5R's Brief Tobacco Interventions in Primary Care*	https://apps.who.int/iris /bitstream/handle/10665 /112835/9789241506953_eng.pdf
Patient Resources		
Centers for Disease Control and Prevention	*Five Reasons Why Calling a Quitline Can Be Key to Your Success* (national portal to a network of state quitlines)	https://www.cdc.gov/tobacco /campaign/tips/quit-smoking /quitline/index.html?s_cid =OSH_misc_M150
American Cancer Society	Cancer Helpline: 800-227-2345 Educational resources, email-based tobacco cessation program	https://www.cancer.org/healthy /stay-away-from-tobacco/great -american-smokeout.html

(continues)

| TABLE 16.11 | Evidence-Based Resources for Treating Tobacco Use | *(continued)* |

Organization	Description	URL
American Lung Association	*Freedom From Smoking*® tobacco cessation program	https://www.lung.org/quit-smoking/join-freedom-from-smoking/about-freedom-from-smoking
BreatheFree 2.0	Evidence-based smoking cessation program	https://www.breathefree2.com/
CHEST Foundation	Video game: *Smoke Out: Tobacco Pirates*	https://appadvice.com/app/smoke-out-tobacco-pirates/1546616873
Mayo Clinic BecomeAnEX	Advice, tips, interactive tools, text messages, support community	https://www.becomeanex.org
National Cancer Institute	NCI Quitline: 877-448-7848 Educational materials, resources, assistance in creating a personalized quit plan, live chat	https://smokefree.gov
Nicotine Anonymous	A 12-step program for nicotine addiction	https://www.nicotine-anonymous.org
QuitAssist	Resources for quitting smoking, quitting success stories	https://www.quitassist.com
SmokefreeVET	Tools, tips, free text message program for daily advice and support	https://veterans.smokefree.gov
U.S. Department of Health and Human Services	Educational materials and quit tools	https://betobaccofree.hhs.gov
U.S. Food and Drug Administration	Educational materials and quitting smoking resources	https://www.fda.gov/tobacco-products/public-health-education/health-effects-tobacco-use
WHO	*A Guide for Tobacco Users to Quit*	https://apps.who.int/iris/handle/10665/112833

Summary

Tobacco use is the leading cause of preventable disease, disability, and death in the United States (CDC, n.d.-g). The current recommendation is for clinicians to ask all adults about tobacco use, advise them to stop using tobacco, and provide behavioral interventions for cessation (U.S. Preventive Services Task Force, 2021). APPs play an essential role in health promotion by implementing tobacco use screening and counseling in various healthcare settings. The 5As model provides a guide for patient conversations: (1) ask about tobacco use, (2) advise quitting, (3) assess readiness to quit, (4) assist in the quit attempt, and (5) arrange for follow-up (Fiore et al., 2008). Treatment approaches for the quit plan should be individualized and based on recognized clinical guidelines, such as *Treating Tobacco Use and Dependence: 2008 Update.* The APP should collaborate with patients to design individualized quit plans that include pharmacotherapy, behavioral counseling, and lifestyle strategies. Many insurance payers reimburse tobacco use intervention.

Acronyms

5As: ask, advise, assess, assist, arrange

5Rs: relevance, risks, rewards, roadblocks, repetition

ACS: American Cancer Society

AHA: American Heart Association

AHRQ: Agency for Healthcare Research and Quality

APP: advanced practice provider

A-SMART: adopt a healthy diet, stress less, move often, avoid alcohol, rest more, and treat tobacco use

CDC: Centers for Disease Control and Prevention

CO: carbon monoxide

EC: electronic cigarettes

ENDS: electronic nicotine delivery systems

FDA: U.S. Food and Drug Administration

HHS: U.S. Department of Health and Human Services

MI: motivational interviewing

NCI: National Cancer Institute

NRT: nicotine replacement therapy

OTC: over the counter

RYO: roll your own

STAR: *set* a quit date, *tell* others, *anticipate* challenges, and *remove* tobacco products from the environment

TTM: transtheoretical model

WHO: World Health Organization

References

Agency for Healthcare Research and Quality. (2012a). *Five major steps to intervention (The "5 A's").* https://www.ahrq.gov/prevention/guidelines/tobacco/5steps.html

Agency for Healthcare Research and Quality. (2012b). *Patients not ready to make a quit attempt now (The "5 R's").* https://www.ahrq.gov/prevention/guidelines/tobacco/5rs.html

Al-Ibrahim, M. S., & Gross, J. Y. (1990). Tobacco use. In H. K. Walker, W. D. Hall, & J. W. Hurst (Eds.), *Clinical methods: The history, physical, and laboratory examinations* (3rd ed.). Butterworths. https://www.ncbi.nlm.nih.gov/books/NBK362

American Cancer Society. (2020, October 28). *Health risks of smoking tobacco.* https://www.cancer.org/cancer/cancer-causes/tobacco-and-cancer/health-risks-of-smoking-tobacco.html

American Heart Association. (n.d.). *How smoking and nicotine damage your body.* Retrieved March 22, 2022, from https://www.heart.org/en/healthy-living/healthy-lifestyle/quit-smoking-tobacco/how-smoking-and-nicotine-damage-your-body

Australian Tobacco Harm Reduction Association. (n.d.). *What is tobacco harm reduction?* Retrieved March 22, 2022, from https://www.athra.org.au/what-is-tobacco-harm-reduction

Babb, S., Malarcher, A., Schauer, G., Asman, K., & Jamal, A. (2017). Quitting smoking among adults—United States, 2000–2015. *Morbidity and Mortality Weekly Report, 65*(52), 1457–1464. http://dx.doi.org/10.15585/mmwr.mm6552a1

Benowitz, N. L. (2010). Nicotine addiction. *New England Journal of Medicine, 362*(24), 2295–2303. https://doi.org/10.1056/NEJMra0809890

Blount, B. C., Karwowski, M. P., Shields, P. G., Morel-Espinosa, M., Valentin-Blasini, L., Gardner, M. S., Braselton, M., Brosius, C. R., Caron, K. T., Chambers, D., Corstvet, J., Cowan, E., De Jesús, V. R., Espinosa, P., Fernandez, C., Holder, C., Kuklenyik, Z., Kusovschi, J. D., Newman, C., . . . Pirkle, J. L. (2020). Vitamin E acetate in bronchoalveolar-lavage fluid associated with EVALI. *New England Journal of Medicine, 382*(8), 697–705. https://doi.org/10.1056/NEJMoa1916433

Boudreaux, E. D., Sullivan, A., Abar, B., Bernstein, S. L., Ginde, A. A., & Camargo, C. A., Jr. (2012). Motivation rulers for smoking cessation: A prospective observational examination of construct and predictive validity. *Addiction Science & Clinical Practice*, 7(1), 8. https://doi.org/10.1186/1940-0640-7-8

Calafat, A. M., Polzin, G. M., Saylor, J., Richter, P., Ashley, D. L., & Watson, C. H. (2004). Determination of tar, nicotine, and carbon monoxide yields in the mainstream smoke of selected international cigarettes. *Tobacco Control*, 13(1), 45–51. https://doi.org/10.1136/tc.2003.003673

Campaign for Tobacco-Free Kids. (2021a, December 21). *Raising cigarette taxes reduces smoking, especially among kids (and the cigarette companies know it)*. https://www.tobaccofreekids.org/assets/factsheets/0146.pdf

Campaign for Tobacco-Free Kids. (2021b, December 15). *The path to tobacco addiction starts at very young ages.* https://www.tobaccofreekids.org/assets/factsheets/0127.pdf

Center of Excellence for Health Systems Improvement. (n.d.). *Documenting, coding, and billing for tobacco dependence treatment: A guide to maximizing reimbursement.* Retrieved March 22, 2022, from https://tobaccofreeny.org/images/hsi/Resources/Documenting-Coding-Billing-For-Tobacco-Dependence-Treatment.pdf

Centers for Disease Control and Prevention. (n.d.-a). *Cigarette smoking in the U.S.* Retrieved March 22, 2022, from https://www.cdc.gov/tobacco/data_statistics/fact_sheets/fast_facts/cigarette-smoking-in-the-us.html

Centers for Disease Control and Prevention. (n.d.-b). *Current cigarette smoking among adults in the United States.* Retrieved March 22, 2022, from https://www.cdc.gov/tobacco/data_statistics/fact_sheets/adult_data/cig_smoking/index.htm

Centers for Disease Control and Prevention. (n.d.-c). *Electronic cigarettes.* Retrieved March 22, 2022, from https://www.cdc.gov/tobacco/basic_information/e-cigarettes/index.htm

Centers for Disease Control and Prevention. (n.d.-d). *History of the surgeon general's reports on smoking and health.* Retrieved March 22, 2022, from https://www.cdc.gov/tobacco/data_statistics/sgr/history/index.htm

Centers for Disease Control and Prevention. (n.d.-e). *Office on Smoking and Health (OSH).* Retrieved March 22, 2022, from https://www.cdc.gov/tobacco/about/osh/index.htm?s_cid=osh-stu-home-nav-001

Centers for Disease Control and Prevention. (n.d.-f). *Smoking and tobacco use: Fast facts.* Retrieved March 22, 2022, from https://www.cdc.gov/tobacco/data_statistics/fact_sheets/fast_facts/index.htm

Centers for Disease Control and Prevention. (n.d.-g). *Tobacco use.* Retrieved March 22, 2022, from https://www.cdc.gov/chronicdisease/resources/publications/factsheets/tobacco.htm

Centers for Disease Control and Prevention. (n.d.-h). *Tobacco use by youth is rising: E-cigarettes are the main reason.* Retrieved March 22, 2022, from https://www.cdc.gov/vitalsigns/youth-tobacco-use

Centers for Disease Control and Prevention. (2018). *Smoking is down, but almost 38 million American adults still smoke.* https://www.cdc.gov/media/releases/2018/p0118-smoking-rates-declining.html

Centers for Disease Control and Prevention. (2019, February 11). *Data visualization: Tobacco product use among high school students (2018).* CDC Vital signs. https://stacks.cdc.gov/view/cdc/75893

Chaiton, M., Diemert, L., Cohen, J. E., Bondy, S. J., Selby, P., Philipneri, A., & Schwartz, R. (2016). Estimating the number of quit attempts it takes to quit smoking successfully in a longitudinal cohort of smokers. *BMJ Open*, 6(6), e011045. https://doi.org/10.1136/bmjopen-2016-011045

Cheng, C. E., Makredes, M., & Kimball, A. B. (2018, June 25). *Smokeless tobacco lesions.* Medscape. https://emedicine.medscape.com/article/1077117-overview#a5

Cornelius, M. E., Loretan, C. G., Wang, T. W., Jamal, A., & Homa, D. M. (2020). Tobacco product use among adults—United States, 2020. *Morbidity and Mortality Weekly Report*, 71(11), 397–405. http://dx.doi.org/10.15585/mmwr.mm7111a1

Creamer, M. R., Wang, T. W., Babb, S., Cullen, K. A., Day, H., Wills, G., Jamal, A., & Neff, L. (2019). Tobacco product use and cessation indicators among adults—United States, 2018. *Morbidity and Mortality Weekly Report*, 68(45), 1013–1019. https://www.cdc.gov/mmwr/volumes/68/wr/mm6845a2.htm

Cullen, K. A., Gentzke, A. S., Sawdey, M. D., Chang, J. T., Anic, G. M., Wang, T. W., Creamer, M. R., Jamal, A., Ambrose, B. K., & King, B. A. (2019). E-cigarette use among youth in the United States, 2019. *Journal of the American Medical Association*, 322(21), 2095–2103. https://doi.org/10.1001/jama.2019.18387

Cummings, K. M., & Proctor, R. N. (2014). The changing public image of smoking in the United States: 1964–2014. *Cancer Epidemiology, Biomarkers, & Prevention*, 23(1), 32–36. https://doi.org/10.1158/1055-9965.EPI-13-0798

Dawkins, L. (2013). Why is it so hard to quit? *The Psychologist*, 26(5), 332–335. https://www.researchgate.net/publication/287639914_Why_is_it_so_hard_to_quit_smoking

Dubuc, B. (n.d.). *How drugs affect neurotransmitters.* The Brain from Top to Bottom. Retrieved March 22, 2022, from https://thebrain.mcgill.ca/flash/i/i_03/i_03_m/i_03_m_par/i_03_m_par_nicotine.html

Ferrara, P., Shantikumar, S., Cabral Veríssimo, V., Ruiz-Montero, R., Masuet-Aumatell, C., Ramon-Torrell, J. M., & the EuroNet MRPH Working Group on Electronic Cigarettes and Tobacco Harm Reduction. (2019). Knowledge about e-cigarettes and tobacco harm reduction among public health residents in

Europe. *International Journal of Environmental Research and Public Health, 16*(12), 2071. https://doi.org/10.3390/ijerph16122071

Fiore, M. C., Jaén, C. R., Baker, T. B., Bailey, W. C., Benowitz, N. L., Curry, S. J., Dorfman, S. F., Froelicher, E. S., Goldstein, M. G., Healton, C. G., Henderson, P. N., Heyman, R. B., Koh, H. K., Kottke, T. E., Lando, H. A., Mecklenberg, R. E., Mermelstein, R. J., Mullen, P. D., Orleans, C. T., . . . Wewers, M. E. (2008). *Treating tobacco use and dependence: 2008 Update.* U.S. Department of Health and Human Services. Public Health Service.

Geletko, K. W., Graves, K., Lateef, H., & Harman, J. (2022). Tobacco cessation counseling and medications provided by physicians to tobacco users during primary care visits. *Journal of Primary Care & Community Health, 13.* https://doi.org/10.1177/21501319221093115

Heatherton, T. F., Kozlowski, L. T., & Frecker, R. C. (1991). The Fagerström Test for Nicotine Dependence: A revision of the Fagerström Tolerance Questionnaire. *British Journal of Addiction 86,* 1119–1127. https://cde.drugabuse.gov/instrument/d7c0b0f5-b865-e4de-e040-bb89ad43202b

Heckman, C. J., Egleston, B. L., & Hofmann, M. T. (2010). Efficacy of motivational interviewing for smoking cessation: A systematic review and meta-analysis. *Tobacco Control, 19*(5), 410–416. https://doi.org/10.1136/tc.2009.033175

Hughes, J. R., Keely, J., & Naud, S. (2004). Shape of the relapse curve and long-term abstinence among untreated smokers. *Addiction, 99*(1), 29–38. https://doi.org/10.1111/j.1360-0443.2004.00540.x

Hrabovsky, S. (2018). *Body, social and material connections as ways of knowing: A reflection of the adult smoker's experiences when learning about and using an electronic cigarette.* Adult Education Research Conference, Victoria, BC, Canada. https://newprairiepress.org/aerc/2018/papers/10

Hrabovsky, S., Yingst, J. M., Veldherr, S., Hammett, E., & Foulds, J. (2017). Measurement of exhaled breath carbon monoxide in clinical practice: A study of levels in Central Pennsylvania community members. *Journal of the American Association of Nurse Practitioners, 29*(6), 310–315. https://doi.org/10.1002/2327-6924.12460

Instituting Smoke-Free Public Housing, 24 C.F.R. § 965.653. (2018). https://www.govinfo.gov/content/pkg/CFR-2018-title24-vol4/pdf/CFR-2018-title24-vol4.pdf

Jain, P., Danaei, G., Manson, J. E., Robins, J. M., & Hernán, M. A. (2020). Weight gain after smoking cessation and lifestyle strategies to reduce it. *Epidemiology, 31*(1), 7–14. https://doi.org/10.1097/EDE.0000000000001106

Kligerman, S., Raptis, C., Larsen, B., Henry, T. S., Caporale, A., Tazelaar, H., Schiebler, M. L., Wehrli, F. W., Klein, J. S., & Kanne, J. (2020). Radiologic, pathologic, clinical, and physiologic findings of electronic cigarette or vaping product use-associated lung injury (EVALI): Evolving knowledge and remaining questions. *Radiology, 294*(3), 491–505. https://doi.org/10.1148/radiol.2020192585

Lindson-Hawley, N., Thompson, T. P., & Begh, R. (2015). Motivational interviewing for smoking cessation. *Cochrane Database of Systematic Reviews.* https://doi.org/10.1002/14651858.CD006936.pub3

Miller, W., & Rollnick, S. (2013). *Motivational interviewing: Helping people change* (3rd ed.). Guilford Press.

National Association of Attorneys General. (n.d.). *The Master Settlement Agreement.* Retrieved March 22, 2022, from https://www.naag.org/our-work/naag-center-for-tobacco-and-public-health/the-master-settlement-agreement

National Cancer Institute. (n.d.-a). *Alcohol and smoking.* Retrieved July 31, 2022, from https://smokefree.gov/challenges-when-quitting/cravings-triggers/alcohol-smoking

National Cancer Institute. (n.d.-b). *Harms of cigarette smoking and health benefits of quitting.* Retrieved March 22, 2022, from https://www.cancer.gov/about-cancer/causes-prevention/risk/tobacco/cessation-fact-sheet

Nutt, D. J., Phillips, L. D., Balfour, D., Curran, H. V., Dockrell, M., Foulds, J., Fagerstrom, K., Letlape, K., Milton, A., Polosa, R., Ramsey, J., & Sweanor, D. (2014). Estimating the harms of nicotine-containing products using the MCDA approach. *European Addiction Research, 20*(5), 218–225. https://doi.org/10.1159/000360220

Omolaoye, S., El Shahawy, O., Skosana, B. T., Boillat, T., Loney, T., & du Plessis, S. S. (2022). The mutagenic effect of tobacco smoke on male fertility. *Environmental Science and Pollution Research, 29,* 62055–62066. https://doi.org/10.1007/s11356-021-16331-x

Prochaska, J. O., & DiClemente, C. C. (1983). Stages and processes of self-change of smoking: Toward an integrative model of change. *Journal of Consulting and Clinical Psychology, 51*(3), 390–395. https://doi.org/10.1037//0022-006x.51.3.390

Rodgman, A., & Perfetti, T. (2013). *The chemical components of tobacco and tobacco smoke* (2nd ed.). CRC Press.

SRNT Subcommittee on Biochemical Verification. (2002). Biochemical verification of tobacco use intervention. *Nicotine & Tobacco Research, 4*(2), 149–159. https://doi.org/10.1080/14622200210123581

Steinberg, M. B., Schmelzer, A. C., Richardson, D. L., & Foulds, J. (2008). The case for treating tobacco dependence as a chronic disease. *Annals of Internal Medicine, 148*(7), 554–556. https://doi.org/10.7326/0003-4819-148-7-200804010-00012

U.S. Department of Health and Human Services. (n.d.). *Smoking cessation: A report of the surgeon general: Smoking cessation by the numbers.* Retrieved March 22, 2022, from https://www.hhs.gov/surgeongeneral/reports-and-publications/tobacco/2020-cessation-sgr-infographic-by-the-numbers/index.html

U.S. Department of Health and Human Services. (2014). *The health consequences of smoking—50 years of progress. A report of the surgeon general.* https://www.ncbi.nlm.nih.gov/books/NBK179276

U.S. Food and Drug Administration. (2020, May 28). *Products, ingredients, & components.* https://www.fda.gov/tobacco-products/products-guidance-regulations/products-ingredients-components

U.S. Food and Drug Administration. (2021). *What it's like to quit smoking.* https://www.fda.gov/tobacco-products/health-information/quitting-smoking-closer-every-attempt

U.S. Food and Drug Administration. (2022a, June 29). *E-cigarettes, vapes, and other electronic nicotine delivery systems (ENDS).* https://www.fda.gov/tobacco-products/products-ingredients-components/vaporizers-e-cigarettes-and-other-electronic-nicotine-delivery-systems-ends

U.S. Food and Drug Administration. (2022b, June 23). *FDA news release: FDA denies authorization to market JUUL products.* https://www.fda.gov/news-events/press-announcements/fda-denies-authorization-market-juul-products

U.S. Preventive Services Task Force. (2021, January 19). *Final recommendation statement: Tobacco cessation in adults, including pregnant persons: Interventions.* https://www.uspreventiveservicestaskforce.org/uspstf/recommendation/tobacco-use-in-adults-and-pregnant-women-counseling-and-interventions

World Health Organization. (2014). *A guide for tobacco users to quit.* https://apps.who.int/iris/handle/10665/112833

World Health Organization. (2020, December 8). *WHO launches year-long campaign to help 100 million people quit tobacco.* https://www.who.int/news/item/08-12-2020-who-launches-year-long-campaign-to-help-100-million-people-quit-tobacco

Wyatt, J. (2016, May 16). *Clinical conversations about cannabis: Using elicit–provide–elicit.* Higher Education Center for Alcohol and Drug Misuse Prevention and Recovery. https://hecaod.osu.edu/clinical-conversations-about-cannabis-using-elicit-provide-elicit

Xu, X., Shrestha, S. S., Trivers, K. F., Neff, L., Armour, B. S., & King, B. A. (2021). U.S. healthcare spending attributable to cigarette smoking in 2014. *Preventive Medicine, 150,* 106529. https://doi.org/ https://doi.org/10.1016/j.ypmed.2021.106529

Yingst, J. M., Hrabovsky, S., Hobkirk, A., Trushin, N., Richie, J. P., Jr., & Foulds, J. (2019). Nicotine absorption profile among regular users of a pod-based electronic nicotine delivery system. *Journal of the American Medical Association Network Open, 2*(11), 15494. https://doi.org/10.1001/jamanetworkopen.2019.15494

Yingst, J. M., Veldheer, S., Hrabovsky, S., Nichols, T. T., Wilson, S. J., & Foulds, J. (2015). Factors associated with electronic cigarette users' device preferences and transition from first generation to advanced generation devices. *Nicotine & Tobacco Research, 17*(10), 1242–1246. https://doi.org/http://dx.doi.org/10.1093/ntr/ntv052

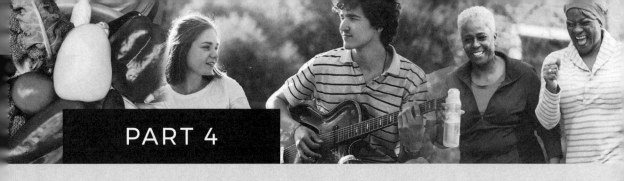

PART 4

The Practice of Health Promotion for Preventing and Managing Chronic Disease

© Kathleen Gail/Shutterstock; © StoryTime Studio/Shutterstock; © kali9/Getty Images

Pre-Obesity and Obesity Prevention and Management

Loureen Downes, PhD, APRN, FNP-BC, DipACLM, FAANP, NBC-HWC
Sonya King, DNP, ARNP, FNP-BC
Rachel Mack, MPAS, PA-C

Contradictory as it seems, malnutrition is a crucial contributor to obesity.

Madeleine M. Kunin

OBJECTIVES

This chapter will enable the reader to:

1. Discuss the incidences and prevalence of pre-obesity and obesity.
2. Examine the pathophysiology of obesity.
3. Describe energy homeostasis and weight regulation.
4. Demonstrate knowledge of pre-obesity and obesity risk and etiology.
5. Examine the health consequences of pre-obesity and obesity.
6. Identify valid measures to evaluate pre-obesity and obesity.
7. Apply practical obesity-centered history and physical exam skills.
8. Utilize evidence-based treatment guidelines to develop a person-centered obesity management plan.
9. Apply A-SMART and behavioral lifestyle interventions to pre-obesity and obesity management.

Overview

Pre-obesity (also known as overweight) and obesity are the world's most significant public health threats, reaching epidemic proportions, and ranked as the fifth most common causes of mortality globally (Ritchie & Roser, 2017; World Health Organization [WHO], 2021). This fundamentally results from excess energy balance attributed to multiple factors such as genetics, personal behavior, environment, and social determinants of health. Obesity is

© Kathleen Gail/Shutterstock; © StoryTime Studio/Shutterstock; © kali9/Getty Images

not only a disease but also a risk factor implicated in many of the leading causes of mortality (WHO, 2021). It is primarily an acquired disease that is highly influenced by lifestyle behaviors, such as poor nutrition, overeating, and sedentary habits, which make pre-obesity and obesity prevention realistic, though challenging (Bischoff et al., 2017; WHO, 2021). Due to the complex etiology of pre-obesity and obesity, many factors must be considered when assessing and managing these conditions. This chapter provides an overview of the pathophysiology, etiology, and strategies for preventing and managing pre-obesity and obesity using a lifestyle management approach. It aims to offer the advanced practice provider (APP) the knowledge, skills, and practical evidence-informed strategies to care for patients with pre-obesity and obesity.

Definition of Pre-Obesity and Obesity

Among the various definitions, pre-obesity and obesity are defined as an "abnormal or excessive fat accumulation that may impair health" (WHO, 2021). Over the years, there have been debates regarding classifying obesity as a disease. According to De Lorenzo et al. (2020), in 1998, obesity was declared a disease by the National Institutes of Health and in 2008 and 2013, endorsed as a disease by The Obesity Society and the American Medical Association, respectively. In 2018, The Obesity Society confirmed that obesity is unequivocally a chronic disease (Jastreboff et al., 2019). The Obesity Medicine Association (OMA) defines obesity as a chronic disease (Bays et al., 2021). See **Table 17.1** for the definitions of obesity from various organizations. In this chapter, pre-obesity represents overweight, and excess weight is used interchangeably with pre-obesity/obesity.

Effect of Pre-Obesity and Obesity

Pre-obesity and obesity are emergent public health concerns that predispose adults to chronic diseases. According to the Global Burden of Disease study conducted in 2017, nearly 5 million premature deaths in 2017 were attributed to obesity (Ritchie & Roser, 2017). This was equivalent to almost four times the number of individuals who died due to motor vehicle accidents and nearly five times those who succumbed to HIV/AIDs in 2017. Globally, over 1.9 billion adults aged 18 and older have excess weight, including 650 million who are obese (WHO, 2021). In addition, more than 340 million children and adolescents were

Table 17.1 Definitions of Obesity

Organization	Definition
World Health Organization	"Overweight and obesity are defined as abnormal or excessive fat accumulation that may impair health" (WHO, 2021).
The Obesity Society	"Obesity is a multi-causal chronic disease recognized across the lifespan resulting from long-term positive energy balance with development of excess adiposity that over time leads to structural abnormalities, physiological derangements, and functional impairments" (Jastreboff et al., 2019, p. 8).
Obesity Medicine Association	"Obesity is defined as a chronic, progressive, relapsing, and treatable multifactorial, neurobehavioral disease, wherein an increase in body fat promotes adipose tissue dysfunction and abnormal fat mass physical forces, resulting in adverse metabolic, biomechanical, and psychosocial health consequences" (Bays et al., 2021).

pre-obese or obese, including 39 million under 5 years old. Worldwide, since 1975, obesity has increased almost threefold in adults and over six- to eightfold in children (5–19 years old), reaching pandemic proportions (Abarca-Gómez et al., 2017; WHO, 2021). Based on the current trends, pre-obesity and obesity are expected to increase to one in two individuals in the United States by 2030 (Ward et al., 2019).

Though pre-obesity and obesity affect all populations, these conditions are increasing in developing countries and disproportionately affecting minority populations in developed countries. For example, in the United States, Hispanics (25.8%) and non-Hispanic Blacks (22%) had higher incidences of obesity compared to non-Hispanic Whites (14.1%) (Hales et al., 2018). In underresourced communities, there tends to be increased availability of low-cost foods with low nutrients, high calories, and high fat and increased sedentary behaviors, resulting in a double burden of obesity and undernutrition in children (WHO, 2021). However, globally, incidences of overweight and obesity exceed underweight. Therefore, APPs must assess minority populations and those from developing countries for risk factors related to pre-obesity and obesity.

Consequences of Pre-Obesity and Obesity

Excess weight is implicated in the leading causes of mortality and decreased life expectancy of populations affecting nearly all body systems in children and adults. Obesity is a risk factor for many chronic diseases, including cardiovascular disease (CVD), type 2 diabetes (T2D), nonalcoholic fatty liver disease, chronic kidney disease, some cancers, various musculoskeletal problems, sleep apnea, poor mental health, and Alzheimer's disease (Blüher, 2019; Chooi et al., 2019). It is interesting to note that the recent World Cancer Research Fund/American Cancer for Research report (2018) identified strong evidence that excess body fat throughout adulthood

correlated with a higher risk of 12 types of cancers by location: mouth, pharynx, larynx, esophagus, stomach, pancreas, gallbladder, liver, colon, breast (during postmenopause), ovaries, endometrium, prostate (advanced), and kidney. Further, obesity promotes an inflammatory cellular environment that stimulates cell growth and influences anti-apoptotic effects to promote the life of cancer cells.

Children who are obese are at risk for premature adverse health outcomes that typically affect adults with obesity. In addition, they may experience bronchial hyperactivity, asthma, shifting of the femoral bone, social isolation, depression, and anxiety (Camacho et al., 2019). Furthermore, children and adolescents who are obese are more likely to be obese in adulthood and may experience teasing and victimization behaviors due to their weight (Grossman et al., 2017). See **Figure 17.1** and **Figure 17.2** for the common health consequences of obesity in children and adults, respectively.

The *Canadian Adult Obesity Clinical Practice Guidelines* (Rueda-Clausen et al., 2020) and Sharma (2010) describe the many consequences of being overweight or obese across four components described as the four Ms: mental, mechanical, metabolic, and monetary. For example, *mental* represents the cognitive and emotional effect of obesity, and *mechanical* relates to factors such as osteoarthritis, sleep apnea, and gastroesophageal reflux. The *metabolic* consequences include T2D, hypertension (HTN), gout, cardiac dysfunction, and cancer. *Monetary* effects of obesity are related to food, occupation, and disability. Refer to the *Canadian Adult Obesity Clinical Practice Guidelines* for a comprehensive description of the mental, mechanical, metabolic, and monetary consequences of obesity (Rueda-Clausen et al., 2020).

Obesity and Mortality

Several epidemiological studies have explored the association between obesity and

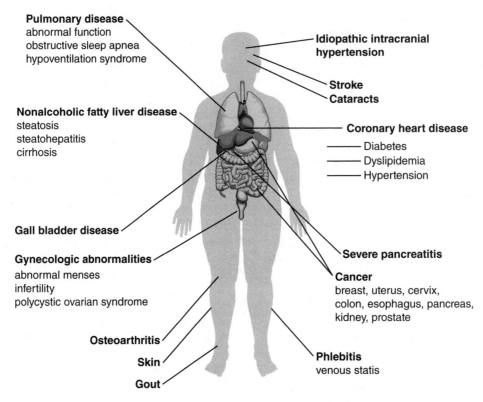

Pulmonary disease
abnormal function
obstructive sleep apnea
hypoventilation syndrome

Idiopathic intracranial hypertension

Stroke
Cataracts

Nonalcoholic fatty liver disease
steatosis
steatohepatitis
cirrhosis

Coronary heart disease
——— Diabetes
——— Dyslipidemia
——— Hypertension

Gall bladder disease

Gynecologic abnormalities
abnormal menses
infertility
polycystic ovarian syndrome

Severe pancreatitis

Cancer
breast, uterus, cervix,
colon, esophagus, pancreas,
kidney, prostate

Osteoarthritis

Skin

Gout

Phlebitis
venous statis

Figure 17.1 Health consequences of childhood obesity.

mortality (Nimptsch et al., 2019). Specifically, in the Prospective Studies Collaboration with 894,576 participants, mortality after adjustment for variables such as smoking was the lowest for those with body mass index (BMI) values of 22.5 to 25 kg/m² (MacMahon et al., 2009). The researchers indicated that every 5 kg/m² increase in BMI correlated with 30% higher all-cause mortality (120% higher diabetes, 80% higher kidney, and 10% higher neoplastic mortality). In another study, the European Prospective Investigation into Cancer and Nutrition, with a sample of 359,387 participants, general adiposity (measured as BMI) and abdominal adiposity (measured as waist circumference [WC] and waist–hip ratio [WHR]) were associated with increased risk of death. However, higher abdominal adiposity was more strongly related to the risk

of death with lower BMI levels, suggesting that abdominal obesity is a better predictor of mortality in individuals with normal BMI (Pischon et al., 2008).

Similarly, a study with a large cohort of nearly 2 million people indicated that most causes of death occurred in BMI ranges classified as underweight, overweight, or obese (Bhaskaran et al., 2018). The highest mortality rates for conditions such as cancer, heart disease, and respiratory diseases were found in individuals who were obese; the lowest risk of death occurred at 21 to 25 kg/m² (Bhaskaran et al., 2018). It is important to note that although there is a significant risk of ill health with excess weight, there are individuals with excess weight without pertinent health conditions (Rueda-Clausen et al., 2020). For these individuals, the recommendation is to

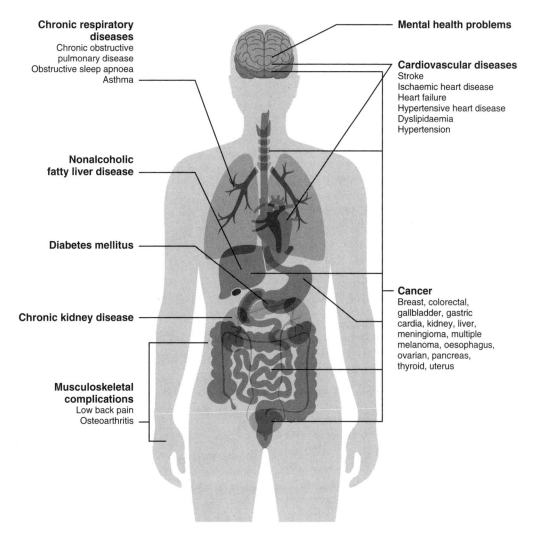

Chronic respiratory diseases
Chronic obstructive pulmonary disease
Obstructive sleep apnoea
Asthma

Nonalcoholic fatty liver disease

Diabetes mellitus

Chronic kidney disease

Musculoskeletal complications
Low back pain
Osteoarthritis

Mental health problems

Cardiovascular diseases
Stroke
Ischaemic heart disease
Heart failure
Hypertensive heart disease
Dyslipidaemia
Hypertension

Cancer
Breast, colorectal, gallbladder, gastric cardia, kidney, liver, meningioma, multiple melanoma, oesophagus, ovarian, pancreas, thyroid, uterus

Figure 17.2 Health consequences of obesity for adults.

World Health Organization. (2022). *WHO European Regional Obesity Report 2022*. Fig 1.10, Medical conditions associated with obesity. WHO Regional Office for Europe. https://apps.who.int/iris/bitstream/handle/10665/353747/9789289057738-eng.pdf

encourage healthy behaviors to prevent additional weight gain and to decrease the progression of relevant complications.

Cost of Obesity

Obesity and associated complications create a significant financial burden on the U.S. economy. According to Waters and Graf (2018) of the Milken Institute, the economic burden of chronic diseases in the United States from

complications of pre-obesity and obesity resulted in $480.7 billion in direct health care and $1.24 trillion in indirect costs. Obesity as a risk factor contributes the most to the cost of chronic diseases in America, nearly 50% of the total cost (Waters & Graf, 2018). Additionally, obesity decreases productivity and increases absenteeism and disability—many complications related to obesity significantly influence the cost of health care at the individual and population levels.

Pathophysiology of Obesity

The pathogenesis of obesity is complex and includes biological, behavioral, and environmental factors. These and many other factors contribute to the energy imbalance resulting in obesity. Regulating energy intake and energy expenditure (EE) is the main phenomenon by which energy balance is obtained (Gadde et al., 2018). In a review of seminal studies about obesity, Gadde et al. (2018) concluded that the physiological process associated with obesity included primarily two corresponding features: energy homeostasis and nutrition.

The three factors contributing to energy balance are energy intake, EE, and energy storage (Kadouh & Acosta, 2017). EE involves three metabolic mechanisms, resting metabolic rate (RMR), food thermogenesis, and physical activity EE. *RMR* is the energy required to maintain essential body organs at rest and is related to fat-free mass, the components of the body that do not accumulate fat, such as the muscles, water content, vital organs, and bones. *Food thermogenesis* includes all energy expended in eating, digesting, and metabolizing food. *Physical activity* is expended with daily living, including but not limited to intentional physical exertion. Physical activity is the most varied of the three EE mechanisms because it is relative to the duration of the movement (Westerterp, 2018). Therefore, energy intake that exceeds EE over time leads to a positive energy balance and significantly contributes to excess body weight (Oussaada et al. 2019).

Body weight is well ordered for survival during times of food abundance and starvation. Therefore, a slight increase in energy balance can add up over time to substantial weight gain. A daily excess of as little as 20 calories (comparable to 1 teaspoon of sugar) greater than EE can result in about 1 kilogram (2.2 pounds) of fat per year, which, if sustained over 20 years, would result in

about 20 kilograms of weight gain (Boron & Boulpaep, 2017, as cited in Oussaada et al., 2019).

Though it is well established that obesity results from an imbalance between energy intake and EE (Kadouh & Acosta, 2017; WHO, 2021), it is crucial that APPs explore the contributing factors to energy balance and not merely focus on energy in and out, which puts the blame solely on the individual. If underlying factors are not addressed and the focus is only on behavior, patients may experience shame and weight bias, which may ultimately defy the efforts of the APP to promote weight loss (Kadouh & Acosta, 2017; Tomiyama, 2019). The following sections will highlight the association among biological, behavioral, and environmental factors and excess weight.

Biological Factors

The biological factors associated with obesity include genes, epigenetics, brain–gut axis, neuroendocrine conditions, medications, and the gut microbiome (Kadouh & Acosta, 2017). One or more of these factors interact with environmental and behavioral factors to promote the expression of obesity. Clinicians should be aware of the multiple biological factors influencing obesity as they make treatment decisions. This section describes the most salient biological factors to increase the knowledge, skills, and attitude of the APP caring for patients with obesity.

Genes and Obesity

Genome-wide association studies have identified 140 genes relevant to adiposity (Fall et al., 2017). Genes are the blueprints given at birth, instructing the body to respond to environmental changes (Yanovski & Yanovski, 2018). The relationship between genetics and obesity is complex, genome-wide research is ongoing, and more evidence is needed to support genetic testing in the clinical setting to predict obesity risk (Loos & Yeo, 2021). The genetic implications of obesity are based on the type of gene involved (Huvenne et al., 2016), such as the more common polygenic or the rare monogenic. Rare genetic variations are monogenic obesity and are identified as syndromic or oligogenic obesity, related to mutations in the gene coding the leptin receptor and many components of the melanocortin pathway.

Syndromic and oligogenic obesity have different characteristics. *Syndromic* is severe early-onset obesity associated with other phenotypes, including mental retardation and malformations of features and organs; the most commonly known syndromic obesity are Prader-Willi and Bardet-Biedl (Huvenne et al., 2016). *Oligogenic* obesity is associated with variation in the severity of obesity attributed to 2% to 3% of adults and children who are obese. It is relatively dependent on environmental elements and nonexistent of a specific phenotype. Overall, monogenic obesity affects a tiny subset of the population worldwide, ranging from less than 10 to 100 patients worldwide (Huvenne et al., 2016). Congenital leptin deficiency causes hyperphagia in infants who, at birth, had weight ranges within the normal limits, resulting in severe obesity within the first months

of life (Yanovski & Yanovski, 2018). If identified through genetic testing, individuals with leptin deficiency may be treated with leptin to decrease obesity (Yanovski & Yanovski, 2018).

The rare forms of monogenic obesity differ from the most common form, polygenic obesity. *Polygenic* obesity is highly correlated to "obesogenic" lifestyle factors, including overeating, lack of physical activity, and stress (Huvenne et al., 2016). One of the genes associated with polygenic obesity is the fat mass and obesity-associated (FTO) gene (Hess & Brüning, 2014). Of all the known genes, FTO is the most strongly associated with BMI in children and adults, irrespective of gender. There are ongoing studies to elucidate the genetic contribution to BMI. See **Table 17.2** for differences in characteristics of monogenic and polygenic obesity.

To further elucidate the influence of the FTO gene on obesity, researchers conducted a study with 359 healthy males with normal BMI levels to determine how those with high-risk FTO genes and those with low-risk FTO genes modulate the neural and hormone responses to eating and food images (Karra et al., 2013). The study results identified that men with the high-risk FTO gene had more

Table 17.2 Characteristics of Monogenic and Polygenic Obesity

Characteristics	Monogenic	Polygenic
Onset of obesity	Early, severe	Common obesity
Genetic contribution	High	Modest
Mutation	Single gene mutation	Hundreds of variants or many genes
Genetic effect	Large	Small effect in each variant
Frequency	Rare	Common
Penetrance	High	Low
Environmental influence	None	High
Gene name (examples)	Leptin, melanocortin 4 receptor	

Data from Loos, R. J. F., & Yeo, G. S. (2021). The genetics of obesity: From discovery to biology. *Nature Reviews Genetics, 23*(2), 120–133. https://doi.org/10.1038/s41576-021-00414-z

of the hunger hormone ghrelin after eating than men with the low-risk FTO gene. Additionally, the FTO gene increased more rapidly after eating, indicating that the men with the high-risk FTO gene did not appropriately decrease ghrelin after meals. The researchers also identified that men with high-risk FTO genes had an increased response in the brain's reward center and the hypothalamus, which regulates appetite, resulting in a desire to eat more. These results provide insightful findings on the influence of the FTO genotype on the complex regulation of metabolism at the physiological level.

The influence of healthy lifestyle behaviors on the genetic tendency to develop obesity is highlighted by a meta-analysis of over 200,000 adults with the FTO gene (Graff et al., 2017). Those who were physically active reduced the odds of being obese by about 30% compared to inactive adults. According to a recent study, increased vegetable and fruit intake can mitigate elevated BMI in individuals genetically susceptible to obesity (Wang et al., 2019). Thus, environmental factors that promote healthy eating and physical activity may alleviate the polygenic effects of obesity.

These findings highlight the importance of multifactorial lifestyle behaviors in attenuating the risk of obesity.

Genetic Obesity Risk Index

In 2002, researchers tested a classic model to detect the genetic risk of obesity in individuals to help guide treatment (Thirby & Randall, 2002). The findings revealed that 85% of bariatric surgery candidates had a history suggesting a genetic risk for morbid obesity and 15% indicated an exceedingly strong *genetic obesity risk index*. The two most likely factors to correlate with multifactorial genetic risk are familial history and age of onset of obesity. See the following box for the classic genetic obesity risk index questionnaire and scoring.

Epigenetics and Obesity

Epigenetics is the effect of behaviors and environment on gene expression and can turn genes on and off (National Human Genome Research Institute, 2022). Epigenetics vary with age due to the usual developmental process and in response to behavioral and

---

Genetic Obesity Risk Index Screening Questionnaire

Patient Instructions: Answer the following four questions to see whether genetics can be the reason for your weight gain. For measurement purposes, pre-obese/overweight means having a BMI of 25–29.9; obese is a BMI of 30–39.9, and very obese is a BMI of ≥ 40. BMI calculators are available online and are calculated based on weight and height.

1. Were either or both of your parents obese or very obese for most of their lives?

	Points	
	Obese	**Very Obese**
Neither/don't know/no	0	0
Yes, one parent	7	14
Yes, both parents	14	28

2. Do you have any second-degree relatives who have been obese most of their lives?
   Score 2 points for every first-degree relative with obesity up to a maximum of 10 points.

3. How would you describe the average BMI of your siblings?

	Points
No siblings with obesity (BMI <30)	0
Average sibling with obesity (BMI ≥30)	6
Average sibling is very obese (BMI ≥40)	12

4. When did you first become pre-obese/overweight and/or obese?

	Points	
	Pre-Obese/Overweight	**Obese**
Never	0	0
Before age 10	20	30
Before age 20	10	20
Before age 30	5	10

Sum the points.

Total score_____

Interpreting your score

<20: Your weight problem does not appear to be significantly related to genetics. This means it is related to lifestyle and could be solved with committed lifestyle change.

20–50: There appears to be a moderate hereditary component to your weight problem. This means you may find losing weight more challenging than people you know. You may need help from a dietitian, nutritionist, health professional with expertise in weight management, or health coach.

30–100: There appears to be a significant hereditary component to your weight problem. This means you need additional help and closer attention from a dietitian or professional in weight management. With the proper approach and a long-range plan, you should be able to overcome your inherited start.

Data from Rossner, S., Egger, G., & Binns, A. (2017). Overweight and obesity: The epidemic's underbelly. In G. Egger, A. Binns, S. Rossner, & M. Sagner (Eds.), *Lifestyle medicine: Lifestyle, the environment and preventive medicine in health and disease* (3rd ed., pp 131–132). Academic Press.

environmental factors. There is evidence that prenatal behavior and ecological conditions can affect the epigenetics of offspring. Among the salient epigenetic contributions to excess weight in first- and second-generation offspring is the effect of maternal nutrition and weight status before conception and during pregnancy (Chen et al., 2021; Kadouh & Acosta, 2017). Additionally, there is evidence that poor paternal nutrition in animal models and humans increases the risk of excess weight (Ozanne, 2015). A review of the findings of studies regarding men and women whose mothers during pregnancy experienced the Dutch famine from 1944 to 1945 revealed that undernutrition increased the risk of chronic conditions, including obesity (Roseboom, 2019). A study identified that mothers with increased intake of pro-inflammatory foods were more likely to have children at increased risk of overweight and obesity (Chen et al., 2021). A pro-inflammatory diet includes a lower intake of fruits, vegetables, and nuts/seeds/legumes and higher intakes of red and processed meats and sugar-sweetened beverages. These findings have clinical significance for APPs to help prospective mothers increase their intake of a high-quality diet that promotes an anti-inflammatory body state and overall weight management.

The environmental influence on epigenetics may commonly influence obesity development, as demonstrated by the findings of obesity from a population with the same genetics but with different ecological exposure. For example, 60% of Pima Indians in Arizona are obese compared to 20% of the genetically similar Pima Indians in Sierra Madre, Mexico, two regions with marked environmental differences in access to food and physical activity levels (Schulz et al., 2006). The U.S. Pima Indians reported having a high percentage of calories from fat, lower fiber intake, and significantly lower occupational and leisure physical activity levels than the Pima Indians in Mexico. These results indicate an evident influence of the environment on obesity (Yanovski & Yanovski, 2018). However, even among individuals surrounded by obese-enhancing factors, there is variability among those who will become obese (Yanovski & Yanovski, 2018). These differences may result from environmental, socioeconomic, psychological, and gene–environmental connections or genetics and epigenetics.

The expression of genes varies across tissue type and time sequence and can also be influenced by *DNA methylation*, a physiological process of adding a methyl group to DNA. This is done by DNA methyltransferase and is a heritable (epigenetic) modification leading to malignancy, arteriosclerosis, CVD, and chromosomal defect neurological disorders such as Prader-Willi syndrome (Kandi & Vadakedath, 2015). Genetic defects can influence methylation, inflammation, nutrition, physical activity, and aging, among many other factors (Fall et al., 2017). These factors can modulate genetics and epigenetics to promote obesity and obesity-related diseases (Fall et al., 2017), as reflected in **Figure 17.3**. An epigenetic predisposition to develop obesity can be prevented or treated through a consistent efficacious plan that includes nutrition, movement, and behavior approaches (OMA, 2018; Rohde, 2019).

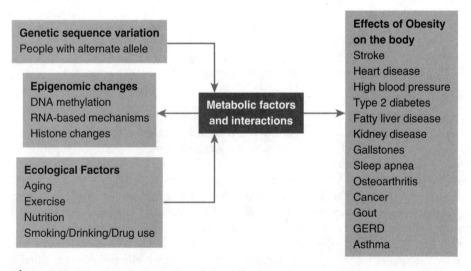

Figure 17.3 Genetic and epigenetic variation influences gene expression.

Brain–Gut Axis and Obesity

The brain is the most significant player in excess weight and energy balance (Lau & Wharton, 2020). The brain–gut axis is impaired in people with obesity compared to normal-weight individuals (Kadouh & Acosta, 2017). The following section will describe the neurobiology of obesity as described in the *Canadian Adult Obesity Clinical Practice Guidelines* (Lau & Wharton, 2020). A broad overview of three areas of the brain—the hypothalamus, mesolimbic area, and cognitive lobe, all of which regulate weight—will provide a basic understanding of the neurobiology of obesity.

Hypothalamus Role in Energy Homeostasis. The hypothalamus plays a vital role in energy homeostasis by controlling energy intake and expenditure (Lau & Wharton, 2020). The arcuate nucleus of the hypothalamus, also referred to as the hunger center, controls eating habits. Signals from hormonal and neuronal activity in the gut, adipose tissue, and peripheral organs activate neurons in the arcuate nucleus to stimulate the feeling of hunger and trigger behaviors to seek food. When there is access to food, there is a downregulation of the activity of the neurons. Many other factors influence appetite control in the arcuate nucleus, including the individual's nutritional state, sensing for nutrients, taste, smell, and food preferences.

Mesolimbic System. The mesolimbic dopamine pathway drives motivation and incentive to repeat pleasurable activities such as eating, known as hedonic eating (Lau & Wharton, 2020). *Hedonic eating* occurs when a satiated person eats food mainly because of its tasty reward rather than for nutritional need (Meye & Adan, 2014). It is associated with the sight, smell, and taste of food and under ideal conditions controls a person's response to natural rewards such as food. Some individuals with obesity have a malfunctioning mesolimbic dopamine system, leading to increased anticipation (wanting) of food, which results in a need to overeat to fulfill the level of expectation (Bello et al., 2010, and Volkow et al., 2010, as cited in Lau & Wharton, 2020). Multiple factors may trigger excess food intake.

In addition to overeating as a response to emotions, mood disorders can promote unhealthy eating behaviors (Singh, 2014). In some situations, excessive eating, particularly foods high in simple carbohydrates that affect the feel-good hormones of serotonin and the reward system, may be used as self-medication to improve symptoms of atypical depression. Other neuropsychological health conditions influencing excessive eating include attention deficit disorder, sleep disorders, chronic pain, anxiety disorders, addictions, seasonal affective disorders, and cognitive disorders (Singh, 2014). Medications, hormone management, and cognitive behavior therapy counseling may control serotonin dysregulation and treat obesity. This accentuates the need for an interprofessional healthcare team to manage overweight and obesity.

Cognitive Lobe and Executive Functioning. The cognitive lobe is responsible for mental skills such as working memory, flexible thinking, and self-control, also referred to as executive functioning (Yang et al., 2018). Working memory manages relevant incoming stimuli and updates the information in memory as needed. Flexible thinking shifts attention or mental rules when situationally appropriate, and self-control suppresses impulsiveness. The cognitive lobe functions best under optimum states, such as adequate rest, decreased stress, and proper social support (Lau & Wharton, 2020). Therefore, overeating when one feels fatigued and stressed at the end of the day is not unusual. Encouraging mindful eating may increase awareness of factors triggering poor eating habits. Individuals who are obese may have a malfunctioning connection between the cognitive lobe and other parts of the brain resulting in a lack of control over eating. For example, when faced with the choice between eating a donut or an apple, individuals with impaired executive function may choose the donut even with the knowledge of the ill effects and that it will hinder their weight loss goal.

Influence of Hormones on Appetite

Several hormones are major players in maintaining homeostasis, including leptin, ghrelin, and insulin (Adamska-Patruno et al., 2018). Leptin and ghrelin are the hormones most associated with satiety and appetite (Yeung & Tadi, 2022). In simple terms, *leptin* is released from adipocytes (fat cells), sending signals to the hypothalamus. The primary purpose of leptin is to maintain body weight by controlling the desire to eat. Leptin, the satiety hormone, deters hunger when the body is at an optimum function, so the body does not desire to eat when it does not need energy. Leptin positively correlates to a person's amount of adiposity. As adiposity increases, leptin levels will increase, and if a person decreases the proportion of body fat, the leptin levels will decrease (Obradovic et al., 2021). However, when individuals are obese, they will have excess leptin levels, resulting in leptin resistance. With *leptin resistance*, there is decreased satiety and an increase in appetite. Hence, overeating and craving may occur, resulting in difficulty maintaining weight loss.

In obese patients, central leptin and insulin resistance develop from excess high-fat foods, caloric surplus, and increasing adiposity (Timper & Brüning, 2017). Furthermore, these factors and a dietary increase in saturated fats contribute to hypothalamic inflammation. Hence, obesity contributes to insulin and leptin resistance in the peripheral and central nervous systems (Timper & Brüning, 2017). Together, these disruptions contribute to hypothalamic inflammation and impairment of the insulin and leptin pathways, leading to increased hunger and exacerbating the development of obesity (Timper & Brüning, 2017).

Ghrelin is an appetite stimulant secreted mainly from the mucosa of the stomach fundus and pancreatic cells (Verdeş et al., 2017). The function of ghrelin is to stimulate appetite and prepare the body to eat, and it has been called the hunger hormone. Ghrelin influences short-term food intake by increasing levels before eating and decreasing levels with food intake.

In a recent study to evaluate the ratio of leptin and ghrelin in men based on meals with various macronutrients, researchers determined differences in men of normal weight compared to men who were pre-obese/obese (Adamska-Patruno et al., 2018). In normal-weight men, the leptin/ghrelin ratio was more favorable after a high-carbohydrate fat-free meal than the high-fat normal amount of carbohydrate meal. Additionally, the study results indicated that compared to individuals with normal weight, males with pre-obesity and obesity had a significantly elevated leptin/ghrelin ratio in a fasting state and after eating each meal. These results provide clinical relevance that a high carbohydrate meal may be more favorable when offering nutrition counseling to men of normal weight. In contrast, in men with pre-obesity or obesity, lower carbohydrate meals may be preferable. In individuals with pre-obesity/obesity, it is ideal to have an elevated leptin/ghrelin ratio to promote satiety and decrease appetite stimulation to improve health outcomes through weight loss.

Endocrine Function of Adipocytes

The physiological link between obesity and chronic diseases is due to the endocrine function of adipocytes in adipose tissue, particularly visceral or abdominal adipose tissue, which secretes cytokines and adipokines (Nimptsch et al., 2019). Also, adiposity results in a disproportional accumulation of adipocytes associated with increased secretion of pro-inflammatory cytokines (e.g., interleukin-1β, interleukin-6, and tumor necrosis factor α) and adipokines (e.g., leptin and resistin) and a decrease in anti-inflammatory adipokines such as adiponectin (Forny-Germano et al., 2019; Nimptsch et al., 2019). The increased release of pro-inflammatory substances and the reduction of anti-inflammatory substances during obesity result in the body's being in a steady state of low-grade inflammation, which leads to insulin resistance, T2D, HTN, coronary artery disease, some cancers, and arthritis, among many other health consequences of obesity (Forny-Germano et al., 2019; Odegaard & Chawla, 2013).

Medications

Many prescribed medications are known to have an obesogenic, or weight-promoting, effect (Rueda-Clausen et al., 2020). **Table 17.3** provides a list of commonly used obesogenic medications across various drug classes and alternative medicines to consider. APPs must consider the implications of medications when evaluating and treating patients with or at risk for pre-obesity and obesity.

Microbiome and Obesity

The role of the microbiome in obesity is not fully understood (Aoun et al., 2020). However, evidence supports that the microbiota promotes digestion and metabolism. A more diverse gut microbiota is favorable to lean weight and may have a protective effect on weight gain in healthy individuals. In contrast, diets high in processed fat and carbohydrates and low in whole-plant foods decrease the variety of the gut microbiome. Dietary eating patterns high in fiber promote a diverse gut microbiome (Aoun et al., 2020). Based on studies using mice, there is emerging evidence that fecal microbiota transplant from lean mice to obese mice resulted in more weight loss and prevention of weight gain in the long term (Thaiss et al., 2016). The results of studies using fecal microbiota transplants with humans have revealed mixed results, but this has the potential to change the future management of obesity (Thaiss et al., 2016).

Behavioral Factors

Behavioral elements encompass high-caloric intake, stress, physical inactivity, alcohol use, inadequate sleep, and former smokers. Besides the rare types of obesity that originate from genetic causes or factors that negatively impair EE, individual lifestyle behaviors are vital in triggering the interaction between biological and environmental influences to produce a state of obesity (Kadouh & Acosta, 2017). Many individuals' choices affect how the environment will determine their weight status. Lifestyle behaviors such as sedentary habits and sleep patterns are ultimately personal choices. Environmental factors promoting healthy options will deter poor decisions, making the healthy choice easy. A brief description of the effect of selected behaviors on weight status will be described next.

Dietary Patterns and Excess Weight

Long-standing evidence supports that dietary patterns high in processed foods, including refined sugars and fats, are linked with excess weight. In a 4-year longitudinal prospective study, researchers identified the relationship between multiple lifestyle behaviors and weight gain over the long term in men and women who were not obese (Mozaffarian et al., 2011). The study results revealed that weight gain was considerably related to eating potato chips, potatoes, beverages sweetened with sugar, unprocessed red meat, and processed meat and was inversely related to eating vegetables, whole grains, fruits, nuts, and yogurt. The results regarding the effect of food on weight are supported by Smith et al. (2015). These researchers argue that the heterogeneity between food and weight change indicates differences in how foods determine satiety, resting EE, microbiome, liver fat content, and other metabolic factors.

Further, Smith et al. (2015) indicate that varied foods of similar caloric value support that not all calories equivalently affect health

Table 17.3 Common Weight-Promoting Medications

Classification	Anticonvulsants	Antidepressants	Antihyperglycemics	Antihypertensive	Antipsychotics	Corticosteroid
Weight-Promoting Medications	Valproic Acid *** Carbamazepine*** Gabapentin***	**Tricyclics** Amitriptyline*** Doxepin*** Imipramine** Nortriptyline** **Atypical** Mirtazapine** **MAOIs** Phenelzine*** Tranylcypromine*** **SSRIs** Sertraline* Paroxetine** Citalopram*** Escitalopram** Fluoxetine***	**Insulins** Insulin** **Thiazolidinedione** Pioglizaone** **Sulfonylureas** Glipizide* Glyburide** Glimepiride**	Clonidine* Propranolol* Metoprolol* Atenolol**	Haloperidol** Loxapine** Clozapine** Risperidone** Olanzapine** Quetiapine*	Prednisone*** Prednisolone*** Cortisone***
Medication substitutes for weight-promoting medications	Topiramate Zonisamide Lamotrigine	Bupropion Nefazodone Duloxetine Venlafaxine Desvenlafaxine Trazodone Levomilnacipran Vilazodone Vortioxetine Selegiline (topical MAOIs) Fluvoxamine (variable weight effect)	Metformin **DPP4i** (alogliptin, linagliptin, sitagliptin, axagliptin) **GLP-1** (exenatide, liraglutide, dulaglutide, semaglutide) **AGI** (acarbose, miglitol) **SGLT-2 analogs** (canagliflozin, dapagliflozin, empagliflozin) +Metformin combination	Prazosin ACEi ARBs Diuretics CCBs (may cause fluid retention)	Ziprasidone Lurasidone Aripiprazole	Budesonide NSAIDs

DPP4i: Inhibitors of dipeptidyl peptidase 4; GLP-1: Glucagon-like peptide-1 receptor agonists; NSAIDs: Nonsteroidal anti-inflammatory drugs: SGLT-2: Sodium glucose co-transporter 2; AGI: Alpha-glucosidase inhibitor; ACEi: Angiotensin-converting inhibitors; ARBs: Angiotensin II receptors blockers; CCBs: Calcium channel blockers; MAOIs: Monoamine oxidase inhibitors; SSRIs: Selective serotonin reuptake inhibitors;+Combination therapy is less likely to cause weight gain; * up to 5 kg weight gain; ** 5–10 kg weight gain; *** more than 10 kg weight gain.

and weight. Some calories may increase weight, and others may promote weight loss. For example, nuts were thought to promote weight gain since they are high in calories per portion size; however, both Mozaffarian et al. (2011) and Smith et al. (2015) identified a decrease in weight with eating nuts, similar to Tan et al. (2014).

Stress and Obesity

Both stress and obesity are ubiquitous issues in society and are interrelated in a cyclical pattern (Tomiyama, 2019). Stress is a well-known contributor to decision-making and affects many lifestyle behavior patterns, resulting in poor eating behaviors. Most recently, Americans have attributed the COVID-19 pandemic as a source of stress for one-third of the adult population affecting fundamental decisions about what to eat (American Psychological Association, 2021). Notably, parents with children under 18, compared to those without children, reported experiencing more stress than before the pandemic.

Chronic or repeated acute stressors are associated with obesity through interactions that span cognition, physiology, biochemistry, and behaviors (Tomiyama, 2019). Stress impairs the cognitive process of self-regulation, which would influence behaviors that prevent obesity, such as dietary choices and physical activity. Impaired self-regulation may then lead to unhealthy behaviors. Further, stress consistently activates many physiological systems, such as activation of the hypothalamic-pituitary-adrenal axis, leading to increased cortisol levels known to promote eating and fat deposition with an emphasis in the abdominal area. There is evidence that the stress-obesity-stigma-stress cycle results from the stigma of excess weight, leading to an increase in stress, which exacerbates weight gain through an interplay of physiology and behaviors (Tomiyama, 2019). A detailed discussion of stress and its relationship to obesity is beyond the scope of this chapter. However, addressing stress as an upstream causal factor in obesity would be effective and valuable (Tomiyama, 2019).

Physical Inactivity and Obesity

Physical inactivity is linked to excess weight (Park et al., 2020). It may be exacerbated by conditions that encourage prolonged sitting, such as working on the computer, playing video games, and excessive TV watching. In particular, sedentary time is associated with increased WC. It is essential to highlight a classic finding that a 10% increase in physical inactivity increased WC by 1.2 in. (Healy et al., 2008). According to the WHO (2022), by 2030, nearly 500 million individuals will develop chronic conditions such as obesity and obesity-related disorders due to physical inactivity if there are no urgent public health measures to promote physical activity globally.

Alcohol and Obesity

Until recently, the prevailing belief was that drinking in moderation was safe. However, most recently, evidence has linked not only excessive drinking with poor health outcomes (Traversy & Chaput, 2015) but also drinking in small amounts. Drinking less than a standard alcoholic drink increased the risk of obesity in a study of 27 million (European Association for the Study of Obesity, 2020). The study defined a standard drink as 14 g (0.6 oz) of alcohol per day, equivalent to 5 oz of wine and 8 oz of beer. This is consistent with the definition of a standard drink by the Centers for Disease Control and Prevention (n.d.).

Compared to nondrinkers, men and women who consumed between 50% and 100% of a standard drink were 22% and 3% more likely to develop obesity, respectively (European Association for the Study of Obesity, 2020). However, the odds increased considerably for obesity for men (34%) and women (22%) who drank more than two drinks compared to those who did not drink. Furthermore, researchers identified an increased risk of illness and death related to nonalcoholic fatty and alcoholic fatty liver disease in individuals who were overweight or obese and who drank more than 14 g per week (Inan-Eroglu et al., 2022). Individuals in the normal range did not have the same response to drinking alcohol. Evidence is emerging that alcohol contributes to obesity, and individuals who are already overweight may increase their risk of liver disease by drinking even small amounts (Inan-Eroglu et al., 2022). Inconclusive evidence exists regarding intake and obesity. The preponderance of evidence taken as a whole suggests that even when consumed in small quantities, alcohol may be a risk factor for obesity in some individuals.

Sleep and Obesity

There is evidence that insufficient and too much sleep can similarly affect weight status. A plethora of evidence indicates that inadequate sleep is associated with increased weight, particularly in children, adolescents, and younger adults (Bonanno et al., 2019; Li et al., 2017; Wu et al., 2014). Individuals who consistently slept less than 7 hours were more likely to have excess weight (Cooper et al., 2018). However, sleeping 9 or more hours was also associated with excess weight (Theorell-Haglow et al., 2014). Also, the relationship between sleep deprivation and increased weight is bidirectional, and it may be challenging to determine what came first, as in the chicken or the egg. Likewise, insomnia can be a barrier to physical activity, and a lack of physical activity can cause sleep impairment (Tomiyama, 2019). Additionally, insufficient sleep is associated with the increased hunger hormone ghrelin, the decreased satiety hormone leptin, and enhanced hedonic signaling—the drive to eat for pleasure without being hungry (Cooper et al., 2018).

Other hormonal imbalances resulting from sleep deficiency include increased cortisol levels and decreased growth hormone, both associated with obesity (Fry, 2022). Further, less than ideal sleep impairs the metabolism of food. The mechanism for long sleep duration and obesity needs further investigation. Still, research findings support an association with factors such as poor sleep quality, physical inactivity, unhealthy food intake, an imbalance between the sleep–wake cycle, or disease comorbidities such as depression and HTN (Tan et al., 2018). Assessing patients for short and prolonged sleep is essential to obesity management.

Tobacco Use and Obesity

It is well known that quitting smoking tends to be associated with weight gain, but this is not conclusive. In a study to determine the relationship between smoking and obesity, the results indicated that former heavy smokers were more likely to be obese than former light smokers (Dare et al., 2015). However, heavy smokers who were younger and those who lived in the most affluent areas were more likely to be obese than those who never smoked. Interestingly, the study revealed that the risk of weight gain after quitting smoking was time limited. Former smokers after 20 years were at the same risk of obesity as those who had never smoked. The APP should put interventions in place to assist patients who quit smoking to prevent weight gain.

Environmental Factors

Environmental determinants of obesity include food abundance, food insecurity, built environment, socioeconomic status, culture, and bias (Kadouh & Acosta, 2017). Though an individual may have a biological tendency toward obesity, it is usually manifested due to an interplay with an obesogenic environment. There are two primary factors of an obesogenic environment. One is an overabundance of foods, and the other is the built environment. Fox et al. (2019) support the theory that modernization has led to economic advances that have promoted the transition from lower-calorie, plant-based diets to processed foods and meats high in calories, resulting in excess weight and ill health. With uncontrolled urban expansion, the built environment has resulted in increased use of cars for transportation, making walking less appealing (Kadouh & Acosta, 2017). It is well established that dietary patterns high in animal meat protein and processed foods and an environment that promotes sedentary behaviors, such as driving, have directly correlated to the rise in overweight and obesity (Fox et al., 2019; Kadouh & Acosta, 2017). Most environmental factors are modifiable through government policies that promote access to healthy foods and areas for recreation and play.

Assessment of Pre-Obesity and Obesity

Many types of measures are available to determine adiposity, with varying utility. There are direct quantitative measures to assess total body adipose tissue, including dual-energy X-ray absorptiometry (DEXA) and bioelectrical impedance (Garvey et al., 2016). However, these direct measures are costly and require specialized personnel; they are not practical for clinical settings and are typically reserved for research. Therefore, measurements of obesity in this chapter will focus on those feasible for the clinical practice or community setting.

There is a long-standing debate about which anthropometric measurement—BMI, WC, or WHR—is the best predictor of disease risk in adults, including CVD, T2D, and all-cause mortality. BMI and WC are interrelated. However, WC is an independent predictor of risk factors and illness beyond BMI (National Heart, Lung, and Blood Institute [NHLBI], n.d.). WC approximates visceral adipose tissue and is the most common and easiest measurement of abdominal obesity (Garvey et al., 2016). Elevated BMI, WC, and WHR values usually indicate an increased risk of CVD, T2D, and all-cause mortality. Individuals with a normal BMI but large WC or WHR are at higher risk of health problems than those with WC or WHR levels within the normal ranges (Huxley, 2010). In general, BMI and WC demonstrate the most substantial evidence for anthropometric criteria for diagnosing pre-obesity and obesity in the clinical setting (Garvey et al., 2016). See **Table 17.4**

Table 17.4 Level of Evidence for Anthropometric Criteria for the Assessment of Pre-Obesity and Obesity in the Clinical Setting

Anthropomorphic Criteria	*Recommendation Grade
BMI to confirm excess adiposity and diagnose pre-obesity or obesity.	A
Other adiposity measurements such as dual-energy X-ray absorptiometry (DEXA) and bioelectrical impedance. Air/water displacement plethysmography may be used at the clinician's discretion if BMI and physical exam results are equivocal or additional evaluation is required.	C
WC should be measured in all patients with BMI <35 kg/m^2 to determine adiposity-related disease risk.	A

* Grades may be interpreted as being based on strong (Grade A), intermediate (Grade B), weak (Grade C), or no (Grade D) scientific substantiation.

Data from Garvey, W. T., Mechanick, J. I., Brett, E. M., Garber, A. J., Hurley, D. L., Jastreboff, A. M., Nadolsky, K., Pessah-Pollack, R., & Plodkowski, R. (2016). American Association of Clinical Endocrinologists and American College of Endocrinology comprehensive clinical practice guidelines for medical care of patients with obesity. *Endocrine Practice, 22,* 1–203. https://doi.org/10.4158/EP161365.GL

for the evidence supporting anthropometric standards to assess weight status in the clinical setting.

Body Mass Index

In adults and children 6 years and older, BMI is the most common clinical measure of weight status and risk associated with weight in the clinical setting, even though it has limitations. For adults, height and weight screening to calculate BMI should be conducted annually or more frequently (Jensen et al., 2014). In children, BMI is calculated the same as in adults, but the weight status for children is based on age- and sex-specific BMI percentiles (U.S. Preventive Services Task Force [USPSTF], 2017). Using BMI measurements to determine weight status and disease risk varies depending on ethnic groups and muscular development (Rueda-Clausen et al., 2020). As such, BMI measures may miscalculate obesity in certain conditions or groups, such as volume overload, sarcopenia, ascites, athletes, and populations of a more petite body frame. For example, Bill, a 49-year-old bodybuilder with a BMI of 33, may not be at the same disease risk as Rick, a 65-year-old adult with sarcopenia who does minimal exercise and has a BMI of 30. Bill, the bodybuilder, has more muscle mass and will weigh more; therefore, APPs should consider other factors related to body structure when interpreting BMI. Though BMI is limited, it continues to be a helpful screening measurement for individuals and populations. Screening patients for excess weight using BMI should be a routine part of most healthcare encounters. WC should be added to the assessment to identify the risk of increased visceral adiposity and the associated health risk. See **Table 17.5** for the BMI formulas in metric and imperial English.

Waist Circumference

WC is positively associated with abdominal adiposity and is a reliable measure to

Table 17.5 Body Mass Index Formula

Unit	Formula
Metric	BMI = weight (kg)/height (m^2)
Imperial English	BMI = weight (lb)/[height (in.)]^2 x 703

determine abdominal fat content before and during weight loss treatment. *Central obesity* is defined as a WC >40 in. (>102 cm) in men and >35 in. (>88 cm) in women (NHLBI, n.d.). WC is considered more beneficial for individuals with BMI <24.9 or BMI 25.0 to 29.9 than for individuals who are obese on the BMI scale (NHLBI, n.d.). Measuring the WC at BMI values ≥35 may not add a predictive value of disease risk or change the management (NHLBI, n.d.).

However, WC may be more predictive of disease risk in older adults and ethnic groups with a shorter stature, including Asian Americans or individuals of Asian descent. Additionally, WC may provide pertinent information regarding the efficacy of weight loss treatment for long-term follow-up. In some patients, central adiposity changes may be initially more noticeable than BMI. Continuing with the scenario regarding Bill and Rick, Bill, the bodybuilder, has a WC of 36 in., and Rick has a WC of 43 in. Rick is at increased risk of cardiometabolic disorders based on the two measurements. WC within the high-risk categories is correlated with an increased risk of T2D, dyslipidemia, HTN, and CVD (NHLBI, n.d.).

Shape Matters

Over six decades ago, a French physician, Jean Vague, identified that body shape could predict disease risk (Harvard T. H. Chan School of Public Health, n.d.). Individuals shaped like an apple or with a larger waist had an increased risk of early heart disease and death than those shaped like a pear, who had a smaller waist or carried more weight around their hips and thighs (Harvard T. H. Chan School of Public

Table 17.6 Weight Classifications by BMI, WC, and Associated Risk

Weight Classification Category	Underweight	Normal	Overweight (Pre-obesity)	Obesity Class I	Obesity Class II	Obesity Class III (Morbid Obesity)
BMI (kg/m^2)	< 18.5	18.5–24.9	25.0–29.9	20.0–34.9	35.0–39.9	≥ 40
Comorbidity Risk	Low, but can lead to other health issues	Average	Increased	Moderate	Severe	Very severe
WC and Comorbidity Risk Men: ≥ 40 in. (102 cm) Female: ≥ 35 in. (88 cm)	-----	-----	High	Very High	Very High	Extremely High

*In individuals of South, Southeast, or East Asian ethnicity, comorbidity risk is observed at lower BMI levels and WC (e.g., Pre-obesity BMI 23-27.9, Obesity BMI >28, men WC ≥ 33 in. [≥ 85 cm], female WC ≥ 31in. [≥ 74–80 cm])

Health, n.d.). In overweight individuals, having a large waist may indicate an additional risk of health problems compared to someone with a normal waist measurement. The Nurses' Health Study, one of the largest longitudinal studies that has followed individuals to determine the association of abdominal obesity with chronic disease mortality, supports this relationship (Zhang et al., 2008). When the study began, over 44,000 healthy female volunteers enrolled. After a decade and a half, women with a WC of 35 in. or more had nearly two times the risk of death from heart disease than those with the lowest WC of <28 in.

Furthermore, the study results revealed that women with the largest waists had a higher risk of death from cancer or any cause than women with smaller waists (Zhang et al., 2008). The risk increased consistently with every inch added to the waist. Women with normal BMI were at high risk if they had more waist adiposity. Women with a BMI <24.9 and a WC of ≥35 in. had triple the risk of death from CVD compared to women with a normal

BMI and whose waist was <35 in. WC is an important indicator of disease risk that should be used in the clinical setting to inform the management of patients (see **Table 17.6**).

Obesity in Children and Adolescents

Obesity in children and adolescents is an age-gender–specific BMI ≥95th percentile. According to the USPSTF (2017), every child and adolescent is at risk for obesity and should be screened. Risk factors comprise parents who are obese, insufficient nutrition, low levels of physical activity, inadequate sleep, sedentary behaviors, ethnic minority, and families with limited resources. There is moderate evidence to support that children and adolescents who are obese should be referred to or provided comprehensive, intensive behavioral intervention. See **Table 17.7** for BMI-for-age weight status categories and corresponding percentiles. The BMI percentile cutoff for obesity in children defines a level that a child is at

Table 17.7 Children and Adolescents Weight Status and Percentile Range

Weight Status	Percentile Range
Underweight	Less than the 5th percentile
Healthy weight	5th percentile to less than the 85th percentile
Overweight	85th percentile to less than the 95th percentile
Obesity	95th percentile or greater

Centers for Disease Control and Prevention. (2023). *Defining child BMI categories*. https://www.cdc.gov/obesity/childhood/defining.html

higher risk of developing significant obesity-related health complications, as reflected in Figure 17.1.

Comprehensive Obesity Assessment

The assessment of obesity requires a comprehensive approach to determine the underlying factors associated with an imbalance in energy homeostasis. It is imperative that APPs not only focus on treating the consequences of obesity but also determine the contributing factors and underlying diseases that promote obesity (van der Valk et al., 2019). Assessment of people with obesity should consider multiple factors, as with any chronic illness. These include vital signs with anthropometrics, a comprehensive review of medications to identify those who are obesogenic (see Table 17.3), a detailed obesity-centered medical history (see **Table 17.8**), an obesity-focused physical exam (see **Table 17.9**), and relevant laboratory and diagnostic testing (see **Table 17.10**). Assessing any physical, mental, and psychosocial limitations is vital. Other recommended measures are fasting glucose or hemoglobin A1C levels, a lipid panel to evaluate for metabolic risk factors, and possibly alanine aminotransferase to screen for nonalcoholic fatty liver disease (Rueda-Clausen et al., 2020). The ultimate goal of the assessment is to determine the root causes of excess weight in a nonjudgmental manner and to develop effective management strategies that are person centered.

Lifestyle Management of Pre-Obesity and Obesity

Pre-obesity and obesity necessitate a multi-faceted management plan; as such, there is no one-size-fits-all approach (Fitch & Bays, 2022). Management will depend on the underlying cause and should be individualized. This chapter will focus primarily on behavioral management that comprises the A-SMART (adopt healthy eating, stress less, move often, avoid alcohol, rest more, and treat tobacco use) lifestyle behaviors supported by the OMA (n.d.) pillars of eating habits, activity level, and behavior. The OMA pillar related to medication is beyond the scope of this chapter; however, indications for considering medications in an obesity management program when lifestyle behaviors are ineffective will be identified. Also, a person-centered strategy in conjunction with an interprofessional team is required for optimum outcomes. APPs are well suited to work with stakeholders to develop and implement strategies to manage pre-obesity and obesity that may address upstream issues to decrease the incidences of pre-obesity and obesity in the most likely affected individuals.

Pre-obesity and obesity should be managed as a long-standing chronic condition that involves an interprofessional team approach (Gonzalez-Campoy et al., 2013). Primordial,

Table 17.8 Components of an Obesity-Centered Medical History

History Component

Weight
- Age at onset of obesity and previous attempts to lose or gain weight and outcome
- Assess satisfaction with current weight

Nutrition
- Determine the ability to comprehend nutrition facts
- Assess caloric intake
- Identify dietary restrictions (gluten intolerance, vegan, vegetarian, lactose intolerance, food allergies

Physical Activity
- Determine routine physical activity habits
- Assess barriers (e.g., pain in joints, personal or environmental factors) to being active
- Assess facilitators of physical activity

Mental Health Disorders
- Conduct mental health screening (e.g., Physical Health Questionnaire-9 and General Anxiety Disorder Assessment), trauma, and hyperactivity

Substance Abuse
- Evaluate
- Tobacco use
- Alcohol use
- Opiates and street drug use
- Stimulants (e.g. coffee)
- Sweetened beverages

Abuse
- Assess for physical, mental, and sexual abuse

Sleep
- Screen for adherence to recommended hours of sleep, use of prescribed or over-the-counter sleep aids
- Assess for symptoms of sleep apnea (snoring, daytime fatigue)

Medications
- Identify use of medications that can increase weight

Social
- Determine shift work (e.g. night shift), support systems
- Financial support, health insurance coverage, and availability of facilities for physical activity such as parks, walking, or bike trails.
- Determine the level of functional ability (e.g., activity of daily living and instrumental activities of daily living

Family
- Determine family history of overweight/obesity or related complications (particularly, parents and siblings)

Interpersonal Assessment
Assess:
- Readiness to change

For a comprehensive outline of recommended components of an obesity-centered medical history, please see: Rueda-Clausen, C. F., Poddar, M., Lear, S. A., Poirier, P., & Sharma, A. M. (2020). Assessment of people living with obesity. *The Canadian Adult Obesity Clinical Practice Guidelines.* https://obesitycanada.ca /guidelines/assessment/

Table 17.9 Obesity Focused Physical Exam

Evaluation	Findings	Complication/Recommendations
Anthropometrics	Weight, BMI, Waist Circumference, neck circumference, Mallampati score	Metabolic syndrome (WC), Obstructive Sleep Apnea
Vital signs	Blood pressure, heart rate	Hypertension
General Exam	Physical activity	Disability resulting from excess weight
Skin	Acanthosis nigricans, hirsutism, acne Xanthelasmata	Insulin resistance, polycystic ovarian syndrome (hormonal testing) Hyperlipidemia
Cardiovascular	Heart Sound (S3), heart rate and rhythm, peripheral edema	Heart Failure/consider BMI interpretation
Respiratory	Wheezing, prolonged expiratory phase, rales	Asthma
Gastrointestinal	Liver enlargement, firm	Non-Alcoholic fatty liver disease
Musculoskeletal	High muscle mass, weakness, decreased range of motion in joints, swelling, tenderness, and crepitus in joints	Consider interpretation of BMI, osteoarthritis, sarcopenia (joint-x-ray)
Endocrine	Hyper/hypothyroid findings, signs of hypercortisolism	Hypo/hyperthyroidism (TSH), Cushing disease (salivary and 24-hr urine cortisol)

Khattak ZE, Zahra F. Evaluation of Patients With Obesity. [Updated 2023 Apr 27]. In: StatPearls [Internet]. Treasure Island (FL): StatPearls Publishing; 2023 Jan-. Available from: https://www.ncbi.nlm.nih.gov/books/NBK576399/

Table 17.10 Obesity-Related Laboratory and Diagnostic Test

Laboratory and Diagnostic Tests	Complications
Fasting glucose, HbA1C, 2hrs OGTT	Prediabetes, metabolic syndrome, Diabetes
Lipid Profile: Total cholesterol, triglycerides, high-density lipoproteins (HDL), low-density lipoproteins (LDL), non-HDL	Dyslipidemia Metabolic syndrome Cardiovascular disease risk
Complete Metabolic Panel (eGFR)	Renal impairment, electrolyte abnormality
Liver function tests: Transamines (AST, ALT); hepatic imaging, biopsy	Non-alcoholic fatty liver disease
Thyroid Function Tests: TSH, T3, T4	Hypo/hyperthyroidism

Table 17.11 Definition, Goals, and Methods for Phases of Prevention in Obesity

Phase of Intervention	Definition and Goals	Method of Prevention
Primordial	Prevent childhood obesity.	■ Provide prenatal, early childhood lifestyle counseling with an emphasis on nutrition and physical activity.
Primary	Prevent the development of overweight and obesity.	■ Educate the public. ■ Develop built environments that promote healthy behaviors (e.g. physical activity). ■ Promote healthy eating and regular physical activity.
Secondary	Prevent future weight gain and the development of weight-related complications in patients with overweight or obesity.	■ Screen using BMI. ■ Diagnose using BMI and evaluation for complications. ■ Treat with lifestyle/behavior intervention ± weight loss medications.
Tertiary	Treat with weight loss therapy to eliminate or lessen weight-related complications and prevent disease progression.	■ Treat with lifestyle/behavior intervention plus weight loss medications if warranted. ■ Consider bariatric surgery.
Quaternary	Avoid weight-enhancing treatments (e.g., medications that are obesogenic).	■ Review medications.

Data from Garvey, W. T., Mechanick, J. I., Brett, E. M., Garber, A. J., Hurley, D. L., Jastreboff, A. M., Nadolsky, K., Pessah-Pollack, R., & Plodkowski, R. (2016). American Association of Clinical Endocrinologists and American College of Endocrinology comprehensive clinical practice guidelines for medical care of patients with obesity. *Endocrine Practice, 22*, 1–203. https://doi.org/10.4158/EP161365.GL

primary, secondary, tertiary, and quaternary prevention measures should be employed for the best outcomes (see **Table 17.11**). There is strong evidence that lifestyle behavior modifications that include physical activity, nutrition, and behavioral therapy interventions create the most effective changes related to obesity prevention and maintaining long-term weight loss (Vallis et al., 2020).

Evidence-Based Guidelines

Various organizations have developed evidence-based clinical practice guidelines for managing patients with pre-obesity and obesity, for example, the American College of Cardiology/American Heart Association Task Force (Jensen et al., 2014), Obesity Canada and the Canadian Association of Bariatric Physicians and Surgeons (Wharton et al., 2020), and the Department of Veterans Affairs/Department of Defense (U.S. Department of Veterans Affairs, 2020). These guidelines are extensive and readily available on the internet. Among the many weight loss treatment options, including popular diets, cutting-edge medications, and surgery, the role of lifestyle behavior change may be overlooked. However, for any weight loss treatment to be optimally effective, it must address the cognitive and behavioral factors through lifestyle management principles and techniques (Wadden et al., 2020). All the guidelines relevant to pre-obesity and obesity comprise changing behaviors that affect the energy balance using decreased caloric intake and increased EE.

The *Clinical Practice Guideline for Multicomponent Behavioral Treatment of Obesity and Overweight in Children and Adolescents* (American Psychological Association, 2018) provides behavioral evidence-based recommendations for interventions to treat overweight and obesity in children and adolescents ages 2 to 18. The consensus is that managing overweight and obesity in children and adolescents should include parental or guardian involvement with a minimum of 26 contact hours of a multicomponent behavioral intervention. This has demonstrated effectiveness, mainly when initiated in young children who are pre-obese or obese. Several organizations, including the American Heart Association (Kelly et al., 2013) and the American Academy of Nutrition and Dietetics (Hoelscher et al., 2013), have published recommendations that support family involvement, dietary changes, and an increase in physical activity to decrease overweight or obesity as first-line treatment. Though the guidelines endorse medications or bariatric surgery as options for treatment, they caution that only a few drugs are approved for pediatric obesity, and bariatric surgery should be considered only for selective adolescents with psychological and medical complications resulting from obesity. Furthermore, the USPSTF (2017) found inadequate evidence regarding medication management in this age group. A discussion regarding medications and surgery for the treatment of obesity is beyond the scope of this chapter.

Starting the Conversation

Conversations about weight can be challenging for patients and providers because weight is a sensitive and complex issue. APPs must use people-first language to avoid labeling patients by their weight status, which promotes bias (Gallagher et al., 2021). The term *patient with obesity* is preferred to *obese patient* because it decreases stigma and may positively influence the patient–provider relationship. Providers often cite barriers to discussing obesity with patients, such as a lack of comfort with starting the conversation, lack of training, and insufficient tools to help patients recognize obesity (Petrin et al., 2017). Despite providers' barriers to discussing weight, patients expect their providers to guide them regarding weight loss strategies. Adult patients who receive overweight or obesity counseling from primary care providers are four times more likely to make an effort to lose weight than patients who do not get weight management guidance (Rose et al., 2013). However, three-fourths of adults with pre-obesity and half of those with class 1 obesity have not received weight management counseling from a provider (Guglielmo et al., 2018). Guidance on effective conversation starters regarding pre-obesity and obesity in the clinical setting may help to overcome these barriers.

To address this issue, organizations have developed guidelines to enhance effective conversations with patients to treat obesity. Recently, the Strategies to Overcome and Prevent (STOP) Obesity Alliance (Gallagher et al., 2021) convened a dozen representatives from primary care and obesity professional organizations, such as the American Association of Nurse Practitioners and the American Academy of Physician Assistants, to develop *Weight Can't Wait: Guide for the Management of Obesity in the Primary Care Setting* (STOP Obesity Alliance, 2020), which offers guidance for primary care providers to speak with patients about weight. The guide provides practical approaches to caring for patients with obesity in the pre-encounter, encounter, and post-encounter period of a primary care visit. The collection of information to start a weight-related conversation happens in the *pre-encounter* period. During the pre-encounter, providers obtain patients' permission to discuss their weight, address weight bias, diagnose

Health Promotion Research Study

Whole-Food Plant-Based Lifestyle Program and Obesity

Background: Most weight loss strategies are adequate for the short term but fail to sustain weight loss. This study aimed to determine whether a whole-food plant-based (WFPB) lifestyle program would result in long-term weight loss.

Methodology: Researchers examined the obesity measures for 151 healthy community-living adults who participated in an ongoing study over a short (0.5 up to 2 years), medium (2 years to up to 5 years), or long (5 to 10 years) time frame. The WFPB lifestyle program included nutrition education, a physical activity component, and support.

Results: The body composition changes were favorable for all time frames and genders. For all participants, there were significant mean decreases in BMI (-2.5 kg/m^2), body mass (-7.1 kg), and percent body fat (-6.4%; $p < .001$ for all). Participants with BMI within the normal range increased from baseline to 16.5% for females and 26.2% for males. For each of the three time frame groups, the number of participants in the normal BMI range increased by 25% (short), 16% (medium), and 16% (long). The proportion of participants whose body fat percentage decreased to normal was 20%, 39%, and 18% for the short, medium, and long time frame groups, respectively. Females had more significant decreases in all indices in the long-term versus short-term program. Most (85.6%) children 18 years and under whose parents were in the program adopted the WFPB lifestyle compared to only 28% of adult children. For females, energy intake was 1,842 ± 539 calories per day, and males consumed 2,618 ± 726 calories per day. Overall, participants were physically active, with good sleep quality and low perceived stress.

Implications for Advanced Practice: Overall, the effect of a WFPB lifestyle program on obesity measures demonstrated a significant decrease in BMI, body mass, and body fat in the individuals who participated in the short, medium, and long time frame groups. Females had more favorable outcomes in the long-term program compared to the short-term program. This study is unique because the beneficial effects were realized within the initial 2 years and sustained over the long term (5–10 years). Additionally, most of the participants' offspring adopted healthy eating and physical activity habits, which may ultimately decrease the incidence of obesity in the next generation. APPs should assist patients ready to lose weight in planning a multicomponent program that includes WFPB foods, physical activity, and a support group for sustainable weight loss.

Reference: Jakše, B., Jakše, B., Pinter, S., Pajek, J., & Fidler Mis, N. (2020). Whole-food plant-based lifestyle program and decreased obesity. *American Journal of Lifestyle Medicine, 16*(3), 1–11. https://doi.org/10.1177/1559827620949205

obesity, and include patients in decision-making (Gallagher et al., 2021).

Further, this guide includes a modified 5As (assess, advise, agree, assist, arrange) counseling framework by adding a sixth *A* (ask) to underscore that seeking permission from the patient to begin the conversation about weight is paramount to enhance the patient–provider experience (see **Table 17.12** for features of the 6As counseling framework). The patients' decision to pursue treatment for their weight determines the *post-encounter* clinic visit. If there is interest, the APP provides patients with a plan summary and schedules a return visit to assess progress. If there is no interest in pursuing treatment for weight, the APP respects the

Table 17.12 6As Counseling Framework

6As	Features
Ask	The APP asks permission to discuss weight, actively listens, acknowledges concerns, and includes the term preferred by patients to discuss their weight (e.g., overweight, unhealthy weight, elevated BMI).
Assess	The APP reviews the prescreen data (e.g., BMI, 24-hour diet recall, weight trajectory), assesses weight-related health concerns, ascertains a weight-centered history (see Table 17.8), and conducts an obesity-centered physical exam (see Table 17.9).
Advise	If patients are interested in discussing weight, the APP starts the shared decision-making process to establish the next steps. If patients are not interested in discussing their weight, the APP should respect their decision and express an openness in discussing the issue in the future (assess readiness at each encounter).
Agree	If patients agree to having a conversation about weight, then their queries and needs prompt the APP's responses. The APP collaborates with patients in specific, measurable, attainable, relevant, and time-bound (SMART) goal setting.
Assist	The APP assists patients by presenting treatment options, including intensive lifestyle intervention and referral to the interprofessional healthcare team as needed (registered dietitian, licensed social worker, certified lifestyle medicine or obesity medicine providers, and behavioral health specialist). The APP should refer as appropriate for treatment options such as anti-obesity medications and bariatric surgery.
Arrange	The APP arranges the coordination of care as appropriate. Providers unable to deliver intensive lifestyle medicine intervention that leads to significant weight loss should refer patients, organize care, and provide follow-up as needed.

Data from Gallagher, C., Corl, A., & Dietz, W. H. (2021). Weight can't wait: A guide to discussing obesity and organizing treatment in the primary care setting. *Obesity, 29*(5), 821–824. https://doi.org/10.1002/OBY.23154

patients' decision and specifies availability for future conversations. **Figure 17.4** represents an algorithm with a suggested provider script to counsel patients with obesity. The guide can be found online and offers practical approaches for starting the conversation that will lead to effective discussions and management of patients with obesity.

Further tips for starting the conversation about weight in the primary care setting are provided by the National Institute of Diabetes and Digestive and Kidney Diseases (2017) and the STOP Obesity Alliance (2020). An abbreviated list of conversation-starter questions and clinician tips can be found in **Table 17.13**. For a detailed list of questions to consider when discussing weight with patients, refer to *Weight Can't Wait: Guide for the Management of Obesity in the Primary Care Setting* (STOP Obesity Alliance, 2020).

Options for Stages of Obesity Treatment

All evidence-based clinical practice guidelines for managing patients with pre-obesity and obesity use lifestyle behavior as the first line of treatment. However, lifestyle treatment options alone may not be effective for obese patients experiencing obesity-related chronic diseases. Nonetheless, no treatment options can be effective without lifestyle measures. The

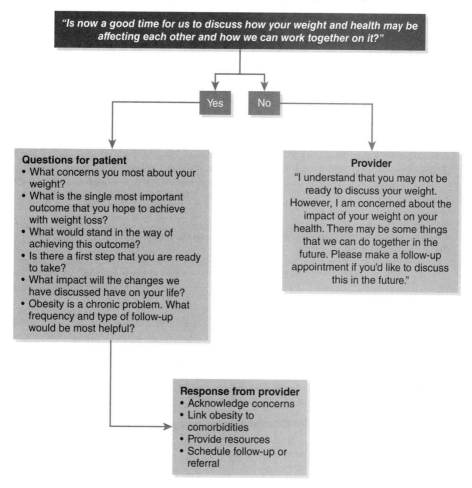

Figure 17.4 Sample questions for the patient encounter.

Edmonton Obesity Staging System (Sharma & Kushner, 2009) provides a seminal framework to guide treatment options for obesity. It considers BMI, psychopathology, metabolic and physical comorbidities, and complications in treating obesity (Sharma & Kushner, 2009). It is a simple clinical staging system that allows clinicians to consider factors beyond BMI associated with excess weight and provides

guidance for treatment measures. **Figure 17.5** lists the description and management for each stage from zero to 4.

Establishing Weight Loss Goals

The APP should work with patients to create realistic and achievable goals to help realize

Table 17.13 Conversation-Starter Questions

Questions	Clinician Tips
"How are you feeling about your weight currently?" "May I discuss your health with you, including your weight?"	Before initiating screening or assessing obesity, ask patients for permission to discuss their weight and determine anthropometric values. Before discussing their weight, discuss the health issues related to excess weight. Patients prefer terms such as *weight* (first) or *BMI* (second) and are opposed to the terms *fatness, excess fat,* and *obesity.* Be sensitive to variations in cultural differences about weight, patterns of food intake, and practices.
"Are you concerned about your weight at this time?"	If patients are not interested in addressing weight, address other health concerns and ask if you can speak with them about their weight at another time.
"Would you be interested in changing lifestyle behaviors to improve your health?"	Determine readiness to begin making the change.
"I would like to learn more about your current lifestyle behaviors. What do you eat and drink on a typical day for breakfast, lunch, and dinner?"	Take an inventory of any food, drink, or snack over the past 24 hours.
"What does 'healthy eating' mean to you?"	Helps to determine person-centered care
"Do you eat only when hungry or for other reasons, such as feeling stressed or bored?"	Identifies emotional eating so interventions can be individualized
"When is the best time of day or evening for you to be active?"	Start with the health benefits of physical activity consistently, even for a short period.
"What types of activities do you enjoy? Do you prefer doing activities alone, with someone else, or in a group?"	Intervention can be customized based on group or individual activities.
"How much time do you spend sitting? Would you want to work some physical activity into your day?"	Identify sedentary behaviors and readiness for physical activity.

National Institute of Diabetes and Digestive and Kidney Diseases. (2017). *Talking with patients about weight loss: Tips for primary care providers.* https://www.niddk.nih.gov/health-information/professionals/clinical-tools-patient-management/weight-management/talking-adult-patients-tips-primary-care-clinicians

sustainable weight loss efforts (Vallis et al., 2020). Goals that aim to improve overall health, functionality, and quality of life, not just decreased weight, will promote long-term behavior changes. Assessing patients' reasons for losing weight and their goals allows the APP to understand where to shift the focus of the conversation, identify specific challenges related to their goals, and provide encouragement when there is progress toward meeting the goals. Because obesity is a chronic condition, it will require lifelong management.

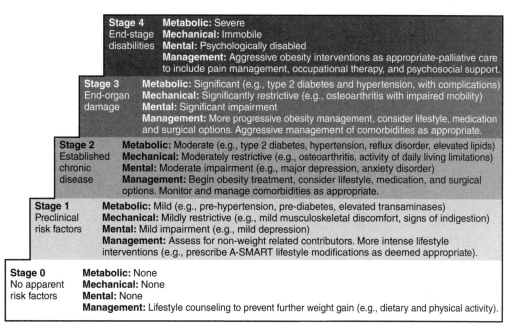

Figure 17.5 Edmonton Obesity Staging System

Health Promotion Case Study: Obesity

Case Description: C.M. is a 42-year-old male with the chief complaint of weight gain. One month ago, he was seen in the clinic for a routine physical and blood work and was noted to have increasing lipids. He was counseled on lifestyle modifications and is seeking more counseling. He has tried multiple diets and supplements in the past and has been unable to lose significant weight or keep it off. He is seeking assistance for weight loss to have more energy and to keep up with his kids for years to come.

- Past medical history: Gastroesophageal reflux disease, prediabetes, hyperlipidemia.
- Medications: Famotidine 20 mg daily, Lipitor 10 mg daily.
- Allergies: No known allergies.
- Social history: Works during the day as a realtor. Divorced with two children and one dog.
- Vital signs: BP 118/74 mmHg left arm, heart rate 76 bpm, respirations 16 bpm, temperature 98.4°F, O_2 saturation 98% on room air, weight 287.7 lb, height 70 in., BMI 41.28 kg/m².
- Review of systems: He is currently asymptomatic with occasional reflux, especially after large meals and dining out. All other systems are negative.
- Physical exam: The physical exam was unremarkable.
- Labs: Recent blood work last month. CBC is unremarkable; CMP with elevated glucose at 160 mg/dL, otherwise unremarkable; hemoglobin A1C 5.8%; total cholesterol 237 mg/dL; triglycerides 439 mg/dL; high-density lipoprotein 34 mg/dL; very-low-density lipoprotein 78 mg/dL; low-density lipoprotein 125 mg/dL; thyroid-stimulating hormone 1.230 uIU/mL.

(continues)

Health Promotion Case Study: Obesity *(continued)*

Lifestyle Vital Signs

- Adopt healthy eating: He eats a lot of meat, dairy, and eggs and gets takeout several nights a week, as he does not have much time to cook. He eats fruits and vegetables once a day. He drinks 3–4 sodas a week.
- Stress less: States work is stressful at times.
- Move often: He recently joined a gym and started exercising for 30 minutes twice a week, a combination of walking and weight lifting.
- Avoid alcohol: He drinks 2–3 alcoholic drinks on the weekend and does not use drugs.
- Rest more: Not assessed.
- Treat tobacco use: He has never smoked.

Critical Thinking Questions

- Based on Table 17.8, what additional medical history do you want to obtain, and why?
- Are there any additional lifestyle questions you want to ask?
- Based on Table 17.9, what additional objective data do you want to assess, and why?
- What additional laboratory data are needed, if any?
- What lifestyle management strategies would you suggest for weight loss based on the A-SMART lifestyle behaviors?
- Write person-centered A-SMART lifestyle prescriptions using SMART goal setting.
- Find research or evidence-informed guidelines to support lifestyle management decisions.

Recommendation: Use the 6As counseling framework (Gallager et al., 2021), for example, *ask* for permission to discuss weight; *assess* pre-encounter data, weight-centered history, and weight-centered physical exam; *advise* as appropriate; *agree* on treatment using goal-setting strategies; *assist* using A-SMART lifestyle behaviors as a guide; and *arrange* follow-up.

Helping patients realize this will allow them to reframe their mindset to create sustainable lifestyle modifications, behaviors, and habits so as not to increase the risk of regaining weight with short-term fixes (Vallis et al., 2020).

Patients often wonder what their ideal weight should be, which is commonly determined using the BMI scale. Because BMI does have limitations, it is suggested to use the concept of *best weight*, which is the weight that patients can attain and maintain while still living their healthiest and most enjoyable life. The weight loss journey can be a period of discovering a person's best weight (Vallis et al., 2020).

Identifying a realistic weight loss goal is essential when clinicians have determined that patients are ready to make lifestyle changes to attain these goals. Generally, a 1 to 2 lb weight loss per week is expected, with a goal of 5% to 10% weight loss from baseline within 6 months to reduce risk factors. However, with weight reduction more substantial than 1 to 2 lb per week, there is a more significant benefit, but patients should be encouraged that even a 5% weight loss can achieve health benefits (Jensen et al., 2014). For example, a goal for a patient with a starting baseline weight of 200 lb would be to lose 10 lb (5%) to 20 lb (10%) within 6 months. These benefits include reduced CVD risk factors, improved lipid profiles, reduced hemoglobin A1C, reduced risk of developing T2D, and reduced risk of obesity-related complications (Lau & Wharton, 2020).

Strategies for Weight Loss

A successful weight loss program is multifaceted and includes lifestyle and psychological strategies. Interventions to adopt A-SMART lifestyle behaviors will enhance weight loss. The first three behaviors (adopt healthy eating, stress less, and move often) will be highlighted in this section. See **Table 17.14** for a summary of the A-SMART action plan for obesity management. In particular, an individualized weight loss or management program that includes both a reduction in calories and an increase in physical activity has been demonstrated to be more effective than only calorie reduction or physical activity (U.S. Department of Health and Human Services [HHS], 2018; Vallis et al., 2020). Psychological strategies that will ensure successful outcomes include setting SMART goals, self-monitoring (using a journal to track food intake, physical activity, and weight), and problem-solving (Vallis et al., 2020). Effective weight management interventions will require an interprofessional healthcare team.

Table 17.14 A-SMART Recommendations with Grade and Level of Evidence

Lifestyle Modification	Recommendation	Grade of Evidence
Adopt healthy eating	Medical nutrition counseling for overweight and obesity should aim to decrease fat mass and correct adipose tissue dysfunction. Include families, particularly with children. The goal of weight loss is 5–10% annually until the ideal body weight is achieved.	Grade A Best Evidence Rating Level (BEL) = 1
Stress less	Spend time in recreation or play, stress reduction, and happiness, including using social support and developing coping skills for overall disease prevention.	Grade A BEL = 1
Move often	Implement a lifestyle intervention to obtain a 7% weight loss and a minimum of 150 minutes per week or the equivalent of 150 minutes of aerobic activity to decrease obesity-related diabetes.	Grade A BEL = 1
Avoid alcohol	Advise patients to avoid alcohol. But for those who consume alcohol, if they are of legal age and without contraindications to alcohol, the guidelines recommend daily intake of ≤1 drink (0.6 oz of pure alcohol) for women and ≤2 drinks for men. Alcohol should not be increased for any supposed beneficial effect.	Grade D BEL = 4
Rest more	Advise patient to obtain at least 6 hours of sleep nightly for disease prevention (ideally 7–8 hours/night). Encourage sleep hygiene practices.	Grade A BEL = 1
Treat tobacco use	Provide treatment for tobacco use. Tobacco use may not contribute to obesity, but it is well established that avoiding it supports a healthy lifestyle.	Grade not available

Data from Gonzalez-Campoy, J. M., St. Jeor, S. T., Castorino, K., Ebrahim, A., Hurley, D., Jovanovic, L., Mechanick, J. I., Petak, S. M., Yu, Y. H., Harris, K., Kris-Etherton, P., Kushner, R., Molini-Blandford, M., Nguyen, Q. T., Plodkowski, R., Sarwer, D. B., & Thomas, K. T. (2013). Clinical practice guidelines for healthy eating for the prevention and treatment of metabolic and endocrine diseases in adults: Cosponsored by the American Association of Clinical Endocrinologists/the American College of Endocrinology and The Obesity Society. *Endocrine Practice, 19*(SUPPL. 3), 1–82. https://doi.org/10.4158/EP13155.GL

Nutritional Strategies for Weight Loss

Individuals living with obesity should receive person-centered medical nutrition therapy (MNT), preferably from a dietitian or provider with experience in obesity management, to optimize weight outcomes (Brown et al., 2022). There is a myriad of evidence-based MNTs effective in improving health outcomes as described in the *Canadian Adult Obesity Clinical Practice Guidelines: Medical Nutrition Therapy in Obesity Management* (Brown et al., 2022). Overall, there is no one-size-fits-all eating approach for weight management. It should be noted that the best dietary pattern for managing weight is one that can be sustained over the long term. Therefore, APPs must consult with patients to develop an individualized eating plan because effective weight loss and maintenance depend on patients' long-standing adherence to a healthy nutritional regimen (Kim, 2021).

Nutritional strategies for weight loss depend on multiple factors, including the pattern, time, quality, and quantity of food intake (Kim, 2021). Reduced caloric intake was identified as the fundamental and most important weight loss factor in the scientific literature (Jenson et al., 2014; Kim, 2021). Further considerations to optimize weight loss are avoiding late-night eating and eating the largest meal of the day at breakfast (Kim, 2021). Additionally, guidelines recommend daily energy intake lower than needed for energy balance, usually 1,200 to 1,500 calories for women and 1,500 to 1,800 calories for men as well as an energy deficit of 500 to 750 calories per day, or an energy deficit of 30%, and approaches as needed to decrease caloric intake by restricting or eliminating particular foods or prescribing selected foods such as whole-plant foods, many of which are naturally lower in calories (Jensen et al., 2014).

In a recent review to determine the best dietary plan for weight loss, the Mediterranean diet, which emphasizes vegetables, fruits, whole grains, and healthy fats, was the most reliable for weight loss (Dinu et al., 2020). This was in comparison to low-fat, high-protein, intermittent energy restriction and vegetarian eating plans. Accordingly, the American College of Lifestyle Medicine (n.d.) recommends eating primarily a variety of minimally processed vegetables, fruits, whole grains, legumes, nuts, and seeds to treat, reverse, and prevent lifestyle-related chronic diseases, such as obesity. Further, patients in the initial stages of adapting to a plant-based dietary plan to decrease weight and improve health outcomes may find it more amenable to sustain adding healthy foods rather than avoiding foods. APPs may use the free online Full Plate Living Nutrition Program to teach the principle of adding high-fiber plant-based foods to increase satiety and ultimately manage weight (Full Plate Living, n.d.).

Stress and Weight Management

Stress management and coping skills should be included in a program to treat individuals with excess weight. A small, randomized controlled trial that included a stress management component to a lifestyle intervention on weight loss revealed successful outcomes after an 8-week program (Xenaki et al., 2018). The intervention had relaxation breathing exercises, progressive muscle relaxation techniques, and guided visualization, all of which decreased perceived stress and depression and improved dietary habits. Patients should be encouraged to assess for emotional triggers that spark the urge to eat even when they may not be physiologically hungry and put cues in place to eat mindfully to avoid overeating. Practical tips to offer patients regarding mindful eating include eating when hungry but before being voraciously hungry, avoiding distractions while eating, breathing deeply five times before starting a meal, eating slowly, taking small bites, stopping eating when feeling full, and having healthy snacks available when leaving home (Daniel, 2018). It is well known that physical activity can alleviate stress and enhance weight loss. Therefore, physical activity is a crucial component of a weight loss program.

Physical Activity and Weight Loss and Maintenance

Physical activity or exercise is essential to achieving and maintaining weight loss goals, particularly in conjunction with other strategies. A review of studies by Cox (2017) to determine the role of physical activity in weight management found that individuals were more likely to lose weight and sustain weight loss if they participated in physical activity for at least 1 hour per day. This finding is in keeping with the recommendation from the 2018 Physical Activity Guidelines (HHS, 2018) that some individuals will need 300 minutes or more per week of physical activity to lose weight. Further, a systematic review (Jakicic et al., 2019) expanded on the evidence that informed the development of the 2018 Physical Activity Guidelines and found that physical activity above 150 minutes of moderate to vigorous intensity per week tempered weight gain in adults. The review indicated that obesity was significantly decreased in a graded manner based on the incremental increase in vigorous physical activity per week. The effect of the association of physical activity on obesity in adults varied by age—as age increased, the effect of physical activity on obesity decreased.

Weight loss as a result of physical activity alone may be insufficient for individuals who are obese (Jakicic et al., 2019). Nevertheless, APPs should routinely assess physical activity and guide patients who can be physically active to integrate intentional movement into their routine behaviors to attenuate weight gain. For weight loss, individuals should do at least 150 to 300 minutes of moderate-intensity or 75 to 150 minutes of vigorous-intensity physical activity per week or a comparable mixture of moderate- and vigorous-intensity aerobic physical exercise (HHS, 2018). However, some movement is better than none (Bays et al., 2021). Patients should be encouraged to include resistance training as an adjunct to their overall physical activity habits but not as the sole activity for weight management.

Multicomponent Interventions for Overweight and Obesity

The Look AHEAD (Action for Health in Diabetes) landmark study particularly underscores the effect of a multicomponent approach to weight management (Look AHEAD Research Group, 2014). Look AHEAD is a randomized controlled trial with over 5,000 individuals with obesity and diabetes. The intensive lifestyle intervention group was prescribed 1,200 to 1,800 calories daily, with no more than 30% of calories from fat (less than 10% from saturated fat) and no less than 15% from protein. Also, participants in the study were prescribed at least 175 minutes of unsupervised moderate-intensity physical activity per week and individual and group counseling at varying intervals. In year 1, participants in the intensive lifestyle intervention had an average

---

Health Promotion Activity: Assess Edmonton's Obesity Stage and Genetic Risk

Reread the obesity case study of C.M.

- Calculate the obesity risk index score, and determine the Edmonton Obesity Staging System stage for C.M.
- What additional information is needed from C.M. to complete the Genetic Obesity Risk Index Screening Questionnaire?

weight loss from baseline of 8.5% ± 0.2% compared with 0.6% ± 0.2% for the comparison group. Even at 8 years, half of those who followed the dietary and physical activity prescriptions had at least a 5% decrease in weight (Look AHEAD Research Group, 2014). Those who achieved the weight loss goals increased physical activity, decreased caloric intake, monitored their weight, and attended counseling sessions.

Interprofessional Approach

Obesity is a chronic systemic condition that requires an interprofessional approach (Bischoff et al., 2017) for prevention and management to ensure the best possible long-term outcome. The root causes of overweight and obesity are multifactorial, as are the treatment approaches and referral needs. The interprofessional healthcare team members who may be required to address the many components of pre-obesity and obesity include psychiatrists, psychologists, behavioral therapists, registered dieticians, exercise physiologists, endocrinologists, health coaches, and bariatric surgeons. A thorough history and physical exam may also reveal comorbidities or obesity-related complications that could require referral to cardiology, endocrinology, dermatology, orthopedist, sleep specialists, physical therapists, occupational therapists, physiotherapy, and other medical specialists (Bischoff et al., 2017).

The APP should consult with a specialist in obesity medicine and an interprofessional team if patients cannot achieve significant and long-term weight loss with behavior modifications alone. Weight loss medications are recommended for those with a BMI of at least 30 or a BMI of 27 with at least one obesity-related comorbidity (Jensen et al., 2014). Bariatric surgery is considered for those with a BMI of at least 40 or a BMI of 35 with obesity-related comorbidities and no response to lifestyle interventions.

Summary

Pre-obesity and obesity are serious public health threats related to energy imbalance that results in excess adiposity. In particular, obesity is not just a disease but also a risk factor for many leading causes of disability, death, and chronic conditions, such as cardiac disease, T2D, osteoarthritis, cancer, and mental disorders. Overall, excess weight can be caused by physiological (genes, epigenetics, brain–gut axis, neuroendocrine conditions, medications, and the gut microbiome), behavioral (high-calorie intake, physical inactivity, alcohol use, former smokers, and inadequate sleep), and environmental (food abundance, food insecurity, built environment, socioeconomic status, culture, and bias) factors. The multifactorial causes of pre-obesity and obesity require an interprofessional team and a comprehensive approach that includes an extensive history and a physical exam to determine the underlying factors associated with the imbalance in energy homeostasis used to guide treatment. The BMI and waist measurements are objective adiposity measurements and should be included routinely in the clinical setting to diagnose and manage treatment progress. Conversations about obesity are complex, and clinicians should use evidence-informed counseling tactics that include first-person language and seek permission to discuss weight. This will ultimately decrease the risk of bias and enhance person-centered treatment plans that likely lead to adherence. Practical weight management includes evidence-informed approaches such as the A-SMART lifestyle behaviors, emphasizing a person-centered approach that supports a plant-based diet and increased physical activity. Finally, since obesity is a multifactorial chronic disease, it will require multicomponent treatments and an interprofessional team of healthcare providers to attain sustainable weight loss goals. See **Table 17.15** for evidence-based resources for assessing, diagnosing, and treating pre-obesity and obesity.

TABLE 17.15	Evidence-Based Resources for Pre-Obesity and Obesity

Resources	URL
Alcohol Calorie Calculator	https://www.rethinkingdrinking.niaaa.nih.gov/Tools/Calculators/calorie-calculator.aspx
American Association of Clinical Endocrinologists and American College of Endocrinology Clinical Practice Guidelines for Medical Care of Patients with Obesity	https://www.endocrinepractice.org/article/S1530-891X(20)44630-0/fulltext
2013 AHA/ACC/TOS Guideline for the Management of Overweight and Obesity in Adults	https://www.ahajournals.org/doi/epub/10.1161/01.cir.0000437739.71477.ee
BMI Calculator	https://www.hepatitisc.uw.edu/page/clinical-calculators/bmi
Canadian Adult Obesity Clinical Practice Guidelines	https://obesitycanada.ca/guidelines/chapters
Clinical Practice Guideline for the Treatment of Obesity and Overweight in Children and Adolescents	https://www.apa.org/obesity-guideline
Fibrosis-4 Calculator	https://www.hepatitisc.uw.edu/page/clinical-calculators/fib-4
Weight Can't Wait: Guide for the Management of Obesity in the Primary Care Setting	https://stoppublichealth9.drupal.gwu.edu/sites/g/files/zaxdzs4356/files/2022-02/wcw-guide-for-the-management-of-obesity-in-the-primary-care-setting.pdf
National Weight Control Registry	http://nwcr.ws/default.htm
Medical Nutrition Therapy in Obesity Management	https://obesitycanada.ca/wp-content/uploads/2022/10/Medical-Nutrition-Therapy_22_FINAL.pdf
VA/DoD Clinical Practice Guideline for the Management of Adult Overweight and Obesity	https://www.healthquality.va.gov/guidelines/CD/obesity/VADoDObesityCPGFinal5087242020.pdf

Acronyms

6As: ask, assess, advise, agree, assist, arrange
APP: advanced practice provider
A-SMART: adopt healthy eating, stress less, move often, avoid alcohol, rest more, and treat tobacco use
BMI: body mass index

CVD: cardiovascular disease
DNA: deoxyribonucleic acid
EE: energy expenditure
FTO: fat mass and obesity-associated gene
HHS: U.S. Department of Health and Human Services

HIV/AIDs: human immunodeficiency virus/acquired immunodeficiency syndrome

HTN: hypertension

MNT: medical nutrition therapy

NHLBI: National Heart, Lung, and Blood Institute

OMA: Obesity Medicine Association

RMR: resting metabolic rate

SMART: specific, measurable, attainable, relevant, time-bound

STOP: Strategies to Overcome and Prevent

T2D: type 2 diabetes

USPSTF: U.S. Preventive Services Task Force

WC: waist circumference

WFPB: whole food plant based

WHO: World Health Organization

WHR: waist–hip ratio

References

Abarca-Gómez, L., Abdeen, Z. A., Hamid, Z. A., Abu-Rmeileh, N. M., Acosta-Cazares, B., Acuin, C., Adams, R. J., Aekplakorn, W., Afsana, K., Aguilar-Salinas, C. A., Agyemang, C., Ahmadvand, A., Ahrens, W., Ajlouni, K., Akhtaeva, N., Al-Hazzaa, H. M., Al-Othman, A. R., Al-Raddadi, R., Al Buhairan, F., . . . Ezzati, M. (2017). Worldwide trends in body-mass index, underweight, overweight, and obesity from 1975 to 2016: A pooled analysis of 2416 population-based measurement studies in 128.9 million children, adolescents, and adults. *The Lancet, 390*(10113), 2627–2642. https://doi.org/10.1016/S0140-6736(17)32129-3

Adamska-Patruno, E., Ostrowska, L., Goscik, J., Pietraszewska, B., Kretowski, A., & Gorska, M. (2018). The relationship between the leptin/ghrelin ratio and meals with various macronutrient contents in men with different nutritional status: A randomized crossover study. *Nutrition Journal, 17*(1), 1–7. https://doi.org/10.1186/s12937-018-0427-x

American College of Lifestyle Medicine. (n.d.). *Dietary position statement.* Retrieved November 6, 2022, from https://lifestylemedicine.org/overview

American Psychological Association. (2018). *Clinical practice guideline for multicomponent behavioral treatment of obesity and overweight in children and adolescents.* https://www.apa.org/about/offices/directorates/guidelines/obesity-clinical-practice-guideline.pdf

American Psychological Association. (2021). *Stress and decision-making during the pandemic.* https://www.apa.org/news/press/releases/stress/2021/october-decision-making

Aoun, A., Darwish, F., & Hamod, N. (2020). The influence of the gut microbiome on obesity in adults and the role of probiotics, prebiotics, and synbiotics for weight loss. *Preventive Nutrition and Food Science, 25*(2), 113. https://doi.org/10.3746/PNF.2020.25.2.113

Bays, H. E., McCarthy, W., Burridge, K., Tondt, J., Karjoo, S., Christensen, S., Ng, J., Golden, A., Davisson, L., & Richardson, L. (2021). *Obesity algorithm 2021: Important principles for the effective treatment of patients with obesity* (e-book). https://obesitymedicine.org

Bhaskaran, K., dos-Santos-Silva, I., Leon, D. A., Douglas, I. J., & Smeeth, L. (2018). Association of BMI with overall and cause-specific mortality: A population-based cohort study of 3.6 million adults in the UK. *The Lancet Diabetes & Endocrinology, 6,* 944–953. https://doi.org/10.1016/S2213-8587(18)30288-2

Bischoff, S. C., Boirie, Y., Cederholm, T., Chourdakis, M., Cuerda, C., Delzenne, N. M., Deutz, N. E., Fouque, D., Genton, L., Gil, C., Koletzko, B., Leon-Sanz, M., Shamir, R., Singer, J., Singer, P., Stroebele-Benschop, N., Thorell, A., Weimann, A., & Barazzoni, R. (2017). Towards a multidisciplinary approach to understand and manage obesity and related diseases. *Clinical Nutrition, 36*(4), 917–938. https://doi.org/10.1016/J.CLNU.2016.11.007

Blüher, M. (2019). Obesity: Global epidemiology and pathogenesis. *Nature Reviews Endocrinology, 15,* 288–298. https://doi.org/10.1038/s41574-019-0176-8

Bonanno, L., Metro, D., Papa, M., Finzi, G., Maviglia, A., Sottile, F., Corallo, F., & Manasseri, L. (2019). Assessment of sleep and obesity in adults and children: Observational study. *Medicine, 98*(46), e17642. https://doi.org/10.1097/MD.0000000000017642

Brown, J., Clarke, C., Johnson Stoklossa, C., & Sievenpiper, J. (2022). *Canadian adult obesity clinical practice guidelines: Medical nutrition therapy in obesity management.* https://obesitycanada.ca/wp-content/uploads/2022/10/Medical-Nutrition-Therapy_22_FINAL.pdf

Camacho, W. J. M., Díaz, J. M. M., Ortiz, S. P., Ortiz, J. E. P., Camacho, M. A. M., & Calderón, B. P. (2019). Childhood obesity: Aetiology, comorbidities, and treatment. *Diabetes/Metabolism Research and Reviews, 35*(8), e3203. https://doi.org/10.1002/DMRR.3203

Centers for Disease Control and Prevention. (n.d.). *Alcohol use and your health.* Retrieved December 6, 2022, from https://www.cdc.gov/alcohol/fact-sheets/alcohol-use.htm

Centers for Disease Control and Prevention. (2023). *Defining child BMI categories.* https://www.cdc.gov/obesity/childhood/defining.html

Chen, L. W., Aubert, A. M., Shivappa, N., Bernard, J. Y., Mensink-Bout, S. M., Geraghty, A. A., Mehegan, J., Suderman, M., Polanska, K., Hanke, W., Jankowska, A., Relton, C. L., Crozier, S. R., Harvey, N. C., Cooper, C., Hanson, M., Godfrey, K. M., Gaillard, R., Duijts, L., . . . Phillips, C. M. (2021). Maternal dietary quality, inflammatory potential and childhood adiposity: An individual participant data pooled analysis of seven European cohorts in the ALPHABET consortium. *BioMed Central Medicine*, *19*(1). https://doi.org/10.1186/s12916-021-01908-7

Chooi, Y. C., Ding, C., & Magkos, F. (2019). The epidemiology of obesity. *Metabolism: Clinical and Experimental*, *92*, 6–10. https://doi.org/10.1016/j.metabol.2018.09.005

Cooper, C. B., Neufeld, E. V., Dolezal, B. A., & Martin, J. L. (2018). Sleep deprivation and obesity in adults: A brief narrative review. *British Medical Journal Open Sport & Exercise Medicine*, *4*(1), 392. https://doi.org/10.1136/BMJSEM-2018-000392

Cox, C. E. (2017). Role of physical activity for weight loss and weight maintenance. *Diabetes Spectrum*, *30*(3), 157. https://doi.org/10.2337/DS17-0013

Daniel, S. (2018, August 9). *Mindful eating and treating obesity*. Obesity Medicine Association. https://obesitymedicine.org/mindful-eating

Dare, S., Mackay, D. F., & Pell, J. P. (2015). Relationship between smoking and obesity: A cross-sectional study of 499,504 middle-aged adults in the UK general population. *PLoS ONE*, *10*(4). https://doi.org/10.1371/journal.pone.0123579

De Lorenzo, A., Romano, L., Di Renzo, L., Di Lorenzo, N., Cenname, G., & Gualtieri, P. (2020). Obesity: A preventable, treatable, but relapsing disease. *Nutrition*, *71*, 110615. https://doi.org/10.1016/j.nut.2019.110615

Dinu, M., Pagliai, G., Angelino, D., Rosi, A., Bresciani, L., Ferraris, C., Guglielmetti, M., Godos, J., Nucci, D., Meroni, E., Landini, L., Martini, D., & Sofi, F. (2020). Effects of popular diets on anthropometric and cardiometabolic parameters: An umbrella review of meta-analyses of randomized controlled trials. *Advances in Nutrition*, *11*(4), 815–833. https://doi.org/10.1093/advances/nmaa006

Ebbeling C. B., Pawlak D. B., & Ludwig D. S. (2002). Childhood obesity: Public-health crisis, common sense cure. *The Lancet*, *360*(9331), 473–482. https://doi.org/10.1016/S0140-6736(02)09678-2

European Association for the Study of Obesity. (2020, September 2). *Even light alcohol consumption linked to higher risk of obesity and metabolic syndrome in study of 27 million adults*. The European and International Congress on Obesity Conference [News release]. https://www.eurekalert.org/news-releases/605322

Fall, T., Mendelson, M., & Speliotes, E. K. (2017). Recent advances in human genetics and epigenetics of adiposity: Pathway to precision medicine? *Gastroenter-ology*, *152*(7), 1695–1706. https://doi.org/10.1053/J.GASTRO.2017.01.054

Fitch, A. K., & Bays, H. E. (2022). Obesity definition, diagnosis, bias, standard operating procedures (SOPs), and telehealth: An Obesity Medicine Association Clinical Practice Statement (CPS) 2022. *Obesity Pillars*, *1*, 100004. https://doi.org/10.1016/J.OBPILL.2021.100004

Forny-Germano, L., De Felice, F. G., & Do Nascimento Vieira, M. N. (2019). The role of leptin and adiponectin in obesity-associated cognitive decline and Alzheimer's disease. *Frontiers in Neuroscience*, *13*(JAN), 1027. https://doi.org/10.3389/FNINS.2018.01027/BIBTEX

Fox, A., Feng, W., & Asal, V. (2019). What is driving global obesity trends? Globalization or "modernization"? *Global Health*, *15*(32). https://doi.org/10.1186/s12992-019-0457-y

Fry, A. (2022, April 18). *Obesity and sleep*. Sleep Foundation. https://www.sleepfoundation.org/physical-health/obesity-and-sleep

Full Plate Living. (n.d.). *Full plate living nutrition programs*. Retrieved November 23, 2022, from https://www.fullplateliving.org

Gadde, K. M., Martin, C. K., Berthoud, H. R., & Heymsfield, S. B. (2018). Obesity: Pathophysiology and management. *Journal of the American College of Cardiology*, *71*(1), 69–84. https://doi.org/10.1016/j.jacc.2017.11.011

Gallagher, C., Corl, A., & Dietz, W. H. (2021). Weight can't wait: A guide to discussing obesity and organizing treatment in the primary care setting. *Obesity*, *29*(5), 821–824. https://doi.org/10.1002/OBY.23154

Garvey, W. T., Mechanick, J. I., Brett, E. M., Garber, A. J., Hurley, D. L., Jastreboff, A. M., Nadolsky, K., Pessah-Pollack, R., & Plodkowski, R. (2016). American Association of Clinical Endocrinologists and American College of Endocrinology comprehensive clinical practice guidelines for medical care of patients with obesity. *Endocrine Practice*, *22*, 1–203. https://doi.org/10.4158/EP161365.GL

Gonzalez-Campoy, J. M., St Jeor, S. T., Castorino, K., Ebrahim, A., Hurley, D., Jovanovic, L., Mechanick, J. I., Petak, S. M., Yu, Y. H., Harris, K., Kris-Etherton, P., Kushner, R., Molini-Blandford, M., Nguyen, Q. T., Plodkowski, R., Sarwer, D. B., & Thomas, K. T. (2013). Clinical practice guidelines for healthy eating for the prevention and treatment of metabolic and endocrine diseases in adults: Cosponsored by the American Association of Clinical Endocrinologists /the American College of Endocrinology and The Obesity Society. *Endocrine Practice*, *19*(Suppl. 3), 1–82. https://doi.org/10.4158/EP13155.GL

Graff, M., Scott, R. A., Justice, A. E., Young, K. L., Feitosa, M. F., Barata, L., Winkler, T. W., Chu, A. Y., Mahajan, A., Hadley, D., Xue, L., Workalemahu, T.,

Heard-Costa, N. L., den Hoed, M., Ahluwalia, T. S., Qi, Q., Ngwa, J. S., Renström, F., Quaye, L., . . . Kilpeläinen, T. O. (2017). Genome-wide physical activity interactions in adiposity—A meta-analysis of 200,452 adults. *PLoS Genetics*, *13*(4), 130. https://doi .org/10.1371/JOURNAL.PGEN.1006528

Grossman, D. C., Bibbins-Domingo, K., Curry, S. J., Barry, M. J., Davidson, K. W., Doubeni, C. A., Epling, J. W., Kemper, A. R., Krist, A. H., Kurth, A. E., Landefeld, C. S., Mangione, C. M., Phipps, M. G., Silverstein, M., Simon, M. A., & Tseng, C. W. (2017). Screening for obesity in children and adolescents: US Preventive Services Task Force recommendation statement. *Journal of the American Medical Association*, *317*(23), 2417–2426. https://doi.org/10 .1001/jama.2017.6803

Guglielmo, D., Hootman, J. M., Murphy, L. B., Boring, M. A., Theis, K. A., Belay, B., Barbour, K. E., Cisternas, M. G., & Helmick, C. G. (2018). Health care provider counseling for weight loss among adults with arthritis and overweight or obesity—United States, 2002–2014. *Morbidity and Mortality Weekly Report*, *67*(17), 485–490. https://doi.org/10.15585 /MMWR.MM6717A2

Hales, C. M., Fryar, C. D., Carroll, M. D., Freedman, D. S., Aoki, Y., & Ogden, C. L. (2018). Differences in obesity prevalence by demographic characteristics and urbanization level among adults in the United States, 2013–2016. *Journal of the American Medical Association*, *319*(23), 2419–2429. https://doi.org/10.1001 /jama.2018.7270

Harvard T. H. Chan School of Public Health. (n.d.). *Obesity prevention source*. Retrieved April 14, 2023, from https://www.hsph.harvard.edu/obesity -prevention-source/obesity-definition/abdominal -obesity

Healy, G. N., Wijndaele, K., Dunstan, D. W., Shaw, J. E., Salmon, J., Zimmet, P. Z., & Owen, N. (2008). Objectively measured sedentary time, physical activity, and metabolic risk: The Australian Diabetes, Obesity and Lifestyle Study (AusDiab). *Diabetes Care*, *31*(2), 369–371. https://doi.org/10.2337/DC07-1795

Hess, M. E., & Brüning, J. C. (2014). The fat mass and obesity-associated (FTO) gene: Obesity and beyond? *Biochimica et Biophysica Acta - Molecular Basis of Disease*, *1842*(10), 2039–2047. https://doi.org/10.1016 /j.bbadis.2014.01.017

Hoelscher, D. M., Kirk, S., Ritchie, L., & Cunningham-Sabo, L. (2013). Position of the Academy of Nutrition and Dietetics: Interventions for the prevention and treatment of pediatric overweight and obesity. *Journal of the Academy of Nutrition and Dietetics*, *113*(10), 1375–1394. https://doi.org/10.1016/j .jand.2013.08.004

Huvenne, H., Dubern, B., Clément, K., & Poitou, C. (2016). Rare genetic forms of obesity: Clinical approach and current treatments in 2016. *Obesity Facts*, *9*(3), 158–173. https://doi.org/10.1159/000445061

Huxley, R., Mendis, S., Zheleznyakov, E., Reddy, S., & Chan, J. (2010). Body mass index, waist circumference and waist:hip ratio as predictors of cardiovascular risk—A review of the literature. *European Journal of Clinical Nutrition*, *64*, 16–22. https://doi.org/10.1038 /ejcn.2009.68

Inan-Eroglu, E., Huang, B. H., Ahmadi, M. N., Johnson, N., El-Omar, E. M., & Stamatakis, E. (2022). Joint associations of adiposity and alcohol consumption with liver disease-related morbidity and mortality risk: Findings from the UK Biobank. *European Journal of Clinical Nutrition*, *76*(1), 74–83. https://doi .org/10.1038/s41430-021-00923-4

Jakicic, J. M., Powell, K. E., Campbell, W. W., Dipietro, L., Pate, R. R., Pescatello, L. S., Collins, K. A., Bloodgood, B., & Piercy, K. L. (2019). Physical activity and the prevention of weight gain in adults: A systematic review. *Medicine & Science in Sports & Exercise*, *51*(6), 1262–1269. https://doi.org/10.1249 /MSS.0000000000001938

Jakše, B., Jakše, B., Pinter, S., Pajek, J., & Fidler Mis, N. (2020). Whole-food plant-based lifestyle program and decreased obesity. *American Journal of Lifestyle Medicine*, *16*(3), 1–11. https://doi.org/10.1177/15598276 20949205

Jastreboff, A. M., Kotz, C. M., Kahan, S., Kelly, A. S., & Heymsfield, S. B. (2019). Obesity as a disease: The Obesity Society 2018 position statement. *Obesity*, *27*(1), 7–9. https://doi.org/10.1002/oby.22378

Jensen, M. D., Ryan, D. H., Apovian, C. M., Ard, J. D., Comuzzie, A. G., Donato, K. A., Hu, F. B., Hubbard, V. S., Jakicic, J. M., Kushner, R. F., Loria, C. M., Millen, B. E., Nonas, C. A., Pi-Sunyer, F. X., Stevens, J., Stevens, V. J., Wadden, T. A., Wolfe, B. M., & Yanovski, S. Z. (2014). 2013 AHA/ACC/TOS guideline for the management of overweight and obesity in adults: A report of the American College of Cardiology/American Heart Association Task Force on Practice Guidelines and The Obesity Society. *Circulation*, *129*(25), S102–S138. https://doi.org/10.1161/01 .CIR.0000437739.71477.EE

Kadouh, H. C., & Acosta, A. (2017). Current paradigms in the etiology of obesity. *Techniques in Gastrointestinal Endoscopy*, *19*(1), 2–11. https://doi.org/10.1016/j .tgie.2016.12.001

Kandi, V., & Vadakedath, S. (2015). Effect of DNA methylation in various diseases and the probable protective role of nutrition: A mini-review. *Cureus*, *7*(8), e309. https://doi.org/10.7759/cureus.309

Karra, E., O'Daly, O. G., Choudhury, A. I., Yousseif, A., Millership, S., Neary, M. T., Scott, W. R., Chandarana, K., Manning, S., Hess, M. E., Iwakura, H., Akamizu, T., Millet, Q., Gelegen, C., Drew, M. E., Rahman, S., Emmanuel, J. J., Williams, S. C. R., Rüther, U. U., . . .

Batterham, R. L. (2013). A link between FTO, ghrelin, and impaired brain food-cue responsivity. *Journal of Clinical Investigation, 123*(8), 3539–3551. https://doi.org/10.1172/JCI44403

Kelly, A. S., Barlow, S. E., Rao, G., Inge, T. H., Hayman, L. L., Steinberger, J., Urbina, E. M., Ewing, L. J., & Daniels, S. R. (2013). Severe obesity in children and adolescents: Identification, associated health risks, and treatment approaches: A scientific statement from the American Heart Association. *Circulation, 128*(15), 1689–1712. doi:10.1161/cir.0b013e3182a5cfb3

Khattak ZE, Zahra F. Evaluation of Patients With Obesity. [Updated 2023 Apr 27]. In: StatPearls [Internet]. Treasure Island (FL): StatPearls Publishing; 2023 Jan-. Available from: https://www.ncbi.nlm.nih.gov/books/NBK576399/

Kim, J. Y. (2021). Optimal diet strategies for weight loss and weight loss maintenance. *Journal of Obesity & Metabolic Syndrome, 30*(1), 20–31. https://doi.org/10.7570/jomes20065

Lau, D. C. W., & Wharton, S. (2020). The science of obesity. *Canadian Adult Obesity Clinical Practice Guidelines,* 1–7. https://obesitycanada.ca/guidelines/science

Li, L., Zhang, S., Huang, Y., & Chen, K. (2017). Sleep duration and obesity in children: A systematic review and meta-analysis of prospective cohort studies. *Journal of Paediatrics and Child Health, 53*(4), 378–385. https://doi.org/10.1111/JPC.13434

Look AHEAD Research Group. (2014). Eight-year weight losses with an intensive lifestyle intervention: The Look AHEAD Study. *Obesity, 22*(1), 5–13. https://doi.org/10.1002/OBY.20662

Loos, R. J. F., & Yeo, G. S. H. (2021). The genetics of obesity: From discovery to biology. *Nature Reviews Genetics, 23*(2), 120–133. https://doi.org/10.1038/s41576-021-00414-z

Luig, T., Anderson, R., Sharma, A. M., & Campbell-Scherer, D. L. (2018). Personalizing obesity assessment and care planning in primary care: Patient experience and outcomes in everyday life and health. *Clinical Obesity, 8*(6), 411. https://doi.org/10.1111/COB.12283

MacMahon, S., Baigent, C., Duffy, S., Rodgers, A., Tominaga, S., Chambless, L., De Backer, G., De Bacquer, D., Kornitzer, M., Whincup, P., Wannamethee, S. G., Morris, R., Wald, N., Morris, J., Law, M., Knuiman, M., Bartholomew, H., Davey Smith, G., Sweetnam, P., . . . Whitlock, G. (2009). Body-mass index and cause-specific mortality in 900 000 adults: Collaborative analyses of 57 prospective studies. *Lancet, 373*(9669), 1083–1096. https://doi.org/10.1016/S0140-6736(09)60318-4

Meye, F. J., & Adan, R. A. H. (2014). Feelings about food: The ventral tegmental area in food reward and emotional eating. *Trends in Pharmacological Sciences, 35*(1), 31–40. https://doi.org/10.1016/j.tips.2013.11.003

Mozaffarian, D., Hao, T., Rimm, E. B., Willett, W. C., & Hu, F. B. (2011). Changes in diet and lifestyle and long-term weight gain in women and men. *New England Journal of Medicine, 364*(25), 2392. https://doi.org/10.1056/NEJMOA1014296

National Heart, Lung, and Blood Institute. (n.d.). *Aim for a healthy weight.* Retrieved August 29, 2022, from https://www.nhlbi.nih.gov/health/educational/lose_wt/risk.htm

National Human Genome Research Institute. (2022). *Epigenetics.* https://www.genome.gov/genetics-glossary/Epigenetics

National Institute of Diabetes and Digestive and Kidney Diseases. (2017). *Talking with patients about weight loss: Tips for primary care providers.* https://www.niddk.nih.gov/health-information/professionals/clinical-tools-patient-management/weight-management/talking-adult-patients-tips-primary-care-clinicians

Nimptsch, K., Konigorski, S., & Pischon, T. (2019). Diagnosis of obesity and use of obesity biomarkers in science and clinical medicine. *Metabolism: Clinical and Experimental, 92,* 61–70. https://doi.org/10.1016/j.metabol.2018.12.006

Obesity Medicine Association. (n.d.). *What is obesity medicine?* Retrieved July 7, 2022, from https://obesitymedicine.org

Obesity Medicine Association. (2018, July 23). *Obesity and genetics: Nature and nurture.* https://obesitymedicine.org/obesity-and-genetics

Obradovic, M., Sudar-Milovanovic, E., Soskic, S., Essack, M., Arya, S., Stewart, A. J., Gojobori, T., & Isenovic, E. R. (2021). Leptin and obesity: Role and clinical implication. *Frontiers in Endocrinology, 12.* https://doi.org/10.3389/fendo.2021.585887

Odegaard, J. I., & Chawla, A. (2013). Pleiotropic actions of insulin resistance and inflammation in metabolic homeostasis. *Science, 339*(6116), 172–177. https://doi.org/10.1126/SCIENCE.1230721/ASSET/1BD8FCE1-C0C9-4606-9465-330B1AF968BD/ASSETS/GRAPHIC/339_172_F3.JPEG

Oussaada, S. M., van Galen, K. A., Cooiman, M. I., Kleinendorst, L., Hazebroek, E. J., van Haelst, M. M., ter Horst, K. W., & Serlie, M. J. (2019). The pathogenesis of obesity. *Metabolism: Clinical and Experimental, 92,* 26–36. https://doi.org/10.1016/j.metabol.2018.12.012

Ozanne, S. E. (2015). Epigenetic signatures of obesity. *New England Journal of Medicine, 372*(10), 973–974. https://doi.org/10.1056/nejmcibr1414707

Park, J. H., Moon, J. H., Kim, H. J., Kong, M. H., & Oh, Y. H. (2020). Sedentary lifestyle: Overview of updated evidence of potential health risks. *Korean Journal of Family Medicine, 41*(6), 365–373. https://doi.org/10.4082/KJFM.20.0165

Petrin, C., Kahan, S., Turner, M., Gallagher, C., & Dietz, W. H. (2017). Current attitudes and practices of obesity counseling by health care providers. *Obesity Research & Clinical Practice, 11*(3), 352–359. https://doi.org/10.1016/J.ORCP.2016.08.005

Pischon, T., Boeing, H., Hoffmann, K., Bergmann, M., Schulze, M. B., Overvad, K., van der Schouw, Y. T., Spencer, E., Moons, K. G. M., Tjønneland, A., Halkjaer, J., Jensen, M. K., Stegger, J., Clavel-Chapelon, F., Boutron-Ruault, M.-C., Chajes, V., Linseisen, J., Kaaks, R., Trichopoulou, A., . . . Riboli, E. (2008). General and abdominal adiposity and risk of death in Europe. *New England Journal of Medicine, 359*(20), 2105–2120. https://doi.org/10.1056/NEJMOA0801891/SUPPL_FILE/NEJM_PISCHON_2105SA1.PDF

Ritchie, H., & Roser, M. (2017). *Obesity.* Our World in Data. https://ourworldindata.org/obesity

Rohde, K., Keller, M., la Cour Poulsen, L., Blüher, M., Kovacs, P., & Böttcher, Y. (2019). Genetics and epigenetics in obesity. *Metabolism: Clinical and Experimental, 92,* 37–50. https://doi.org/10.1016/j.metabol.2018.10.007

Rose, S. A., Poynter, P. S., Anderson, J. W., Noar, S. M., & Conigliaro, J. (2013). Physician weight loss advice and patient weight loss behavior change: A literature review and meta-analysis of survey data. *International Journal of Obesity, 37*(1), 118–128. https://doi.org/10.1038/ijo.2012.24

Roseboom, T. J. (2019). Epidemiological evidence for the developmental origins of health and disease: Effects of prenatal undernutrition in humans. *Journal of Endocrinology, 242*(1), T135–T144. https://doi.org/10.1530/JOE-18-0683

Rossner, S., Egger, G., & Binns, A. (2017). Overweight and obesity: The epidemic's underbelly. In G. Egger, A. Binns, S. Rossner, & M. Sagner (Eds.), *Lifestyle medicine: Lifestyle, the environment and preventive medicine in health and disease* (3rd ed., pp 131–132). Academic Press.

Rueda-Clausen, C. F., Poddar, M., Lear, S. A., Poirier, P., & Sharma, A. M. (2020). *Canadian adult obesity clinical practice guidelines: Assessment of people living with obesity.* https://obesitycanada.ca/wp-content/uploads/2021/05/6-Obesity-Assessment-v6-with-links.pdf

Sharma, A. M. (2010). M, M, M & M: A mnemonic for assessing obesity. *Obesity Reviews, 11*(11), 808–809. https://doi.org/10.1111/j.1467-789X.2010.00766.x

Sharma, A. M., & Kushner, R. F. (2009). A proposed clinical staging system for obesity. *International Journal of Obesity, 33*(3), 289–295. https://doi.org/10.1038/IJO.2009.2

Schulz, L. O., Bennett, P. H., Ravussin, E., Kidd, J. R., Kidd, K. K., Esparza, J., & Valencia, M. E. (2006). Effects of traditional and Western environments on prevalence of type 2 diabetes in Pima Indians in Mexico and the U.S. *Diabetes Care, 29*(8), 1866–1871. https://doi.org/10.2337/DC06-0138

Singh, M. (2014). Mood, food, and obesity. *Frontiers in Psychology, 5,* 925. https://doi.org/10.3389/fpsyg.2014.00925

Smith, J. D., Hou, T., Hu, F. B., Rimm, E. B., Spiegelman, D., Willett, W. C., & Mozaffarian, D. (2015). A comparison of different methods for evaluating diet, physical activity, and long-term weight gain in 3 prospective cohort studies. *Journal of Nutrition, 145*(11), 2527–2534. https://doi.org/10.3945/jn.115.214171

Strategies to Overcome and Prevent (STOP) Obesity Alliance. (2020, October). *Weight can't wait: Guide for the management of obesity in the primary care setting.* https://stoppublichealth9.drupal.gwu.edu/sites/g/files/zaxdzs4356/files/2022-02/wcw-guide-for-the-management-of-obesity-in-the-primary-care-setting.pdf

Tan, S. Y., Dhillon, J., & Mattes, R. D. (2014). A review of the effects of nuts on appetite, food intake, metabolism, and body weight. *American Journal of Clinical Nutrition, 100* (Suppl. 1), 412S–422S. https://doi.org/10.3945/AJCN.113.071456

Tan, X., Chapman, C. D., Cedernaes, J., & Benedict, C. (2018). Association between long sleep duration and increased risk of obesity and type 2 diabetes: A review of possible mechanisms. *Sleep Medicine Reviews, 40,* 127–134. https://doi.org/10.1016/J.SMRV.2017.11.001

Thaiss, C. A., Itav, S., Rothschild, D., Meijer, M. T., Levy, M., Moresi, C., Dohnalová, L., Braverman, S., Rozin, S., Malitsky, S., Dori-Bachash, M., Kuperman, Y., Biton, I., Gertler, A., Harmelin, A., Shapiro, H., Halpern, Z., Aharoni, A., Segal, E., & Elinav, E. (2016). Persistent microbiome alterations modulate the rate of post-dieting weight regain. *Nature, 540*(7634), 544–551. https://doi.org/10.1038/nature20796

Theorell-Haglöw, J., Berglund, L., Berne, C., & Lindberg, E. (2014). Both habitual short sleepers and long sleepers are at greater risk of obesity: A population-based 10-year follow-up in women. *Sleep Medicine, 15*(10), 1204–1211. https://doi.org/10.1016/J.SLEEP.2014.02.014

Thirby, R. C., & Randall, J. (2002). A genetic "Obesity Risk Index" for patients with morbid obesity. *Obesity Surgery, 12*(1), 25–29. https://doi.org/10.1381/096089202321144531

Timper, K., & Brüning, J. C. (2017). Hypothalamic circuits regulating appetite and energy homeostasis: Pathways to obesity. *Disease Models & Mechanisms, 10*(6), 679. https://doi.org/10.1242/DMM.026609

Tomiyama, A. J. (2019). Stress and obesity. *Annual Review of Psychology, 70,* 703–718. https://doi.org/10.1146/annurev-psych-010418-102936

Traversy, G., & Chaput, J.-P. (2015). Alcohol consumption and obesity: An update. *Current Obesity Reports, 4*(1), 122–130. https://doi.org/10.1007/S13679-014-0129-4

U.S. Department of Health and Human Services. (2018). *Physical activity guidelines for Americans.* https://health.gov/our-work/nutrition-physical-activity/physical-activity-guidelines

U.S. Department of Veterans Affairs. (2020). *VA/DoD clinical practice guideline for the management of adult overweight and obesity.* https://www.healthquality.va.gov/guidelines/CD/obesity/VADoDObesityCPGFinal5087242020.pdf

U.S. Preventive Services Task Force. (2017). *Obesity in children and adolescents: Screening.* https://www.uspreventive servicestaskforce.org/uspstf/recommendation/obesity -in-children-and-adolescents-screening

Vallis, M., Macklin, D., & Russell-Mayhew, S. (2020). *Effective psychological and behavioural interventions in obesity management.* https://obesitycanada.ca/wp-content /uploads/2021/07/10-Psych-Interventions-2-v7-with -links-1.pdf

van der Valk, E. S., van den Akker, E. L. T., Savas, M., Kleinendorst, L., Visser, J. A., van Haelst, M. M., Sharma, A. M., & van Rossum, E. F. C. (2019). A comprehensive diagnostic approach to detect underlying causes of obesity in adults. *Obesity Reviews*, *20*(6), 795–804. https://doi.org/10.1111/OBR.12836

Verdeș, G., Duță, C. C., Popescu, R., Mitulețu, M., Ursoniu, S., & Lazăr, O. F. (2017). Correlation between leptin and ghrelin expression in adipose visceral tissue and clinical-biological features in malignant obesity. *Romanian Journal of Morphology and Embryology*, *58*(3), 923–929.

Wadden, T. A., Tronieri, J. S., & Butryn, M. L. (2020). Lifestyle modification approaches for the treatment of obesity in adults. *American Psychologist*, *75*(2), 235–251. https://doi.org/10.1037/amp0000517

Wang, T., Heianza, Y., Sun, D., Zheng, Y., Huang, T., Ma, W., Rimm, E. B., Manson, J. E., Hu, F. B., Willett, W. C., & Qi, L. (2019). Improving fruit and vegetable intake attenuates the genetic association with long-term weight gain. *American Journal of Clinical Nutrition*, *110*(3), 759–768. https://doi.org/10.1093/AJCN/NQZ136

Ward, Z. J., Bleich, S. N., Cradock, A. L., Barrett, J. L., Giles, C. M., Flax, C., Long, M. W., & Gortmaker, S. L. (2019). Projected U.S. state-level prevalence of adult obesity and severe obesity. *New England Journal of Medicine*, *381*(25), 2440–2450. https://doi .org/10.1056/NEJMsa1909301

Waters, H., & Graf, M. (2018). *The costs of chronic disease in the U.S.* Milken Institute. https://milkeninstitute .org/sites/default/files/reports-pdf/ChronicDiseases -HighRes-FINAL.pdf

Westerterp, K. R. (2018). Exercise, energy balance and body composition. *European Journal of Clinical Nutrition*, *72*(9), 1246–1250. https://doi.org/10.1038 /s41430-018-0180-4

Wharton, S., Lau, D. C. W., Vallis, M., Sharma, A. M., Biertho, L., Campbell-Scherer, D., Adamo, K., Alberga, A., Bell, R., Boulé, N., Boyling, E., Brown, J., Calam, B., Clarke, C., Crowshoe, L., Divalentino, D., Forhan, M.,

Freedhoff, Y., Gagner, M., . . . Wicklum, S. (2020). Obesity in adults: A clinical practice guideline. *Canadian Medical Association Journal*, *192*(31), E875–E891. https://doi.org/10.1503/CMAJ.191707

World Cancer Research Fund/American Cancer for Research. (2018). *Diet, nutrition, physical activity and cancer: A global perspective.* https://www.wcrf.org/wp-content /uploads/2021/02/Summary-of-Third-Expert-Report -2018.pdf

World Health Organization. (2021, June 9). *Obesity and overweight.* https://www.who.int/news-room/fact-sheets /detail/obesity-and-overweight

World Health Organziation. (2022). *Global status report on physical activity 2022.* https://apps.who.int/iris/rest /bitstreams/1473751/retrieve

World Health Organization. (2022). *WHO European Regional Obesity Report 2022.* Fig 1.10, Medical conditions associated with obesity. WHO Regional Office for Europe. https://apps.who.int/iris/bitstream/handle /10665/353747/9789289057738-eng.pdf

Wu, Y., Zhai, L., & Zhang, D. (2014). Sleep duration and obesity among adults: A meta-analysis of prospective studies. *Sleep Medicine*, *15*(12), 1456–1462. https:// doi.org/10.1016/J.SLEEP.2014.07.018

Xenaki, N., Bacopoulou, F., Kokkinos, A., Nicolaides, N. C., Chrousos, G. P., & Darviri, C. (2018). Impact of a stress management program on weight loss, mental health and lifestyle in adults with obesity: A randomized controlled trial. *Journal of Molecular Biochemistry*, *7*(2), 78–84. https://www.ncbi.nlm.nih.gov/pmc/articles /PMC6296480/#__ffn_sectitle

Yang, Y., Shields, G. S., Guo, C., & Liu, Y. (2018). Executive function performance in obesity and overweight individuals: A meta-analysis and review. *Neuroscience and Biobehavioral Reviews*, *84*(2), 225–244. https://doi.org/10.1016/j.neubiorev.2017.11.020

Yanovski, S. Z., & Yanovski, J. A. (2018). Toward precision approaches for the prevention and treatment of obesity. *Journal of the American Medical Association*, *319*(3), 223–224. https://doi.org/10.1001/jama.2017.20051

Yeung, A. Y., & Tadi, P. (2022). *Physiology, obesity neurohormonal appetite and satiety control.* StatPearls. https:// www.ncbi.nlm.nih.gov/books/NBK555906

Zhang, C., Rexrode, K. M., van Dam, R. M., Li, T. Y., & Hu, F. B. (2008). Abdominal obesity and the risk of all-cause, cardiovascular, and cancer mortality. *Circulation*, *117*(13), 1658–1667. https://doi.org/10.1161 /CIRCULATIONAHA.107.739714

CHAPTER 18

Lifestyle Management of Insulin Resistance and Type 2 Diabetes

Lilly Tryon, DNP, APRN, FNP-BC, DipACLM, NBC-HWC, ACSM-EP
Jenna Gigliotti, MPAS, PA-C
Rachel Mack, MPAS, PA-C

No disease that can be treated by diet should be treated with any other means.

Maimonides

OBJECTIVES

This chapter will enable the reader to:

1. Discuss the incidence, prevalence, and impact of prediabetes and type 2 diabetes.
2. Define diabetes, prediabetes, and insulin resistance.
3. Examine the underlying mechanisms of glucose metabolism and insulin resistance.
4. Identify valid measures to evaluate insulin resistance and type 2 diabetes.
5. Review the current literature and considerations around lifestyle modification in preventing, treating, and reversing insulin resistance and type 2 diabetes.
6. Apply A-SMART prescriptions for diabetes prevention, treatment, and reversal.

Overview

Diabetes is one of the 21st century's fastest-rising health emergencies and poses a significant challenge for clinicians worldwide (International Diabetes Federation [IDF], 2021). This chronic metabolic condition occurs when the body doesn't produce or effectively use insulin (IDF, 2021), resulting in the inability of the cells to utilize glucose as fuel. Consequently, elevated blood glucose levels damage the blood vessels, nerves, eyes, kidneys, and heart (World Health Organization [WHO], 2022).

In 1980, there were 108 million people worldwide living with diabetes (WHO, 2022). That number has since skyrocketed to 537 million in 2021 (IDF, 2021). Additionally,

© Kathleen Gail/Shutterstock; © StoryTime Studio/Shutterstock; © kali9/Getty Images

the IDF reports that 45% of people had undiagnosed diabetes, and an estimated 541 million people had impaired glucose tolerance (prediabetes) in 2021. At the current trend, the IDF estimates that the number of people worldwide living with diabetes will rise to 643 million (11.3%) by 2030 and climb to 783 million (12.2%) by 2045. The growing number of diabetes-related deaths placed diabetes on the WHO's list of the top 10 leading causes of death in 2019 (WHO, 2020).

In the United States, the statistics are also concerning. The Centers for Disease Control and Prevention (CDC) 2022 National Diabetes Statistics Report estimated that in 2019, 37.3 million people (11.3% of the U.S. population) were living with diabetes (CDC, 2022). Another 96 million people aged 18 years or older have prediabetes (38.0% of the adult U.S. population), 90% of whom are unaware. Diabetes was the eighth leading cause of death in the United States in 2020, with an age-adjusted death rate of 14.8% (Murphy et al., 2021).

The *Healthy People 2030* goal is to "reduce the burden of diabetes and improve quality of life for all people who have, or are at risk for, diabetes" (U.S. Department of Health and Human Services, n.d.). Most diabetes and related complications can be prevented and treated with proven, achievable lifestyle changes (CDC, n.d.-b). There is also evidence to support the remission of type 2 diabetes (IDF, 2021). The U.S. Preventive Services Task Force (2021) recommends screening for prediabetes and diabetes, with subsequent referral to intensive lifestyle intervention (e.g., a healthful diet and physical activity) for those who screen positive. The Community Preventive Services Task Force (2017) also recommends a combined diet and physical activity program for diabetes prevention. Yet Wu et al. (2018) found that lifestyle management was addressed at only 22.8% of provider visits with people having prediabetes, a population at high risk for diabetes progression. These findings highlight the urgent need for advanced practice providers (APPs) to be equipped to integrate effective evidence-informed lifestyle concepts into health promotion and disease prevention strategies for diabetes prevention and treatment.

Defining Diabetes and Prediabetes

Diabetes is a chronic metabolic disease characterized by hyperglycemia resulting from the body's inability to make or use insulin (ElSayed et al., 2023a). There are three main types of diabetes: gestational diabetes, type 1 diabetes, and type 2 diabetes. *Gestational diabetes* is hyperglycemia that occurs only during the second or third trimester of pregnancy in women without a medical history of diabetes. Hyperglycemia in pregnancy affects approximately one in six pregnancies and can lead to babies that are large for gestational age and increased risk of pregnancy and birth complications (IDF, 2021). *Type 1 diabetes* is thought to be caused by an autoimmune reaction that destroys the insulin-producing β-cells in the pancreas. *Type 2 diabetes* (T2D) accounts for the vast majority (over 90%) of diabetes worldwide (IDF, 2021) and is due to a non-autoimmune progressive β-cell dysfunction and insulin resistance. This chapter will focus on T2D and prediabetes (which often leads to T2D) because this comprises the majority of cases.

Prediabetes is a term used to describe a condition in which the blood glucose level is elevated but does not yet meet the criteria for diabetes (IDF, 2021). Although below the diabetes diagnostic threshold, prediabetes indicates a higher risk for developing diabetes and cardiovascular disease (CVD) and should prompt additional screening for cardiovascular risk factors (American Diabetes Association [ADA], 2022). Alternative terms for prediabetes include *impaired fasting glucose* and *impaired glucose tolerance*, both of which refer to the testing methods for determining prediabetes (Nathan et al., 2007). Impaired fasting glucose (IFG) is diagnosed with a fasting blood glucose (FBG) of 100 to 125 mg/dL, and impaired glucose tolerance (IGT) is based on a 2-hour blood glucose of 140 to 199 mg/dL after ingesting 75 g of oral glucose. An HbA1c of 5.7% to 6.4% may also be considered prediabetes. Each of these tests indicates an inability of the body's cells to adequately respond to insulin in glucose metabolism, known as insulin resistance (IR), resulting in chronic hyperglycemia (IDF, 2021). Diagnosis of T2D, IGT, and IFG is based on one or more of the following tests: FBG, oral glucose tolerance test, HbA1c, and random blood glucose in the presence of symptoms. **Table 18.1** outlines the diagnostic criteria using these tests.

Effect of Type 2 Diabetes

T2D can affect people of every age, sex, race/ethnicity, socioeconomic status, education level, and world region. Globally as of 2021, total diabetes prevalence increased as age increased, starting with a prevalence of 2.2% in those aged 20 to 24 up to 24.0% in those aged 74 to 79 (IDF, 2021). The prevalence was slightly higher in men (10.8%) than in women (10.2%) aged 20 to 79 and higher in urban areas (12.1%) than in rural areas (8.3%). Diabetes prevalence has risen more rapidly in low- and middle-income countries than in higher-income countries (WHO, 2022).

The United States, which ranks fourth for the highest number of adults aged 20 to 79

Table 18.1 Diagnostic Criteria for Diabetes

Test	T2D	Impaired Glucose Tolerance (IGT)	Impaired Fasting Glucose (IFG)
	Should be diagnosed if *one or more* of the following criteria are met.	Should be diagnosed if *both* of the following criteria are met.	Should be diagnosed if the *first or both* of the following are met.
Fasting blood glucose	126 mg/dL (≥7.0 mmol/L)	126 mg/dL (<7.0 mmol/L)	110–125 mg/dL* (6.1–6.9 mmol/L)
2-hour blood glucose after 75 g of oral glucose load (oral glucose tolerance test, or OGTT)	200 mg/dL (≥11.1 mmol/L)	140–199 mg/dL (7.8–11.0 mmol/L)	140 mg/dL (<7.8 mmol/L)
Hemaglobin A1C (HbA1c)	6.5% ≥48 mmol/mol	5.7–6.4% (39–47 mmol/mol)	5.7–6.4% (39–47 mmol/mol)
Random blood glucose, in the presence of symptoms of hyperglycemia	200 mg/dL (≥11.1 mmol/L)		

The ADA criteria for diagnosis of IFG is an FBG between 100 and 125 mg/dL (5.6–6.9 mmol/L).

Data from International Diabetes Federation. (2021). *IDF diabetes atlas 2021* (10th ed.). https://diabetesatlas.org/atlas/tenth-edition and ElSayed, N. A., Aleppo, G., Aroda, V. R., Bannuru, R. R., Brown, F. M., Bruemmer, D., Collins, B. S., Hilliard, M. E., Isaacs, D., Johnson, E. L., Kahan, S., Khunti, K., Leon, J., Lyons, S. K., Perry, M. L., Prahalad, P., Pratley, R. E., Seley, J. J., Stanton, R. C., & Gabbay, R. A. on behalf of the American Diabetes Association. (2023a). 2. Classification and diagnosis of diabetes: Standards of care in diabetes—2023. *Diabetes Care, 46*(Supplement 1), S19–S40. https://doi.org/10.2337/dc23-S002

with diabetes (behind China, India, and Pakistan), has a similar distribution (CDC, 2022; IDF, 2021). The data from 2017 through 2020 showed that the total diabetes (diagnosed and undiagnosed) estimated crude prevalence increased with age (4.8% in ages 18–44 to 29.2% in ages 65 and older) and men were affected more than women (15.4% vs. 14.1%, respectively). Age-adjusted data for 2018 to 2019 among those over age 18 showed that the prevalence of diagnosed diabetes was highest in American Indians/Alaskan Natives (14.5%), followed by non-Hispanic Blacks (12.1%), Hispanics (11.8%), non-Hispanic Asians (9.5%), and non-Hispanic Whites (7.4%). It also showed a higher prevalence in those with less than a high school education (13.4%) versus those with more than a high school education (7.1%), which can be an indicator of socioeconomic status. Diagnosed diabetes prevalence ranged from 4.1% to 17.6% across U.S. counties, with a higher prevalence in the Southeast (CDC, 2022).

The effect of these figures is staggering in light of diabetic comorbidities, complications, mortality rates, and healthcare costs.

Comorbidities and Complications

Several *comorbidities*, or separate coexisting disease processes, are associated with diabetes. Some of the most common include obesity, hypertension (HTN), dyslipidemia, metabolic syndrome, non-alcoholic fatty liver disease (NAFLD), chronic kidney disease, and CVD. These comorbidities can also significantly affect the risk of developing complications. Additionally, diabetes and its comorbidities influence the risk of contracting COVID-19 infection, the clinical course, the need for hospitalization and ICU care, and mortality (IDF, 2021). Of those older than 18 diagnosed with diabetes, crude estimates for risk factors associated with diabetes-related complications for 2015 through 2018 included 89.8% had a BMI ≥25 kg/m^2, 69.0% had a blood pressure (BP)

≥140/90 mmHg or were on BP medication, and 44.3% had a non-high-density lipoprotein (non-HDL) level ≥130 mg/dL (CDC, 2022).

Diabetes-related complications range from microvascular to macrovascular and are associated with significant morbidity and mortality (Papatheodorou et al., 2018). Complications include ischemic heart disease and myocardial infarctions, stroke, neuropathy, peripheral arterial disease, lower extremity amputations, nephropathy, retinopathy, blindness, and end-stage renal disease, leading to dialysis. Additional complications include hyperglycemic crisis; hypoglycemia; and increased risk of dental diseases, infections, and birth complications in pregnant women with diabetes (CDC, 2022; IDF, 2021; Papatheodorou et al., 2018). Diabetes remains a leading cause of CVD, lower limb amputation, kidney disease, and blindness in most high-income countries (IDF, 2021).

Mortality Rates

Unfortunately, the majority of those with diabetes have a reduced life expectancy (Wright et al., 2017). Stop and count to eight seconds: one, two, three, four, five, six, seven, eight. In that time frame, approximately one person between the age of 20 and 79 around the world died in 2021 due to diabetes and its complications. This equates to about 6.7 million diabetes-related deaths in 2021, excluding the mortality risks associated with the COVID-19 pandemic. Nearly one-third (32.6%) of those deaths were in those younger than 60. Cardiovascular conditions remain the leading cause of morbidity and mortality in those with diabetes (IDF, 2021).

Economic Effect

The IDF estimates that direct health expenditures worldwide due to diabetes were $966 billion in 2021, with projections of $1.03 trillion in 2030 and $1.05 trillion by 2045 (IDF, 2021). It may come as no surprise that the region with the highest expenditure was estimated to be in the North American/Caribbean region, accounting for 42.9% of the total global diabetes-related health expenditure. Individually, the average medical expenditure of a person with diabetes in the United States in 2017 was $16,752 per year, with $9,601 directly related to diabetes—approximately 2.3 times higher than those without diabetes (ADA, n.d.). The ADA's analysis of the economic costs of diabetes found that diabetes care accounted for one in four healthcare dollars in the United States in 2017. This expenditure did not include indirect costs, such as absenteeism, reduced productivity, inability to work due to disease-related disability, and lost productive capacity due to early mortality. Diabetes imposes a significant economic burden on society.

Reducing the Effect

While this information may sound grim, the good news is that there is abundant hope when it comes to T2D—its comorbidities, complications, and even mortality. T2D can often be prevented with lifestyle modifications, such as those represented by the A-SMART (adopt healthy eating, stress less, move often, avoid alcohol, rest more, and treat tobacco use) model. Many risk factors for diabetic complications are modifiable, including lifestyle factors such as poor diet, physical inactivity, and smoking, and comorbidities such as overweight/obesity, HTN, and high cholesterol. Lifestyle modifications can better manage diabetes and, in many cases, achieve remission. They can also reduce the risk of developing or delay the onset of complications, comorbidities, and even mortality. Lifestyle modifications are potent prescriptions. In combination with medications, when indicated, a lifestyle approach can provide hope and improve the quality of life for those affected by diabetes.

Glucose Metabolism

Before discussing the pathophysiology of T2D, it is helpful to review some of the underlying mechanisms of glucose metabolism, the process by which glucose is processed and used to produce energy. Dietary carbohydrates (CHOs) are the body's primary energy source. They are broken down in the small intestine into glucose molecules, which are then absorbed into the blood for transport throughout the body. There are two types of CHOs: *simple* (referred to as unhealthy, processed, or refined) and *complex* (referred to as healthy, minimally processed, or unprocessed). Simple CHOs like sugar are broken down into glucose very quickly, whereas complex CHOs like starches and fiber are broken down into glucose more slowly. As circulating blood glucose levels rise, insulin is released from the pancreas in a dose-dependent fashion.

Insulin Synthesis and Secretion

Insulin is a peptide hormone secreted by the β-cells of the pancreatic islets of Langerhans. It comprises two peptide chains (A and B chains) linked by two disulphide bonds. Insulin synthesis begins as *pre-proinsulin*, which consists of a signal peptide, the A chain, the B chain, and a connecting peptide known as C-peptide. The signal peptide is then removed, creating *proinsulin*. Enzymes convert proinsulin into insulin (the A and B chains linked by disulfide bonds) by separating it from C-peptide (Wilcox, 2005). **Figure 18.1** provides a visual image of insulin synthesis. Because insulin and C-peptide are released in a 1:1 ratio, measuring C-peptide can be helpful as a marker of insulin production.

Insulin is secreted in response to non-insulin-dependent glucose entry into the β-cells, which triggers a cascade that results in insulin secretion. Insulin can also sometimes be secreted in response to a few other non-nutrient stimuli. The release of insulin into the bloodstream is typically pulsatile and biphasic, with a rapid initial first-phase burst triggered by a stimulus (e.g., increased blood glucose levels after eating) followed by a

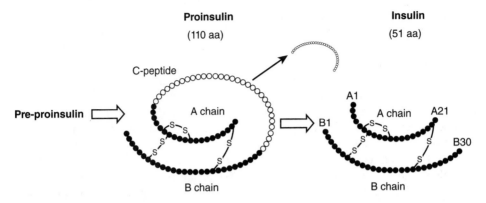

Figure 18.1 Structure of proinsulin and insulin.

Data from Khudhair, H. (2019). *Detection of potential β-cell stress and/or death biomarkers in patients with type 1 diabetes mellitus in Thi-Qar province* [Doctoral thesis]. Southern Technical University – Iraq. https://doi.org/10.13140/RG.2.2.24751.56484

more prolonged and sustained second-phase secretion (Wilcox, 2005).

Blood Glucose Regulation

The insulin response by the pancreas helps to normalize the blood glucose levels by enabling glucose molecules to enter the cells, where they can be used for energy. Insulin binds to insulin receptors on the surface of *myocytes* (muscle cells) and *adipocytes* (fat cells). Once insulin binds to the insulin receptors, a multi-step cascade is triggered, leading to the translocation of *glucose transporter (GLUT) proteins* into the cell wall, which then facilitate glucose uptake into the cells (see **Figure 18.2**). Different subtypes of GLUTs allow different cell types to use glucose according to their specific needs. For example, many brain cells, highly dependent on glucose for cellular energy, have GLUT1, which allows glucose to enter the cells without the need for insulin and even in the presence of very low blood glucose concentrations (like during the fasting state). Meanwhile, most insulin-dependent myocytes and adipocytes have GLUT4, which requires insulin and larger glucose concentrations to facilitate increased intracellular glucose transport (Wilcox, 2005).

In addition to facilitating cellular uptake of glucose into insulin-dependent tissues,

insulin helps to regulate the metabolism of CHO, protein (PRO), and lipids and promotes the division and growth of cells, among other activities. Insulin also regulates blood glucose concentrations, along with other counterregulatory hormones like glucagon. *Glucagon* is secreted by the α-cells of the pancreatic islets of Langerhans and helps to increase low blood glucose levels through pathways such as glycogenolysis and gluconeogenesis (Wilcox, 2005).

Just enough insulin is secreted during the fasting (basal) state to allow for glucose to enter into cells to be used for energy, but *lipolysis* (the breakdown of fats to be used for energy) and *gluconeogenesis* (the creation of new glucose from non-CHO precursors to be used for energy) are limited. This basal insulin secretion accounts for over 50% of daily insulin secretion and helps to maintain normal FBG levels (Wilcox, 2005). When a person eats a meal, a bolus of insulin is secreted to enable insulin-dependent hepatic, skeletal muscle, and adipose cells to receive the glucose molecules for energy and other processes.

In the presence of excess energy, these cells create fatty acids and store triglycerides to be used for energy later through lipolysis (e.g., during the fasting state). *Glycogen*, the stored form of glucose, is created and stored in skeletal muscle and hepatic cells. When

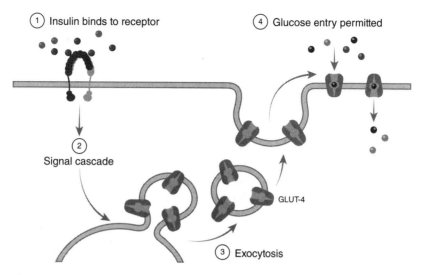

Figure 18.2 Activation of GLUT4 by insulin.

Chaurasiya, A., Shah, A., & Singh, R. (2020). Interaction between oxidative stress and diabetes: A mini-review. *Journal of Diabetes and Metabolic Disorders, 7*(2). https://doi .org/10.15406/jdmdc.2020.07.00201

needed for energy, glycogen can later be stimulated by glucagon for conversion back into glucose via *glycogenolysis*, and the energy from CHOs (rather than fatty acids) is used for muscle contraction. Therefore, insulin promotes the creation and storage of glycogen and lipids while suppressing gluconeogenesis and lipolysis (Wilcox, 2005).

Pathophysiology of Insulin Resistance and Type 2 Diabetes

Understanding the etiology, pathogenesis, characteristics, and clinical consequences of IR and T2D is vital for choosing appropriate and effective strategies for preventing and managing these chronic diseases.

Etiology

The etiology behind IR and T2D, like many other disease processes, is complex and multifactorial. Genetic, environmental, and lifestyle factors all play a role. Genetic factors include over 100 genetic loci that affect the risk of T2D (e.g., genes involved in β-cell growth and development, insulin synthesis, and insulin release). It should be noted that genetic loci, particularly in isolation, contribute only a small degree of risk for the development of T2D. A person may have a genetic predisposition to developing T2D but likely won't unless other environmental and lifestyle factors are in place (Xue et al., 2018). *Epigenetic* changes are modifications to DNA that regulate gene expression. These changes can include switching genes on or off and result from environmental and lifestyle influences, such as body weight, physical activity, diet composition, sleep, stress, substance use, and socioeconomic factors. A review by Van Dijk et al. (2015) reported epigenetic differences between adults with obesity and T2D and healthy controls. They also noted epigenetic changes associated with nutritional, weight loss, and exercise interventions.

Two prominent lifestyle factors that play a significant role in the development of T2D are obesity and decreased physical activity. Unfortunately, these factors are rampant in many

Westernized societies due to high dietary fat intake, high energy consumption, stress, chronic sleep deprivation, and sedentary lifestyles. Overweight and obesity are intimately involved with T2D by playing a role in IR, β-cell glucose sensitivity, inflammation, and intramyocellular lipid deposition. A-SMART strategies would also be helpful because diet composition, physical activity, and other healthy lifestyle behaviors play a significant role in obesity and the underlying mechanisms of T2D. Fortunately, weight loss can reverse these underlying mechanisms. Regular exercise also increases tissue sensitivity to insulin, even if weight is not lost. If regular exercise brings about weight loss, the β-cell function can also be improved (Cerf, 2013; Riddell, 2022; Robertson & Udler, 2021).

While the various factors contributing to IR and T2D may make it difficult to determine the exact underlying cause for individual patients, it does not mean a well-rounded approach to T2D prevention and management (with a heavy focus on environmental and lifestyle factors) will be unsuccessful. On the contrary, it will likely be quite effective. A position statement from the American College of Lifestyle Medicine (ACLM) on lifestyle medicine and T2D remission attests that there is enough evidence to support the *reversal* of diabetes through intensive lifestyle interventions (Kelly et al., 2020).

Pathogenesis

T2D is characterized by IR, impairment of insulin secretion, and hyperglycemia. During IR, the insulin signaling pathways in the skeletal muscle, fat, and hepatic cells no longer stimulate the changes needed to take up glucose from the blood. The cells become resistant, or no longer responsive, to insulin. Skeletal muscle is most affected by IR. Some studies suggest that IGT is associated with higher rates of skeletal muscle IR and that IFG is associated with more hepatic IR (Abdul-Ghani et al., 2006).

The reduced effectiveness of insulin to bind with the insulin receptors on the cell membranes leads to hyperglycemia, and the β-cells of the pancreas work harder to produce more insulin in response. The pancreas will compensate for some time, but the overproduction of insulin can eventually result in β-cell exhaustion and failure, leading to further impairment of insulin secretion. Chronic IR and hyperinsulinemia can lead to hyperglycemia, which leads to T2D. Chronic hyperglycemia can also cause oxidative stress and chronic inflammation, further aggravating tissue insensitivity to insulin and β-cell dysfunction. Thus, hyperglycemia creates a vicious cycle that can exacerbate both IR and impaired insulin secretion, leading to a worsening metabolic state and glucose tolerance. Oxidative stress and chronic inflammation also play a role in diabetic complications and numerous other disease processes (Cerf, 2013; IDF, 2021; Robertson & Udler, 2021).

Mechanisms for the Development of Insulin Resistance

Since IR is one of the characteristics of T2D and precedes its development, it is essential to understand the many factors contributing to IR. These include physical activity levels; stress levels; amount of food eaten; type of food eaten; nutrients and phytochemicals consumed; amount of sleep; substances used; and excess adipose tissue, particularly visceral or intra-abdominal fat, which also correlates with fat in the liver (Wilcox, 2005). One of the major culprits of IR is diet because it is a significant contributor to T2D and often the one with the most confusion surrounding it. Several dietary concepts offer explanations of the development of IR and T2D, including the carbohydrate–insulin model, intramyocellular lipids, and the type of fat and CHO in the diet.

Carbohydrate–Insulin Model of Type 2 Diabetes

In the *carbohydrate–insulin model of T2D*, insulin itself is thought to be the culprit because it has become known as a fat-storage hormone since it promotes the creation and storage of lipids (and glycogen). Therefore, this model avoids excess CHO intake, often without differentiation between unhealthy processed CHO and healthy complex CHO from whole-plant foods. The reasoning is that CHOs cause increased blood glucose levels, which lead to increased insulin secretion, which causes increased fat storage with downregulation of insulin receptors, which leads to increased weight gain, IR, and the development of diabetes (Wilcox, 2005). Following this reasoning, the solution is to eat foods that don't cause the release of much insulin, such as low-CHO, high-fat, and high-PRO foods. This perspective is why some healthcare professionals recommend that patients with T2D eat a low-CHO, or ketogenic, diet; avoid CHO-rich foods like fruit; and count CHOs to control blood sugars and lower HbA1c.

However, while these mechanisms play a role in diabetes, this view overlooks a critical piece of the dietary puzzle. High-fat diets, particularly those high in saturated fatty acids (SFAs) and trans fatty acids (TFAs), are strongly associated with IR, β-cell dysfunction, and the development of obesity (Cerf, 2013; Kahn et al., 2014; Wilcox, 2005). Furthermore, scientific evidence over many years has shown that a high-fat diet causes IR (Boden, 2003; Hernández et al., 2017; Koska et al., 2016; Luukkonen et al., 2018). Therefore, people with T2D who transition to a low-CHO, high-PRO, high-fat diet can worsen T2D and increase their risk for complications and mortality, particularly when animal products are the primary source of PRO and fat (Kosinski & Jornayvaz, 2017; Li et al., 2015; Mc-Macken & Shah, 2017; Sears & Perry, 2015).

Intramyocellular Lipids and Insulin Resistance

Another proposed mechanism for the development of IR is the presence of excess intramyocellular lipids (i.e., fats stored in muscle cells) due to SFA intake (Li et al., 2015; Sears & Perry, 2015). When the intake of energy (i.e., calories) exceeds the body's immediate needs, the body stores the excess. The ideal location for storing excess fatty acids is the adipose tissue, a specialized connective tissue that stores and releases energy as needed, insulates the body, cushions vital organs, and secretes hormones. However, the adipocytes can only hold so much before becoming overexpanded. This overexpansion creates inflammation, leading to IR in the adipocytes. The excess fatty acids then build up in other tissues, such as skeletal muscle and hepatic cells, which are not designed to store large quantities of fat like the adipose tissue can. This explains how a high intake of SFA leads to excess intramyocellular lipids that normally should not be present in large quantities in these muscle cells (Li et al., 2015; Sears & Perry, 2015).

While it is normal for some fat to be stored in skeletal muscle cells to be used for energy (e.g., during the fasting state or exercise), too many intramyocellular lipids can cause IR and the inability for the cell to utilize glucose properly. This can happen through several mechanisms, including inhibited insulin signaling caused by toxic lipid metabolites (e.g., diacylglycerol, ceramides), interference of insulin-stimulated glucose metabolism, and increased cellular stress and inflammation. Excess intramyocellular lipids are problematic because skeletal muscle is responsible for most of the body's disposal of glucose after meals. Therefore, skeletal muscle IR plays a significant role in the pathogenesis of T2D. The chronic overexpansion of adipose cells and spilling over of fatty acids that leads to excess intramyocellular lipids and IR can also explain a mechanism for the link between obesity and IR (Wilcox, 2005). The accumulation of excess fatty acids, also known as lipotoxicity, is also associated with NAFLD.

Type of Fat and Carbohydrate Matters

Not only does the *amount* of fat intake matter, but more importantly, the *type* of fat intake (particularly SFA) contributes to IR (Li et al., 2015; Sears & Perry, 2015). Eating foods high in SFA has been shown to increase the amount of intramyocellular lipids and lipid metabolites. However, this is not true for polyunsaturated fatty acids (PUFAs) and monounsaturated fatty acids (MUFAs), which are protective against IR. SFAs are found predominantly in animal products, whereas most plant foods contain unsaturated fats or smaller quantities of SFAs. TFAs, which may also contribute to IR, have now been banned by the U.S. Food and Drug Administration. However, they can still sometimes be found in processed food, baked goods, and fried foods.

As in fat intake, the type of CHO consumed is significant. Excess simple CHO consumption can contribute to fat storage in tissues not designed to store large quantities of fat, although CHOs play a lesser role. As noted previously, a significant difference between simple and complex CHOs is how quickly they are broken down into glucose. This misunderstanding of CHO is where the confusion lies when low-CHO diets are recommended for patients with diabetes. While it is always beneficial to decrease the intake of sugar and other processed CHOs, reducing the intake of complex CHOs from whole-plant foods is a mistake, as will be further discussed later in this chapter.

Impaired Insulin Secretion

Another key characteristic of T2D is the impairment of insulin secretion by the β-cells. Over time, the β-cells can no longer produce enough insulin to keep up with the demand caused by IR. It has also been noted that those with T2D appear to have a decrease in β-cell mass. Excess fatty acids (e.g., SFAs from the diet and fatty acids spilling out of the over-expanded adipocytes) not only cause intramyocellular lipotoxicity leading to IR but are also toxic to the β-cells and can cause β-cell death. While the exact mechanism is still under study, researchers think that fatty

acid–induced stress to the endoplasmic reticulum of the β-cells triggers β-cell dysfunction and apoptosis through crosstalk with the mitochondrial pathway (Cerf, 2013; Chang-Chen et al., 2008).

Gut Microbiome and Fiber Consumption

A relatively new and fascinating area of research also links the gut microbiome to IR and the development of T2D (Zhu & Goodarzi, 2020). There are about 100 trillion bacteria that comprise each person's gut microbiome, which means there is roughly 100 times more genetic information found in the gut microbiome than in the human genome. The gut microbiome plays an essential role in normal physiology, the pathophysiology of various disease processes (e.g., T2D and obesity), and regulating gene expression. The gut microbiome's effect on a person's health depends on the species of bacteria present, which is determined by factors such as diet, stress, medications, and sleep. Certain types of bacteria are pathogenic, whereas others are beneficial. While there are multiple proposed mechanisms linking dietary intake to gut microbiota to IR, one such mechanism has to do with short-chain fatty acids.

Short-chain fatty acids (SCFAs) are metabolites produced by the gut microbiota through the anaerobic fermentation of nondigestible complex CHOs, such as dietary fiber and resistant starch. Nondigestible CHOs, also known as prebiotics, are the preferred food source for beneficial gut microbes to flourish and create SCFAs. SCFAs have multiple beneficial effects throughout the body, including decreasing intestinal permeability, increasing fatty acid oxidation/energy expenditure (which promotes weight loss), improving insulin sensitivity, promoting satiety, reducing inflammation, and mediating multiple signaling pathways involved in maintaining good health.

Interestingly, animal product consumption is linked to the overgrowth of pathogenic bacteria, decreased SCFA production, increased inflammation, and increased IR. One reason for these adverse effects is that animal products have no fiber. Dietary fiber, found in plant foods, is associated with reduced risk of T2D, heart disease, digestive problems, HTN, stroke, obesity, and certain cancers. Unfortunately, only 5% of the American population consumes the recommended daily intake of fiber, although the majority of the population believes that they are meeting recommendations. Thus, APPs should educate patients on the benefits provided by adequate fiber consumption as an important health promotion strategy for T2D prevention and management and for improving overall health (Kahn et al., 2014; Quagliani & Felt-Gunderson, 2016; Saad et al., 2016; Sharma & Tripathi, 2019).

Chronic Inflammation

Another hallmark of T2D is chronic, systemic inflammation, particularly in insulin-target tissues, such as adipose tissue, liver, skeletal muscle, and the β-cells (Rohm et al., 2022; Tsalamandris et al., 2019). This inflammation is both caused by hyperglycemia and contributes to hyperglycemia, setting up a self-perpetuating, destructive cycle. Chronic hyperglycemia promotes the production of free radicals, oxidative stress, activation of inflammatory response pathways, and persistent low-grade inflammation that leads to IR, β-cell dysfunction, impaired insulin secretion, glucose intolerance, and T2D. Inflammatory markers associated with T2D include tumor necrosis factor alpha (TNF-α), interleukin-6 (IL-6), and C-reactive protein (CRP), among others.

The chronic effects of inflammation in T2D are also contributing factors to some of the major complications, including retinopathy, neuropathy, nephropathy, NAFLD, atherosclerosis, and CVD. Chronic inflammation may also explain the association of T2D with Alzheimer's disease, polycystic ovarian syndrome (PCOS), gout, and rheumatoid arthritis. Although the mechanisms linking inflammation and T2D are beyond the scope of this chapter, a key message is the need for APPs to target an anti-inflammatory diet and lifestyle in health promotion strategies, including regular physical activity, tobacco cessation, and eating a healthy diet containing ingredients with antioxidant potential, such as vegetables and fruits (Teymoori et al., 2021; Wronka et al., 2022).

Role of Lifestyle Modification in Preventing, Managing, and Reversing Type 2 Diabetes

Understanding the underlying mechanisms of T2D leads the APP to appreciate the significance of lifestyle modification for improving insulin sensitivity, reversing IR, and putting T2D into remission. T2D was once thought to be a chronic, progressive condition that was irreversible, and healthcare providers were limited to a disease management approach rather than a curative one (Saudek, 2009). However, a growing body of evidence reveals that improved insulin sensitivity and T2D remission can be achieved without pharmacological interventions (Kelly et al., 2020). As a result, a shift toward treatment that can both prevent T2D and lead to complete remission is advocated by the ACLM as the standard of care for T2D. T2D remission is defined as achieving an HbA1c <6.5% for at least 3 months with no surgery, devices, or active pharmacological therapy for the specific purpose of lowering blood glucose (Rosenfeld et al., 2022).

Preventing Type 2 Diabetes

Fortunately, the same lifestyle recommendations that can help manage T2D and even put it into remission can also help prevent it from occurring in the first place. Over 20 years ago, the Diabetes Prevention Program research found that lifestyle interventions focusing on weight loss and physical activity were more effective than metformin in reducing the incidence of diabetes in people at high risk (Knowler et al., 2002). Dietary patterns have also been shown to play a role in preventing T2D. Vegetarians have been shown to have a lower risk of diabetes than nonvegetarians, with the lowest risk occurring in vegans (Tonstad et al., 2013). These findings could be attributed to lower BMI; increased fiber and plant PRO intake; and a lower intake of SFAs, animal PRO, and heme iron in the vegan and vegetarian groups (Pawlak, 2017). In an extensive 17-year study of the Seventh-day Adventist population, whose members are overall health conscious and follow a wide range of diets from omnivore to vegan, researchers found that those who ate meat, even just once a week, increased their risk of developing diabetes by 29%. Long-term weekly meat intake was associated with a 74% increased odds of developing diabetes compared to vegetarian diets (Vang et al., 2008). The prevalence of diabetes in vegetarians in this population was half that of the omnivores. Additionally, lifestyle modifications in those over age 60, in particular, reduced the risk of T2D by 71% (Yokoyama et al., 2014).

Reducing Type 2 Diabetes Complications

Microvascular and macrovascular complications are unwanted sequelae of diabetes that often reduce the quality and length of life. However, plant-predominant dietary patterns and lifestyle modifications have been shown to reduce the risk of and sometimes even improve microvascular and macrovascular complications of diabetes. The benefits can be seen in complications such as CVD, HTN, and hyperlipidemia and can even extend to chronic kidney disease and neuropathy. The ability to affect all these outcomes makes plant-predominant dietary patterns and lifestyle modifications

vital healing components for those with T2D (McMacken & Shah, 2017).

Dosing Lifestyle Interventions

Just as the causes of IR are numerous, the approach to prevention and treatment must be *comprehensive*. Intensive lifestyle interventions should include a whole-food plant-based dietary pattern that facilitates weight loss (Kelly et al., 2020). Regular physical activity is one way to reduce skeletal muscle IR by increasing the oxidation of the stored fatty acids, thereby getting the intramyocellular lipids out of the cells, increasing glucose transport into the cells, and helping with weight loss (Sears & Perry, 2015). Stress management and reduction, adequate sleep quality, and avoiding risky substances also play essential roles.

Most diabetes treatment guidelines recommend *first* making nutritional and physical activity lifestyle changes before starting pharmacotherapy. For example, the Consensus Statement by the American Association of Clinical Endocrinologists and the American College of Endocrinology on comprehensive T2D management states that "lifestyle optimization is essential for all patients with diabetes" (Garber et al., 2020, p. 108). However, this is not always followed in clinical practice. If diabetes reversal becomes the goal in the management of T2D, as recommended by the Counterpoint Study on the reversibility of T2D (Lim et al., 2011), then APPs should discuss lifestyle interventions with patients early in a shared decision-making process (Kelly et al., 2020; Linke et al., 2022). Pharmacotherapy can be initiated concurrently in higher-risk individuals and adjusted based on patient response to lifestyle efforts (Garber et al., 2020).

Kelly et al. (2020) also emphasize the importance of appropriate *dosing* in the context of lifestyle modification, similar to dosing principles in the use of medications. For example, the lifestyle modifications needed for the remission of T2D must be dosed higher than those used for prevention. Dosing strength was a differentiating factor in the outcomes of the Look AHEAD study intervention, which included 1,200 to 1,800 calories per day, and the DiRECT intervention, which was more intensive at 825 to 853 calories per day (Gregg et al., 2012; Lean et al., 2018). In most cases, failure of lifestyle modification to achieve remission is related to inadequate dosing or the advanced progression of the disease. However, around half of those who are within the first 10 years of T2D diagnosis and make intensive lifestyle changes are able to discontinue medication and return to nondiabetic glucose control (Steven et al., 2016; Taylor et al., 2018).

Type 2 Diabetes Screening and Assessment

Early detection and screening for prediabetes and T2D are needed because early lifestyle intervention can prevent diabetes complications and target organ disease. A brief, online, validated Prediabetes Risk Test developed by the ADA and CDC is helpful for quickly computing age, family history, BP, ethnicity, wellness, gender, and BMI into a risk score (see Table 18.4). A score of 5 or higher (out of 10) suggests that the individual needs further

Health Promotion Research Study

Type 2 Diabetes Remission

Background: T2D has traditionally been viewed as a chronic progressive condition that can be managed but not cured. The frequency of remission of T2D achievable with lifestyle intervention is unclear. Therefore, researchers conducted an ancillary analysis of the Look AHEAD (Action for Health for Diabetes) cohort to determine the association of an intensive lifestyle intervention (ILI) with frequency of partial and complete remission of T2D to prediabetes or normoglycemia.

Methodology: Participants were 4,503 U.S. adults with BMI ≥25 and T2D who were randomized to receive either ILI—weekly group and individual counseling in the first 6 months followed by three sessions per month for the second 6 months and twice-monthly contact and regular refresher group series and campaigns in years 2 to 4 ($n = 2,241$)—or diabetes support and education (DSE)—an offer of three group sessions per year on diet, physical activity, and social support ($n = 2,262$). Remission of diabetes was defined as a transition from meeting diabetes criteria to a prediabetes or nondiabetic level of glycemia (FBG <126 mg/dL and HbA1c <6.5% with no antihyperglycemic medication).

Results: ILI participants lost significantly more weight than DSE participants at year 1 and had greater fitness increases at year 1 and year 4 ($p < .001$). The ILI group was significantly more likely to experience any remission (partial or complete), with prevalences of 11.5% during the first year and 7.3% at year 4, compared with 2.0% for the DSE group at both time points ($p < .001$). Among ILI participants, 9.2%, 6.4%, and 3.5% had continuous, sustained remission for at least 2, at least 3, and 4 years, respectively, compared with 1.7% of DSE participants for at least 2 years, 1.3% for at least 3 years, and 0.5% for 4 years.

Implications for Advanced Practice: Although the absolute diabetes remission rates were modest, an ILI was associated with a greater likelihood of partial remission of T2D compared with DSE. APPs can share these findings with patients with T2D to instill hope and increase motivation for lifestyle change.

Reference: Gregg, E. W., Chen, H., Wagenknecht, L. E., Clark, J. M., Delahanty, L. M., Bantle, J., Pownall, H. J., Johnson, K. C., Safford, M. M., Kitabchi, A. E., Pi-Sunyer, F. X., Wing, R. R., Bertoni, A. G., & Look AHEAD Research Group. (2012). Association of an intensive lifestyle intervention with remission of type 2 diabetes. *JAMA, 308*(23), 2489–2496. https://doi.org/10.1001/jama.2012.67929

screening. Recognized risk factors for prediabetes and T2D are included in **Table 18.2**, which also summarizes the criteria for screening for diabetes or prediabetes in asymptomatic adults.

Based on the presence of risk factors, the APP should order a random plasma glucose, FBG, OGTT, or HbA1c (see Table 18.1). Additional tests to consider, or for further follow-up, include a comprehensive metabolic panel (to assess liver and kidney function), lipid panel, urine microalbumin,

C-peptide, and fasting insulin. C-peptide and fasting insulin levels can help estimate how much IR is occurring. Analyzing how much insulin is being secreted, in combination with glucose levels, gives the APP a way of determining the severity of the patient's IR and diabetes. The HOMA2 calculator, developed by the University of Oxford (see Table 18.4), uses FBG and fasting insulin or C-peptide to calculate a patient's β-cell function, insulin sensitivity, and IR. This information can give the APP an idea

Table 18.2 Criteria for Screening for Diabetes or Prediabetes in Asymptomatic Adults

Criteria	Screening Frequency
All adults ≥35 years	Every 3 years if normal. More frequently based on initial results and risk status.
Those with overweight or obesity (BMI ≥25 kg/m^2 or ≥23 kg/m^2 in Asian American individuals) who have one or more of the following risk factors: ■ First-degree relative with diabetes ■ High-risk race/ethnicity (e.g., African American, Latino, Native American, Asian American, Pacific Islander) ■ History of CVD ■ HTN (≥140/90 mmHg or on medication for HTN) ■ HDL cholesterol level <35 mg/dL (0.90 mmol/L) and/or a triglyceride level >250 mg/dL (2.82 mmol/L) ■ Individuals with PCOS ■ Physical inactivity ■ Other clinical conditions associated with IR (e.g., severe obesity, acanthosis nigricans)	Yearly
People with prediabetes (A1C ≥5.7% [39 mmol/mol], IGT, or IFG)	Yearly
People who were diagnosed with gestational diabetes mellitus	Every 3 years
People with HIV	Every 3 years if normal. More frequently based on initial results and risk status.

Data from ElSayed, N. A., Aleppo, G., Aroda, V. R., Bannuru, R. R., Brown, F. M., Bruemmer, D., Collins, B. S., Hilliard, M. E., Isaacs, D., Johnson, E. L., Kahan, S., Khunti, K., Leon, J., Lyons, S. K., Perry, M. L., Prahalad, P., Pratley, R. E., Seley, J. J., Stanton, R. C., Gabbay, R. A. on behalf of the American Diabetes Association. (2023). 2. Classification and diagnosis of diabetes: Standards of care in diabetes—2023. *Diabetes Care, 46*(Supplement 1), S19–S40. https://doi.org/10.2337/dc23-S002

of how early the patient is in the course of the disease, the strength of the pancreas, and whether the patient is a good candidate for lifestyle intervention. Additional assessments can include a foot exam, retinal exam, sleep study, and Fibroscan (for assessing the presence of liver fibrosis), as indicated.

Starting the Conversation

Diagnosing patients with T2D or reviewing results showing that their T2D is poorly controlled or progressing can be overwhelming and foreboding to them. To ease the conversation, the APP may wish to start the discussion about diabetes with *hope*. Patients' prior experiences with T2D often consist of observing diabetes progression and complications in loved ones. APPs can share recent evidence that T2D can significantly improve and even be reversed with lifestyle modification (Kelly et al., 2020). IR can be dramatically reduced, and complications can also be avoided (McMacken & Shah, 2017).

After communicating hope, the APP should offer ongoing support and remind patients that it will be a team effort to improve their insulin sensitivity or reverse their T2D. The APP's role is to equip them with the knowledge, tools, and skills necessary to achieve and sustain lifestyle modification. Although it may take considerable time and effort for patients to make lifestyle changes, the rewards of improved health and quality of life will be worth the effort. After the APP starts the conversation with hope, they can segue into assessing patients' readiness for change, reviewing their current dietary and lifestyle habits, identifying knowledge gaps, and exploring their reasons for making lifestyle changes. Examples of questions to continue this conversation include the following:

- "Research shows that diet and lifestyle change can improve and even reverse diabetes. Would you like to learn more about how you can implement these lifestyle changes?"
- "What do you know about how to lower your risk for diabetes (or improve your diabetes)?"
- "Many healthcare providers have helped patients decrease or eliminate their diabetes medications by adopting a plant-predominant diet and other healthy lifestyle habits. Are you interested in learning what that would look like?"
- "So you want to learn how to eat healthier to improve your insulin resistance. What is *your* reason why you want to make dietary changes? It is important to establish your 'why' before making goals and lifestyle changes."

Motivational interviewing techniques can be beneficial when facilitating lifestyle change conversations and centering recommendations around patients' motivation for change. This person-centered approach will make goal setting and action planning more meaningful and achievable. Some patients may not be ready to commit to making changes, but planting the seed of the power of lifestyle modification can be enough of a start, with continued encouragement at follow-up visits. For patients ready for change, the APP can share the concept of SMART goals to help them translate lifestyle prescriptions into actions that are specific, measurable, attainable, relevant, and time-bound. Most patients will have a higher success rate if they initially set only one or two goals instead of attempting too many goals simultaneously and losing attention or willpower. With the concept of dosing lifestyle medicine, the APP can offer suggestions for the most potent lifestyle interventions, keeping the conversation collaborative and person centered. Encouraging patients to enlist a friend or family member to join them in making lifestyle improvements can provide added support and accountability.

A-SMART Prescriptions to Address Insulin Resistance and Type 2 Diabetes

Medications prescribed to patients with T2D work by making muscle and adipose tissue more sensitive to insulin, decreasing the production of glucose by the liver, and increasing insulin production by the pancreas. While often effective and necessary for managing hyperglycemia, they don't address the root causes of prediabetes and T2D and may not prevent diabetic complications. Since the standard of care includes a comprehensive lifestyle approach as first-line treatment, APPs must become proficient at prescribing lifestyle prescriptions for preventing and reversing T2D. Moreover, since lifestyle prescriptions for the prevention and management of T2D overlap with general principles applicable to all populations (Forouhi et al., 2018), there is a solid argument for integrating lifestyle concepts into every health promotion intervention (see **Figure 18.3**).

The A-SMART (adopt health eating, stress less, move often, avoid alcohol, rest more, and treat tobacco use) framework is an excellent way to ensure a comprehensive treatment approach and the best possible outcomes for patients with prediabetes or T2D. The following sections review diabetes-specific lifestyle prescriptions. These recommendations are summarized in **Table 18.3**.

Adopt Healthy Eating

Diet quality plays a fundamental role in insulin resistance. Thus, nutrition therapy is recommended for all patients with prediabetes and T2D (Davies et al., 2022; Evert et al., 2019). Food intake significantly influences glycemia and offers a wide range of opportunities for individualizing the nutritional prescription based on comorbidities, metabolic status (e.g., lipid function, insulin sensitivity, renal function), personal and cultural preferences, access to healthy foods, and readiness to change.

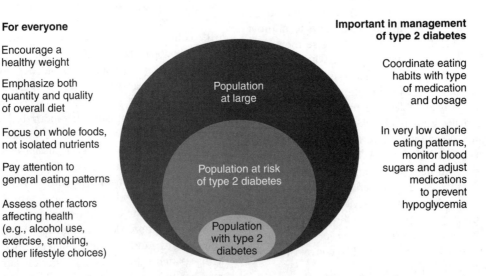

For everyone

Encourage a healthy weight

Emphasize both quantity and quality of overall diet

Focus on whole foods, not isolated nutrients

Pay attention to general eating patterns

Assess other factors affecting health (e.g., alcohol use, exercise, smoking, other lifestyle choices)

Important in management of type 2 diabetes

Coordinate eating habits with type of medication and dosage

In very low calorie eating patterns, monitor blood sugars and adjust medications to prevent hypoglycemia

Population at large

Population at risk of type 2 diabetes

Population with type 2 diabetes

Figure 18.3 Lifestyle considerations for different populations for prevention and management of T2D.

Table 18.3 A-SMART Lifestyle Prescriptions for Prediabetes and T2D

Lifestyle Component	Prescription
Adopt healthy eating	Move toward a plant-predominant dietary pattern, emphasizing nonstarchy vegetables, whole fruits, whole grains, and legumes. Minimize added sugars, refined grains, and ultra-processed foods. Avoid foods with a CHO-to-fiber ratio of greater than 10:1. Avoid artificial sweeteners. Shift away from animal PRO toward plant-based PROs. Eliminate processed meats. Decrease total dietary fat, and choose healthier unsaturated fats over SFAs and TFAs. Eat breakfast regularly. "Eat breakfast like a king, lunch like a prince, and dinner like a pauper." Observe a daily fast of at least 14 hours between dinner and breakfast. Achieve and maintain a healthy weight. The goal of weight loss is 5–10% annually until the ideal body weight is achieved.
Stress less	Use stress management techniques, such as deep breathing, self-care practices, social support, and coping skills. Participate in a mindfulness-based stress reduction or cognitive behavioral therapy program.
Move often	Perform at ≥150 minutes of moderate- to vigorous-intensity aerobic physical activity, spread over at least 3 days per week with no more than 2 consecutive days without exercise. Physical activity can also be accumulated in bouts of ≥10 minutes throughout the day. Move often, and decrease the amount of time spent in daily sedentary behavior by interrupting prolonged sitting with brief activity breaks of 1–5 minutes every 30 minutes for blood glucose benefits. Perform light- to moderate-intensity physical activity for 30–45 minutes after finishing the largest meal of the day. Supplement with two or three resistance, flexibility, and/or balance sessions.
Avoid alcohol	Avoid alcohol. For those who consume alcohol, recommend one drink per day for women and two drinks per day for men. Monitor blood glucose levels.
Rest more	Advise patients to obtain at least 6 hours of sleep daily (ideally 7–8 hours). Encourage sleep hygiene practices.
Treat tobacco use	Assess for tobacco use and address it through brief counseling and pharmacological therapy.

Move Toward a Plant-Predominant Dietary Pattern

The Western diet is characterized by high intakes of refined sugars, animal fats, processed meats, refined grains, high-fat dairy products, and salt (Malesza et al., 2021). The APP should assess where patients are on the dietary spectrum and encourage movement toward a plant-predominant dietary pattern for better diabetes outcomes. While the ADA recognizes that a variety of eating patterns can help to manage diabetes, it emphasizes that healthcare providers focus on three key factors: (1) emphasize nonstarchy vegetables, (2) minimize added sugars and refined grains, and (3) choose whole foods over highly processed foods to the extent possible (Evert et al., 2019). Due to the chronicity of T2D, it is also important to collaborate with patients in choosing a *sustainable* eating pattern.

An Expert Consensus Statement from the American College of Lifestyle Medicine concluded that "diet as a primary intervention for T2D is most effective in achieving remission when emphasizing whole, plant-based foods with minimal consumption of meat and other animal products" (Rosenfeld et al., 2022, p. 349). Several studies have looked at the benefits of consuming more of a whole-food plant-predominant eating pattern that is naturally lower in fats and higher in fiber and complex CHOs (Orlich et al., 2013). This is in contrast to the standard recommendation of a low-CHO, high-fat, and high-PRO diet. While the latter, high in animal products, may have short-term benefits such as weight loss, it has been associated with long-term adverse health outcomes, such as increased BP, IR, inflammation, risk of CVD, and even increased mortality (Fung et al., 2010; Levine et al., 2014; Noto et al., 2013; Song et al., 2016).

On the other hand, a low-fat, whole-food plant-predominant diet is highly beneficial for preventing and treating T2D and reducing the burden and cost of complications and treatment (Linke et al., 2022). In a large systematic review and meta-analysis of more than 300,000 participants from nine major prospective studies, Qian et al. (2019) examined the association between plant-predominant dietary patterns and the risk of T2D. They found a 30% lower risk for T2D in those eating plant-predominant diets, even after adjusting for BMI, physical activity, total calorie intake, and other confounding variables. They also noted a positive dose–response (i.e., the more plant based the diet, the lower the risk of T2D).

In another systematic review and meta-analysis of 20 randomized controlled trials to evaluate the effectiveness of 6 or more months of various dietary patterns in the management of T2D, Papamichou et al. (2019) concluded that "mounting evidence supports the view that vegan, vegetarian, and Mediterranean dietary patterns should be implemented in public health strategies in order to better control glycemic markers in individuals with type 2 diabetes" (p. 531). The Dietary Approach to Stop Hypertension (DASH) eating pattern shares many similarities with vegan/vegetarian and Mediterranean dietary patterns, but its glycemic effect needs further study (Benson & Hayes, 2020).

Plant-based diets are helpful for managing T2D because they significantly reduce IR and improve weight, HbA1c, psychological health, and quality of life (Cerf, 2013; Toumpanakis et al., 2018). A low-fat, plant-based diet is also associated with significant improvements in diabetic neuropathy symptoms (Bunner et al., 2015). Additionally, a meta-analysis of vegetarian and vegan dietary patterns found beneficial effects on BP, cardiovascular health, weight, lipids, and consumption of nutrients compared to omnivorous diets. The person with T2D is at increased risk for CVD, so a plant-based diet that simultaneously reduces IR and lowers CVD risk factors is significant (McMacken & Shah, 2017). Possible mechanisms of the HbA1c-lowering effects of vegetarian/vegan dietary patterns include decreases in energy, total fat, and cholesterol consumption and increases in CHO and fiber consumption (Yokoyama et al., 2014). In another 24-week study with a randomized, open, parallel design, Kahleova et al. (2011) compared a vegetarian diet with a conventional diabetic diet. The researchers concluded that "a vegetarian diet alone or in combination with exercise is more effective in increasing insulin sensitivity, reducing the volume of visceral fat, and improving plasma concentrations of adipokines and oxidative stress markers than a conventional diabetic diet with or without the addition of exercise" (p. 558).

Assess Dietary Composition

No ideal mix of macronutrients (i.e., CHO, PRO, fat) has been identified for patients with diabetes. Notwithstanding, the APP should still assess dietary composition and intake due to the underlying mechanisms explained earlier. Based on patients' current diet pattern and understanding of macronutrients, patient education may be needed to help them make healthier food choices. With this foundational knowledge, patients should be encouraged to focus on foods, not on isolated nutrients.

Choose Healthy Carbohydrates. As the predominant fuel source for the human body, CHOs are not the enemy in prediabetes and diabetes. The critical distinction that is often missed is that the insulin responses to different CHOs are different. Insulin response varies based on the *type* of CHO consumed (i.e., high-fiber complex CHO vs. simple sugars) and the *form* of CHO consumed (i.e., whole-plant foods vs. processed foods). When CHOs are digested, absorbed, and broken down into glucose in a slower fashion, the insulin secretion rate is usually lower. This concept is the basis for the *glycemic index*, a value assigned to foods based on how quickly and how high those foods cause increases in blood glucose levels. Complex CHO from whole, unprocessed foods that contain fiber take longer to break down than simple, processed CHO, thus having a less dramatic effect on blood glucose levels and a more favorable insulin response (Wilcox, 2005).

Increase Dietary Fiber From Unprocessed Plant Foods. Another concern about the Western diet is its lack of fiber. Ninety-five percent of Americans have dietary fiber intakes significantly below the Institute of Medicine's daily intake recommendations (Quagliani & Felt-Gunderson, 2016). For the person with prediabetes or T2D, adequate fiber intake is essential because fiber improves postprandial glucose response, increases satiety,

lowers calorie density, and lowers overall calorie intake by 10% to 18% for every 14 grams of fiber added per day (Howarth et al., 2001; Lattimer & Haub, 2010). Furthermore, an increasing number of studies support the role of fiber in microbiota diversity and production of SCFAs, which increase incretin hormones, such as GLP-1; increase insulin sensitivity; regulate cytokines to decrease inflammation; and improve mitochondrial function for oxidizing fat (Nogal et al., 2021; Portincasa et al., 2022).

The foods highest in dietary fiber are from unprocessed plant foods, such as vegetables, whole fruits, whole grains, and legumes. In the systematic review by Schwingshackl et al. (2017), every serving of whole grains was linked to a 13% decreased risk of T2D. The benefit of whole grains may have to do with the effects of fiber to lower calorie density, increase satiety, and improve postprandial glucose response. One daily serving of fruit (whole, not fruit juice, dried fruit, or canned fruit with sugar) is associated with a 12% reduced risk of developing T2D. Similarly, people with T2D who consumed one serving of fruit three times per week were associated with a 28% reduced risk of microvascular complications, 13% reduced risk of macrovascular complications, and 17% reduced risk of all-cause mortality (Du et al., 2017). Pulses, or cooked dried legumes, such as lentils, garbanzos, and beans, are also integral to preventing and managing T2D. A single pulse serving of ¾ to 1 cup significantly reduces postprandial blood glucose response, and long-term pulse consumption of 5 cups per week appears to improve glycemic control (Ramdath et al., 2016).

Avoid Sugar, Refined Carbohydrates, and Processed Foods. Sugar and other sweeteners are primary ingredients in many foods in the Western diet and are often hidden in beverages and processed foods. The average American consumes about 17 teaspoons of added sugar daily (Bowman et al., 2020). Meng et al. (2021) conducted a meta-analysis on the consumption of sugar-sweetened beverages (SSB) and artificially sweetened beverages (ASB) and found increased risks for T2D, CVD, and all-cause mortality.

Isolated fructose is found in SSB and foods with added sugars, whereas fructose is found in whole fruit, in combination with fiber, antioxidants, and other beneficial nutrients. Isolated fructose, especially combined with excess calories, contributes to IR by two pathways: (1) weight gain, leading to obesity and IR; and (2) excess fructose metabolized by the liver into fat, leading to fatty liver and increased fat storage in skeletal muscle cells (Basciano et al., 2005). However, fructose found in whole fruit doesn't have the same effect, as noted in research by Du et al. (2017) previously discussed. Ironically, artificial sweeteners have also been associated with negative effects on blood glucose, triggering the pancreas to secrete insulin and contributing to IR and weight gain (Pearlman et al., 2017). Artificial sweeteners can also negatively affect the gut microbiome, contributing to IR via dysbiosis (Mathur et al., 2020).

Likewise, refined CHOs and ultra-processed foods are widespread in the Western diet and have also been associated with an increased risk of T2D (Jannasch et al., 2017; Srour et al., 2020), among other risks. While a single focus of moving toward a more plant-predominant diet will automatically decrease the intake of processed foods and increase fiber-rich foods, another approach is to avoid foods with a CHO-to-fiber ratio of greater than 10:1 (Hashimoto et al., 2018).

Favor Plant Over Animal Protein. Another nutrition prescription to consider is to shift the source of PRO in the diet. In the large EPIC-InterACT case-cohort study, researchers found a 22% increased risk of diabetes for women consuming the highest quintile of PRO intake (109 g/day), adjusted for BMI and other risk factors (van Nielen et al., 2014). High total PRO intake was associated with a 13% higher incidence of T2D for every 10-gram increment after adjustment for energy, research center,

sex, T2D risk factors, and dietary factors. The association was attributable to animal PRO. Malik et al. (2016) found the same relationship: those consuming the highest quintile of animal PRO experienced a 13% increased risk of T2D.

When comparing diets with different PRO sources, Vang et al. (2008) found that omnivores eating meat once or more a week had a 34% increased risk of T2D compared with those who ate a vegan diet, even after adjusting for BMI. A decade later, Chiu et al. (2018) also found that a higher intake of animal PRO was associated with an increased risk of T2D while a higher intake of vegetable PRO was associated with a modestly reduced risk. Changing from an omnivorous to a vegetarian diet was associated with a 53% reduced risk of developing T2D.

Hosseinpour-Niazi et al. (2015) replaced six servings of red meat with legumes each week for 8 weeks but kept calories the same. They found significant decreases in FBG, fasting insulin, and triglycerides in those who consumed the legume-based PRO. A risk-benefit analysis from a shift toward more plant PRO in the diet shows that the benefit seems incremental. Replacing about 35% of total PRO with plant PRO instead of animal PRO significantly lowered HbA1c, FBG, and fasting insulin (Viguiliouk et al., 2015). In a model substituting only 5% of dietary calories from plant PRO instead of animal PRO, the researchers found a 23% decreased risk of T2D (Malik et al., 2016).

Avoid Processed Meats. When shifting away from animal PROs, an excellent place to start is to eliminate processed meats, such as bacon, sausage, hot dogs, and lunch meats. Processed meats are one of the primary foods associated with T2D. Each additional daily 50 grams of processed meat was strongly associated with a 37% increased diabetes risk (Schwingshackl et al., 2017). Kim et al. (2015) identified several potential mechanisms that may contribute to this risk, including SFAs, sodium, advanced glycation end products (AGEs), nitrates/nitrites, heme iron, trimethylamine N-oxide (TMAO), branched-chain amino acids (BCAAs), and endocrine disruptor chemicals (EDCs).

Decrease Dietary Fat. As noted earlier, fat accumulation in skeletal muscle and liver cells is a primary cause of IR (Shulman, 2014). By consuming less dietary fat, particularly SFAs, patients can decrease intracellular fat and increase insulin sensitivity (Yokoyama et al., 2014). In a small 12-week pilot study, the use of a low-fat, vegetarian diet in patients with T2D was associated with significant reductions in FBG and body weight, even without recommendations for exercise or other lifestyle changes (Nicholson et al., 1999).

Barnard et al. (2009) compared a low-fat plant-based diet without calorie restriction to a conventional reduced-calorie diet for T2D in a population of people who had T2D for over 8 years, on average. The researchers found better glycemic control, lipid reduction, and weight loss with the plant-based diet. The vegan diet group ate about 10% fat, 15% PRO, and 75% CHO in the form of vegetables, fruits, whole grains, and legumes while avoiding animal products and fatty foods and favoring low glycemic index foods. Their portion sizes and food/energy intake were unrestricted. In contrast, the ADA diet group ate about 15% to 20% PRO, 60% to 70% CHO, and <7% SFA and were prescribed a 500 to 1,000 kcal energy deficit primarily through portion control. Lower lipid concentrations in the vegan diet group are significant since the leading cause of death in people with diabetes is coronary artery disease (Barnard et al., 2009).

In addition to focusing on a low-fat dietary pattern, the APP should recommend that patients choose healthier unsaturated fats over SFAs and TFAs. Wanders et al. (2019) conducted a meta-analysis of 13 randomized controlled trials and found that different fats have different effects on IR. Plant-derived PUFAs significantly lowered measures of IR

(via HOMA-IR) compared with SFAs (primarily from animal fats), even when calories were kept constant. Furthermore, a dose–response relationship was identified. This may explain why some studies show a higher risk of T2D when consuming a low-CHO diet. The higher intake of animal fats and PRO in the diet may exacerbate IR, despite the short-term effect of lower FBG levels due to decreased consumption of CHO.

Interestingly, in some studies, a high-CHO, low-fat diet showed no benefit over a low-CHO, high-fat diet for patients with T2D (Guldbrand et al., 2012; Shai et al., 2008; Westman et al., 2008). A closer review of the research methodology reveals that these studies often consider a fat content of 25% to 35% fat as low-fat in the high-CHO, low-fat group (and usually contained a high intake of animal foods and SFAs). As a result, the higher fat intake and SFAs would have negatively affected IR, so any intake of CHO caused higher blood glucose levels. These findings led researchers to conclude that high-CHO, low-fat diets are not more beneficial than low-CHO, high-fat diets. However, comparing individuals prescribed a vegan diet focused predominately on complex carbohydrate whole-plant food consumption with about 10% energy from fat, to those prescribed a conventional diet with less than 7% fat, high carbohydrate foods, the outcomes were similar for reduced HbA1c and medication needs (Barnard et al., 2009; McMacken & Shah, 2017). Furthermore, low-CHO diets have been linked to a higher risk of T2D (Bao et al., 2016; de Koning et al., 2011; Schulze et al., 2008; Snorgaard et al., 2017; van Wyk et al., 2016).

It is understandable to see a decrease in blood glucose levels when consuming a low-CHO, high-fat diet because the individual is not eating the foods (i.e., CHO) that raise blood glucose levels. Still, since the underlying IR isn't being addressed, these patients will not be able to tolerate CHO consumption without blood glucose spikes. Low-CHO, high-fat diets treat a symptom of IR (e.g., high blood glucose levels) rather than the underlying mechanism—IR. In contrast, those who eat high-CHO, low-fat diets emphasizing whole-plant foods address the underlying IR. Intracellular lipids decrease, insulin sensitivity improves, and patients are thus better able to tolerate CHO intake.

Meal Timing

The timing of food intake also plays a role in insulin sensitivity and glycemic control. Mekary et al. (2012) showed that skipping breakfast can increase the risk for T2D by 21% compared with individuals who ate breakfast daily. In another study, Kahleova et al. (2014) found that eating fewer, larger meals twice a day (e.g., a hearty breakfast and lunch) improved body weight, hepatic fat, FBG, C-peptide, and glucagon levels in individuals with T2D compared with eating six small meals daily (e.g., breakfast, lunch, dinner, and three snacks), even though the macronutrient ratios were the same in both groups. These results support the saying, "Eat breakfast like a king, lunch like a prince, and dinner like a pauper."

A few small studies have shown the benefits of intermittent fasting (IF), the practice of alternating periods of eating and fasting, for improving insulin sensitivity and promoting weight loss. A review by Albosta and Bakke (2021) found IF to be an effective nonpharmacological treatment option for T2D, resulting in reduced body weight, decreased FBG, decreased fasting insulin, and improved IR. However, further research is needed to delineate the effects of IF from weight loss. APPs need to caution diabetic patients about the risk of hypoglycemia (Cho et al., 2019) and should consider titration of diabetic medication during periods of fasting.

Time-restricted feeding (TRF) is a form of IF that involves limiting daily food intake to a period of 10 hours or less, followed by a daily fast of at least 14 hours between dinner and breakfast the following morning. TRF can be practiced with or without reducing calorie intake and losing weight. Early time-restricted feeding (eTRF) is a form of IF that involves eating earlier in the day to align with circadian rhythms in metabolism (human metabolism is optimized for morning food intake). Researchers found that eTRF decreases postprandial insulin, increases insulin sensitivity, improves β-cell function, and lowers BP and oxidative stress (Sutton et al., 2018).

Achieve and Maintain a Healthy Weight

Achieving and maintaining a healthy weight has long been a recommended strategy for preventing and treating T2D, likely because of the association of adiposity with IR. A weight loss of greater than 5% appears necessary for beneficial effects on HbA1c, lipids, and BP (Franz, 2017). Furthermore, those who achieved 10% or greater weight loss in the 5 years after T2D diagnosis had a significantly higher likelihood of remission (Dambha-Miller et al., 2020). In the DiRECT study, researchers found a strong correlation between weight loss and diabetes remission in a dose–response relationship. Forty-six percent of participants achieved remission to a nondiabetic state without antidiabetic drugs (Lean et al., 2018).

The ADA and American Association of Clinical Endocrinologists recommend that "all patients should strive to attain and maintain an optimal weight through a primarily plant-based meal plan high in polyunsaturated and monounsaturated fatty acids, with limited intake of saturated fatty acids and avoidance of trans fats" (Garber et al., 2020, p. 109). The increased fiber intake of whole-plant foods can slow the rate at which glucose is absorbed, increase satiety, promote weight loss, decrease inflammation, and increase the production of SCFAs, all of which can affect insulin signaling and sensitivity. Even without reducing portion sizes, these dietary patterns are associated with lower energy intake and weight loss. Weight loss is known to reduce HbA1c; however, a high complex CHO, low-fat diet has been shown to improve glycemic control even without weight loss (McMacken & Shah, 2017; Yokoyama et al., 2014). These studies are encouraging for patients with T2D because they emphasize the benefit and freedom that a whole-food plant-predominant dietary pattern can provide: targeting and improving the underlying mechanisms of T2D and its complications and comorbidities, all while enjoying a variety of delicious foods, in many cases even without the need to decrease portion sizes or feel hungry. However, dietary strategies for weight loss should be individualized since a critical factor in the effectiveness of any diet is adherence over time (Forouhi et al., 2018).

Adherence to Plant-Predominant Dietary Patterns

It is a misconception that patients find it challenging to adhere to plant-predominant dietary patterns, such as the Mediterranean, vegetarian, and vegan diets. On the contrary, studies have found that when a healthcare provider suggests adopting these dietary patterns, patients find adherence *easier* (Storz, 2022). Patients were also *more* compliant with these plant-predominant dietary patterns than with diets focusing on CHO counting and limiting portion sizes. APPs should not be hesitant to recommend plant-predominant eating patterns to patients or withhold information believing that patients may not be willing to make dietary changes. Patients highly value their healthcare provider's recommendations, and it is the provider's responsibility to provide patients with all available information about their condition and treatment options so that they can make informed decisions (McMacken & Shah, 2017; Pawlak, 2017).

Stress Less

Psychological stress activates the renin-angiotensin-aldosterone system, the hypothalamic-pituitary-adrenal axis (HPA), and the sympathetic adrenomedullary system—each pathway contributing to oxidative stress, which

induces IR (Onyango, 2018). Stress also triggers biological responses, such as the release of glucose and lipids into the circulation, that can exacerbate IR. There seems to be a bidirectional relationship between diabetes and depression. Psychological distress, such as depression and anxiety, is associated with an increased risk of progression from prediabetes to diabetes (Deschênes et al., 2016). This finding underscores the value of screening for depression and anxiety in patients with prediabetes. On the other hand, stress and depression in patients with T2D are associated with poor glycemic control and an increased risk of cardiovascular complications (Fung et al., 2018).

The stress response is also a known barrier associated with decreased engagement in healthy behaviors, increased unhealthy lifestyle behaviors, and reduced adherence to T2D treatment (Gonzalez et al., 2008; Wallace et al., 2022). Therefore, providing stress management interventions, such as deep breathing, self-care practices, and group-based stress management training, can support the patients' ability to adhere to intensive lifestyle interventions. Adding a mindfulness-based stress reduction program to conventional diabetes education was associated not only with a reduction in perceived stress but also improvements in BMI and dietary habits that were not seen in the conventional diabetes education program (Ni et al., 2021; Woods-Giscombe et al., 2019). Cogntivite behavioral therapy (CBT) has also been beneficial, significantly reducing HbA1c, FBG, diastolic BP, depression, and anxiety symptoms and improving sleep quality (Li et al., 2022; Ni et al., 2021).

Move Often

Physical activity is essential for improving cardiometabolic health in both prediabetes and T2D. The ADA guidelines recommend that most adults with diabetes be advised to perform at least 150 minutes or more of moderate-to vigorous-intensity aerobic physical activity spread over at least 3 days per week with no more than 2 consecutive days without activity (ElSayed et al., 2023b). Walking daily for at least 30 minutes reduces the risk of T2D by approximately 50% (Hamasaki, 2016). Structured exercise durations of more than 150 minutes per week were associated with an HbA1c reduction of 0.89%, which is thought to be due to exercise improving insulin sensitivity and increasing lean mass (Yanai et al., 2018). Physical activity can also be accumulated in bouts of 10 or more minutes throughout the day. APPs should encourage patients to move often and to decrease the amount of time spent in daily sedentary behavior by interrupting prolonged sitting with brief activity breaks of 1 to 5 minutes' duration every 30 minutes for blood glucose benefits (Chang et al., 2020). Resistance training also appears to be an effective modality.

The timing of exercise is also important. Høstmark et al. (2006) found that postprandial blood glucose levels were appreciably reduced when performing light physical activity for 30 minutes after finishing the meal. Although the blood glucose levels rose again postexercise, the value was lower than that found without physical activity. Another study comparing walking before and after the meal found that postprandial exercise was more effective at lowering the glycemic effect of the meal (Colberg et al., 2009). Exercise can reduce postprandial hyperglycemia by increasing skeletal muscle contraction–mediated glucose uptake (Borror et al., 2018). Therefore, it is recommended that individuals with T2D focus on increasing energy expenditure after the largest meal of the day. Although there are no guidelines for optimal postprandial exercise prescription, Borror et al. (2018) saw the most consistent benefits in long-duration (≥45 minutes) moderate-intensity aerobic exercise. In another study, there was no difference in the improvement of postprandial blood glucose in patients with T2D who performed 30 minutes or 60 minutes of moderate-intensity exercise after dinner (Li et al., 2018). The researchers concluded that although both protocols were

safe, the longer duration could be more effective in lowering 2-hour postprandial glucose. Exercising 30 minutes after dinner might be safer for patients at risk of hypoglycemia.

Avoid Alcohol

People with prediabetes or T2D should follow the same guidelines as those without diabetes for alcohol consumption (ElSayed, 2023b). For women, the recommendation is for no more than one drink per day and for men, no more than two drinks per day (one drink is equal to a 12-oz beer, a 5-oz glass of wine, or 1.5 oz of distilled spirits). Alcohol can contribute to excess calorie intake, hyperglycemia, and weight gain. In addition, patients with T2D who use insulin or insulin secretagogue therapies are at increased risk for hypoglycemia or delayed hypoglycemia. APPs should educate patients about these risks, recommend avoidance of alcohol, and encourage patients who choose to drink alcohol to stay within the recommended guidelines and monitor glucose frequently after drinking.

Rest More

Adequate rest is another key lifestyle component for addressing prediabetes and T2D. People with T2D have an increased prevalence of insomnia, obstructive sleep apnea, and restless leg syndrome, all of which negatively affect sleep (Davies et al., 2022). The association between insufficient sleep duration, sleep restriction, poor sleep quality, and sleep disorders such as insomnia and sleep apnea with diabetes risk, IR, increased food intake, and impaired decision-making is well documented (Antza et al., 2021; Grandner et al., 2016; Koren & Taveras, 2018; Reutrakul & Van Cauter, 2018).

While the causal relationship between sleep and IR is multifactorial (Reutrakul & Van Cauter, 2018; Singh et al., 2022), APPs should emphasize the importance of sleep in preventing and reversing diabetes and its complications. The American Academy of Sleep Medicine and Sleep Research Society recommends 7 to 9 hours of sleep per night to maintain optimal metabolic health (Consensus Conference Panel et al., 2015). APPs should work with patients to implement sleep hygiene strategies to optimize sleep duration and quality. Sleep duration and quality should be assessed at every visit, and a referral should be made for a sleep study if indicated.

Treat Tobacco Use

Tobacco use is associated with the progression of glucose intolerance, development of T2D, worse macrovascular and microvascular complications, and increased risks of total mortality among patients with diabetes (López Zubizarreta et al., 2017; Pan et al., 2015; Śliwińska-Mossoń & Milnerowicz, 2017). In their review of evidence linking tobacco use and diabetes and its complications, Zhu et al. (2017) concluded that urgent action is needed to aid tobacco cessation. The ADA recommends routine assessment of tobacco use in diabetes care and addressing tobacco use through brief counseling and pharmacological therapy (ElSayed et al., 2023b).

Although there is a concern for weight gain with smoking cessation (Tian et al., 2016), recent research has demonstrated that the long-term CVD and health benefits outweigh the short-term effect on weight gain (Clair et al., 2013; Wang et al., 2021). Tobacco users with diabetes may also find it harder to quit tobacco due to interactions between insulin and dopamine that alter the body's reward mechanism (López Zubizarreta et al., 2017). In light of the short-term detrimental effects on body weight and challenges with cessation, APPs should provide close monitoring during cessation attempts.

Type 2 Diabetes Counseling and Education

Upon diagnosing prediabetes or T2D or meeting new patients with these conditions, it can be helpful to begin by assessing what patients know about diabetes and providing education to meet any knowledge gaps. There is often misunderstanding around these concepts, so some myth dispelling may be needed. It is important to explain IR because this is how to address the root cause of diabetes, reverse diabetes, and avoid complications (see **Figure 18.4**). Drawing a simple sketch during the explanation or providing educational materials can be very useful and time saving.

After explaining the root cause of diabetes, the APP can remind patients of the possibility of improving or reversing their diabetes. It is also prudent to explain the risks of untreated prediabetes and the possible complications of poorly managed diabetes—not as a scare tactic but to support informed decision-making. Mainous et al. (2018) found that fewer than 25% of patients with prediabetes were even aware that they were at risk for developing T2D. An awareness of the implications of diabetes can provide a stronger motivation for lifestyle strategies to prevent complications and help patients recognize and address symptoms early if they develop. As the conversation moves toward lifestyle recommendations, it is important to take the time to identify and answer questions.

The ADA (2022) recommends that patients with diabetes focus on consuming an overall healthy eating pattern, with predominant consumption of nutrient-dense high-quality foods (such as whole-plant foods), rather than focusing on specific nutrient intakes (such as high CHO or low fat intake). It just so happens that these overall healthy eating patterns are typically naturally higher in complex CHOs and lower in fats, particularly SFAs and TFAs. While it is valuable for the APP to understand the science behind these specific nutrients and how they affect T2D, it does not need to be the main focus when educating patients. Instead, the emphasis should be on educating about overall healthy, plant-based eating patterns and emphasizing the predominant intake of whole-plant foods.

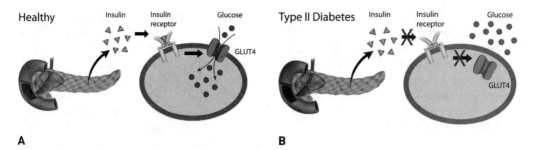

Explanation: When a person eats CHO-rich food, the CHOs are broken down into glucose. The glucose is absorbed into the bloodstream from the small intestine and travels to cells in need of energy. As blood glucose levels increase, insulin is secreted from the pancreas in response. Insulin is like the key that unlocks a door to allow glucose to enter the cell to be used for energy. If the lock is gummed up or blocked, glucose cannot enter the cell and stays in the bloodstream. When insulin is available but not functioning properly, this is called insulin resistance. What gums up the lock? Intramyocellular lipids, or fat stored in muscle cells, block the insulin from working properly, which leads to insulin resistance. The pancreas produces more and more insulin in hopes of getting the glucose into the cells, possibly even to the point of burning itself out. However, suppose intramyocellular lipid levels in the cells are reduced. In that case, the lock will become unblocked, and the insulin key will be able to unlock the doors again and allow glucose to enter the cells.

Figure 18.4 Layperson's explanation of insulin resistance.

Explanation original to the authors. Image retrieved from https://www.dreamstime.com with a search for insulin resistance illustrations. The title of the image is "Insulin Action and Diabetes Types."

A: © Alila Medical Media/Shutterstock; **B:** © Alila Medical Media/Shutterstock

The ADA also recommends that all patients with diabetes participate in diabetes self-management education and support (DSMES). DSMES should be person centered and can be provided individually or in groups. The CDC (n.d.-a) has developed a standardized DSMES curriculum that reflects current evidence and practice guidelines. The recommendation lists four critical time points when the need for DSMES should be evaluated and referrals made as needed (Powers et al., 2020):

1. At diagnosis
2. Annually and/or when not meeting treatment targets
3. When complicating factors (e.g., health conditions, physical limitations, emotional factors, or basic living needs) develop that influence self-management
4. When transitions in life and care occur

Self-Monitoring

Glycemic variability, or fluctuations in blood glucose levels, provides a more sensitive assessment of glycemic health than periodic lab tests. Therefore, self-monitoring of blood glucose (SMBG) can be a useful tool for diabetes self-care, better glycemic control, prevention of hypoglycemia and medication adjustments, and evaluation of the effectiveness of lifestyle changes. Frequency of testing may vary from once a day (e.g., fasting) to multiple times a day (e.g., postprandial, bedtime), to having a continuous glucose monitor (CGM), depending on the patients' severity of diabetes and current medication regimen. APPs should remind patients to log their blood sugar readings and note food intake and physical activity before readings. Technology can be used to track this data in apps that can be shared with the APP.

An additional self-monitoring task to recommend to patients is a daily foot exam to evaluate for broken skin, areas of warmth or redness, and ulcers.

Medication Deprescribing

The pharmacological management of T2D is beyond the scope of this chapter. However, since lifestyle modification targets the root drivers of T2D—IR—it is imperative that both APPs and patients are mindful of the possible rapid improvement in blood sugar (and other markers like BP) with lifestyle change. This is crucial because medications may need to be adjusted to avoid hypoglycemia or hypotension. APPs should review with patients the signs and symptoms of hypoglycemia and hypotension and what to do if they develop. Depending on patients' current blood glucose levels, how motivated they are to improve their lifestyle habits, and what medications they are currently taking, it may be necessary to begin deprescribing some medications before they leave the office to avoid hypoglycemia or hypotensive crisis. Insulin and sulfonylurea medications are two particular classes that may need preemptive deprescribing and very close monitoring. The APP should also review patients' entire medication list and look beyond the more obvious risks of hypoglycemia and hypotension for other medications, such as warfarin, that may be affected by significant dietary and lifestyle changes.

Health Promotion Case Study: Diabetes

Case description: M.A. is a 67-year-old Hispanic female who presented to her primary care APP last month for an annual wellness exam, during which blood work revealed elevated glucose levels. Further testing revealed an HbA1c of 6.2%. She returns for a follow-up visit to review labs and discuss the plan of care.

- Past medical history: HTN.
- Medications: Lisinopril 10 mg daily.
- Allergies: No known drug or food allergies.
- Family history: Parents deceased, both from cardiovascular-related deaths. No family history of diabetes, cancer, or mental disorders.
- Social history: Retired from a management position in the restaurant industry. She is a widow; lives alone in an apartment; and has one child, who lives in another state.
- Vital signs: BP 130/77 mmHg left arm, heart rate 84 bpm, respirations 18 bpm, temperature 98.2°F, O_2 saturation 90% on room air, weight 166.2 lb, height 65 in., BMI 27.7 kg/m^2.
- Review of systems: Reviewed notes from the previous visit, with no changes. Frequently experiences fatigue, headaches, increased sleepiness, and loss of interest in activities. Has gained 5 pounds during the last year. Occasional unproductive cough but denies wheezing and SOB. She states that she often feels "bloated" but denies reflux, changes in stool, and abdominal pain. Denies thoughts of suicide. All other systems are negative.
- Physical exam: PE from the last visit included eye and foot exams with no abnormal findings. Visual exam only at this visit. Well nourished and well developed, in no acute distress. Affect is normal and appropriate. Gait is normal.
- Labs: Recent blood work last month. CBC is unremarkable; CMP with elevated FBG at 116 mg/dL, otherwise unremarkable; HbA1c 6.2%; fasting insulin 26.4 mIU/mL; lipid panel with HDL 43 mg/dL; urine microalbumin 24 mcg/ml.

Lifestyle Vital Signs

- Adopt healthy eating: M.A. eats most of her meals at home. She typically eats a scrambled egg, a slice of toast with jelly, and a glass of orange juice for breakfast. Midmorning, she has a cup of coffee with milk and sugar. Most days, lunch consists of something she can grab quickly, like a ham and cheese sandwich, a soda, and a cookie. For dinner, she prepares simple foods like pasta or soup and finishes the meal with ice cream. She rarely consumes legumes and doesn't

(continues)

Health Promotion Case Study: Diabetes *(continued)*

---

eat many fresh fruits and vegetables because they spoil before she can eat them. Her go-to snack is a handful of corn nuts. She reports a weight gain of about 15 pounds since her daily routine changed at retirement.

- Stress less: M.A. attends church on the weekend and midweek prayer meetings. Outside of church activities, her social interactions are limited to Facebook groups and talking with her son on the phone once a week. Her recreational activities include tending her houseplants, feeding a few neighborhood cats, and crocheting while watching television.

- Move often: Her job in the restaurant industry kept her on her feet all day, but since retiring, she has become largely sedentary. She performs light housework daily but does not engage in regular physical activity.

- Avoid alcohol: She consumes alcohol only on social occasions.

- Rest more: During a typical day, M.A. usually wakes up around 8:00 (or later, "depending on whether I fell asleep in my recliner watching TV"). She frequently naps in the afternoon and retires to bed around midnight. She reports difficulty falling asleep and frequent arousals during the night to use the bathroom.

- Treat tobacco use: She smoked one-half pack of cigarettes daily for 30 years and quit 10 years ago.

Critical Thinking Questions

- Based on the diagnostic criteria in Table 18.1, how would you evaluate M.A.'s glucose levels?

- What additional diagnostic studies or screening might you consider, if any?

- How might you initiate a conversation with M.A. to address diabetes? What questions would you ask? What individualized counseling and educational needs might she have?

- Based on M.A.'s comorbidities and physical assessment, what concerns do you have? What lifestyle modifications would you make to prevent and reverse diabetes? Where would you initially focus, and why?

- Write three person-centered A-SMART lifestyle prescriptions using specific, measurable, attainable, realistic, and time-bound (SMART) goal setting.

- What referrals would you consider for M.A.?

An Interprofessional Approach to Type 2 Diabetes

T2D diagnosis and management typically start in the primary care setting of an outpatient family medicine or internal medicine office. However, an interprofessional approach to managing T2D is essential to providing optimal patient care. Studies have shown that collaborative team care can not only decrease HbA1c and reduce the risk of complications but also improve quality of life, increase patient follow-up and satisfaction, and reduce healthcare costs (McGill et al., 2017).

Interprofessional teams can vary according to professional skills, local resources, and patient needs. Clear and frequent communication and collaboration are the key elements for any size interprofessional team to utilize all team members' knowledge and skills to the fullest extent and ultimately provide the best patient outcomes. It is important to keep patients at the center of decision-making and to have shared goals and approaches among team members to ensure consistency of the message to the patient (McGill et al., 2017; National Diabetes Education Program, 2011). While primary care providers are a source of continual care, the APP may consider collaboration and referral to the following specialists, as needed:

- Endocrinology for medication management for complex patients or patients not responding to typical initiation and titration of medications
- Nephrology for patients with evidence of advanced kidney disease
- Neurology for patients with symptoms of neuropathy
- Cardiology for patients with comorbid cardiac conditions
- Podiatry for routine foot and toenail care
- Ophthalmology for a dilated eye exam to assess and monitor retinopathy
- Certified tobacco treatment specialist for tobacco cessation counseling
- Certified diabetes educator (CDE) for diabetes DSMES
- Registered dietitian nutritionist (RDN) for medical nutrition therapy (MNT) and specific meal planning recommendations
- Behavioral health specialist for psychosocial care
- Exercise specialist for an individualized exercise plan and fitness training
- Social worker to help patients find resources for their medical or financial needs

- Health coach to assist patients in creating an action plan for implementing A-SMART prescriptions and working through barriers to lifestyle change
- Intensive therapeutic lifestyle change programs, such as Mastering Diabetes or Pivio Health (see **Table 18.4**).

Novel approaches to delivering health care should also be considered. Group medical visits benefit the provider by allowing more time to educate patients and answer their questions. Patients also benefit from group medical visits because they can relate to others with diabetes, exchange success tips and stories, and support one another in efforts to manage and reverse diabetes. An online diabetes education and health coaching program demonstrated improved HgA1c and weight (Sarver et al., 2019). Telemedicine can help reach patients with physical or geographic barriers to accessing care. Culinary medicine is an emerging discipline combining basic nutrition information with instruction in practical food-related skills to aid in creating lasting behavioral change (Parks & Polak, 2020).

TABLE 18.4	Evidence-Based Resources for Diabetes
Resources	**URL**
YouTube video by Dr. Beth Motley explaining IR in patient-friendly language (7 minutes)	https://www.youtube.com/watch?v=WT6yZEM5VlA
American Association of Clinical Endocrinologists and American College of Endocrinology on the Comprehensive T2D Management Algorithm – 2020 Executive Summary	https://www.endocrinepractice.org/article/S1530-891X(20)35066-7/fulltext
American Medical Association Prevent Diabetes website (includes tools and resources for healthcare professionals)	https://amapreventdiabetes.org
Centers for Disease Control and Prevention National Diabetes Prevention Program	https://www.cdc.gov/diabetes/prevention/index.html

(continues)

TABLE 18.4	Evidence-Based Resources for Diabetes	*(continued)*

Resources	URL
Centers for Disease Control and Prevention DSMES Toolkit	https://www.cdc.gov/diabetes/dsmes-toolkit/index.html
CDC and ADA, Do I Have Prediabetes? Online screening tool in English and Spanish and a printable version in English	https://doihaveprediabetes.org https://adcouncil-campaigns.brightspotcdn.com/2e/3c/4a863eea4a9795b9ebac123f2e95/prediabetes-printablerisktestenglish.pdf
Healthy People 2030 evidence-based resources related to diabetes	https://health.gov/healthypeople/objectives-and-data/browse-objectives/diabetes/evidence-based-resources
Mastering Diabetes website	https://www.masteringdiabetes.org
National Institute of Diabetes and Digestive and Kidney Diseases, clinical practice tools and patient education materials	https://www.niddk.nih.gov/health-information/professionals/clinical-tools-patient-management/diabetes
Physicians Committee for Responsible Medicine offers free online classes, *Fight Diabetes with Food*, and other resources.	https://www.pcrm.org/health-topics/diabetes
Pivio Health, a comprehensive therapeutic lifestyle change program	https://piviohealth.com
University of Oxford HOMA2 calculator	https://www.dtu.ox.ac.uk/homacalculator

Health Promotion Activity: Explaining Insulin Resistance

Review Figure 18.4 and the YouTube video by Dr. Beth Motley explaining IR (see Table 18.4 for the URL).
Draft an explanation of IR (with a quick sketch) that you could share with a patient in 1–2 minutes. Practice your explanation with a friend or family member. Then use the teach-back method to ask them to repeat the information in their own words. How well did they comprehend IR? What questions did they have? If necessary, adjust your explanation to make it clearer. Practice your revised explanation with a different person.

Summary

T2D is a chronic metabolic disease characterized by IR and hyperglycemia, leading to significant and debilitating complications. The number of people living with prediabetes and diabetes is escalating worldwide, affecting mortality rates and economic burden.

A growing body of evidence reveals that improved insulin sensitivity and T2D remission can be achieved without pharmacological interventions (Kelly et al., 2020; van Ommen et al., 2018). A lifestyle approach can also reduce the risk of diabetes-related complications, comorbidities, and mortality. However, these lifestyle modifications are not addressed at most provider visits with patients having prediabetes.

Foundational to health promotion strategies for prediabetes and diabetes is understanding the underlying mechanisms of glucose metabolism, IR, and T2D. Prominent lifestyle factors that play a role include obesity, decreased physical activity, and diet composition. An intake of excess calories and SFAs, as seen in the Western diet, contributes to intramyocellular lipotoxicity and leads to IR. In addition, animal product consumption and low dietary fiber intake interfere with the gut microbiota's ability to produce SCFAs, which improve insulin sensitivity. Another hallmark of T2D is chronic systemic inflammation, which is also influenced by diet.

APPs should discuss lifestyle interventions with patients early in a shared decision-making process for preventing and reversing diabetes. Motivational interviewing techniques can be beneficial when facilitating lifestyle change conversations and centering recommendations around patients' motivation for change. Education should be offered on the benefits of a comprehensive lifestyle intervention that includes moving toward a plant-predominant dietary pattern, regular physical activity, weight loss, and other lifestyle modifications. In addition to providing A-SMART prescriptions tailored for diabetes prevention, treatment, and reversal, the APP should include an interprofessional team for ongoing patient support.

Acronyms

ACLM: American College of Lifestyle Medicine
ADA: American Diabetes Association
APP: advanced practice provider
A-SMART: adopt healthy eating, stress less, move often, avoid alcohol, rest more, and treat tobacco use
BMI: body mass index
BP: blood pressure
CDE: certified diabetes educator
CGM: continuous glucose monitor
CHO: carbohydrate
CVD: cardiovascular disease
DSMES: diabetes self-management education and support
eTRF: early time-restricted feeding
FBG: fasting blood glucose
GLUT: glucose transporter protein
HbA1c: hemaglobin A1C
HDL: high-density lipoprotein
HTN: hypertension

IDF: International Diabetes Federation
IF: intermittent fasting
IFG: impaired fasting glucose
IGT: impaired glucose tolerance
IR: insulin resistance
MNT: medical nutrition therapy
MUFA: monounsaturated fatty acid
NAFLD: non-alcoholic fatty liver disease
OGTT: oral glucose tolerance test
PRO: protein
PUFA: polyunsaturated fatty acid
RDN: registered dietitian nutritionist
SCFA: short-chain fatty acid
SFA: saturated fatty acid
SMBG: self-monitoring of blood glucose
T2D: type 2 diabetes
TFA: trans fatty acid
TRF: time-restricted feeding
WHO: World Health Organization

References

Abdul-Ghani, M. A., Tripathy, D., & DeFronzo, R. A. (2006). Contributions of beta-cell dysfunction and insulin resistance to the pathogenesis of impaired glucose tolerance and impaired fasting glucose. *Diabetes Care*, *29*(5), 1130–1139. https://doi.org/10.2337/diacare.2951130

Albosta, M., & Bakke, J. (2021). Intermittent fasting: Is there a role in the treatment of diabetes? A review of the literature and guide for primary care physicians. *Clinical Diabetes and Endocrinology*, *7*(1), 3. https://doi.org/10.1186/s40842-020-00116-1

American Diabetes Association. (n.d.). *The cost of diabetes*. Retrieved November 15, 2020, from https://diabetes.org/about-us/statistics/cost-diabetes

American Diabetes Association. (2022). Standards of care in diabetes – 2023. *Diabetes Care*, *46*(Suppl. 1). https://diabetesjournals.org/care/issue/46/Supplement_1

Antza, C., Kostopoulos, G., Mostafa, S., Nirantharakumar, K., & Tahrani, A. (2021). The links between sleep duration, obesity and type 2 diabetes mellitus. *Journal of Endocrinology*, *252*(2), 125–141. https://doi.org/10.1530/JOE-21-0155

Bao, W., Li, S., Chavarro, J. E., Tobias, D. K., Zhu, Y., Hu, F. B., & Zhang, C. (2016). Low carbohydrate-diet scores and long-term risk of type 2 diabetes among women with a history of gestational diabetes mellitus: A prospective cohort study. *Diabetes Care*, *39*(1), 43–49. https://doi.org/10.2337/dc15-1642

Barnard, N. D., Cohen, J., Jenkins, D. J., Turner-McGrievy, G., Gloede, L., Green, A., & Ferdowsian, H. (2009). A low-fat vegan diet and a conventional diabetes diet in the treatment of type 2 diabetes: A randomized, controlled, 74-wk clinical trial. *American Journal of Clinical Nutrition*, *89*(5), 1588S–1596S. https://doi.org/10.3945/ajcn.2009.26736H

Basciano, H., Federico, L., & Adeli, K. (2005). Fructose, insulin resistance, and metabolic dyslipidemia. *Nutrition & Metabolism*, *2*(1), 5. https://doi.org/10.1186/1743-7075-2-5

Benson, G., & Hayes, J. (2020). An update on the Mediterranean, vegetarian, and DASH eating patterns in people with type 2 diabetes. *Diabetes Spectrum*, *33*(2), 125–132. https://doi.org/10.2337/ds19-0073

Boden, G. (2003). Effects of free fatty acids (FFA) on glucose metabolism: Significance for insulin resistance and type 2 diabetes. *Experimental and Clinical Endocrinology & Diabetes*, *111*(3), 121–124. https://doi.org/10.1055/s-2003-39781

Borror, A., Zieff, G., Battaglini, C., & Stoner, L. (2018). The effects of postprandial exercise on glucose control in individuals with type 2 diabetes: A systematic review. *Sports Medicine*, *48*(6), 1479–1491. https://doi.org/10.1007/s40279-018-0864-x

Bowman, S., Clemens, J., Friday, J., & Moshfegh, A. (2020). *Food patterns equivalent intakes from food: Mean amounts consumed per individual, what we eat in America, NHANES 2017–2018, tables 1–4*. https://www.ars.usda.gov/research/publications/publication/?seqNo115=379583

Bunner, A. E., Wells, C. L., Gonzales, J., Agarwal, U., Bayat, E., & Barnard, N. D. (2015). A dietary intervention for chronic diabetic neuropathy pain: A randomized controlled pilot study. *Nutrition & Diabetes*, *5*(5), e158. https://doi.org/10.1038/nutd.2015.8

Centers for Disease Control and Prevention. (n.d.-a). *National standards for DSMES. Standard 6 - curriculum*. Retrieved February 2, 2023, from https://www.cdc.gov/diabetes/dsmes-toolkit/standards/standard6.html

Centers for Disease Control and Prevention. (n.d.-b). *Prevent type 2 diabetes*. Retrieved January 22, 2023, from https://www.cdc.gov/diabetes/prevent-type-2/index.html

Centers for Disease Control and Prevention. (2022). *National Diabetes Statistics Report*. https://www.cdc.gov/diabetes/data/statistics-report/index.html

Cerf, M. E. (2013). Beta cell dysfunction and insulin resistance. *Frontiers in Endocrinology*, *4*, 37. https://doi.org/10.3389/fendo.2013.00037

Chang, C. R., Russell, B. M., Dempsey, P. C., Christie, H. E., Campbell, M. D., & Francois, M. E. (2020). Accumulating physical activity in short or brief bouts for glycemic control in adults with prediabetes and diabetes. *Canadian Journal of Diabetes*, *44*(8), 759–767. https://doi.org/10.1016/j.jcjd.2020.10.013

Chang-Chen, K. J., Mullur, R., & Bernal-Mizrachi, E. (2008). Beta-cell failure as a complication of diabetes. *Reviews in Endocrine & Metabolic Disorders*, *9*(4), 329–343. https://doi.org/10.1007/s11154-008-9101-5

Chiu, T. H. T., Pan, W. H., Lin, M. N., & Lin, C. L. (2018). Vegetarian diet, change in dietary patterns, and diabetes risk: A prospective study. *Nutrition & Diabetes*, *8*(1), 12. https://doi.org/10.1038/s41387-018-0022-4

Cho, Y., Hong, N., Kim, K. W., Cho, S. J., Lee, M., Lee, Y. H., Lee, Y. H., Kang, E. S., Cha, B. S., & Lee, B. W. (2019). The effectiveness of intermittent fasting to reduce body mass index and glucose metabolism: A systematic review and meta-analysis. *Journal of Clinical Medicine*, *8*(10), 1645. https://doi.org/10.3390/jcm8101645

Clair, C., Rigotti, N. A., Porneala, B., Fox, C. S., D'Agostino, R. B., Pencina, M. J., & Meigs, J. B. (2013). Association of smoking cessation and weight change with cardiovascular disease among adults with and without diabetes. *JAMA*, *309*(10), 1014–1021. https://doi.org/10.1001/jama.2013.1644

Colberg, S. R., Zarrabi, L., Bennington, L., Nakave, A., Thomas Somma, C., Swain, D. P., & Sechrist, S. R. (2009). Postprandial walking is better for lowering the glycemic effect of dinner than pre-dinner exercise in type 2 diabetic individuals. *Journal of the American Medical Directors Association, 10*(6), 394–397. https://doi.org/10.1016/j.jamda.2009.03.015

Community Preventive Services Task Force. (2017, February 14). *Putting it all together: Preventing diabetes with clinical and community-based evidence.* https://www.thecommunityguide.org/stories/putting-it-all-together-preventing-diabetes-clinical-and-community-based-evidence.html

Consensus Conference Panel, Watson, N. F., Badr, M. S., Belenky, G., Bliwise, D. L., Buxton, O. M., Buysse, D., Dinges, D. F., Gangwisch, J., Grandner, M. A., Kushida, C., Malhotra, R. K., Martin, J. L., Patel, S. R., Quan, S. F., & Tasali, E. (2015). Joint consensus statement of the American Academy of Sleep Medicine and Sleep Research Society on the recommended amount of sleep for a healthy adult: Methodology and discussion. *Sleep, 38*(8), 1161–1183. https://doi.org/10.5665/sleep.4886

Dambha-Miller, H., Day, A. J., Strelitz, J., Irving, G., & Griffin, S. J. (2020). Behaviour change, weight loss and remission of type 2 diabetes: A community-based prospective cohort study. *Diabetic Medicine, 37*(4), 681–688. https://doi.org/10.1111/dme.14122

Davies, M. J., Aroda, V. R., Collins, B. S., Gabbay, R. A., Green, J., Maruthur, N. M., Rosas, S. E., Del Prato, S., Mathieu, C., Mingrone, G., Rossing, P., Tankova, T., Tsapas, A., & Buse, J. B. (2022). Management of hyperglycemia in type 2 diabetes, 2022. A consensus report by the American Diabetes Association (ADA) and the European Association for the Study of Diabetes (EASD). *Diabetes Care, 45*(11), 2753–2786. https://doi.org/10.2337/dci22-0034

De Koning, L., Fung, T. T., Liao, X., Chiuve, S. E., Rimm, E. B., Willett, W. C., Spiegelman, D., Hu, F. B. (2011). Low-carbohydrate diet scores and risk of type 2 diabetes in men. *American Journal of Clinical Nutrition, 93*(4), 844–850. https://doi.org/10.3945/ajcn.110.004333

Deschênes, S. S., Burns, R. J., Graham, E., & Schmitz, N. (2016). Prediabetes, depressive and anxiety symptoms, and risk of type 2 diabetes: A community-based cohort study. *Journal of Psychosomatic Research, 89*, 85–90. https://doi.org/10.1016/j.jpsychores.2016.08.011

Du, H., Li, L., Bennett, D., Guo, Y., Turnbull, I., Yang, L., Bragg, F., Bian, Z., Yiping, C., Chen, J., Millwood, I. Y., Sansome, S., Ma, L., Huang, Y., Zhang, N., Zheng, X., Sun, Q., Key, T. J., Collins, R., . . . China Kadoorie Biobank Study. (2017). Fresh fruit consumption in relation to incident diabetes and diabetic vascular complications: A 7-y prospective study of 0.5 million Chinese adults. *PLoS Medicine, 14*(4), e1002279. https://doi.org/10.1371/journal.pmed.1002279

ElSayed, N. A., Aleppo, G., Aroda, V. R., Bannuru, R. R., Brown, F. M., Bruemmer, D., Collins, B. S., Hilliard, M. E., Isaacs, D., Johnson, E. L., Kahan, S., Khunti, K., Leon, J., Lyons, S. K., Perry, M. L., Prahalad, P., Pratley, R. E., Seley, J. J., Stanton, R. C., & Gabbay, R. A. on behalf of the American Diabetes Association. (2023a). 2. Classification and diagnosis of diabetes: Standards of care in diabetes—2023. *Diabetes Care, 46*(Suppl. 1), S19–S40. https://doi.org/10.2337/dc23-S002

ElSayed, N. A., Aleppo, G., Aroda, V. R., Bannuru, R. R., Brown, F. M., Bruemmer, D., Collins, B. S., Hilliard, M. E., Isaacs, D., Johnson, E. L., Kahan, S., Khunti, K., Leon, J., Lyons, S. K., Perry, M. L., Prahalad, P., Pratley, R. E., Seley, J. J., Stanton, R. C., Young-Hyman, D., & Gabbay, R. A. (2023b). 5. Facilitating positive health behaviors and well-being to improve health outcomes: Standards of care in diabetes—2023. *Diabetes Care, 46*(Suppl. 1): S68–S96. https://doi.org/10.2337/dc23-S005

Evert, A. B., Dennison, M., Gardner, C. D., Garvey, W. T., Lau, K. H. K., MacLeod, J., Mitri, J., Pereira, R. F., Rawlings, K., Robinson, S., Saslow, L., Uelmen, S., Urbanski, P. B., & Yancy, W. S., Jr. (2019). Nutrition therapy for adults with diabetes or prediabetes: A consensus report. *Diabetes Care, 42*(5), 731–754. https://doi.org/10.2337/dci19-0014

Forouhi, N. G., Misra, A., Mohan, V., Taylor, R., & Yancy, W. (2018). Dietary and nutritional approaches for prevention and management of type 2 diabetes. *BMJ, 361*, k2234. https://doi.org/10.1136/bmj.k2234

Franz, M. J. (2017). Weight management: Obesity to diabetes. *Diabetes Spectrum, 30*(3), 149–153. https://doi.org/10.2337/ds17-0011

Fung, A. C. H., Tse, G., Cheng, H. L., Lau, E. S. H., Luk, A., Ozaki, R., So, T. T. Y., Wong, R. Y. M., Tsoh, J., Chow, E., Wing, Y. K., Chan, J. C. N., & Kong, A. P. S. (2018). Depressive symptoms, co-morbidities, and glycemic control in Hong Kong Chinese elderly patients with type 2 diabetes mellitus. *Frontiers in Endocrinology, 9*, 261. https://doi.org/10.3389/fendo.2018.00261

Fung, T. T., van Dam, R. M., Hankinson, S. E., Stampfer, M., Willett, W. C., & Hu, F. B. (2010). Low-carbohydrate diets and all-cause and cause-specific mortality: Two cohort studies. *Annals of Internal Medicine, 153*(5), 289–298. https://doi.org/10.7326/0003-4819-153-5-201009070-00003

Garber, A. J., Handelsman, Y., Grunberger, G., Einhorn, D., Abrahamson, M. J., Barzilay, J. I., Blonde, L., Bush, M. A., DeFronzo, R. A., Garber, J. R., Garvey, W. T., Hirsch, I. B., Jellinger, P. S., McGill, J. B., Mechanick, J. I., Perreault, L., Rosenblit, P. D., Samson, S., & Umpierrez, G. E. (2020). Consensus statement by the American Association of Clinical Endocrinologists and American College of Endocrinology on the comprehensive type 2 diabetes management algorithm - 2020 executive summary. *Endocrine Practice, 26*(1), 107–139. https://doi.org/10.4158/CS-2019-0472

Gonzalez, J. S., Peyrot, M., McCarl, L. A., Collins, E. M., Serpa, L., Mimiaga, M. J., & Safren, S. A. (2008). Depression and diabetes treatment nonadherence: A meta-analysis. *Diabetes Care, 31*(12), 2398–2403. https://doi.org/10.2337/dc08-1341

Grandner, M. A., Seixas, A., Shetty, S., & Shenoy, S. (2016). Sleep duration and diabetes risk: Population trends and potential mechanisms. *Current Diabetes Reports, 16*(11), 106. https://doi.org/10.1007/s11892-016-0805-8

Gregg, E. W., Chen, H., Wagenknecht, L. E., Clark, J. M., Delahanty, L. M., Bantle, J., Pownall, H. J., Johnson, K. C., Safford, M. M., Kitabchi, A. E., Pi-Sunyer, F. X., Wing, R. R., Bertoni, A. G., & Look AHEAD Research Group. (2012). Association of an intensive lifestyle intervention with remission of type 2 diabetes. *JAMA, 308*(23), 2489–2496. https://doi.org/10.1001/jama.2012.67929

Guldbrand, H., Dizdar, B., Bunjaku, B., Lindström, T., Bachrach-Lindström, M., Fredrikson, M., Ostgren, C. J., & Nystrom, F. H. (2012). In type 2 diabetes, randomisation to advice to follow a low-carbohydrate diet transiently improves glycaemic control compared with advice to follow a low-fat diet producing a similar weight loss. *Diabetologia, 55*(8), 2118–2127. https://doi.org/10.1007/s00125-012-2567-4

Hamasaki, H. (2016). Daily physical activity and type 2 diabetes: A review. *World Journal of Diabetes, 7*(12), 243–251. https://doi.org/10.4239/wjd.v7.i12.243

Hashimoto, Y., Tanaka, M., Miki, A., Kobayashi, Y., Wada, S., Kuwahata, M., Kido, Y., Yamazaki, M., & Fukui, M. (2018). Intake of carbohydrate to fiber ratio is a useful marker for metabolic syndrome in patients with type 2 diabetes: A cross-sectional study. *Annals of Nutrition & Metabolism, 72*(4), 329–335. https://doi.org/10.1159/000486550

Hernández, E. Á., Kahl, S., Seelig, A., Begovatz, P., Irmler, M., Kupriyanova, Y., Nowotny, B., Nowotny, P., Herder, C., Barosa, C., Carvalho, F., Rozman, J., Neschen, S., Jones, J. G., Beckers, J., de Angelis, M. H., & Roden, M. (2017). Acute dietary fat intake initiates alterations in energy metabolism and insulin resistance. *Journal of Clinical Investigation, 127*(2), 695–708. https://doi.org/10.1172/JCI89444

Hosseinpour-Niazi, S., Mirmiran, P., Hedayati, M., & Azizi, F. (2015). Substitution of red meat with legumes in the therapeutic lifestyle change diet based on dietary advice improves cardiometabolic risk factors in overweight type 2 diabetes patients: A cross-over randomized clinical trial. *European Journal of Clinical Nutrition, 69*(5), 592–597. https://doi.org/10.1038/ejcn.2014.228

Høstmark, A. T., Ekeland, G. S., Beckstrøm, A. C., & Meen, H. D. (2006). Postprandial light physical activity blunts the blood glucose increase. *Preventive Medicine, 42*(5), 369–371. https://doi.org/10.1016/j.ypmed.2005.10.001

Howarth, N. C., Saltzman, E., & Roberts, S. B. (2001). Dietary fiber and weight regulation. *Nutrition Reviews, 59*(5), 129–139. https://doi.org/10.1111/j.1753-4887.2001.tb07001.x

International Diabetes Federation. (2021). *IDF diabetes atlas 2021* (10th ed.). https://diabetesatlas.org/atlas/tenth-edition

Jannasch, F., Kröger, J., & Schulze, M. B. (2017). Dietary patterns and type 2 diabetes: A systematic literature review and meta-analysis of prospective studies. *Journal of Nutrition, 147*(6), 1174–1182. https://doi.org/10.3945/jn.116.242552

Kahleova, H., Belinova, L., Malinska, H., Oliyarnyk, O., Trnovska, J., Skop, V., Kazdova, L., Dezortova, M., Hajek, M., Tura, A., Hill, M., & Pelikanova, T. (2014). Eating two larger meals a day (breakfast and lunch) is more effective than six smaller meals in a reduced-energy regimen for patients with type 2 diabetes: A randomised crossover study. *Diabetologia, 57*(8), 1552–1560. https://doi.org/10.1007/s00125-014-3253-5

Kahleova, H., Matoulek, M., Malinska, H., Oliyarnik, O., Kazdova, L., Neskudla, T., Skoch, A., Hajek, M., Hill, M., Kahle, M., & Pelikanova, T. (2011). Vegetarian diet improves insulin resistance and oxidative stress markers more than conventional diet in subjects with type 2 diabetes. *Diabetic Medicine, 28*(5), 549–559. https://doi.org/10.1111/j.1464-5491.2010.03209.x

Kahn, S. E., Cooper, M. E., & Del Prato, S. (2014). Pathophysiology and treatment of type 2 diabetes: Perspectives on the past, present, and future. *Lancet, 383*(9922), 1068–1083. https://doi.org/10.1016/S0140-6736(13)62154-6

Kelly, J., Karlsen, M., & Steinke, G. (2020). Type 2 diabetes remission and lifestyle medicine: A position statement from the American College of Lifestyle Medicine. *American Journal of Lifestyle Medicine, 14*(4), 406–419. https://doi.org/10.1177/1559827620930962

Khudhair, H. (2019). *Detection of potential β-cell stress and/or death biomarkers in patients with type 1 diabetes mellitus in Thi-Qar province* [Doctoral thesis]. Southern Technical University – Iraq. https://doi.org/10.13140/RG.2.2.24751.56484

Kim, Y., Keogh, J., & Clifton, P. (2015). A review of potential metabolic etiologies of the observed association between red meat consumption and development of type 2 diabetes mellitus. *Metabolism: Clinical and Experimental, 64*(7), 768–779. https://doi.org/10.1016/j.metabol.2015.03.008

Knowler, W. C., Barrett-Connor, E., Fowler, S. E., Hamman, R. F., Lachin, J. M., Walker, E. A., Nathan, D. M., & Diabetes Prevention Program Research Group. (2002). Reduction in the incidence of type 2 diabetes with lifestyle intervention or metformin. *New England Journal of Medicine, 346*(6), 393–403. https://doi.org/10.1056/NEJMoa012512

Koren, D., & Taveras, E. M. (2018). Association of sleep disturbances with obesity, insulin resistance and the metabolic syndrome. *Metabolism: Clinical and Experimental*, *84*, 67–75. https://doi.org/10.1016/j.metabol.2018.04.001

Kosinski, C., & Jornayvaz, F. R. (2017). Effects of ketogenic diets on cardiovascular risk factors: Evidence from animal and human studies. *Nutrients*, *9*(5), 517. https://doi.org/10.3390/nu9050517

Koska, J., Ozias, M. K., Deer, J., Kurtz, J., Salbe, A. D., Harman, S. M., & Reaven, P. D. (2016). A human model of dietary saturated fatty acid induced insulin resistance. *Metabolism: Clinical and Experimental*, *65*(11), 1621–1628. https://doi.org/10.1016/j.metabol.2016.07.015

Lattimer, J. M., & Haub, M. D. (2010). Effects of dietary fiber and its components on metabolic health. *Nutrients*, *2*(12), 1266–1289. https://doi.org/10.3390/nu2121266

Lean, M. E., Leslie, W. S., Barnes, A. C., Brosnahan, N., Thom, G., McCombie, L., Peters, C., Zhyzhneuskaya, S., Al-Mrabeh, A., Hollingsworth, K. G., Rodrigues, A. M., Rehackova, L., Adamson, A. J., Sniehotta, F. F., Mathers, J. C., Ross, H. M., McIlvenna, Y., Stefanetti, R., Trenell, M., . . . Taylor, R. (2018). Primary care-led weight management for remission of type 2 diabetes (DiRECT): An open-label, cluster-randomised trial. *Lancet*, *391*(10120), 541–551. https://doi.org/10.1016/S0140-6736(17)33102-1

Levine, M. E., Suarez, J. A., Brandhorst, S., Balasubramanian, P., Cheng, C. W., Madia, F., Fontana, L., Mirisola, M. G., Guevara-Aguirre, J., Wan, J., Passarino, G., Kennedy, B. K., Wei, M., Cohen, P., Crimmins, E. M., & Longo, V. D. (2014). Low protein intake is associated with a major reduction in IGF-1, cancer, and overall mortality in the 65 and younger but not older population. *Cell Metabolism*, *19*(3), 407–417. https://doi.org/10.1016/j.cmet.2014.02.006

Li, Y., Storch, E. A., Ferguson, S., Li, L., Buys, N., & Sun, J. (2022). The efficacy of cognitive behavioral therapy-based intervention on patients with diabetes: A meta-analysis. *Diabetes Research and Clinical Practice*, *189*, 109965. https://doi.org/10.1016/j.diabres.2022.109965

Li, Y., Xu, S., Zhang, X., Yi, Z., & Cichello, S. (2015). Skeletal intramyocellular lipid metabolism and insulin resistance. *Biophysics Reports*, *1*, 90–98. https://doi.org/10.1007/s41048-015-0013-0

Li, Z., Hu, Y., & Ma, J. (2018). Nan fang yi ke da xue xue bao [Effect of moderate exercise for 30 min at 30 min versus 60 min after dinner on glycemic control in patients with type 2 diabetes: A randomized, cross-over, self-controlled study]. *Journal of Southern Medical University*, *38*(10), 1165–1170. https://doi.org/10.3969/j.issn.1673-4254.2018.10.03

Lim, E. L., Hollingsworth, K. G., Aribisala, B. S., Chen, M. J., Mathers, J. C., & Taylor, R. (2011). Reversal of type 2 diabetes: Normalisation of beta cell function in association with decreased pancreas and liver triacylglycerol. *Diabetologia*, *54*(10), 2506–2514. https://doi.org/10.1007/s00125-011-2204-7

Linke, C. S., Kelly, J., Karlsen, M., Pollard, K., & Trapp, C. (2022). Type 2 diabetes prevention and management with a low-fat, whole-food, plant-based diet. *Journal of Family Practice*, *71*(Suppl. 1 Lifestyle), S41–S47. https://doi.org/10.12788/jfp.0252

López Zubizarreta, M., Hernández Mezquita, M. Á., Miralles García, J. M., & Barrueco Ferrero, M. (2017). Tobacco and diabetes: Clinical relevance and approach to smoking cessation in diabetic smokers. *Endocrinologia, Diabetes y Nutricion*, *64*(4), 221–231. https://doi.org/10.1016/j.endinu.2017.02.010

Luukkonen, P. K., Sädevirta, S., Zhou, Y., Kayser, B., Ali, A., Ahonen, L., Lallukka, S., Pelloux, V., Gaggini, M., Jian, C., Hakkarainen, A., Lundbom, N., Gylling, H., Salonen, A., Orešič, M., Hyötyläinen, T., Orho-Melander, M., Rissanen, A., Gastaldelli, A., . . . Yki-Järvinen, H. (2018). Saturated fat is more metabolically harmful for the human liver than unsaturated fat or simple sugars. *Diabetes Care*, *41*(8), 1732–1739. https://doi.org/10.2337/dc18-0071

Mainous, A. G., Mansoor, H., Rahmanian, K. P., & Carek, P. J. (2018). Perception of risk of developing diabetes among patients with undiagnosed prediabetes: The impact of health care provider advice. *Clinical Diabetes*, *37*(3), 221–226. https://doi.org/10.2337/cd18-0050

Malesza, I. J., Malesza, M., Walkowiak, J., Mussin, N., Walkowiak, D., Aringazina, R., Bartkowiak-Wieczorek, J., & Mądry, E. (2021). High-fat, Western-style diet, systemic inflammation, and gut microbiota: A narrative review. *Cells*, *10*(11), 3164. https://doi.org/10.3390/cells10113164

Malik, V. S., Li, Y., Tobias, D. K., Pan, A., & Hu, F. B. (2016). Dietary protein intake and risk of type 2 diabetes in US men and women. *American Journal of Epidemiology*, *183*(8), 715–728. https://doi.org/10.1093/aje/kwv268

Mathur, K., Agrawal, R. K., Nagpure, S., & Deshpande, D. (2020). Effect of artificial sweeteners on insulin resistance among type-2 diabetes mellitus patients. *Journal of Family Medicine and Primary Care*, *9*(1), 69–71. https://doi.org/10.4103/jfmpc.jfmpc_329_19

McGill, M., Blonde, L., Chan, J. C. N., Khunti, K., Lavalle, F. J., Bailey, C. J., & Global Partnership for Effective Diabetes Management. (2017). The interdisciplinary team in type 2 diabetes management: Challenges and best practice solutions from real-world scenarios. *Journal of Clinical & Translational Endocrinology*, *7*, 21–27. https://doi.org/10.1016/j.jcte.2016.12.001

McMacken, M., & Shah, S. (2017). A plant-based diet for the prevention and treatment of type 2 diabetes. *Journal of Geriatric Cardiology*, *14*(5), 342–354. https://doi.org/10.11909/j.issn.1671-5411.2017.05.009

Mekary, R. A., Giovannucci, E., Willett, W. C., van Dam, R. M., & Hu, F. B. (2012). Eating patterns and type 2 diabetes risk in men: Breakfast omission, eating frequency, and snacking. *American Journal of Clinical Nutrition, 95*(5), 1182–1189. https://doi.org/10.3945/ajcn.111.028209

Meng, Y., Li, S., Khan, J., Dai, Z., Li, C., Hu, X., Shen, Q., & Xue, Y. (2021). Sugar- and artificially sweetened beverages consumption linked to type 2 diabetes, cardiovascular diseases, and all-cause mortality: A systematic review and dose-response meta-analysis of prospective cohort studies. *Nutrients, 13*(8), 2636. https://doi.org/10.3390/nu13082636

Murphy, S. L., Kochanek, K. D., Xu, J. Q., & Arias, E. (2021). *Mortality in the United States, 2020.* Centers for Disease Control and Prevention. https://dx.doi.org/10.15620/cdc:112079

Nathan, D. M., Davidson, M. B., DeFronzo, R. A., Heine, R. J., Henry, R. R., Pratley, R., Zinman, B., & American Diabetes Association. (2007). Impaired fasting glucose and impaired glucose tolerance: Implications for care. *Diabetes Care, 30*(3), 753–759. https://doi.org/10.2337/dc07-9920

National Diabetes Education Program. (2011). *Redesigning the health care team: Diabetes prevention and lifelong management.* U.S. Department of Health and Human Services, National Institutes of Health, Centers for Disease Control and Prevention. https://ambiohealth.com/uploads/Redesigning%20the%20Health%20Care%20Team.pdf

Ni, Y. X., Ma, L., & Li, J. P. (2021). Effects of mindfulness-based intervention on glycemic control and psychological outcomes in people with diabetes: A systematic review and meta-analysis. *Journal of Diabetes Investigation, 12*(6), 1092–1103. https://doi.org/10.1111/jdi.13439

Nicholson, A. S., Sklar, M., Barnard, N. D., Gore, S., Sullivan, R., & Browning, S. (1999). Toward improved management of NIDDM: A randomized, controlled, pilot intervention using a lowfat, vegetarian diet. *Preventive Medicine, 29*(2), 87–91. https://doi.org/10.1006/pmed.1999.0529

Nogal, A., Valdes, A. M., & Menni, C. (2021). The role of short-chain fatty acids in the interplay between gut microbiota and diet in cardio-metabolic health. *Gut Microbes, 13*(1), 1–24. https://doi.org/10.1080/19490976.2021.1897212

Noto, H., Goto, A., Tsujimoto, T., & Noda, M. (2013). Low-carbohydrate diets and all-cause mortality: A systematic review and meta-analysis of observational studies. *PloS One, 8*(1), e55030. https://doi.org/10.1371/journal.pone.0055030

Onyango, A. N. (2018). Cellular stresses and stress responses in the pathogenesis of insulin resistance. *Oxidative Medicine and Cellular Longevity, 4321714.* https://doi.org/10.1155/2018/4321714

Orlich, M. J., Singh, P. N., Sabaté, J., Jaceldo-Siegl, K., Fan, J., Knutsen, S., Beeson, W. L., & Fraser, G. E. (2013). Vegetarian dietary patterns and mortality in Adventist Health Study 2. *JAMA, 173*(13), 1230–1238. https://doi.org/10.1001/jamainternmed.2013.6473

Pan, A., Wang, Y., Talaei, M., & Hu, F. B. (2015). Relation of smoking with total mortality and cardiovascular events among patients with diabetes mellitus: A meta-analysis and systematic review. *Circulation, 132*(19), 1795–1804. https://doi.org/10.1161/CIRCULATIONAHA.115.017926

Papamichou, D., Panagiotakos, D. B., & Itsiopoulos, C. (2019). Dietary patterns and management of type 2 diabetes: A systematic review of randomised clinical trials. *Nutrition, Metabolism, and Cardiovascular Diseases, 29*(6), 531–543. https://doi.org/10.1016/j.numecd.2019.02.004

Papatheodorou, K., Banach, M., Bekiari, E., Rizzo, M., & Edmonds, M. (2018). Complications of diabetes 2017. *Journal of Diabetes Research, 2018,* 3086167. https://doi.org/10.1155/2018/3086167

Parks, K., & Polak, R. (2020). Culinary medicine: Paving the way to health through our forks. *American Journal of Lifestyle Medicine, 14*(1), 51–53. https://doi.org/10.1177/1559827619871922

Pawlak, R. (2017). Vegetarian diets in the prevention and management of diabetes and its complications. *Diabetes Spectrum, 30*(2), 82–88. https://doi.org/10.2337/ds16-0057

Pearlman, M., Obert, J., & Casey, L. (2017). The association between artificial sweeteners and obesity. *Current Gastroenterology Reports, 19,* 64. https://doi.org/10.1007/s11894-017-0602-9

Portincasa, P., Bonfrate, L., Vacca, M., De Angelis, M., Farella, I., Lanza, E., Khalil, M., Wang, D. Q., Sperandio, M., & Di Ciaula, A. (2022). Gut microbiota and short chain fatty acids: Implications in glucose homeostasis. *International Journal of Molecular Sciences, 23*(3), 1105. https://doi.org/10.3390/ijms23031105

Powers, M. A., Bardsley, J. K., Cypress, M., Funnell, M. M., Harms, D., Hess-Fischl, A., Hooks, B., Isaacs, D., Mandel, E. D., Maryniuk, M. D., Norton, A., Rinker, J., Siminerio, L. M., & Uelmen, S. (2020). Diabetes self-management education and support in adults with type 2 diabetes: A consensus report of the American Diabetes Association, the Association of Diabetes Care and Education Specialists, the Academy of Nutrition and Dietetics, the American Academy of Family Physicians, the American Academy of PAs, the American Association of Nurse Practitioners, and the American Pharmacists Association. *Diabetes Care, 43*(7), 1636–1649. https://doi.org/10.2337/dci20-0023

Qian, F., Liu, G., Hu, F. B., Bhupathiraju, S. N., & Sun, Q. (2019). Association between plant-based dietary patterns and risk of type 2 diabetes: A systematic review and meta-analysis. *JAMA Internal*

Medicine, 179(10), 1335–1344. https://doi.org/10.1001/jamainternmed.2019.2195

Quagliani, D., & Felt-Gunderson, P. (2016). Closing America's fiber intake gap: Communication strategies from a food and fiber summit. *American Journal of Lifestyle Medicine, 11*(1), 80–85. https://doi.org/10.1177/1559827615588079

Ramdath, D., Renwick, S., & Duncan, A. M. (2016). The role of pulses in the dietary management of diabetes. *Canadian Journal of Diabetes, 40*(4), 355–363. https://doi.org/10.1016/j.jcjd.2016.05.015

Reutrakul, S., & Van Cauter, E. (2018). Sleep influences on obesity, insulin resistance, and risk of type 2 diabetes. *Metabolism: Clinical and Experimental, 84*, 56–66. https://doi.org/10.1016/j.metabol.2018.02.010

Riddell, M. C. (2022). Exercise guidance in adults with diabetes mellitus. *UpToDate.* https://www.uptodate.com/contents/exercise-guidance-in-adults-with-diabetes-mellitus

Robertson, R. P., & Udler, M. S. (2021). Pathogenesis of type 2 diabetes mellitus. *UpToDate.* https://www.uptodate.com/contents/pathogenesis-of-type-2-diabetes-mellitus#H17

Rohm, T. V., Meier, D. T., Olefsky, J. M., & Donath, M. Y. (2022). Inflammation in obesity, diabetes, and related disorders. *Immunity, 55*(1), 31–55. https://doi.org/10.1016/j.immuni.2021.12.013

Rosenfeld, R. M., Kelly, J. H., Agarwal, M., Aspry, K., Barnett, T., Davis, B. C., Fields, D., Gaillard, T., Gulati, M., Guthrie, G. E., Moore, D. J., Panigrahi, G., Rothberg, A., Sannidhi, D. V., Weatherspoon, L., Pauly, K., & Karlsen, M. C. (2022). Dietary interventions to treat type 2 diabetes in adults with a goal of remission: An expert consensus statement from the American College of Lifestyle Medicine. *American Journal of Lifestyle Medicine, 16*(3), 342–362. https://doi.org/10.1177/15598276221087624

Saad, M. J., Santos, A., & Prada, P. O. (2016). Linking gut microbiota and inflammation to obesity and insulin resistance. *Physiology, 31*(4), 283–293. https://doi.org/10.1152/physiol.00041.2015

Sarver, J., Khambatta, C., Barbaro, R., Chavan, B., & Drozek, D. (2019). Retrospective evaluation of an online diabetes health coaching program: A pilot study. *American Journal of Lifestyle Medicine, 15*(4), 466–474. https://doi.org/10.1177/1559827619879106

Saudek, C. D. (2009). Can diabetes be cured? Potential biological and mechanical approaches. *JAMA, 301*(15), 1588–1590. https://doi.org/10.1001/jama.2009.508

Schulze, M. B., Schulz, M., Heidemann, C., Schienkiewitz, A., Hoffmann, K., & Boeing, H. (2008). Carbohydrate intake and incidence of type 2 diabetes in the European Prospective Investigation into Cancer and Nutrition (EPIC)-Potsdam Study. *British Journal of Nutrition, 99*(5), 1107–1116. https://doi.org/10.1017/S0007114507853360

Schwingshackl, L., Hoffmann, G., Lampousi, A., Knüppel, S., Iqbal, K., Schwedhelm, C., Bechthold, A., Schlesinger, S., & Boeing, H. (2017). Food groups and risk of type 2 diabetes mellitus: A systematic review and meta-analysis of prospective studies. *European Journal of Epidemiology, 32*(5), 363–375. https://doi.org/10.1007/s10654-017-0246-y

Sears, B., & Perry, M. (2015). The role of fatty acids in insulin resistance. *Lipids in Health and Disease, 14*, 121. https://doi.org/10.1186/s12944-015-0123-1

Shai, I., Schwarzfuchs, D., Henkin, Y., Shahar, D. R., Witkow, S., Greenberg, I., Golan, R., Fraser, D., Bolotin, A., Vardi, H., Tangi-Rozental, O., Zuk-Ramot, R., Sarusi, B., Brickner, D., Schwartz, Z., Sheiner, E., Marko, R., Katorza, E., Thiery, J., . . . Dietary Intervention Randomized Controlled Trial (DIRECT) Group. (2008). Weight loss with a low-carbohydrate, Mediterranean, or low-fat diet. *New England Journal of Medicine, 359*(3), 229–241. https://doi.org/10.1056/NEJMoa0708681

Sharma, S., & Tripathi, P. (2019). Gut microbiome and type 2 diabetes: Where we are and where to go? *Journal of Nutritional Biochemistry, 63*, 101–108. https://doi.org/10.1016/j.jnutbio.2018.10.003

Shulman, G. I. (2014). Ectopic fat in insulin resistance, dyslipidemia, and cardiometabolic disease. *New England Journal of Medicine, 371*(12), 1131–1141. https://doi.org/10.1056/NEJMra1011035

Singh, T., Ahmed, T. H., Mohamed, N., Elhaj, M. S., Mohammed, Z., Paulsingh, C. N., Mohamed, M. B., & Khan, S. (2022). Does insufficient sleep increase the risk of developing insulin resistance: A systematic review. *Cureus, 14*(3), e23501. https://doi.org/10.7759/cureus.23501

Śliwińska-Mossoń, M., & Milnerowicz, H. (2017). The impact of smoking on the development of diabetes and its complications. *Diabetes & Vascular Disease Research, 14*(4), 265–276. https://doi.org/10.1177/1479164117701876

Snorgaard, O., Poulsen, G. M., Andersen, H. K., & Astrup, A. (2017). Systematic review and meta-analysis of dietary carbohydrate restriction in patients with type 2 diabetes. *BMJ Open Diabetes Research & Care, 5*(1), e000354. https://doi.org/10.1136/bmjdrc-2016-000354

Song, M., Fung, T. T., Hu, F. B., Willett, W. C., Longo, V. D., Chan, A. T., & Giovannucci, E. L. (2016). Association of animal and plant protein intake with all-cause and cause-specific mortality. *JAMA, 176*(10), 1453–1463. https://doi.org/10.1001/jamainternmed.2016.4182

Srour, B., Fezeu, L. K., Kesse-Guyot, E., Allès, B., Debras, C., Druesne-Pecollo, N., Chazelas, E., Deschasaux, M., Hercberg, S., Galan, P., Monteiro, C. A., Julia, C., & Touvier, M. (2020). Ultraprocessed food consumption and risk of type 2 diabetes among participants of the NutriNet-Santé Prospective Cohort. *JAMA Internal*

Medicine, 180(2), 283–291. https://doi.org/10.1001/jamainternmed.2019.5942

Steven, S., Hollingsworth, K. G., Al-Mrabeh, A., Avery, L., Aribisala, B., Caslake, M., & Taylor, R. (2016). Very low-calorie diet and 6 months of weight stability in type 2 diabetes: Pathophysiological changes in responders and nonresponders. *Diabetes Care, 39*(5), 808–815. https://doi.org/10.2337/dc15-1942

Storz, M. A. (2022). Adherence to low-fat, vegan diets in individuals with type 2 diabetes: A review. *American Journal of Lifestyle Medicine, 16*(3), 300–310. https://doi.org/10.1177/1559827620964755

Sutton, E. F., Beyl, R., Early, K. S., Cefalu, W. T., Ravussin, E., & Peterson, C. M. (2018). Early time-restricted feeding improves insulin sensitivity, blood pressure, and oxidative stress even without weight loss in men with prediabetes. *Cell Metabolism, 27*(6), 1212–1221. https://doi.org/10.1016/j.cmet.2018.04.010

Taylor, R., Al-Mrabeh, A., Zhyzhneuskaya, S., Peters, C., Barnes, A. C., Aribisala, B. S., Hollingsworth, K. G., Mathers, J. C., Sattar, N., & Lean, M. E. J. (2018). Remission of human type 2 diabetes requires decrease in liver and pancreas fat content but is dependent upon capacity for β cell recovery. *Cell Metabolism, 28*(4), 547–556. https://doi.org/10.1016/j.cmet.2018.07.003

Teymoori, F., Farhadnejad, H., Mokhtari, E., Sohouli, M. H., Moslehi, N., Mirmiran, P., & Azizi, F. (2021). Dietary and lifestyle inflammatory scores and risk of incident diabetes: A prospective cohort among participants of Tehran lipid and glucose study. *BMC Public Health, 21*(1), 1293. https://doi.org/10.1186/s12889-021-11327-1

Tian, J., Venn, A., Otahal, P., & Gall, S. (2016). The association between quitting smoking and weight gain: A systematic review and meta-analysis of prospective cohort studies. *Obesity Reviews, 17*(10), 1014. https://doi.org/10.1111/obr.12448

Tonstad, S., Stewart, K., Oda, K., Batech, M., Herring, R. P., & Fraser, G. E. (2013). Vegetarian diets and incidence of diabetes in the Adventist Health Study-2. *Nutrition, Metabolism, and Cardiovascular Diseases, 23*(4), 292–299. https://doi.org/10.1016/j.numecd.2011.07.004

Toumpanakis, A., Turnbull, T., & Alba-Barba, I. (2018). Effectiveness of plant-based diets in promoting well-being in the management of type 2 diabetes: A systematic review. *BMJ Open Diabetes Research & Care, 6*(1), e000534. https://doi.org/10.1136/bmjdrc-2018-000534

Tsalamandris, S., Antonopoulos, A. S., Oikonomou, E., Papamikroulis, G. A., Vogiatzi, G., Papaioannou, S., Deftereos, S., & Tousoulis, D. (2019). The role of inflammation in diabetes: Current concepts and future perspectives. *European Cardiology, 14*(1), 50–59. https://doi.org/10.15420/ecr.2018.33.1

U.S. Department of Health and Human Services. (n.d.). *Healthy People 2030: Diabetes*. Office of Disease Prevention and Health Promotion. Retrieved June 11, 2023, from https://health.gov/healthypeople/objectives-and-data/browse-objectives/diabetes

U.S. Preventive Services Taskforce. (2021, August 24). *Final recommendation statement: Prediabetes and type 2 diabetes: Screening*. https://www.uspreventiveservicestaskforce.org/uspstf/recommendation/screening-for-prediabetes-and-type-2-diabetes

Van Dijk, S. J., Tellam, R. L., Morrison, J. L., Muhlhausler, B. S., & Molloy, P. L. (2015). Recent developments on the role of epigenetics in obesity and metabolic disease. *Clinical Epigenetics, 7*, 66. https://doi.org/10.1186/s13148-015-0101-5

Vang, A., Singh, P. N., Lee, J. W., Haddad, E. H., & Brinegar, C. H. (2008). Meats, processed meats, obesity, weight gain and occurrence of diabetes among adults: Findings from Adventist Health Studies. *Annals of Nutrition & Metabolism, 52*(2), 96–104. https://doi.org/10.1159/000121365

van Nielen, M., Feskens, E. J., Mensink, M., Sluijs, I., Molina, E., Amiano, P., Ardanaz, E., Balkau, B., Beulens, J. W., Boeing, H., Clavel-Chapelon, F., Fagherazzi, G., Franks, P. W., Halkjaer, J., Huerta, J. M., Katzke, V., Key, T. J., Khaw, K. T., Krogh, V., . . . InterAct Consortium. (2014). Dietary protein intake and incidence of type 2 diabetes in Europe: The EPIC-InterAct Case-Cohort Study. *Diabetes Care, 37*(7), 1854–1862. https://doi.org/10.2337/dc13-2627

van Ommen, B., Wopereis, S., van Empelen, P., van Keulen, H. M., Otten, W., Kasteleyn, M., Molema, J. J. W., de Hoogh, I. M., Chavannes, N. H., Numans, M. E., Evers, A. W. M., & Pijl, H. (2018). From diabetes care to diabetes cure: The integration of systems biology, eHealth, and behavioral change. *Frontiers in Endocrinology, 8*, 381. https://doi.org/10.3389/fendo.2017.00381

van Wyk, H. J., Davis, R. E., & Davies, J. S. (2016). A critical review of low-carbohydrate diets in people with type 2 diabetes. *Diabetic Medicine, 33*(2), 148–157. https://doi.org/10.1111/dme.12964

Viguiliouk, E., Stewart, S. E., Jayalath, V. H., Ng, A. P., Mirrahimi, A., de Souza, R. J., Hanley, A. J., Bazinet, R. P., Blanco Mejia, S., Leiter, L. A., Josse, R. G., Kendall, C. W., Jenkins, D. J., & Sievenpiper, J. L. (2015). Effect of replacing animal protein with plant protein on glycemic control in diabetes: A systematic review and meta-analysis of randomized controlled trials. *Nutrients, 7*(12), 9804–9824. https://doi.org/10.3390/nu7125509

Wallace, D. D., Barrington, C., Albrecht, S., Gottfredson, N., Carter-Edwards, L., & Lytle, L. A. (2022). The role of stress responses on engagement in dietary and physical activity behaviors among Latino adults living with prediabetes. *Ethnicity & Health*, *27*(6), 1395–1409. https://doi.org/10.1080/13557858.2021.1880549

Wanders, A. J., Blom, W. A. M., Zock, P. L., Geleijnse, J. M., Brouwer, I. A., & Alssema, M. (2019). Plant-derived polyunsaturated fatty acids and markers of glucose metabolism and insulin resistance: A meta-analysis of randomized controlled feeding trials. *BMJ Open Diabetes Research & Care*, *7*(1), e000585. https://doi.org/10.1136/bmjdrc-2018-000585

Wang, X., Qin, L. Q., Arafa, A., Eshak, E. S., Hu, Y., & Dong, J. Y. (2021). Smoking cessation, weight gain, cardiovascular risk, and all-cause mortality: A meta-analysis. *Nicotine & Tobacco Research*, *23*(12), 1987–1994. https://doi.org/10.1093/ntr/ntab076

Westman, E. C., Yancy, W. S., Jr., Mavropoulos, J. C., Marquart, M., & McDuffie, J. R. (2008). The effect of a low-carbohydrate, ketogenic diet versus a low-glycemic index diet on glycemic control in type 2 diabetes mellitus. *Nutrition & Metabolism*, *5*, 36. https://doi.org/10.1186/1743-7075-5-36

Wilcox, G. (2005). Insulin and insulin resistance. *Clinical Biochemist Reviews*, *26*(2), 19–39.

Woods-Giscombe, C. L., Gaylord, S. A., Li, Y., Brintz, C. E., Bangdiwala, S. I., Buse, J. B., Mann, J. D., Lynch, C., Phillips, P., Smith, S., Leniek, K., Young, L., Al-Barwani, S., Yoo, J., & Faurot, K. (2019, August 14). A mixed-methods, randomized clinical trial to examine feasibility of a mindfulness-based stress management and diabetes risk reduction intervention for African Americans with prediabetes. *Evidence-Based Complementary and Alternative Medicine*, *2019*, 3962623. https://doi.org/10.1155/2019/3962623

World Health Organization. (2020, December 9). *The top 10 causes of death*. https://www.who.int/news-room/fact-sheets/detail/the-top-10-causes-of-death

World Health Organization. (2022, September 16). *Diabetes*. https://www.who.int/news-room/fact-sheets/detail/diabetes

Wright, A. K., Kontopantelis, E., Emsley, R., Buchan, I., Sattar, N., Rutter, M. K., & Ashcroft, D. M. (2017). Life expectancy and cause-specific mortality in type 2 diabetes: A population-based cohort study quantifying relationships in ethnic subgroups. *Diabetes Care*, *40*(3), 338–345. https://doi.org/10.2337/dc16-1616

Wronka, M., Krzemińska, J., Młynarska, E., Rysz, J., & Franczyk, B. (2022). The influence of lifestyle and treatment on oxidative stress and inflammation in diabetes. *International Journal of Molecular Sciences*, *23*(24), 15743. https://doi.org/10.3390/ijms232415743

Wu, J., Ward, E., & Lu, Z. K. (2018). Addressing lifestyle management during visits involving patients with prediabetes: Namcs 2013–2015. *Journal of General Internal Medicine*, *34*(8), 1412–1418. https://doi.org/10.1007/s11606-018-4724-z

Xue, A., Wu, Y., Zhu, Z., Zhang, F., Kemper, K. E., Zheng, Z., Yengo, L., Lloyd-Jones, L. R., Sidorenko, J., Wu, Y., eQTLGen Consortium, McRae, A. F., Visscher, P. M., Zeng, J., & Yang, J. (2018). Genome-wide association analyses identify 143 risk variants and putative regulatory mechanisms for type 2 diabetes. *Nature Communications*, *9*, 2941. https://doi.org/10.1038/s41467-018-04951-w

Yanai, H., Adachi, H., Masui, Y., Katsuyama, H., Kawaguchi, H., Hakoshima, M., Waragai, Y., Harigae, T., Hamasaki, H., & Sako, A. (2018). Exercise therapy for patients with type 2 diabetes: A narrative review. *Journal of Clinical Medicine Research*, *10*(5), 365–369. https://doi.org/10.14740/jocmr3382w

Yokoyama, Y., Barnard, N. D., Levin, S. M., & Watanabe, M. (2014). Vegetarian diets and glycemic control in diabetes: A systematic review and meta-analysis. *Cardiovascular Diagnosis and Therapy*, *4*(5), 373–382. https://doi.org/10.3978/j.issn.2223-3652.2014.10.04

Zhu, P., Pan, X. F., Sheng, L., Chen, H., & Pan, A. (2017). Cigarette smoking, diabetes, and diabetes complications: Call for urgent action. *Current Diabetes Reports*, *17*(9), 78. https://doi.org/10.1007/s11892-017-0903-2

Zhu, T., & Goodarzi, M. O. (2020). Metabolites linking the gut microbiome with risk for type 2 diabetes. *Current Nutrition Reports*, *9*(2), 83–93. https://doi.org/10.1007/s13668-020-00307-3

CHAPTER 19

Lifestyle Approaches for Preventing and Improving Cardiovascular Disease

Sheila Hautbois, PA-C, MPAS, MPH, CHES®, DipACLM
Jenifer M. Spadafore, PA-C, MPAS

"Heart disease will affect 1 in 2 adults in the U.S. But most of the time, healthy habits can prevent it."

American College of Cardiology, n.d.

OBJECTIVES

This chapter will enable the reader to:

1. Define cardiovascular disease.
2. Identify the effect of cardiovascular diseases.
3. Review cardiovascular guidelines.
4. Discuss cardiovascular screening and assessment.
5. Review how to start the conversation and counsel about heart health.
6. Apply A-SMART prescriptions to cardiovascular conditions.
7. Compare the roles of the healthcare team members in cardiovascular health.

Overview

Cardiovascular disease (CVD) is essentially any abnormality related to the heart or circulatory system. It is a broader term than heart disease, although the terms are sometimes used interchangeably. CVDs include hypertension (HTN), hyperlipidemia, cerebrovascular disease, peripheral vascular disease, coronary artery disease, arrhythmias, cardiomyopathies, and systolic or diastolic heart failure.

CVD is associated with and affected by other health conditions, including diabetes,

© Kathleen Gail/Shutterstock; © StoryTime Studio/Shutterstock; © kali9/Getty Images

obesity, and gum disease. Certain types of heart disease, such as valvular and congenital heart disease, may not be preventable or treatable with lifestyle changes alone. However, a healthy lifestyle will optimize overall physical health and may delay the worsening of the conditions or help a person be in the best shape to obtain any necessary surgical treatment. Regardless of the presence or type of CVD, the advanced practice provider (APP) can significantly affect health at both personal and population levels by promoting a heart-healthy lifestyle.

Effect of CVD

On average, someone dies of CVD every 36 seconds in the United States (Virani et al., 2021). According to the National Vital Statistics System report for the U.S. Department of Health and Human Services, heart disease was the leading cause of death in the United States from 2015 to 2020 (Ahmad & Anderson, 2021). Approximately 690,882 deaths from heart disease occurred in 2020—more than double the number of deaths from COVID-19. Adding death rates from stroke, CVD claims more lives each year than all forms of cancer and chronic lower respiratory disease combined (Virani et al., 2021). Even more sobering is that these numbers are not improving. Heart disease deaths increased by 4.8% from 2019 to 2020, the largest increase since 2012 (Ahmad & Anderson, 2021).

It is reported that 30.3 million Americans currently live with a diagnosis of heart disease, which includes but is not limited to atherosclerotic cardiovascular disease (ASCVD), heart failure, and atrial fibrillation (AF) (Kochanek et al., 2019). Sadly, CVD and its risk factors are not age specific. The prevalence of cardiovascular risk factors among American high school students includes 31.2% having used any tobacco products and 73.9% not meeting recommended physical activity levels. In youth ages 12 to 19, 36.6% are overweight

or obese, 22.8% have elevated cholesterol, 10.9% have high blood pressure (BP), and 13.8% have diabetes (Virani et al., 2021). The American College of Cardiology (ACC) guidelines place the estimated cost of CVD treatment at greater than $200 billion annually and attribute much of the cost and disease burden to inadequate prevention strategies (Arnett, Blumenthal, et al., 2019).

The Role of Inflammation in Cardiovascular Pathology

ASCVD was once thought to be a function of cholesterol deposition; however, the current understanding is that it is a function of inflammation (Nabel & Braunwald, 2012). Chronic stressors such as HTN, glucose elevation as seen in diabetes, elevated cholesterol levels, smoking, obesity, and physical inactivity are all sources of endothelial insult and dysfunction. Damage to the endothelium triggers a cascade of mechanisms that lead to inflammation, activation of white blood cells and platelets, and deposition of cholesterol plaques and platelets at the site of injury. When the endothelium is damaged, nitric oxide production is reduced. Nitric oxide is a potent vasodilator that protects the endothelium and helps maintain vessel homeostasis. A decrease in nitric acid production can narrow the arterial lumens, decrease perfusion, and damage the endothelial cells. This damage further supports atherosclerosis.

Fortunately, taking measures to decrease inflammation can help reduce and potentially reverse ASCVD. Lifestyle measures such as a healthy dietary pattern, exercise, and restorative behaviors can support nitric oxide production and reduce inflammation. These measures continue to be evaluated, modified, and adopted as means to maintain and improve cardiovascular health.

Current Recommendations for Preventing Cardiovascular Disease

The INTERHEART study (Yusuf et al., 2004) identified nine risk factors that accounted for 90% of the population attributable risks for myocardial infarction in men and 94% in women worldwide. These include abnormal lipids, smoking, HTN, diabetes, abdominal obesity, psychosocial factors, intake of fruits and vegetables, consumption of alcohol, and regular physical activity. The American Heart Association (AHA, 2022) recommends seven of these nine risk factors as components of ideal cardiovascular health in their Life's Essential 8 model: (1) manage blood pressure, (2) control cholesterol, (3) reduce blood sugar, (4) get active, (5) eat better, (6) lose weight, (7) stop smoking, and (8) get adequate sleep (see **Figure 19.1**). Making lifestyle changes to improve these core health behaviors and health factors can help patients achieve ideal cardiovascular health and a lower risk of heart disease.

Studies show that addressing cardiovascular conditions through lifestyle approaches can significantly improve overall health and well-being. For example, the Nurses' Health Study demonstrated a lower rate of cardiovascular events among participants who demonstrated healthy lifestyle practices, including dietary choices, exercise, abstinence from tobacco use, and favorable body mass index (BMI; Bland, 2017). The benefits of a favorable lifestyle can even offset the risk for coronary events by 46% in individuals with high genetic risk factors for CVD (Khera et al., 2016). More importantly, addressing the risk factors for these conditions through lifestyle prescriptions can improve quality of life and disease prevention.

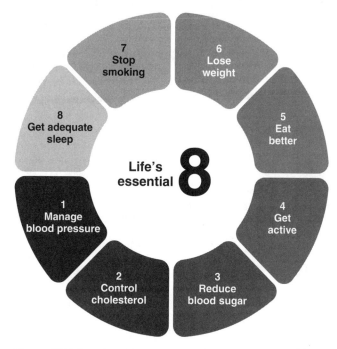

Figure 19.1 American Heart Association Life's Essential 8™.

Data from American Heart Association

Dietary Patterns

Dietary patterns studied in randomized controlled trials and prospective cohorts have exhibited a cardioprotective effect. In the landmark Lifestyle Heart Trial, Ornish et al. (1998) demonstrated improvement in risk factor indices and regression of cardiovascular stenosis after 1 year with a dietary and intensive lifestyle approach independent of medications. The study was extended for four additional years to show that patients can successfully sustain comprehensive lifestyle changes and experience long-term positive effects.

The Dietary Approaches to Stop Hypertension (DASH) diet has been shown to significantly decrease systolic BP (SBP) and diastolic BP (DBP). The DASH diet emphasizes fruits, vegetables, and whole grains. These foods are generally good sources of potassium, magnesium, and calcium, which support the cardiovascular system. The diet also recommends limiting foods high in saturated fat, including fatty meats and full-fat dairy products, and those high in sugar, such as sweets and sugary beverages. A meta-analysis of 30 randomized controlled trials ($n = 5,545$) investigating the BP effects of the DASH diet found that, compared with a control diet, the DASH diet reduced both SBP and DBP (Filippou et al., 2020). The International Society of Hypertension and the ACC/AHA both support the DASH diet as a Class I recommendation for preventing and treating HTN (Unger et al., 2020; Whelton et al., 2018).

Studies on the Mediterranean diet have also shown cardiovascular benefits. The landmark PREDIMED study randomized patients to the Mediterranean diet, which is high in fruits, vegetables, and grains while low in animal protein and dairy products versus a traditional low-fat diet. All subjects were considered high risk regarding their CVD scores. Subjects were followed for 4.8 years. It was noted that those with the Mediterranean diet supplemented with olive oil or nuts had a decrease in cardiovascular risk factor indices and cardiac events compared to the group assigned a low-fat diet (Estruch et al., 2013).

A nutrient-dense vegetarian diet has also been studied in relation to cardiovascular risk factors and disease. Vegetarian diets have demonstrated an ability to decrease CVD mortality and risk for coronary heart disease (CHD) by 40% due to their ability to lower BP, improve cholesterol levels, and reduce platelet aggregation (Kahleova et al., 2018). They are also associated with other improvements in cardiovascular risk factors, such as weight and diabetes management. Through case reports, Esselstyn and Golubic (2014) demonstrated that coronary artery disease could be arrested and reversed with adherence to a whole-food plant-based diet. When patients eliminated meat, dairy, fish, and oils from their diet and increased fruits, vegetables, legumes, and whole grains, they not only experienced regression of coronary artery disease but had a lower incidence of cardiovascular events, decreased symptoms, and improved functional status (Esselstyn et al., 2014). It is important to note that the nutrient quality of plant-based foods is essential since a plant-based diet that consists of highly processed foods (e.g., juices, sweetened beverages, fried potatoes, refined grains, sweets) is associated with a higher CHD risk (Satija et al., 2017).

The AHA recommends adopting a diet low in saturated fats that includes fruits, vegetables, grains, and low-fat protein sources. Additionally, this diet recommends restricting sodium intake to less than 2,300 mg (Arnett, Khera, et al., 2019; Van Horn et al., 2016).

Activity Patterns

Research has found that physical activity is also cardioprotective. Exercise positively influences BP, blood glucose, lipids, endothelial function, and inflammation. Randomized controlled trials have shown a decrease in mortality among patients who participate in moderate physical activity most days of the week. Physical activity is a Class I recommendation for preventing and treating CVD (Arnett, Khera, et al.,

2019). The Physical Activity Guidelines for Americans recommend that adults accumulate at least 150 minutes of moderate-intensity or 75 minutes of vigorous-intensity aerobic activity weekly (U.S. Department of Health and Human Services, 2018).

Combining physical activity with dietary interventions can further improve cardiovascular risk factors. The ENCORE (*Exercise and Nutrition Interventions for Cardiovascular Health*) study randomized patients to the DASH diet alone versus lifestyle modification plus the DASH diet. The primary endpoint measured at 4 months demonstrated a 16-point drop in SBP for those who participated in the combination multimodality study versus diet alone. The secondary endpoint measured at 8 months was a weight loss of approximately 7 kilograms in this same group. This study again demonstrated that multimodality lifestyle interventions, including dietary changes and exercise, are feasible and beneficial for improving HTN and disease risk factors, including obesity (Blumenthal et al., 2010; Hinderliter et al., 2014).

Cardiac rehabilitation, developed in the 1970s for patients with heart disease, is one of the largest sources of information confirming the benefits of physical activity on morbidity and mortality in cardiovascular patients. In addition to exercise training, a structured traditional cardiac rehabilitation program delivers education and counseling on the risk factors of CHD and recommended lifestyle modifications, including diet and stress management. Cardiac rehabilitation is a program endorsed by the Centers for Medicare and Medicaid Services (CMS). It is a Class 1A recommendation for treating patients with heart disease (Aggarwal et al., 2021).

Other Lifestyle Behaviors

Stress reduction with lifestyle modification, specifically mindfulness-based interventions, has also been studied in patients with heart disease. Interventions such as meditation, yoga,

and tai chi positively affect cardiovascular event outcomes (Teng et al., 2020). The benefits of these activities can include a decrease in BP, heart rate, and depression, all of which can contribute to CVD. In a scientific statement in 2017, the AHA endorsed mindfulness-based interventions as adjunctive therapy to guideline-directed treatment (Levine et al., 2017).

In addition to dietary changes and exercise, meditation can decrease BP and the morbidity associated with HTN, including stroke and CVD (Goldstein et al., 2012; Shi et al., 2017). Meditation and mindfulness training are not traditionally used as treatments for HTN since randomized controlled trials have been unable to consistently demonstrate that either can be effective monotherapy. However, the 2020 International Society of Hypertension Global Hypertension Practice Guidelines recognize meditation and mindfulness as part of a healthy lifestyle and beneficial for stress reduction. These guidelines include mindfulness practices, and the society encourages further study on the effect of chronic stress on BP and cardiovascular risk (Unger et al., 2020).

The effect of sleep on cardiovascular health continues to be investigated. Sleep quality and duration, when combined with the evaluation of traditional cardiovascular risk factors, led to more accurate risk prediction for heart disease (Makarem et al., 2020). Studies have suggested that poor sleep can affect cardiovascular risk factors, including an increase in inflammatory markers and BP, and affect diabetes and blood glucose levels (Yan et al., 2021). Sleep duration outside of the recommended 7 to 8 hours of sleep for adults is associated with increased risk for cardiovascular events and mortality (Kwok et al., 2018).

Finally, it is important to consider substance use as a risk factor for CVD. The use of tobacco has long been associated with an increased risk for CVD. Smoking causes 25% of deaths from CVD and contributes to an increased risk for CHD in nonsmokers exposed to secondhand smoke (Office on Smoking and

Health, 2014). Although some cardiovascular benefits to alcohol consumption, particularly wine, have been noted (Haseeb et al., 2017), new evidence suggests that even drinking within the recommended limits increases the risk of death from some forms of CVD (U.S. Department of Agriculture & U.S. Department of Health and Human Services, 2020). Alcohol has also been associated with HTN, decreasing BP initially (up to 12 hours) after consumption and then increasing BP (Tasnim et al., 2020).

Risk Factor Management

Management of cholesterol, a building block of atherosclerotic heart disease, is another essential aspect of prevention. The ACC/AHA clinical practice guidelines on cholesterol management emphasize the importance of lifestyle therapies. The guidelines specifically address diet, weight control, and physical activity as the first-line treatment of disease. Additional medical therapies are recommended based on cholesterol levels and risk for CVD (Grundy et al., 2019).

HTN has been identified as a stimulus for endothelial dysfunction and a risk factor for stroke and CVD. Essentially void of symptoms, HTN is known as the silent killer. Detection of HTN and subsequent treatment can reduce cardiovascular morbidity and mortality (Fryar et al., 2017). The ACC/AHA clinical practice guidelines on managing HTN also discuss lifestyle practice as first-line therapy. Recommendations are for dietary management to include the DASH diet, which highlights sodium restriction, weight loss, and exercise (Cifu & Davis, 2017).

The PREMIER study focused on multifaceted lifestyle practices for BP control. This study included patients with a BP of 120 to 159/80 to 95 mmHg. Participants were randomized to lifestyle and dietary changes in the established guidelines to include a decrease in weight, salt, alcohol consumption, and fat as well as an increase in physical activity.

Additionally, one of the groups was randomized to the DASH diet. The control group received education only. Motivational sessions were incorporated, and participants were encouraged to establish lifestyle modification goals to include increased aerobic activity and decreased alcohol intake. The groups were followed for 18 months. Outcomes suggested that a multifaceted approach to HTN management with lifestyle changes could decrease patient weight, increase physical fitness, and decrease BP (Elmer et al., 2006; Funk et al., 2008).

Cardiovascular Screening and Assessment

Cardiovascular events result from disease that progresses throughout life, starting as early as childhood with changes in coronary risk factors and health (National Heart, Lung, and Blood Institute, 2012). The ACC/AHA published clinical practice guidelines for the prevention of CVD (Arnett, Blumenthal, et al., 2019). Clinical practice guidelines allow providers to order and interpret clinical investigations according to best practice.

The guidelines outline screening for primary prevention of CVD for adults 18 to 75 years of age, including risk factor identification, routine diagnostic testing, and the use of risk assessment pooled cohort tools. Proper use of these tools allows the APP to identify areas of risk and implement preventive education and counseling for patients based on the risk of developing CVD. Adopting and practicing a healthy lifestyle can halt the development of CVD, which is why cardiovascular screening is an important strategy in managing the health and well-being of all adults.

Cardiovascular screening starts with an interview to identify risk factors and areas of concern in a patient's current and future health. Routine symptom assessment, past medical history, and social history can help identify heart disease risk. Risk factors for heart disease include both underlying health conditions and lifestyle practices. Risk factors can be further divided into nonmodifiable versus modifiable elements. Recognized nonmodifiable risk factors include increasing age, gender, and heredity (race, family history of premature heart disease). Modifiable risk factors include tobacco smoke, HTN, hyperlipidemia, diabetes, obesity, physical inactivity, stress, alcohol use, and poor diet (AHA, 2016). Addressing modifiable risk factors can improve and often reverse health conditions known to promote heart diseases such as HTN, dyslipidemia, type 2 diabetes, and obesity.

It is important to take note of risk factors that cannot be modified. African Americans, Mexican Americans, American Indians, native Hawaiians, and some Asian Americans are at higher risk for heart disease. African Americans are also at higher risk for more severe HTN (AHA, 2016). Although men and women can have the same risk factors for CVD, the effect that these risk factors have on disease may vary. For example, although the prevalence of CVD increases with age, the incidence of CVD tends to present 10 years later in women than in men. Furthermore, more women than men live with CVD after age 75. This may be related to the differences in life expectancy between men and women (Mosca et al., 2011).

In addition to a focused interview for traditional risk factors, the guidelines also recommend screening for non-health–related measures that can affect health outcomes (Arnett, Blumenthal, et al., 2019). According to the CMS, failure to address the effect of social determinants of health has undermined prevention measures. As a result, the CMS developed the Accountable Health Communities model to allow practitioners to assess five health-related social needs: housing instability, food insecurity, transportation difficulties, utility assistance needs, and interpersonal safety concerns. By utilizing this model, APPs can identify areas of need and connect with available social services to assist patients in embarking on a more effective healthcare journey (Billioux et al., 2017).

The physical examination can quantify risk factors. Vital signs such as BP, weight, and waist circumference should be routinely assessed. These vitals can identify patients with HTN and obesity. The ACC/AHA recommends that tobacco use screening be addressed at every patient encounter and treated as an additional vital sign given the significant morbidity and mortality associated with its use (Arnett, Khera, et al., 2019).

In addition to the interview, diagnostic testing to include lipid profile, complete blood count, complete metabolic panel, urinalysis, and high sensitivity C-reative should be obtained as part of the screening process beginning at age 20 (Arnett, Blumenthal, et al., 2019). These routine labs provide objective data on cholesterol levels, kidney function, and glucose levels in screening for HTN and diabetes. The high sensitivity C-reactive protein level can identify a state of inflammation that could contribute to cardiovascular risk.

Once objective data are obtained, risk assessment can be done using pooled cohort equations (PCEs), such as the ASCVD Risk Estimator, Framingham Risk Score, and Reynolds Risk Score. The ASCVD estimates a 10-year risk of cardiovascular events for a symptomatic adults. Patients are categorized into low, borderline, intermediate, or high-risk groups. For those in the low-risk group or those adopting or practicing a healthy lifestyle, the tool can monitor progress and predict 30-year risk. The ACC/AHA recommends the use of the ASCVD Risk Estimator, which has been well validated in non-Hispanic White and non-Hispanic Black populations (Lloyd-Jones et al., 2019). In racial/ethnic groups outside this cohort, additional tools such as the Framingham General CVD Risk Profile and the Reynolds Risk Score may assist in calculating risk (Lloyd-Jones et al., 2019). The Reynolds Risk Score includes family history of either parent having a heart attack before age 60 and the hs-CRP as a measure of inflammation.

A coronary artery calcium (CAC) screening is recommended to further quantify CVD risk following calculations with PCEs. This testing modality is felt to be superior to clinical biomarkers because it can noninvasively identify calcifications in the coronary arteries, which in most cases is directly associated with the level of atherosclerotic disease burden (Lloyd-Jones et al., 2019). The Multi-Ethnic Study of Atherosclerosis (MESA) tool can be used once the CAC score is obtained to calculate the potential benefit of pharmacological interventions on CHD risk. This tool is appropriate for Chinese, Hispanic, African American, and White populations between the ages of 45 and 84. Routine follow-up is recommended to monitor treatment and recalculate risk if the patient was initially at low risk; risk recalculation is generally unnecessary once a patient has known coronary calcification per the CAC score.

In summary, the approach to the assessment of the patient for cardiovascular risk includes routine history and physical examination, assessment of health behaviors (e.g., tobacco use, diet, physical activity), and measurement of physiological risk factors (e.g., BP, lipid panel, diabetes screening as appropriate). A PCE, such as the ASCVD Risk Estimator, should be used to assess risk. Clinic appointments, phone calls, and telemedicine visits can keep patients on track with optimal lifestyle management and improved quality of life. APPs should engage all patients in meaningful conversation to discuss risk reduction

Health Promotion Research Study

Primary Prevention of CVD with a Mediterranean Diet

Background: The Mediterranean diet, which emphasizes fruits, vegetables, nuts, and grains, with low dairy and animal protein intake and moderate wine consumption, has long demonstrated benefit in patients at risk of CVD. In 2003, the PREDIMED (Prevención con Dieta Mediterránea) trial was launched to explore the cardioprotective benefits of the Mediterranean diet.

Methodology: The study, conducted in Spain, enrolled 7,447 participants among 169 clinics from 2003–2009. Participants' ages were 55–80 for men and 60–80 for women. Participants were considered high risk for CVD based on risk factors of type 2 diabetes or a combination of smoking, obesity, high low-density lipoprotein (LDL), high-density lipoprotein (HDL), or family history of premature CVD. Participants were divided into the following groups: a Mediterranean diet with extra-virgin olive oil, a Mediterranean diet with mixed nuts, and a low-fat diet control group. Each group filled out surveys and met with dieticians at specified intervals.

Results: Participants were followed for 4.8 years. The primary endpoint was death from a cardiovascular cause, myocardial infarction, or stroke. The study demonstrated superior outcomes in the groups assigned to the Mediterranean diet regardless of supplementation with olive oil or nuts.

Implications for Advanced Practice: This research demonstrated the value of a largely plant-based diet on CVD outcomes. The Mediterranean diet continues to be recommended by the ACC/AHA in guidelines for the prevention of CVD (Arnett, Khera, et al., 2019).

Reference: Data from Estruch, R., Ros, E., Salas-Salvadó, J., Covas, M. I., Corella, D., Arós, F., Gómez-Gracia, E., Ruiz-Gutiérrez, V., Fiol, M., Lapetra, J., Lamuela-Raventos, R. M., Serra-Majem, L., Pintó, X., Basora, J., Muñoz, M. A., Sorlí, J. V., Martínez, J. A., & Martínez-González, M. A. (2018). Primary prevention of cardiovascular disease with a Mediterranean diet supplemented with extra-virgin olive oil or nuts. *New England Journal of Medicine, 378*(25), e34. https://doi.org/10.1056/NEJMoa1800389

through lifestyle management and the potential benefits and risks of pharmaceutical therapies.

Starting the Cardiovascular Conversation

An excellent question for starting a conversation about heart health and cardiovascular risk reduction is, "On a scale of 1–10, with 10 being excellent, how good do you feel your heart health is?" The answer to this question, in addition to cardiovascular screening and test results, can serve as the basis for personalized patient education and counseling for risk reduction. Each patient should be asked what specific concerns they have about their heart health so that the APP can understand and address those concerns and obtain an idea of how the patient perceives their risk.

All patients should be asked about family history of heart disease, especially in birth parents, siblings, and biological children. If a patient's mother or sister had heart disease before age 65 or father or brother before age 55, this is concerning for increased cardiovascular risk (Hajar, 2017). A thorough assessment of family and personal risk factors is necessary for guiding the counseling and education that will follow. The assessment should include a weight history for all patients because having been overweight or obese in the past may have increased inflammation at that time. All female patients should be asked about pregnancy and postpartum experience history. Preeclampsia, gestational diabetes, HTN during pregnancy that did not resolve in the postpartum period, lipids that did not return to baseline after 3 months postpartum, and premature menopause should all be considered cardiovascular risk factors (Alfaddagh et al., 2019). Additional factors to include in initial patient conversations about CVD, as well as monitoring over time, are summarized in **Table 19.1**.

A-SMART Prescriptions to Address Cardiovascular Conditions

The basic healthy lifestyle prescription for all cardiovascular conditions is the same. It can be summarized using the A-SMART lifestyle behaviors: adopt healthy eating, stress less, move often, avoid alcohol, rest more, and treat tobacco use (see **Table 19.2**).

Cardiovascular Counseling and Education

The ABCs of Primary Cardiovascular Prevention is a succinct model for remembering the key areas for counseling (Alfaddagh et al., 2019). Since its original iteration, the model has been expanded to include risk assessment, antiplatelet therapy, BP, cholesterol, cigarette smoking, diabetes, diet and weight, exercise, and economic and social factors and is now known as the ABCDEs (Alfaddagh et al., 2019) (see **Figure 19.2**). Along with diet and weight, hydration must also be addressed. Sleep and stress management should also be discussed since these lifestyle factors affect several of the ABCDEs. When counseling about cigarettes, general questions regarding nicotine or tobacco should be asked rather than specifying "cigarettes" since the drug is available in forms other than cigarettes. Another E to assess and provide resources for is emotional health and support.

When providing counseling and education to patients about cardiovascular risk reduction, motivational interviewing tools will be helpful. Ask permission to discuss body weight since that is a sensitive topic. Using the transtheoretical model to determine stages of change will allow counseling targeted to a patient's specific needs. Stages of change for each

Table 19.1 Conversations About CVD

"Tell me about your . . ."	Goal
BP	120/80 mmHg (SBP up to 140 mmHg may be acceptable in elderly patients)
Resting heart rate	60–100 bpm (lower is acceptable in athletes)
Cholesterol	LDL <100 mg/dL (<70 mg/dL if history of cardiovascular event) Triglycerides <150 mg/dL and no greater than 3 times the HDL HDL >40 mg/dL (males) and >50 mg/dL (females)
Coronary artery calcium score (CAC)	0
Fasting blood sugar	60–100 mg/dL
BMI	18.5–24.9 kg/m^2
Alcohol use	None
Tobacco/nicotine use and history	None
Marijuana, cocaine, or other drug use	None
Physical activity	Cardio, strength, flexibility, and balance exercises each week
Sleep habits	7–9 hours a night for adults, with no snoring If snoring, consider sleep apnea screening
Stress	Good stress management practices and social support system
Oral health and hygiene	Regular dental cleanings twice a year; brushing and flossing daily
Nutrition	Whole-food plant-predominant eating pattern, with appropriate daily caloric intake
Hydration	One-half of body weight in ounces for total fluid intake daily unless on fluid restriction due to heart failure

Table 19.2 A-SMART Lifestyle Prescriptions for CVD

Behavior	Prescription	Considerations
Adopt healthy eating	Limit highly processed foods, fast food, and restaurant foods. The ACC recommends a diet rich in vegetables, fruits, legumes, nuts, whole grains, and fish (Alfaddagh et al., 2019).	Increasing plant foods will naturally increase fiber intake, resulting in improved cholesterol levels.
Stress less	Good stress management options include deep breathing, meditation, prayer, aerobic exercise, adequate sleep, counseling, and support groups.	Referral to a psychologist or coach may be needed.

Behavior	Prescription	Considerations
Move often	APPs should encourage patients to avoid long periods of being sedentary (Alfaddagh et al., 2019). Additionally, patients should engage in at least 150 minutes of moderate-intensity or 75 minutes of vigorous-intensity cardiovascular exercise, two full-body strength training sessions, and flexibility exercises weekly (Alfaddagh et al., 2019).	Everyone can exercise; some patients, such as those who have heart failure with reduced ejection fraction or recent myocardial infarction, may need cardiac rehab to gradually increase intensity and personalize rest periods. Heart rate and BP are monitored in the cardiac rehab setting to ensure an appropriate and safe response to exercise. Some patients may need physical or occupational therapy to learn how to exercise safely and gradually increase exercise tolerance. Patients who are safe to exercise but do not know what to do should be referred to an exercise specialist to help design a safe and effective, progressive, personalized exercise program.
Avoid alcohol	No amount of alcohol consumption is safe for the heart, and abstainers should not start drinking (World Heart Federation [WHF], 2022). Adults without underlying health conditions should be counseled to reduce or eliminate alcohol intake.	Alcohol use increases the risk of AF and HTN (Alfaddagh et al., 2019). It also increases the risk of stroke and cardiovascular events (WHF, 2022).
Rest more	For adults, 7–9 hours per night is recommended. Good sleep hygiene should be practiced.	APPs should perform sleep apnea screening if a patient has any combination of large neck, HTN, snoring, and daytime fatigue.
Treat tobacco use	The goal is cessation, but harm reduction includes cutting back on tobacco use of any kind. Pharmacotherapy plus behavioral therapy is recommended to support cessation (Alfaddagh et al., 2019).	Use of tobacco significantly increases cardiovascular risk, directly and indirectly. Tobacco use directly increases risk of heart failure, AF, blood clots, and atherosclerosis (Kondo et al., 2019). Nicotine is a stimulant, increasing BP and heart rate. Tobacco use also is known to suppress HDL cholesterol and increase insulin resistance.

behavior should be assessed routinely. The APP should ask the patients about their goals and which healthy behaviors they would like to focus on. Then specific support can be offered to patients. Using team-based language, such as "we," helps create an alliance and empower the patients. The team approach helps patients to experience a supportive and partnering relationship with their APP and to feel that the APP is on their side in a coach-like role.

As possible, provide education using a personalized approach with shared decision-making. A healthy lifestyle should be addressed in addition to discussing medications for guideline-directed medical therapy. Patients should be counseled that using medication should not be seen as a failure; often, medications need to be used in conjunction with lifestyle to provide the best results or minimize the risk of recurrence after a cardiovascular

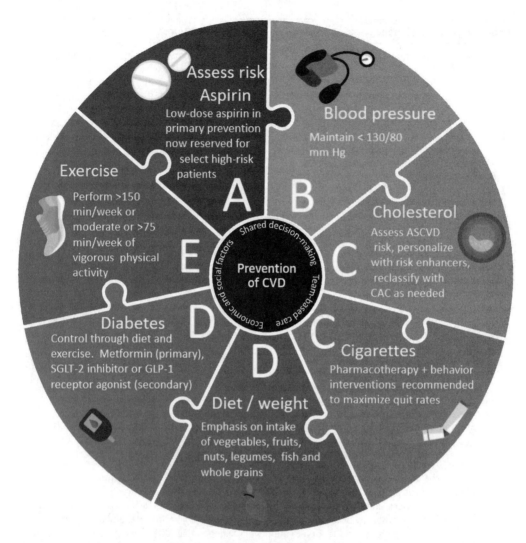

Figure 19.2 ABCDEs of Primary Cardiovascular Prevention: Lifestyle changes and team-based care.

Alfaddagh, A., Arps, K., Blumenthal, R., & Martin, S. S. (2019, March 21). *The ABCs of primary cardiovascular prevention: 2019 update.* American College of Cardiology. https://www.acc.org/latest-in-cardiology/articles/2019/03/21/14/39/abcs-of-primary-cv-prevention-2019-update-gl-prevention

event. Many patients find it helpful to learn that some medications may only be needed short term while lifestyle changes are initiated. Once specific biomarkers have been achieved and sustained, some medications might be discontinued after shared decision-making between patient and provider. The APP should ensure that patients understand they should not abruptly stop medications independently.

Deprescribing medications should be supervised; it may take time to wean patients off medication gradually. Close monitoring needs to happen during that time, and one clinician gatekeeper should be supervising that monitoring, whether it be the primary care provider or the specialist. Either way, the other providers on the patient's care team should be kept informed.

Health Promotion Case Study Addressing CVD in an Adult Male

Case Description: J.B. is a 69-year-old Caucasian male who presents to the primary care clinic to establish care. Recent health concerns include constipation and bloating, for which he has been using MiraLAX without adequate response. He also reports shortness of breath and lower-extremity swelling that has progressively worsened over the past 2 weeks. States that he is okay when sitting quietly but becomes significantly short of breath with any activity. He denies chest pain or pressure. Admits feeling extra heartbeats at times. Denies light-headedness or dizziness.

- Past medical history: Denies. Has not had an established relationship with a healthcare provider.
- Medications: Prilosec and MiraLAX over the counter.
- Allergies: No known drug allergies.
- Social history: Married. Recently retired.
- Vital signs: Blood pressure 106/73 mmHg, heart rate 118 beats per minute, respirations 20 breaths per minute, oxygen saturation 96% on room air, weight 229 pounds (104 kilograms), height 5 feet, 9 inches (182 cm), body mass index 31.4 kilogram/meters^2.
- Physical exam: Alert and oriented to person, place, time, and situation. Well-nourished male. Speaking in complete sentences. HEENT: Head is normocephalic. Non-icteric. Cardiovascular: S1 and S2 audible. Rate tachycardic. Rhythm irregularly irregular. No murmurs. Jugular venous distention not appreciated. Point of maximal impulse laterally displaced. Pulses 2+. RESP: Tachypneic, diminished bases, otherwise clear to auscultation without rales, rhonchi, or wheezing. Abdomen: Soft with adiposity. Bowel sounds: Active in all four quadrants. No tenderness. No guarding. SKIN: Cool and dry. Extremities: Trace nonpitting edema in the lower extremities bilaterally. Neurological: no focal neuro deficits. Psychiatric: Mood normal. Behavior appropriate.
- Labs: Hemoglobin 16.2 g/dL, hematocrit 47.8%, white blood cells 9.1 x 10^9/L, platelets 143 x 10^9/L, sodium 139 mEq/L, potassium 4.1 mEq/L, chloride 101 mEq/L, carbon dioxide 20 mEq/L, fasting blood sugar 135 mg/dL, blood urea nitrogen 61 mg/dL, creatinine 2.9 mg/dL, thyroid stimulating hormone 2.85 mU/L.
- Electrocardiogram: Atrial fibrillation at 118 bpm. No ST or T wave abnormalities.
- Chest X-ray: Cardiomegaly. Diffuse interstitial edema with bilateral pleural effusions.
- Echocardiogram: Enlarged left ventricular chamber EF 25%, mildly dilated left atria.
- Assessment: Atrial fibrillation with a rapid ventricular response; acute decompensated heart failure.

Lifestyle Vital Signs

- Adopt healthy eating: Not assessed.
- Stress less: Not assessed.
- Move often: He has not been exercising due to fatigue and lack of endurance with breathing.
- Avoid alcohol: No alcohol use. No recreational drug use.
- Rest more: His wife indicates that he has been snoring more, for which he is using pillows to prop himself up in bed.
- Treat tobacco use: He denies recent smoking. Thirty-five pack-year history; quit in 2010.

Critical Thinking Questions

1. What other factors would you want to assess?
2. Estimate J.B.'s 10-year ASCVD risk using an online calculator. How does it compare with an optimal ASCVD risk score?

(continues)

Health Promotion Case Study Addressing CVD in an Adult Male   (*continued*)

---

3. How might you start the conversation with J.B. about his cardiovascular risks and the benefits of lifestyle change?

4. Which lifestyle prescriptions would you offer initially to reduce his cardiovascular risks? What would you want to address in future visits?

5. What educational resources might you share with J.B.?

An Interprofessional Approach to Cardiovascular Conditions

APPs and other health professionals may collaborate to help patients with cardiovascular risk factors or conditions. The following professionals may be involved in addition to the primary care provider (physician, or APP), who is responsible for the coordination of the patient's health, handling minor acute concerns, and managing chronic conditions:

- Cardiology specialist: A physician, or APP whose scope is beyond primary care, specializing in the heart and blood vessels. Refer patients with resistant HTN, familial hypercholesterolemia, known ASCVD, AF, and those needing specialized cardiovascular testing and monitoring.

- Electrophysiologist (EP): A clinician whose cardiology subspecialty focuses on electrical issues in the heart. Refer patients with heart rhythm issues, unexplained syncope, ventricular tachycardia, severe bradycardia or Tachy-Brady syndrome, or second- or third-degree heart block on ECG.

- Other specialty providers to consult as needed include the following:
  - Nephrologist: Involve if any suspicion of cardiorenal syndrome or if having trouble managing BP.
  - Endocrinologist: Refer if having trouble managing blood sugars or if adrenal issues are suspected.

- Pulmonologist: Refer to evaluate sleep apnea and shortness of breath with potential pulmonary causes.

- Palliative care specialist: A clinician who specializes in optimizing the quality of life. Provide referral for patients of any age and any stage of a serious illness.

- Health coach: Refer for additional strategies and support for health behavior change.

- Cardiac rehabilitation program: A structured program that delivers supervised physical activity; education on the risk factors of CHD; and counseling on recommended lifestyle modifications, including diet, exercise, and stress management.

- Exercise specialist: Includes kinesiologists, personal trainers, and exercise physiologists, all of whom can develop fitness and exercise programs. Provide referrals for patients who need help creating a safe, progressive exercise program.

- Registered dietician nutritionist (RDN) or certified nutrition specialist (CNS): Specialists in diet and nutritional counseling. Provide referrals for patients with complex dietary needs such as renal diets.

- Psychologist, counselor, or therapist: Specialist in mental, emotional, and behavioral issues. Offer referrals for patients with high stress, anxiety, depression, trauma, or grief and loss.

- Social worker: Can assist with access to community resources as well as counseling and support groups.

TABLE 19.3	Evidence-Based Resources for Cardiovascular Health Promotion

Organization	Resource	URL
American College of Cardiology	ASCVD Risk Estimator Plus	https://tools.acc.org/ascvd-risk-estimator-plus/#!/calculate/estimate
American College of Cardiology	Guidelines and clinical documents	https://www.acc.org/guidelines
American College of Cardiology	CardioSmart: Patient education, tools for shared decision-making	https://www.cardiosmart.org
American Heart Association	Publications and resources for patients and healthcare professionals	https://www.heart.org
Multi-Ethnic Study of Atherosclerosis (MESA)	MESA 10-Year CHD risk with coronary artery calcification	https://www.mesa-nhlbi.org/MESACHDRisk/MesaRiskScore/RiskScore.aspx
National Heart, Lung, and Blood Institute	Publications and resources for patients and healthcare professionals	https://www.nhlbi.nih.gov

Health Promotion Activity: Computing a 10-year ASCVD Risk Score

- Estimate your 10-year atherosclerotic cardiovascular disease (ASCVD) risk score and that of an older relative using the ASCVD Plus app or website (or MESA risk calculator if CAC is known).
- Were you able to compute your risk score? If not, why? Were you at all surprised by the risk score results? What are the biggest factors that could be changed to reduce your future risk? Would your relative's risk score change if any medications were added, and if so, by how much?

Summary

Lifestyle plays a huge role in CVD. All patients should have a cardiovascular risk assessment performed routinely (see **Table 19.3**). APPs should provide counseling and encourage behavior change to optimize modifiable cardiovascular risk factors. The goal is CVD prevention and risk reduction. For those patients who already have CVD, the goal is to improve their quality of life and prevent secondary cardiovascular events. In some cases, CVD can be reversed. In other cases, the focus is on symptom management. In all cases, maximizing quality of life is key. The A-SMART lifestyle behaviors provide a framework for meeting those goals.

Acronyms

ACC: American College of Cardiology
ACC/AHA: American College of Cardiology and the American Heart Association
AF: atrial fibrillation
AHA: American Heart Association
APP: advanced practice provider
ASCVD: atherosclerotic cardiovascular disease
A-SMART: adopt healthy eating, stress less, move often, avoid alcohol, rest more, treat tobacco use

BP: blood pressure
CAC: coronary artery calcium
CHD: coronary heart disease
CVD: cardiovascular disease
DASH: Dietary Approaches to Stop Hypertension
DBP: diastolic blood pressure
HTN: hypertension
PCE: pooled cohort equation
SBP: systolic blood pressure

References

Aggarwal, M., Ornish, D., Josephson, R., Brown, T. M., Ostfeld, R. J., Gordon, N., Madan, S., Allen, K., Khetan, A., Mahmoud, A., Freeman, A. M., & Aspry, K. (2021). Closing gaps in lifestyle adherence for secondary prevention of coronary heart disease. *American Journal of Cardiology, 145*, 1–11. https://doi.org/10.1016/j.amjcard.2021.01.005

Ahmad, F. B., & Anderson, R. N. (2021). The leading causes of death in the US for 2020. *JAMA, 325*(18), 1829–1830. https://doi.org/10.1001/jama.2021.5469

Alfaddagh, A., Arps, K., Blumenthal, R., & Martin, S. S. (2019, March 21). *The ABCs of primary cardiovascular prevention: 2019 update.* American College of Cardiology. https://www.acc.org/latest-in-cardiology/articles/2019/03/21/14/39/abcs-of-primary-cv-prevention-2019-update-gl-prevention

American College of Cardiology. (n.d.). *Stop heart disease before it starts. CardioSmart.* https://www.cardiosmart.org/assets/infographic/stop-heart-disease-before-it-starts

American Heart Association. (2016). *Understand your risks to prevent a heart attack.* https://www.heart.org/en/health-topics/heart-attack/understand-your-risks-to-prevent-a-heart-attack

American Heart Association. (2022). *Life's Essential 8 fact sheet.* https://www.heart.org/en/healthy-living/healthy-lifestyle/lifes-essential-8/lifes-essential-8-fact-sheet

Arnett, D. K., Blumenthal, R. S., Albert, M. A., Buroker, A. B., Goldberger, Z. D., Hahn, E. J., Himmelfarb, C. D., Khera, A., Lloyd-Jones, D., McEvoy, J. W., Michos, E. D., Miedema, M. D., Muñoz, D., Smith, S. C., Virani, S. S., Williams, K. A., Yeboah, J., & Ziaeian, B. (2019). 2019 ACC/AHA Guideline on the Primary Prevention of Cardiovascular Disease: A report of the American College of Cardiology/American Heart Association Task Force on Clinical Practice Guidelines. *Circulation, 140*(11), e596–e646. https://doi.org/10.1161/CIR.0000000000000678

Arnett, D. K., Khera, A., & Blumenthal, R. S. (2019). 2019 ACC/AHA Guideline on the Primary Prevention of Cardiovascular Disease: Part 1, Lifestyle and Behavioral Factors. *JAMA Cardiology, 4*(10), 1043–1044. https://doi.org/10.1001/jamacardio.2019.2604

Billioux, A., Verlander, K., Anthony, S., & Alley, D. (2017, May 30). Standardized screening for health-related social needs in clinical settings: The Accountable Health Communities Screening Tool. *NAM Perspectives.* Discussion Paper, National Academy of Medicine. https://doi.org/10.31478/201705b

Bland, J. S. (2017). Cardiology meets personalized lifestyle medicine. *Integrative Medicine, 16*(6), 12–16.

Blumenthal, J. A., Babyak, M. A., Hinderliter, A., Watkins, L. L., Craighead, L., Lin, P.-H., Caccia, C., Johnson, J., Waugh, R., & Sherwood, J. (2010). Effects of the DASH diet alone and in combination with exercise and weight loss on blood pressure and cardiovascular biomarkers in men and women with high blood pressure: The ENCORE Study. *Archives of Internal Medicine, 170*(2), 126–135. https://doi.org/10.1001/archinternmed.2009.470

Cifu, A. S., & Davis, A. M. (2017). Prevention, detection, evaluation, and management of high blood pressure in adults. *JAMA, 318*(21), 2132–2134. https://doi.org/10.1001/jama.2017.18706

Elmer, P. J., Obarzanek, E., Vollmer, W. M., Simons-Morton, D., Stevens, V. J., Young, D. R., Lin, P.-H., Champagne, C., Harsha, D. W., Svetkey, L. P., Ard, J., Brantley, P. J., Proschan, M. A., Erlinger, T. P., & Appel, L. J. (2006). Effects of comprehensive lifestyle modification on diet, weight, physical fitness, and blood pressure control: 18-month results of a randomized trial. *Annals of Internal Medicine, 144*(7), 485. https://doi.org/10.7326/0003-4819-144-7-200604040-00007

Esselstyn, C., & Golubic, M. (2014). The nutritional reversal of cardiovascular disease: Fact or fiction? Three case reports. *Experimental and Clinical Cardiology, 20*(7), 1901–1908.

Esselstyn, C. B., Jr., Gendy, G., Doyle, J., Golubic, M., & Roizen, M. F. (2014). A way to reverse CAD? *Journal of Family Practice, 63*(7), 356–364.

Estruch, R., Ros, E., Salas-Salvadó, J., Covas, M. I., Corella, D., Arós, F., Gómez-Gracia, E., Ruiz-Gutiérrez, V., Fiol, M., Lapetra, J., Lamuela-Raventos, R. M., Serra-Majem, L., Pintó, X., Basora, J., Muñoz, M. A., Sorlí, J. V., Martínez, J. A., & Martínez-González, M. A. (2013). Primary prevention of cardiovascular disease with a Mediterranean diet. *New England Journal of Medicine, 368*(14), 1279–1290. https://doi.org/10.1056/NEJMoa1200303

Estruch, R., Ros, E., Salas-Salvadó, J., Covas, M. I., Corella, D., Arós, F., Gómez-Gracia, E., Ruiz-Gutiérrez, V., Fiol, M., Lapetra, J., Lamuela-Raventos, R. M., Serra-Majem, L., Pintó, X., Basora, J., Muñoz, M. A., Sorlí, J. V., Martínez, J. A., & Martínez-González, M. A. (2018). Primary prevention of cardiovascular disease with a Mediterranean diet supplemented with extra-virgin olive oil or nuts. *New England Journal of Medicine, 378*(25), e34. https://doi.org/10.1056/NEJMoa1800389

Filippou, C. D., Tsioufis, C. P., Thomopoulos, C. G., Mihas, C. C., Dimitriadis, K. S., Sotiropoulou, L. I., Chrysochoou, C. A., Nihoyannopoulos, P. I., & Tousoulis, D. M. (2020). Dietary Approaches to Stop Hypertension (DASH) diet and blood pressure reduction in adults with and without hypertension: A systematic review and meta-analysis of randomized controlled trials. *Advances in Nutrition, 11*(5), 1150–1160. https://doi.org/ 10.1093/advances/nmaa041

Fryar, C. D., Ostchega, Y., Hales, C. M., Zhang, G., & Kruszon-Moran, D. (2017, October). *Hypertension prevalence and control among adults: United States, 2015–2016*. Centers for Disease Control and Prevention. https://www.cdc.gov/nchs/data/databriefs/db289.pdf

Funk, K. L., Elmer, P. J., Stevens, V. J., Harsha, D. W., Craddick, S. R., Lin, P.-H., Young, D. R., Champagne, C. M., Brantley, P. J., McCarron, P. B., Simons-Morton, D. G., & Appel, L. J. (2008). PREMIER—A trial of lifestyle interventions for blood pressure control: Intervention design and rationale. *Health Promotion Practice, 9*(3), 271–280. https://doi.org/10.1177/1524839906289035

Goldstein, C. M., Josephson, R., Xie, S., & Hughes, J. W. (2012). Current perspectives on the use of meditation to reduce blood pressure. *International Journal of Hypertension, 2012*, 1–11. https://doi.org/10.1155/2012/578397

Grundy, S. M., Stone, N. J., Bailey, A. L., Beam, C., Birtcher, K. K., Blumenthal, R. S., Braun, L. T., de Ferranti, S., Faiella-Tommasino, J., Forman, D. E., Goldberg, R., Heidenreich, P. A., Hlatky, M. A., Jones, D. W., Lloyd-Jones, D., Lopez-Pajares, N., Ndumele,

C. E., Orringer, C. E., Peralta, C. A., . . . Yeboah, J. (2019). 2018 AHA/ACC/AACVPR/AAPA/ABC/ACPM/ADA/AGS/APhA/ASPC/NLA/PCNA Guideline on the Management of Blood Cholesterol: A report of the American College of Cardiology/American Heart Association Task Force on Clinical Practice Guidelines. *Circulation, 139*, e1082–e1143. https://doi.org/10.1161/CIR.0000000000000625

Hajar, R. (2017). Risk factors for coronary artery disease: Historical perspectives. *Heart Views, 18*(3), 109–114. https://doi.org/10.4103/heartviews.heartviews_106_17

Haseeb, S., Alexander, B., & Baranchuk, A. (2017). Wine and cardiovascular health: A comprehensive review. *Circulation, 136*(15), 1434–1448. https://doi.org/10.1161/CIRCULATIONAHA.117.030387

Hinderliter, A. L., Sherwood, A., Craighead, L. W., Lin, P.-H., Watkins, L., Babyak, M. A., & Blumenthal, J. A. (2014). The long-term effects of lifestyle change on blood pressure: One-year follow-up of the ENCORE study. *American Journal of Hypertension, 27*(5), 734–741. https://doi.org/10.1093/ajh/hpt183

Kahleova, H., Levin, S., & Barnard, N. (2018). Vegetarian dietary patterns and cardiovascular disease. *Progress in Cardiovascular Diseases, 61*(1), 54–61. https://doi.org/10.1016/j.pcad.2018.05.002

Khera, A. V., Emdin, C. A., Drake, I., Natarajan, P., Bick, A. G., Cook, N. R., Chasman, D. I., Baber, U., Mehran, R., Rader, D. J., Fuster, V., Boerwinkle, E., Melander, O., Orho-Melander, M., Ridker, P. M., & Kathiresan, S. (2016). Genetic risk, adherence to a healthy lifestyle, and coronary disease. *New England Journal of Medicine, 375*, 2349–2358. https://doi.org/ 10.1056/NEJMoa1605086

Kochanek, K. D., Murphy, S. L., Xu, J., & Arias, E. (2019, June 24). Deaths: Final data for 2017. *National Vital Statistics Report, 68*(9), 1–77. Centers for Disease Control and Prevention. https://www.cdc.gov/nchs/data/nvsr/nvsr68/nvsr68_09-508.pdf

Kondo, T., Nakano, Y., Adachi, S., & Murohara, T. (2019). Effects of tobacco smoking on cardiovascular disease. *Circulation Journal, 83*(10), 1980–1985. https://doi.org/10.1253/circj.CJ-19-0323

Kwok, C. S., Kontopantelis, E., Kuligowski, G., Gray, M., Muhyaldeen, A., Gale, C. P., Peat, G. M., Cleator, J., Chew-Graham, C., Loke, Y. K., & Mamas, M. A. (2018). Self-reported sleep duration and quality and cardiovascular disease and mortality: A dose-response meta-analysis. *Journal of the American Heart Association, 7*(15), e008552. https://doi.org/ 10.1161/JAHA.118.008552

Levine, G. N., Lange, R. A., Bairey-Merz, C. N., Davidson, R. J., Jamerson, K., Mehta, P. K., Michos, E. D., Norris, K., Ray, I. B., Saban, K. L., Shah, T., Stein, R., Smith, S. C., American Heart Association Council on Clinical Cardiology, Council on Cardiovascular and Stroke Nursing, & Council on Hypertension.

(2017). Meditation and cardiovascular risk reduction: A scientific statement from the American Heart Association. *Journal of the American Heart Association*, 6, e002218. https://doi.org/10.1161/JAHA.117.002218

Lloyd-Jones, D. M., Braun, L. T., Ndumele, C. E., Smith, S. C., Jr., Sperling, L. S., Virani, S. S., & Blumenthal, R. S. (2019). Use of risk assessment tools to guide decision-making in the primary prevention of atherosclerotic cardiovascular disease. *Journal of the American College of Cardiology*, 73(24), 3153–3167. https://doi.org/10.1016/j.jacc.2018.11.005

Makarem, N., Castro-Diehl, C., St-Onge, M., Redline, S., Shea, S., Lloyd-Jones, D., Ning, H., & Aggarwal, B. (2020). Abstract 36: The role of sleep as a cardiovascular health metric: Does it improve cardiovascular disease risk prediction? Results from the Multi-Ethnic Study of Atherosclerosis. *Circulation*, 141(Suppl 1). https://doi.org/10.1161/circ.141.suppl_1.36

Mosca, L., Barrett-Connor, E., & Wenger, N. K. (2011). Sex/gender differences in cardiovascular disease prevention: What a difference a decade makes. *Circulation*, 124(19), 2145–2154. https://doi.org/10.1161/CIRCULATIONAHA.110.968792

Nabel, E. G., & Braunwald, E. (2012). A tale of coronary artery disease and myocardial infarction. *New England Journal of Medicine*, 366(1), 54–63. https://doi.org/10.1056/NEJMra1112570

National Heart, Blood, and Lung Institute. (2012, October). *Expert panel on integrated guidelines for cardiovascular health and risk reduction in children and adolescents, summary report.* https://www.nhlbi.nih.gov/files/docs/peds_guidelines_sum.pdf

Office on Smoking and Health. (2014). *The health consequences of smoking—50 years of progress: A report of the Surgeon General.* Centers for Disease Control and Prevention, National Center for Chronic Disease Prevention and Health Promotion. https://www.ncbi.nlm.nih.gov/books/NBK179276

Ornish, D. M., Scherwitz, L. W., Billings, J. H., Gould, L. M., Merritt, T. A., Sparler, S., Armstrong, W. T., Ports, T. A., Kirkeeide, R. L., Hogeboom, C., & Brand, R. J. (1998). Intensive lifestyle changes for reversal of coronary heart disease. *JAMA*, 280(23), 2001–2007. https://doi.org/10.1001/jama.280.23.2001

Satija, A., Bhupathiraju, S. N., Spiegelman, D., Chiuve, S. E., Manson, J. E., Willett, W., Rexrode, K. M., Rimm, E. B., & Hu, F. B. (2017). Healthful and unhealthful plant-based diets and the risk of coronary heart disease in U.S. adults. *Journal of the American College of Cardiology*, 70(4), 411–422. https://doi.org/10.1016/j.jacc.2017.05.047

Shi, L., Zhang, D., Wang, L., Zhuang, J., Cook, R., & Chen, L. (2017). Meditation and blood pressure: A meta-analysis of randomized clinical trials.

Journal of Hypertension, 35(4), 696–706. https://doi.org/10.1097/HJH.0000000000001217

Tasnim, S., Tang, C., Musini, V. M., & Wright, J. M. (2020). Effect of alcohol on blood pressure. *Cochrane Database of Systematic Reviews*, 7(7), CD012787. https://doi.org/10.1002/14651858.CD012787.pub2

Teng, Y., Yang, S., Chen, Y., Guo, Y., Hu, Y., Zhang, P., Cao, J., Zhang, X., Chen, Y., Jiang, C., Liu, T., & Zeng, F. (2020). Review of clinical trials on the effects of tai chi practice on primary hypertension: The current state of study design and quality control. *Evidence-Based Complementary and Alternative Medicine*, 2020, Article 6637489, 1–9. https://doi.org/10.1155/2020/6637489

Unger, T., Borghi, C., Charchar, F., Khan, N. A., Poulter, N. R., Prabhakaran, D., Ramirez, A., Schlaich, M., Stergiou, G. S., Tomaszewski, M., Wainford, R. D., Williams, B., & Schutte, A. E. (2020). 2020 International Society of Hypertension Global Hypertension Practice Guidelines. *Hypertension*, 75(6), 1334–1357. https://doi.org/10.1161/HYPERTENSIONAHA.120.15026

U.S. Department of Agriculture & U.S. Department of Health and Human Services. (2020). *Dietary guidelines for Americans, 2020–2025* (9th ed.). www.dietaryguidelines.gov

U.S. Department of Health and Human Services. (2018). *Physical activity guidelines for Americans* (2nd ed.). https://health.gov/sites/default/files/2019-09/Physical_Activity_Guidelines_2nd_edition.pdf

Van Horn, L., Carson, J. A. S., Appel, L. J., Burke, L. E., Economos, C., Karmally, W., Lancaster, K., Lichtenstein, A. H., Johnson, R. K., Thomas, R. J., Vos, M., Wylie-Rosett, J., & Kris-Etherton, P. (2016). Recommended dietary pattern to achieve adherence to the American Heart Association/American College of Cardiology (AHA/ACC) Guidelines: A scientific statement from the American Heart Association. *Circulation*, 134, e505–e529. https://doi.org/10.1161/CIR.0000000000000462

Virani, S. S., Alonso, A., Aparicio, H. J., Benjamin, E. J., Bittencourt, M. S., Callaway, C. W., Carson, A. P., Chamberlain, A. M., Cheng, S., Delling, F. N., Elkind, M. S. V., Evenson, K. R., Ferguson, J. F., Gupta, D. K., Khan, S. S., Kissela, B. M., Knutson, K. L., Lee, C. D., Lewis, T. T., . . . American Heart Association Council on Epidemiology and Prevention Statistics Committee and Stroke Statistics Subcommittee. (2021). Heart disease and stroke statistics—2021 update: A report from the American Heart Association. *Circulation*, 143(8), e254–e743. https://doi.org/10.1161/CIR.0000000000000950

Whelton, P. K., Carey, R. M., Aronow, W. S., Casey, D. E., Jr., Collins, K. J., Himmelfarb, C. D., DePalma, S. M., Gidding, S., Jamerson, K. A., Jones, D. W., MacLaughlin, E. J., Munter, P., Ovbiagele, P., Smith, S. C., Jr., Spencer, C. C., Stafford, R. S., Taler, S. J., Thomas, R.

J., Williams, K. A., Sr., . . . Wright, J. T., Jr. (2018). 2017 ACC/AHA/AAPA/ABC/ACPM/AGS/APhA/ASH/ASPC/NMA/PCNA Guideline for the prevention, detection, evaluation, and management of high blood pressure in adults: Executive summary: A report of the American College of Cardiology/American Heart Association Task Force on Clinical Practice Guidelines. *Hypertension*, *71*(6), 1269–1324. https://doi.org/10.1161/HYP.0000000000000066

World Heart Federation. (2022). *The impact of alcohol consumption on cardiovascular health: Myths and measures. A World Heart Federation policy brief.* https://world-heart-federation.org/wp-content/uploads/WHF-Policy-Brief-Alcohol.pdf

Yan, B., Yang, J., Zhao, B., Fan, Y., Wang, W., & Ma, X. (2021). Objective sleep efficiency predicts cardiovascular disease in a community population: The Sleep Heart Health Study. *Journal of the American Heart Association*, *10*(7), e016201. https://doi.org/10.1161/JAHA.120.016201

Yusuf, S., Hawken, S., Ôunpuu, S., Dans, T., Avezum, A., Lanas, F., McQueen, M., Budaj, A., Pais, P., Varigos, J., Lisheng, L., & INTERHEART Study Investigators. (2004). Effect of potentially modifiable risk factors associated with myocardial infarction in 52 countries (the INTERHEART study): Case-control study. *Lancet*, *364*(9438), 937–952. https://doi.org/10.1016/S0140-6736(04)17018-9

CHAPTER 20

Reducing Chronic Pain Through Lifestyle Behaviors

Connie R. Kartoz, PhD, RN, MS, FNP-BC

Although the world is full of suffering, it is also full of the overcoming of it.

Helen Keller

OBJECTIVES

This chapter will enable the reader to:

1. Identify the most common causes of chronic pain in the United States.
2. Recognize the effect on quality of life for patients with chronic pain.
3. Complete holistic patient and family assessments for those experiencing chronic pain.
4. Identify A-SMART goals for patient care related to activity level, sleep, and counseling.
5. Engage with an interprofessional team in the care of individuals with chronic pain.
6. Create holistic, nonpharmacological, and person-centered plans of care to improve the quality of life for patients experiencing chronic pain.

Overview

Chronic pain affects 50 million adults in the United States, nearly one in five adults (Dahlhamer et al., 2018), and results in costs of $635 billion per year (National Center for Complementary and Integrative Health, 2020). Some patients experience chronic pain related to a well-defined condition such as rheumatoid arthritis (RA) while others struggle with discomfort from poorly understood conditions such as fibromyalgia. For many of these patients, pharmacological or surgical solutions are insufficient to control pain, or they lead to substantial adverse effects, such as opioid addiction. Given that the United States has a National Pain Strategy calling for interprofessional and holistic interventions (Interagency Pain Research Coordinating Committee [IPRCC], 2016), advanced practice providers (APPs)

© Kathleen Gail/Shutterstock; © StoryTime Studio/Shutterstock; © kali9/Getty Images

need to be knowledgeable about chronic pain and evidence-informed interventions to reduce the burden on individuals, families, and communities. This chapter aims to provide information about select chronic pain conditions, professional guidelines for patients with chronic pain, and evidence-informed lifestyle management strategies for reducing the morbidity resulting from chronic pain states.

Definition of Chronic Pain

Definitions of chronic pain are varied. The International Association for the Study of Pain (IASP) provides a broad definition of *pain*: "An unpleasant sensory and emotional experience associated with, or resembling that associated with, actual or potential tissue damage" (IASP, 2021, Definition of Pain, para. 1). *Chronic pain* is defined as pain lasting more than three months (Treede et al., 2019). The IPRCC (2016) further adds that pain should be experienced more than half the days.

The International Classification of Diseases 11 (ICD-11) contains a new diagnostic category for chronic pain (see **Table 20.1**). This new classification identifies chronic pain as a disease entity and identifies seven diagnostic codes for chronic pain (Treede et al., 2019). Within the definition and classification of chronic pain, APPs may consider differentiating between existing pain and pain that significantly affects function. *High impact chronic pain* is defined as pain that results in a "substantial restriction of participation in work, social, and self-care activities for six months or more" (IPRCC, 2016, p. 11). Based on these new diagnostic categories, APPs will recognize the broad and complex nature of chronic pain.

Epidemiology

The National Health Interview Survey indicates chronic pain affects 20% of the U.S. population, with approximately 8% of adults

Table 20.1 ICD-11 Diagnosis Codes for Chronic Pain

Code	Description
MG30.0	Chronic primary pain
MG30.1	Chronic cancer pain
MG30.2	Chronic postsurgical and posttraumatic pain
MG30.3	Chronic musculoskeletal pain
MG30.4	Chronic visceral pain
MG30.5	Chronic neuropathic pain
MG30.6	Chronic headache and orofacial pain

Data from Treede, R.-D., Rief, W., Barke, A., Aziz, Q., Bennett, M. I., Benoliel, R., Cohen, M., Evers, S., Finnerup, N. B., First, M. B., Giamberardino, M. A., Kaasa, S., Korwisi, B., Kosek, E., Lavand'homme, B., Nicholas, M., Perrot, S., Scholz, J., Schug, S., . . . Wang, S. (2019). Chronic pain as a symptom or a disease: The IASP Classification of Chronic Pain for the International Classification of Diseases (ICD-11). *PAIN, 160*(1), 19–27. https://doi.org/10.1097/j.pain.0000000000001384

in the United States experiencing high impact chronic pain (Dahlhamer et al., 2018). A considerable variety of noncancerous conditions cause chronic pain, with chronic widespread pain (CWP) being one of the most commonly experienced conditions within chronic pain conditions, affecting approximately 10% of the U.S. population (Mansfield et al., 2016). The 2016 survey of outpatient office visits demonstrates that chronic pain conditions are some of the most common reasons for seeking care. After respiratory conditions (9.6% of office visits), musculoskeletal concerns are the second most common reason for seeking primary care, accounting for 8.3% of visits (Rui & Okeyode, 2016).

Chronic pain is similarly noted as a common reason to seek care worldwide. A global systematic review exploring reasons to seek primary care reported back pain and headache in the top 10 reasons to access care

(Finley et al., 2018). Older adults have an apparent higher prevalence, with estimates approaching 30% at age 50 (Grol-Prokopczyk, 2017). Women, those living in rural areas, and individuals living in poverty also have a higher prevalence of chronic pain. Other groups with higher prevalence are non-Hispanic Whites and veterans (Dahlhamer et al., 2018; Kim et al., 2020). Additional risk factors for chronic pain include a previous history of chronic pain, life stressors, physical inactivity, psychological comorbidities, and impaired sleep (Generaal et al., 2017; Lindell & Grimby-Eckman, 2022; Schneiderhan & Orizondo, 2017).

Pathophysiology

While a multiplicity of pathologies cause chronic pain, including inflammatory and noninflammatory arthritis, headaches, neuropathic pain, and other musculoskeletal multifocal conditions such as low back pain (LBP) and CWP, there is no single clear etiology for chronic pain syndromes. Some of the most common conditions for primary care chronic pain visits include osteoarthritis (OA) (1.3% of visits), RA (0.6%), migraine (0.5%), and LBP (0.3%) (Rui & Okeyode, 2016). The variation in causes of chronic pain limits a comprehensive discussion of the pathophysiology of each specific condition. However, such understanding may become available because the new ICD-11 contains a unique classification for chronic pain, suggesting a unifying pathophysiology and experience (Treede et al., 2015).

Normal Pain Response

Pain perception, a conscious process, is only part of the human response to noxious stimuli. In acute pain, a stimulus affects a receptor, which then causes an impulse to travel via the afferent pathway through the spinal cord to the central nervous system. Nociceptive and non-nociceptive nerve fibers are involved in the transmission of the impulse.

Thus begins the balancing act of signal transmission (e.g., nociceptive fibers) and the pain arc, which in acute pain serves to direct automated and more complex responses to pain. Inhibitory responses, which inhibit nerve cell firing along the path, are part of that arc. The reflex arc occurs first at the spinal cord level and can direct rapid and automated responses such as jerking a hand away from noxious stimuli (see **Figure 20.1**). Inflammatory substances such as serotonin, prostaglandins, and bradykinins are released in the periphery at this point as well.

In the central nervous system, pain is processed in three dimensions, sensory, affective, and cognitive, and involves the immune, endocrine, and nervous systems (Berger & Zelman, 2016). The sensory component of pain includes the typical APP assessment of "intensity, location, quality, and duration" (Dlugasch & Story, 2021, p. 668). The affective dimension becomes quite important in chronic pain and includes the overall level of *unpleasantness* for a person and the response to the pain. Several components mitigate pain intensity, one being activation in the midbrain and medulla, which results in the release of inhibitory neurotransmitters such as serotonin, epinephrine, and norepinephrine. Finally, the cognitive dimension includes considerations of culture, the meaning of pain to the individual, and the context in which the pain is experienced (Dlugasch & Story, 2021).

Chronic Pain Response

For those with chronic pain or pain that continues over time, the well-established acute pain arc becomes damaged (Berger & Zelman, 2016). Nociceptive and slower C fibers repeatedly fire in chronic pain, causing sensitization and enhanced perception of pain (Dlugasch & Story, 2021). Researchers are now beginning to understand that dysfunction can span all the body systems that regulate pain (i.e., immune, endocrine, and nervous systems). For example, there is evidence of

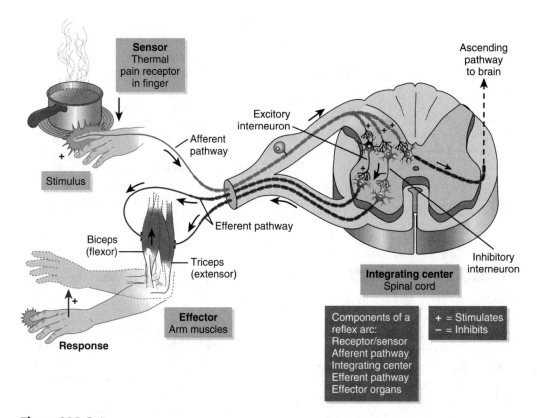

Figure 20.1 Reflex arc.

Data from Dlugasch, L., & Story, L. (2021). *Applied pathophysiology for the advanced practice nurse.* Jones & Bartlett Learning

hypothalamic-pituitary-adrenal (HPA) axis dysfunction and chronically elevated cortisol levels, leading to depression, weight gain, and hyperglycemia (Berger & Zelman, 2016).

Chronic pain states often include entities that involve nerve cells. Diabetic neuropathy and CWP have different etiologies but share common pathophysiological processes. Patients with painful polyneuropathy have elevated inflammatory cytokines, such as tumor necrosis factor alpha (TNF-α), interleukin 2 (IL-2), and interleukin 10 (IL-10). In contrast, those with chronic pain states such as CWP have lower levels of the anti-inflammatory cytokine interleukin 4 (IL-4) (Sommer et al., 2018). Novel cellular research suggests that miRNA (microRNA material, which does not code for proteins) may play a role in chronic pain such as migraine and arthritis (Sommer et al., 2018), thus reflecting an

increasingly accepted view that immune system imbalance contributes to chronic inflammation and pain. The involvement of genetic material in the development of chronic pain is supported by studies that find an increased incidence of CWP among twins (Vehof et al., 2014).

Biopsychosocial Model

While the cellular explanations may provide treatment targets for the future, it may be more helpful to consider and evaluate patients with chronic pain using established functional models of pain. The biopsychosocial model of pain includes considerations of pain's biological, psychological, and social underpinnings (Paice, 2016). The National Pain Strategy suggests that this is the optimal model for evaluating and caring for patients with chronic pain (IPRCC, 2016). In this model, the APP should consider the pathophysiology of the pain condition (e.g., cartilage damage in OA) and the biological effect of treatments (e.g., surgery) and pharmacological agents the patient takes. Psychological influences on pain include anxiety, anger, depression, and sleep disorders (Barrett & Chang, 2016). Finally, social effects on pain include the level of social support, which can include financial support (Paice, 2016). An additional component of the response to pain emanates from early social learning about how one should respond to pain (Berger & Zelman, 2016) and thus connects the cultural component to the experience of chronic pain. The following section includes a more detailed discussion of these biopsychosocial influences on chronic pain.

The patient's psychological state may increase the risk of chronic pain (Schneiderhan & Orizondo, 2017). Because depression and anxiety are common comorbidities (IPRCC, 2016; National Center for Complementary and Integrative Health, 2020), APPs should recognize that the psychological state of the patient with chronic pain is important to consider. Patients with chronic pain often demonstrate difficulty with emotional regulation and may have higher levels of catastrophizing about pain and lower levels of pain acceptance (Aaron et al., 2020). These psychological responses have a complex effect on pain levels, quality of life (QOL), and functionality yet are amenable to treatment (Craner et al., 2017).

The context, social, and family settings in which patients with chronic pain exist affect and are affected by chronic pain. The greater the levels of perceived pain, the more a patient's interactions with recreation and work are reduced (IPRCC, 2016). Not surprisingly, such withdrawal from routine activities negatively affects the family system (Boone & Kim, 2019). As with social functioning and engagement, families in which a member is dealing with chronic pain have higher levels of conflict, which may increase pain levels. Spouses may experience role strain because they take on more responsibilities for individuals who may not work. Non-spouse family members' levels of depression and functioning also affect a patient's pain level (Boone & Kim, 2019).

An additional layer is that of one's culture. Patients' cultural background can affect nearly all aspects of the pain experience, including how they communicate pain, beliefs about their pain, and coping methods (Sharma et al., 2018). How others around the patients respond to them and provide (or do not provide) empathy also relates to cultural learnings. In a meta-analysis of qualitative studies about the lived experience of older adults living with arthritic pain, Chen et al. (2020) noted that an expectation of bearing one's pain and not expressing or complaining about it might transcend varied ethnic backgrounds yet is common in the cultural milieu of the elderly. In our multicultural society, individuals working to manage a chronic pain state may encounter one set of expectations at home, another in their local community, and yet another in a work environment. Examples of cultural influence are wide ranging. The intersection of culture and stress can be seen in immigrant populations, where both qualitative and quantitative data suggest that immigrants may be at additional risk for lower QOL and higher levels of pain compared to their counterparts living in the country of origin (Kim et al., 2020; Nyen & Tviet, 2018). Latino manual workers frequently report musculoskeletal pain, affecting 17% of non-farmworkers and 7% of farmworkers in a sample (n = 445) of North Carolina manual laborers (Tribble et al., 2016).

Effect of Chronic Pain

For individuals with chronic pain, the effect on their life is broad, interconnected, and substantive. The overall QOL is reduced, and there are several comorbidities, especially for their mental health. Finally, even mortality rates are increased for patients with a chronic pain diagnosis (Nijs et al., 2020).

Quality of Life

Multiple studies support that, overall, QOL is adversely affected by chronic pain. Health-related quality of life (HRQOL) is noted by the Centers for Disease Control and Prevention to be a broad-ranging concept that includes positive and negative dimensions of life (CDC, 2020). It involves physical health, such as discomfort, and mental health, such as mood and energy. This concept reflects the biopsychosocial model of pain in consideration of physical, emotional, personal, and social effects on daily living. Improving HRQOL is a common, fundamental, and recommended goal in caring for those with chronic pain (IPRCC, 2016).

In a medium-sized study of 591 patients with chronic pain and 150 without chronic pain in the midwestern United States, Kawai et al. (2017) found that about 25% of patients with chronic pain noted difficulty with daily activities, including work. In a small sample ($n = 85$) of patients with new-onset chronic low back pain (CLBP), all patients had lower than normal/optimal scores on QOL measures (Majlesi, 2019). In a Brazilian sample ($n = 132$) of patients with CLBP, QOL was also lower than standard averages. Emotion-related QOL and fear of movement due to pain were significantly inversely correlated ($r = -0.41$, $p < 0.01$) (Comachio et al., 2018). These findings suggest that reduced QOL is cross-cultural. Because of the heterogeneity of the causes of chronic pain, the literature is difficult to generalize, which supports the need for individual and holistic patient assessments.

Comorbidities

Individuals experiencing chronic pain often have several psychiatric and medical comorbidities. It is unclear whether these conditions are caused by or are a result of pain, but the APP must be aware of the increase in the prevalence of these comorbidities, then screen for them and intervene as necessary. Data are somewhat limited regarding the effect on pain itself, but the APP will recognize that

addressing these comorbid conditions should improve QOL. Depression, anxiety, and substance abuse are associated with chronic pain (Barrett & Chang, 2016; Tribble et al., 2016). Patients with a chronic pain diagnosis were found to have higher rates of obesity and sleep difficulty in a large Norwegian study, and the presence of these comorbidities predicted continuing chronic pain (Mundal et al., 2014). Unfortunately, data also suggest that chronic pain is associated with increased mortality risk (MRR 1.22, 95% CI 0.93–1.60) (Smith et al., 2014). Results from a large retrospective study of suicide decedents from 18 states identified that nearly 10% of those who died by suicide had evidence of chronic pain (Petrosky et al., 2018).

Opioid Addiction

Another unfortunate comorbidity is opioid addiction. Palermo and Kerns (2020) discuss the now well-understood harmful whirlwind of a medical model of care and the availability of opioids as elements leading to this crisis, which significantly affected patients in chronic pain. Although reducing pain was a laudable clinical goal, the evidence now suggests that while opioids may reduce acute pain, in chronic pain, such treatment may increase pain and is associated with addiction and suicide (U.S. Department of Health and Human Services [HHS], 2019; Palermo & Kerns, 2020). The person-centered A-SMART (adopt healthy eating, stress less, move often, avoid alcohol, rest more, and treat tobacco use) interventions align with national strategies to provide compassionate, evidence-informed care that reduces opioid prescribing and emphasizes a nonpharmacological approach (Dowell et al., 2019).

Chronic Pain Guidelines

There are three categories of guidelines available to the APP in assessing and managing patients with chronic pain. The first relates to the rational and safe prescribing of medication (which is beyond the scope of this chapter). For example, the CDC provides a guideline for safely prescribing opioids for patients who need these medications (Dowell et al., 2016). As important as the safe use of prescribing opioids is the tapering, or deprescribing, of opioids. The CDC pocket guide suggests considering a taper when opioid use seems to be imparting a limited benefit, is associated with signs of a substance use disorder, or there is an overdose event. A person-centered plan includes a slow decrease in dose by 10% per month and the inclusion of interprofessional team members such as psychology and social workers (CDC, n.d.). An interprofessional group has recently published recommendations for nonsteroidal anti-inflammatory drug (NSAID) use in patients with hypertension, cardiovascular, renal, or gastrointestinal comorbidities (Szeto et al., 2020).

Other guidelines are disease or body location specific. For example, the North American Spine Society (NASS, 2020) provides guidelines for LBP. These guidelines incorporate input from an interprofessional panel, and the recommendations are holistic and cover the assessment of patients through treatment. Grade A recommendations for assessment include consideration of psychosocial factors and work status. Cognitive behavioral therapy (CBT) and physical therapy with patient education about preventive care hold a Grade A recommendation. Acupuncture is also a recommended intervention in CLBP. Additionally, lifestyle interventions such as aerobic exercise should be part of the plan of care (NASS, 2020).

Another disease-specific guideline from the American College of Rheumatology covers OA of the hand, hip, and knee (Kolasinski et al., 2020). It is similarly holistic and interprofessional, reflecting the biopsychosocial model of pain. Exercise and weight loss benefit patients with knee and hip OA. Physical therapy and activity programs that utilize a range of modalities, such as tai chi, taping, acupuncture, orthotics, and bracing, carry a strong

recommendation. As with other pain guidelines, patient education for self-management improves the QOL and reduces pain (Kolasinski et al., 2020).

Finally, guidelines and guiding principles are available for treating chronic pain from any source. HHS (2019) provides a comprehensive, interprofessional set of recommendations for pain management. While there are considerations for psychological counseling and physical activities such as tai chi and yoga, these recommendations lack a detailed discussion of other lifestyle interventions. The recommendations are broad and include national goals for research and dissemination priorities. One core recommendation is for the development of self-care management programs that can be delivered in a wide range of communities and settings and that include information for patients about the pathophysiology of pain, are culturally appropriate, and are available in a variety of languages. Additional goals include documenting and addressing disparities in care and improving access to interprofessional programs (HHS, 2019). See **Table 20.5** at the end of the chapter for links to some of the available guidelines and resources for chronic pain conditions.

Starting the Conversation

APPs must recognize that patients in chronic pain have been living with a painful condition for at least six months. Likely, individuals and families have had multiple encounters with the healthcare system, and these encounters may be less than fully satisfying (Hadi et al., 2017). Gruß et al. (2020) reported findings from a mixed-methods study that suggest excellent communication skills by primary care providers can lead to high patient care satisfaction. Nonjudgmental listening and education were associated with higher satisfaction, even when pain persisted. According to Calabrese (2020), the evidence supporting empathy

Health Promotion Research Study

Lifestyle Interventions for Chronic Pain

Background: The objective of this study was to develop a lifestyle-based intervention program for individuals with chronic pain and then evaluate patient benefits.

Methodology: The program included nine weekly educational sessions covering content related to nutrition, activity levels, and CBT. This randomized controlled trial enrolled 279 participants. The outcomes included level of pain, QOL, depression, and anxiety scales.

Results: The intervention group had improvement across all measures, as indicated by the effect size of the benefit. The largest effect size (0.79) was found in the mental health measures of reduced anxiety and depression scores.

Implications for Advanced Practice: This study demonstrates that holistically derived programs are feasible and have good outcomes for patients with chronic pain. The focus on lifestyle interventions supports the interventions noted in this chapter.

Reference: Morales, F. A., Jimenez, M. J. M., Morales, A. J. M., Vegara, R. M., Mora, B. A. M., Aranda, G. M., & Canca, S. J. C. (2021). Impact of a nurse-led intervention on quality of life in patients with chronic non-malignant pain: An open randomized controlled trial. *Journal of Advanced Nursing, 77*(1), 255–265. https://doi.org/10.1111/jan.14608

within the patient encounter is expanding and suggests that active listening and empathy likely improve the QOL and reduce pain levels in rheumatology patients. Thus, the first step in assessing a patient with chronic pain is to listen. Additional data suggest that the quality of the patients' relationship in terms of confidence in their providers may also improve response to interventions (Lee et al., 2020).

Once APPs establish that patients are living with chronic pain, they should ask if the patients want to discuss it further during this or a future visit. Patients may be seeing multiple clinicians and may not be interested in further discussing their pain. A holistic approach to assessment will allow the APP to understand if possible lifestyle interventions are likely to reduce pain, improve QOL, and increase function. The APP should be mindful that patients may not be ready to implement such changes. Following principles of motivational interviewing techniques may help clinicians maintain a trusting and respectful patient–provider relationship, laying the groundwork for future encounters and interventions. For patients who may be ready to discuss how lifestyle interventions can affect their experience of pain, a simple question such as *What do you know about the effect of lifestyle factors, such as diet, stress, exercise, sleep, and use of tobacco and alcohol, on your chronic pain?* can open the door to deeper discussions and identify patients willing to engage in lifestyle modification for pain reduction and improvement in QOL.

Chronic Pain Assessment

Because of the complexity and individuality of chronic pain, a comprehensive, holistic, and family-centered assessment is essential to create a mutually derived plan of care for the patient (HHS, 2019; NASS, 2020). Chronic pain often coexists with multiple medical and psychiatric conditions such as substance abuse and depression, indicating that the APP must assess mental and physical health in patients with a complaint of pain lasting more than six months (Barrett & Chang, 2016; NASS,

2020). A comprehensive mental health assessment will also include consideration of substance use. Previous use or misuse and family history are risk factors for substance use disorder (HHS, 2020). This type of comprehensive health assessment represents the core of what APPs need to understand to create a plan of care. Still, additional components are likely necessary to reduce pain substantially and increase patients' QOL.

The APP is encouraged to include some functional assessments (Ballantyne & Sullivan, 2016). APPs who regularly see large numbers of patients with chronic pain may wish to consider some specific measures (e.g., Brief Pain Inventory) to include as options within their electronic health record system. Assessment tools can be both quantitative and qualitative. APPs working on evidence-informed practice or research projects will want to select highly reliable and valid measures.

Pain Measures

The most familiar quantitative evaluation of pain is the pain scale, often implemented as the fifth vital sign. The familiarity of having patients rate pain on a 0 to 10 scale may be comforting to the APP. However, there is little data to suggest that this is a useful monitoring tool to evaluate the effectiveness of interventions, and more holistic assessments are encouraged (HHS, 2020). The CDC's Health-Related Quality of Life (HRQOL) measure is a free tool that can be incorporated into an electronic health record (CDC, 2020). The NASS (2020) notes that using the HRQOL helps identify patients with acute back pain who may progress to a chronic state.

The Brief Pain Inventory (BPI) is a widely used scale to measure pain quality, quantity, and effect on daily functions (Cleeland et al., 1996). It was designed for patients with cancer, but the BPI also has wide usage in pain research. The BPI is available in two formats: the BPI Long Form, which may require more time than allotted in a busy primary care setting, and the BPI Short Form, which contains 11 questions and has been validated for use with several noncancer conditions. Krebs et al. (2009) provide a reliable and valid three-question measure that assesses pain intensity and interference with activity. It may be better suited for time-pressured primary care settings (see **Figure 20.2**).

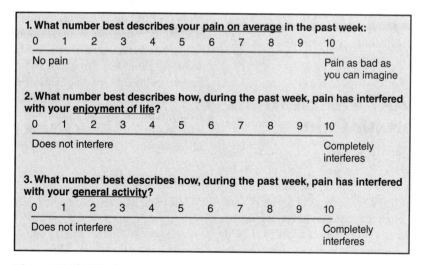

Figure 20.2 PEG, shortened Brief Pain Inventory questionnaire.

Krebs, E. E., Lorenz, K. A., Bair, M. J., Damush, T. M., Wu, J., Sutherland, J. M., Asch, S. M., & Kroenke, K. (2009). Development and initial validation of the PEG, a three-item scale assessing pain intensity and interference. *Journal of General Internal Medicine, 24*(6), 733–738. https://doi.org/ 10.1007/s11606-009-0981-1

Disease-Specific Assessments

In addition to scales and measures to explore the biopsychosocial effect of chronic pain without regard to a specific diagnosis, disease-specific assessment tools are available to the APP. The American College of Rheumatology created diagnostic criteria for fibromyalgia in 2010 (Häuser et al., 2012) that incorporate the number of painful body areas and a score for somatic symptoms. Patients can indicate how many of 19 possible body sites in which they have pain and grade symptoms of fatigue, unrefreshed sleep, and cognition difficulty on a 0 to 3 scale. Diagnostic criteria require a widespread pain index (number of body sites) of at least seven and a somatic symptom score of at least five (Häuser et al., 2012). However, APPs can use this scale to provide a quick, valid, and reliable assessment of pain and some measures of its effect on QOL. This assessment can also be used at a follow-up visit to evaluate the effectiveness of interventions.

When completing a pain assessment, the key point is that the APP must consider more than a scale rating of pain intensity. It is essential to include comprehensive questions about the overall effect on QOL, functionality, and the patient's family and social settings as well as seeking to identify comorbidities that may contribute to or affect pain.

A-SMART Prescriptions for Chronic Pain

Once the APP has partnered with the patient and family and completed a holistic assessment of the effect of pain on the patient's function, the mutual development of a plan of care can begin. Shared decision-making should be the cornerstone of this plan, and APPs should continue to nurture a therapeutic relationship (Schneiderhan & Orizondo, 2017). While pharmacological agents may be utilized, lifestyle changes represent a core component

of the plan of care that is more likely to enhance function and QOL than pharmacological agents (Nijs et al., 2020; Schneiderhan & Orizondo, 2017). These interventions should be individualized based on patient needs and interests. Furthermore, it is recommended that lifestyle interventions be implemented within an overall holistic and multimodal plan for patient wellness (Nijs et al., 2020). The lifestyle approach to the patient experiencing chronic pain discussed in this chapter uses the A-SMART interventions represented in **Table 20.2**.

Adopt Healthy Eating

As noted throughout this text, a healthy eating pattern has a wide-ranging beneficial effect on overall health. This section aims to guide specific recommendations for individuals dealing with chronic pain. Also, as previously noted, there is substantial heterogeneity in causes of chronic pain, some of which may have specific and evidence-informed dietary guidelines (e.g., RA) and others (e.g., CWP) for which there are no known specific nutritional interventions beyond a healthy eating pattern. A recent systematic review notes a wide range of dietary interventions studied for patients with chronic pain, some targeting specific nutrients and others with an anti-inflammatory focus. Nearly half of these studies demonstrate reduced pain, but more research is needed before specific interventions can be easily applied (Field et al., 2021). In general, healthy eating supports overall health and well-being, matching the treatment goals for those with chronic pain.

Weight Loss

While weight loss is beneficial for anyone whose body mass index exceeds 25 kg/m², some specific benefits can be noted in painful chronic conditions. For LBP, there is insufficient evidence for particular nutrition (NASS, 2020); however, weight loss may result in reduced pain levels. National OA guidelines

Table 20.2 A-SMART Prescriptions for Chronic Pain

Lifestyle Vital Sign	Interventions	Strength of Evidence* Organizational Recommendation
Adopt healthy eating	Mediterranean diet, anti-inflammatory diet	High-quality evidence and strong recommendation in OA of hand, knee, and hip for weight loss (Kolansinski et al., 2020); low-level evidence in overall pain; no national recommendations for overall pain
Stress less	Cognitive behavioral therapy (CBT), mindfulness, music therapy	Moderate for benefit in reducing depression and anxiety; improves QOL; conditional recommendation for OA (Kolansinski et al., 2020) Low-quality evidence for music (Crawford et al., 2014)
	Support groups	Low level of evidence
Move often	Physical therapy, yoga, tai chi, walking	High-quality evidence in OA of hand, knee, and hip; low-level evidence in overall pain; moderate evidence in fibromyalgia (Lawford et al., 2016)
Avoid alcohol	Screen all patients; alcohol interacts with opioids and other pain medication; reduce use	Moderate evidence supports reduced use (Caniglia et al., 2020)
Rest more	Insomnia CBT	Moderate evidence in OA (Kolansinski et al., 2020) and chronic pain in midlife adults (Koffel et al., 2019)
Treat tobacco use	Screen all patients for tobacco use; tobacco cessation	High-quality evidence in RA; tobacco cessation reduces risk in RA and assists in disease control (Chang et al., 2014)

*GRADE—high, moderate, low, and very low quality as per Guyatt, G. H., Oxman, A. D., Vist, G. E., Kunz, R., Falck-Ytter, Y., Alonso-Coello, P., Schünemann, H. J., & GRADE Working Group. (2008). GRADE: An emerging consensus on rating quality of evidence and strength of recommendations. *BMJ, 336*(7650), 924–926. https://doi.org/10.1136/bmj.39489.470347.AD

recommend weight loss for knee and hip OA, with benefits for weight loss of as little as 5% of body weight (Kolasinski et al., 2020). Because chronic pain may be augmented by high levels of pro-inflammatory states (e.g., central obesity), efforts to reduce weight are suggested (Bjørklund et al., 2019).

Specific Nutrients

A more detailed discussion of nutritional specifics to reduce chronic pain demonstrates the many unanswered questions for researchers and clinicians. There is some consensus that adequate intake of specific nutrients, such as vitamin D, selenium, magnesium, zinc, and curcumin, may decrease pain (Bjørklund et al., 2019). Tryptophan, a precursor amino acid for serotonin synthesis, may also reduce pain levels. Nutritional intake is difficult to achieve without supplementation (Casale et al., 2021). Magnesium is now used as a supplement in migraine and chronic pain. Rich dietary sources include whole grains, nuts, and leafy green vegetables (Casale et al., 2021).

Anti-Inflammatory Diet

Much more complex relationships surround information about foods that might decrease inflammatory mediators or increase the release of anti-inflammatory mediators such as IL-10. Diets rich in fiber, flavonoids such as those found in berries and other vegetables, and curcuminoids (e.g., turmeric) have some evidence to reduce inflammatory mediators and pain. Indeed, in a systematic review, Wu et al. (2020) found that for older adults, the Mediterranean diet reduces levels of C-reactive protein and IL-6. The Mediterranean diet encourages the eating of fish, vegetables, whole grains, legumes, and nuts while limiting the intake of high-fat foods such as red meat, hard cheeses, and fried foods (American Heart Association, n.d.). Given its ease of use and improvements for overall health, the Mediterranean diet provides a sound underpinning of principles for patients with chronic pain syndromes.

Stress Less

Stress management encompasses a myriad of possible interventions for APPs to offer patients. This section will discuss broad interventions ranging from psychotherapies such as CBT to mindfulness activities and art-type therapies.

Psychological Therapies

Because patients living with chronic pain have a substantial risk of depression and anxiety, referral to a therapist should be a standard component of management. A holistic assessment should help the APP consider specific patients' needs. Chronic pain often begins with acute pain from injury or surgery, which may have emanated from a trauma. The APP should continue to have a trauma-informed focus for the plan of care. In a systematic review, Barrett and Chang (2016) noted that CBT, acceptance and commitment therapy, and interpersonal psychotherapy have a small to moderate effect in reducing chronic pain. A brief description of these therapies is found in **Table 20.3**. These modalities are also beneficial for coexisting depressive symptoms. CBT is recommended for CLBP and OA of the hand, knee, and hip (Kolasinski et al., 2020; NASS, 2020).

Table 20.3 Types of Psychotherapy for Chronic Pain

Therapy	Description	Resources
Acceptance and commitment therapy	Utilizes elements of mindfulness. The goal is to help patients accept what is and learn to live fully despite challenges.	https://www.psychotherapy.net /article/Acceptance-and -Commitment-Therapy-ACT
Cognitive behavioral therapy	Treatment focuses on helping patients understand the connections among thoughts, feelings, and behaviors.	https://www.abct.org/get-help /symptoms-and-treatments
Interpersonal therapy	Based on the theory that depression and the resultant relationship challenges emanate from a biological predisposition. Therapy works to reduce the likelihood that relational issues trigger the biological tendency.	https://psychcentral.com/lib /interpersonal-therapy-ipt#what -is-ipt

Mindfulness, Meditation, and Relaxation

Patients in chronic pain often have a sustained activation of the HPA axis and increased cortisol levels, for which mindfulness activities can be helpful (Koncz et al., 2020). However, in a systematic review of the benefit of mindfulness in patients with chronic pain, Hilton et al. (2017) noted low-quality evidence indicating that this intervention will decrease pain. As with many of the other interventions noted in this chapter, there seems to be benefits for QOL and depression symptoms, thus making this intervention important for patients with these concerns (Hilton et al., 2017). Additional mindful interventions include a gratitude practice, during which patients note elements of their life they are grateful for, such as a sunny day. In a Portuguese sample of patients with fibromyalgia, gratitude practice contributed to reduced pain and fatigue and improved sleep (Yuan et al., 2021).

In addition to face-to-face education and practice of mindfulness and meditation skills, the COVID-19 pandemic has pushed many of these resources online. In a systematic review, Mikolasek et al. (2018) found that virtual mindfulness training had mixed results for decreasing pain (two of four studies showed benefit) but no harm in controlled trials. Further, the authors concluded that electronic mindfulness programs showed benefits for improving overall health and psychological problems such as depression.

Music

The use of music and music therapy may reduce pain and improve the QOL for individuals with chronic pain. However, the evidence in this area is relatively small. In a systematic review of all art therapies and chronic pain, Crawford et al. (2014) noted just four studies with adequate quality for inclusion. A search of more recent articles (Academic Search Premier, 2014–2021) identified just 17 articles regarding music therapy and chronic pain. At the time, Crawford et al. (2014) concluded that music therapy could be used as a treatment modality to reduce pain with a small to moderate effect size. In a small pilot study, Usui et al. (2020) demonstrated that listening to classical music for 15 minutes reduced pain scores and showed brain function changes on fMRI.

Another pilot study ($n = 23$) compared meditation and music in reducing knee OA pain and found that both reduced pain. Of the two, meditation was more likely to improve sleep (Innes et al., 2018). A more recent trial of a 12-week vocal music program found improved QOL and pain (Low et al., 2020). These small studies highlight the importance of engaging patients with chronic pain in their treatment and matching their interests to interventions. APPs can use these simple strategies to help patients mitigate pain and improve QOL. An essential consideration of music and music therapy in working with patients with chronic pain is that the interventions can be individualized, inexpensive, and unlikely to harm.

Social Connections

The relationship between chronic pain and social connection is bidirectional and complex (Allen et al., 2020; Hirsch et al., 2016). Lower levels of QOL in patients with chronic pain indicate difficulty carrying out routine activities that provide social connections (McMurty et al., 2020). Once an individual has chronic pain, it becomes more challenging to engage in social activities, and this lack of social connection may further increase pain. On the other hand, social support and connectedness may act as mediators to reduce pain and improve function (Stevens et al., 2020). Because social connectedness is bidirectional, patients with chronic pain may benefit from providing help to others as much as receiving help. The provision of help to others is correlated with lower levels of pain interference in daily functioning (Nguyen et al., 2020).

The extent to which interventions that increase social connection can reduce pain is less well known. In a small ($n = 54$) study, Koebner et al. (2019) enrolled patients with chronic pain in an art museum tour. Results indicated that the activity reduced both pain perception and feelings of social isolation. Because the benefits of social connectedness are widespread for health, APPs consider the social world of patients with chronic pain when planning care. However, there is limited evidence for APPs to suggest that patients will have lower levels of pain based on increasing their social connections. But given the emphasis on improving functionality and QOL in patients with chronic pain, such interventions are merited.

Move Often

National recommendations for exercise indicate adults should get 150 minutes of moderate activity per week (Physical Activity Guidelines Advisory Committee, 2008). For individuals with chronic pain, this may be an incredibly daunting goal. Indeed, Majlesi (2019) reports that among patients with CLBP, over half of them indicated low levels of physical activity. Barriers include fear of reinjury, pain catastrophizing, and anxiety (Booth et al., 2017).

Even though exercise and physical fitness may be difficult for patients with chronic pain, and despite some mixed evidence that such activities will reduce pain or improve QOL, the goal for patients with chronic pain is to move (HHS, 2019). In a recent Cochrane review, Puljak and Chiara (2019) noted that the limited evidence suggests small to moderate benefits in reducing pain and increasing functionality for patients with mild to moderate pain levels. Findings supporting improvement in QOL measures are more variable.

In a study of women with fibromyalgia ($n = 419$), researchers found that light activity was associated with reduced pain and fatigue (Estévez-López et al., 2015). A systematic review of seven studies exploring the benefits of walking in patients with LBP concluded that walking (especially outside) is at least as beneficial as other types of exercise interventions, such as physical therapy and light weights (Lawford et al., 2016). The authors of this study noted that walking was one of the most affordable options. However, for patients who live in communities that may not be safe for outdoor walking, APPs should provide alternatives to walking outside, such as indoor malls or internet-based programs that promote walking in the home.

Other disease-specific guidelines concur with some of the difficulties in prescribing exercise for patients with chronic pain. In OA of the hands, knees, and hips, exercise has benefits, but the specifics of which kind of activity, for how long, and in what setting are not yet apparent in the literature. The OA guidelines echo other guidelines and researchers in that exercise suggestions should be individualized and based on patient ability and preference (Kolasinski et al., 2020). An example is the recommendation of aquatic exercise in OA, which may increase range of motion (ROM) (and thus function) and provide overall aerobic fitness in patients for whom weight-bearing activities are painful (Kolasinski et al., 2020). Such exercise may be cost prohibitive for some patients and not preferred by patients who do not know how to swim. Aquatic therapy can be prescribed as part of a physical therapy prescription.

An additional issue related to increasing physical activity is that patients living with chronic pain may have other comorbidities, such as depression, anxiety, sleep disruption, and obesity in addition to the common medical conditions of diabetes and hypertension, for which exercise is beneficial. Therefore, APP efforts to increase patient physical activity and exercise are likely to benefit overall health.

Tai Chi and Yoga

Research into the benefits of tai chi, yoga, and other mind–body exercise practices is still relatively young. As there are a plethora of chronic pain syndromes and specific populations experiencing such pain, studies regarding a specific group of patients (e.g., Hispanic women under 40 with CWP) may be difficult to locate. One meta-analysis of the effect of tai chi on community-dwelling elders with chronic conditions (not limited to painful conditions) identified only 12 studies of sufficient quality and found some substantial heterogeneity among those studies. However, the analysis demonstrated that tai chi had a small but significant effect on increasing QOL and reducing depressive symptoms (Choo et al., 2020). Tai chi is strongly recommended for knee and hip OA (Kolasinski et al., 2020). Overall, these interventions can be found in a variety of settings, from free online classes to classes at local YMCAs and senior centers to private one-on-one coaching. The conclusion is that tai chi and yoga may be especially beneficial in chronic musculoskeletal pain conditions (HHS, 2019).

Physical Therapy and Water Therapy

Physical therapy may provide a range of benefits in patients with chronic pain conditions. Physical therapy evaluation and treatment plans incorporate components of the A-SMART principles and can assist the APP in using measurable outcomes. A referral for a physical therapy evaluation may be an excellent place to begin for individuals with chronic pain. APPs can also order ROM exercises as a good beginning for patients who have been immobile or sedentary. A standard physical therapy report will include precise measurements of joint ROM with short- and long-term goals. Knowing the starting functional capability, APPs can begin to develop an interprofessional plan of care.

The APP should complete a careful assessment of pain locations, limitations in ROM, and muscle strength and consider realistic expectations of body function for patients. Further, it is important to understand the evidence related to the causative factor for chronic pain because exercise prescriptions may need to be carefully tailored for each unique patient situation. In addition to prescribing traditional physical therapy, APPs can consider aquatic therapies for patients whose conditions are worsened by weight-bearing activity. OA is an example of a condition that responds well to water-based therapy (Kolasinski et al., 2020).

Avoid Alcohol

Excessive alcohol use is a common finding in patients with chronic pain (Alford et al., 2016). Alcohol has a muscle relaxant and anxiolytic effect, so patients with muscular sources of chronic pain and who experience anxiety related to their chronic pain may feel better after an alcoholic drink, thus reinforcing alcohol use and putting patients at risk for addiction. Alcohol also makes people tired and may ease insomnia symptoms related to the initiation of sleep, but as the night wears on, alcohol disrupts sleep (Inkelis et al., 2020). Finally, alcohol is processed through the liver, as are many medications patients use to manage chronic pain. Benzodiazepines and alcohol together can increase the risk for falls, injury, and liver damage. NSAIDs and steroids combined with alcohol increase the risk of gastrointestinal bleeding (Mayes-Burnett, 2020). Some patients with chronic rheumatological causes for their pain, such as RA or systemic lupus erythematosus, may take methotrexate, which should not be combined with alcohol (Burchum & Chung, 2020).

Unfortunately, while alcohol may provide short-term relief from pain, it is a depressant and can worsen mood. Individuals with anxiety disorders are also found to have increased rates of alcohol use (Caniglia et al., 2020). While national recommendations suggest that a daily alcohol limit of one drink for women and two drinks for men may not adversely affect health (U.S. Department of Agriculture, 2020), a core question for patients with chronic pain is whether reducing any amount of drinking will decrease pain and improve QOL. The Veterans Aging Cohort Study found that 44% of 1,491 veterans with chronic pain reported problematic drinking patterns. Those who reduced alcohol use reported less pain interference with activities one and two years later. Anxiety symptoms also decreased, although there was only a small reduction in depression symptoms (Caniglia et al., 2020).

Consequently, APPs should make alcohol intake a routine part of assessing patients with chronic pain and recommend reducing alcohol intake to at or below recommended levels to improve QOL. Brief screening for alcohol use can be done by asking patients the four CAGE questions: (1) Has anyone suggested you *cut down* on your drinking? (2) Is anyone *annoyed* by your drinking? (3) Do you feel *guilty* about your drinking? and (4) Have you ever had an alcoholic drink in the morning as an *eye-opener*? (Ewing, 1984). One study suggests that the 10-question Alcohol Use Disorder Identification Tool (AUDIT), along with serum measurement of gamma-glutamyl transferase, is significantly more sensitive than the CAGE questions (Kandaswamy & Rengaramanujem, 2019). Efforts to help patients reduce alcohol use will be best accomplished by utilizing shared decision-making and motivational interviewing strategies. Referrals to Alcoholics Anonymous and counseling, as well as detoxification, may also be required. Long after reduction or abstinence, APPs should also attend to relapse prevention during follow-up visits.

Rest More

Poor sleep quality and quantity are risk factors for chronic pain and are more common in patients with chronic pain conditions (Generaal

et al., 2017). Impaired sleep is associated with worse outcomes in back pain (NASS, 2020). Some randomized controlled trial data indicate interventions to improve sleep reduce pain in middle-aged adults (Koffel et al., 2019). Still, there are no data to determine specific intervention levels as helpful. Thus, the relationship between sleep and pain is complex, with problematic sleep increasing pain and vice versa (Haack et al., 2020). Sleep problems may be particularly important to consider in the setting of chronic musculoskeletal complaints and headaches. Impaired sleep causes a multiplicity of abnormalities across many systems. Most significant for patients with chronic pain, poor sleep causes dysregulation of the HPA axis and leads to higher cortisol levels (which may increase obesity). Impaired sleep promotes a relative pro-inflammatory state that includes higher levels of inflammatory cytokines, such as IL-6 (Haack et al., 2020).

Patients with chronic pain must be assessed for sleep habits as part of the initial encounter. While chronic pain and sleep difficulty are complexly intertwined, APPs must also holistically evaluate sleep problems and not assume that chronic pain and sleep problems are related for a particular patient. Specifically, sleep studies to diagnose common conditions such as sleep apnea are essential. Medications such as corticosteroids, commonly prescribed in inflammatory conditions, are well known to disrupt sleep. Finally, as part of core sleep hygiene, an assessment of caffeine intake is also necessary.

Once possible differential diagnoses have been eliminated, CBT for insomnia (iCBT) is a well-supported intervention that improves sleep and reduces pain in patient populations such as those with OA and fibromyalgia (Haack et al., 2020). iCBT includes education about sleep hygiene, the core of helping patients repair disordered sleeping. Online iCBT is available and is beneficial and affordable. Though beyond the scope of lifestyle interventions, readers should note that for inflammatory autoimmune disorders such as inflammatory bowel disease, RA, and ankylosing spondylitis, biological pharmaceutical agents that lower inflammatory mediators such as TNF-α and IL-6 are associated with improved sleep (Haack et al., 2020). Thus, patient education and support to improve medication adherence for patients prescribed these therapies can help enhance restorative rest.

Treat Tobacco Use

Tobacco use is similar to sleep disruption in that the two are intertwined, and research has not fully described the relationship. However, there are some important known concerns. For example, smoking increases the risk of RA and makes it more challenging to treat (Chang et al., 2014; Deane & Holers, 2021). In a survey of over 12,000 patients with chronic pain at the Stanford Pain Clinic, those who smoke reported increased pain on QOL measures and increased rates of depression, anxiety, and sleep dysfunction (Khan et al., 2019). Unfortunately, treating nicotine addiction in patients with chronic pain is challenging because smoking provides a short-term analgesic effect.

Additionally frustrating is that for patients with chronic pain, it is unclear if quitting or reducing nicotine consumption reduces pain (Khan et al., 2019). However, for patients with RA, quitting does reduce disease activity and thus pain (Roelsgaard et al., 2020). Furthermore, nicotine cessation is essential for cardiovascular health regardless of pain level. A plan for nicotine cessation in patients with chronic pain should be mutually created and with as much clear patient education as possible. Promising or suggesting that patients will have reduced pain (patients with RA excepted) if they quit is not supported by the evidence. APPs may wish to help patients select other lifestyle interventions to support overall well-being (e.g., sleep hygiene and exercise) before beginning smoking cessation efforts.

Chronic Pain Management Counseling and Education

Education regarding chronic pain and its management is commonly incorporated into the treatment plan for patients with chronic pain. In a recent systematic review, Louw et al. (2016) reported that for patients with musculoskeletal pain, patient education with a neuroscience focus has several benefits, including reduced pain, increased function, increased movement, and reduced anxiety and depression. Indeed, patient education is part of the national care recommendation for OA (Kolasinski et al., 2020). Topics to be covered are wide ranging and include pathophysiology, psychosocial factors, medication side effects, goal setting, positive thinking, and how to engage in the A-SMART behaviors (Kolasinski et al., 2020; Louw et al., 2016). APPs will recognize the extensive nature of the information that can benefit a patient and reasonably wonder how to implement such education within the typical 15-minute office visit.

Fortunately, evidence suggests several alternative methods and platforms for educating patients. The IPRCC (2016), in its National Pain Strategy, provides an excellent overview of public education messages related to pain. The APP should be aware of these messages in the role of patient care advocate. This messaging can also be provided during one-on-one patient encounters. Such principles include the idea that chronic pain is a manageable yet complex condition that may require an interprofessional team to meet the goal to "alleviate pain and restore function" (IPRCC, 2016, p. 77). Gokhale et al. (2020) reported that group and individual education offerings have similar efficacy in reducing pain and increasing function. Flynn et al. (2018) utilized psychiatric technicians in an interprofessional and holistic chronic pain intervention to provide education.

The internet and other electronic resources such as apps can also provide patient education (Mikolasek et al., 2018). Digital health education is still a relatively newer area of research, and there are many variables to consider before recommending an app (Ross et al., 2020). A recent study evaluated 19 apps for patients with chronic pain for completeness of content, quality, and availability of research findings. The results indicated that only three were reasonably comprehensive (Devan et al., 2019). None had research findings related to outcomes in chronic pain. The wide variety of platforms and providers who

---

Health Promotion Case Study Addressing Chronic Pain in an Adult Female

Case description: L.J. is a 41-year-old female who presents for an annual physical. Her chief complaint is pain most days of the week.

- Past medical history: Diagnosed four years ago with amplified pain syndrome, fibromyalgia, and CWP. She has seen a rheumatologist, a physiatrist, and an orthopedist since her symptoms began five years ago. Her past medical history is otherwise unremarkable.

- Current medications: Pregablin 75 mg BID; naproxen sodium 500 mg BID PRN; tramadol/acetaminophen 37.5/325 mg, 2 PO every 6 hours PRN severe pain, which she takes about 1–2 times per month.

- Social history: She is married with two children, ages 7 and 10. Works in retail. She and her husband split shifts to reduce the need for outside care for the children. He works a 7–3 shift, and she works afternoons and evenings three days per week plus Saturdays.

- Vital signs: Height 64 in., weight 168 lb, BP 130/82 mmHg left arm, temperature 97.9°F, heart rate 84 bpm, respiratory rate 14/min, pain 4/10.

- Physical exam: Casually dressed and clean, with no makeup, restricted affect, and somewhat labile, tearing when she discusses how exhausted she is much of the time. Her cardiopulmonary exam is unremarkable. The musculoskeletal exam reveals trigger point tenderness in her trapezius bilaterally and in her upper thighs, but otherwise there is full strength. Her neurological exam shows +2/4 reflexes and good sensation to sharp and dull with intact cranial nerves and intact cerebellar function.

Lifestyle Vital Signs

- Adopt healthy eating: Not assessed.
- Stress less: Not assessed.
- Move often: States that she is on her feet most of her work shift. Reports minimal exercise due to low and upper back pain and exhaustion.
- Avoid alcohol: Drinks 1–2 glasses of wine about once per week.
- Rest more: Reports poor sleep.
- Treat tobacco use: Nonsmoker.
- BMI 28.8 kg/m².

Critical Thinking Questions

- What additional subjective and objective data related to lifestyle behaviors do you want to assess and why?
- What lifestyle management strategies would you consider for optimizing L.J.'s health outcomes?
- What referrals to other providers and internet resources will you consider?

can offer such education should lead the APP to work in a person-centered manner, using shared decision-making and assessing which option the patient prefers and which will give the most benefit.

The American Chronic Pain Association is a patient education and support organization. Its website offers a multiplicity of resources, including education on pathophysiology; treatment information; and opioid use, abuse, and overdose. Lifestyle management materials include free relaxation and meditation audio files and instructions for self-advocacy. Additionally, there is a comprehensive tool kit for clinicians that includes reference materials and listings of organizations that support patients in chronic pain (e.g., the Lupus Foundation and the American Council for Headache Education). Professional organizations across the care continuum are also listed, ranging from the American Music Therapy Association to the Association for Applied and Therapeutic Humor.

Interprofessional Approach to Chronic Pain

The reader will note that many of the interventions discussed in this chapter require collaborations with other healthcare professionals. Disciplines involved in team-based care vary but commonly include pain specialists, pharmacists, physical therapists, primary care providers, psychologists, psychiatrists, nurses, occupational therapists, and social workers (Murphy et al., 2021). There are many examples of interprofessional programs for rehabilitation from chronic pain (Flynn et al., 2018). Evidence suggests that pain can be lowered and QOL improved and that patient satisfaction is good with such programs (Coffey et al., 2019; Crouch et al., 2020). Indeed, the Pain Management Best Practices Inter-Agency Task Force Report suggests an interprofessional team approach (HHS, 2019).

Interprofessional care benefits begin with provider education and extend to end of program outcomes. Simply attending an online interactive educational program about chronic pain allowed professionals to understand better the skills and abilities of other professionals (Zhao et al., 2020). A multiprogram assessment of nine Veterans Affairs interprofessional programs demonstrated reduced pain, less pain catastrophizing, and improved sleep (Murphy et al., 2021). Challenges with interprofessional programs and specialty clinics include cost and wait times, leading some centers to create stepped care programs involving a variety of professions at each step. Patients enter the program with self-education modules about chronic pain and the biopsychosocial elements affecting pain. They may then progress to group education programs delivering CBT and group yoga. Only if all of those measures fail to reduce pain and improve QOL will a patient be referred to a pain care specialist (Bell et al., 2020).

APPs should identify local interprofessional programs or be knowledgeable of offerings from health insurance companies. For example, the New Jersey Division of Pensions and Benefits provides a digital and remote program for physical therapy for free to plan members, Hinge Health (https://www.hingehealth.com/for/newjersey1). The program offers free electronic monitors, apps, and phone support. Where programs do not exist, APPs can help coordinate an interprofessional team with clinicians who may agree on shared patient- and family-centered treatment goals such as improved QOL, reduced opioid use, and increased daily functioning. A team composed of a primary care APP, counseling professional, physical therapist, and pain management specialist may serve patients well. Occupational therapists, social workers, dentists, and integrative health practitioners may also be beneficial, depending on the causative diagnosis (HHS, 2019). For APPs practicing in rural or remote locations, many of these services can be provided virtually, with good evidence of benefit.

Comprehensive Care Process

Treating patients with chronic pain can be challenging. However, a care process that includes comprehensive assessment, an interprofessional approach, and a person-centered plan of care using A-SMART interventions can guide the APP. An overview of this process is found in **Table 20.4**. Since chronic pain can last from three months to many years, it is important to recognize the need for regular reassessment, modification of the plan, and long-term support.

Table 20.4 Overview of the Care Process in Chronic Pain

Action	Components
Assess	▪ Pain quality, effect on daily function ▪ Mental health, substance use ▪ Sleep, relationships, work, habits ▪ QOL
Create interprofessional team	▪ Psychology, psychiatry ▪ Physical therapy, occupational therapy ▪ Pain specialists ▪ Pharmacy ▪ Social work
Enact plan	▪ Person centered ▪ Use motivational interviewing ▪ Select A-SMART interventions
Reassess	▪ Successes ▪ Pain level, effect, and QOL ▪ Ineffective strategies
Modify	▪ Increase goals ▪ New or revised A-SMART interventions ▪ Additional interprofessional team members
Maintain	▪ Follow up frequently ▪ Support

Summary

Patients with chronic pain endure a wide array of effects on daily living and often have a lower QOL. Armed with the information in this chapter, APPs can adopt an A-SMART approach to caring for these patients, offering evidence-informed interventions that can reduce the burden of chronic pain for patients and their families. Such care begins by understanding the complex and multisystem physiological processes involved in chronic pain, including the immune, endocrine, and nervous systems. The multifactorial causes of chronic pain indicate that a holistic and interprofessional approach is well suited to improve a patient's QOL.

The care process for the patient with chronic pain begins by providing a nonjudgmental, comprehensive chronic pain assessment. This assessment can be guided by several evidence-informed tools, including the BPI short or long forms. The APP may add several members to the interprofessional team, including physical and occupational therapists, psychological therapists, pharmacists, pain management specialists, social workers, and specialist physicians (e.g., rheumatologists, physiatrists).

Motivational interviewing principles help the APP establish a trusting patient–provider relationship and create mutual goals with patients and families. A-SMART strategies and patient education via the internet and other electronic resources offer patients affordable and accessible options for managing chronic pain through lifestyle interventions. A person-centered approach guides the APP in helping patients choose which lifestyle behaviors to address first. Interventions with good evidence for improving the lived experience of patients

TABLE 20.5	Evidence-Based Resources for Chronic Pain	
Organization	**Resource**	**URL**
American Chronic Pain Association	Patient education, lifestyle management materials, clinician tool kit, lists of organizations that support patients in chronic pain	https://www.acpanow.com
American College of Rheumatology	Patient/caregiver information on amplified musculoskeletal pain syndrome (AMPS)	https://www.rheumatology.org /I-Am-A/Patient-Caregiver /Diseases-Conditions/Amplified -Musculoskeletal-Pain-Syndrome -AMPS
American College of Rheumatology	Patient/caregiver information on rheumatoid arthritis	https://www.rheumatology.org /I-Am-A/Patient-Caregiver/Diseases -Conditions/Rheumatoid-Arthritis
American College of Rheumatology/Arthritis Foundation	2019 Guideline for the Management of Osteoarthritis of the Hand, Hip, and Knee	https://www.rheumatology.org /Portals/0/Files/Osteoarthritis -Guideline-Early-View-2019.pdf
Centers for Disease Control and Prevention	Pocket Guide: Tapering Opioids for Chronic Pain	https://www.cdc.gov/drugoverdose /pdf/clinical_pocket_guide_tapering -a.pdf
Centers for Disease Control and Prevention	Health-Related Quality of Life (HRQOL) Methods and Measures	https://www.cdc.gov/hrqol/methods .htm
MD Anderson Center	Brief Pain Inventory (BPI), Short Form	https://www.mdanderson.org /research/departments-labs -institutes/departments-divisions /symptom-research/symptom -assessment-tools/brief-pain -inventory.html
National Fibromyalgia Association	Patient-led advocacy and support groups	https://www.fmaware.org
National Institutes of Health Interagency Pain Research Coordinating Committee	National Pain Strategy (released March 2016)	https://www.iprcc.nih.gov/sites /default/files/documents /NationalPainStrategy_508C.pdf
National Institute of Neurological Disorders and Stroke	Back pain information	https://www.ninds.nih.gov/health -information/disorders/back-pain? search-term=Pain

(continues)

TABLE 20.5	Evidence-Based Resources for Chronic Pain	*(continued)*
Organization	**Resource**	**URL**
North American Spine Society	2020 Guidelines for Low Back Pain	https://www.spine.org/Portals /0/assets/downloads/Research ClinicalCare/Guidelines/LowBack Pain.pdf
U.S. Department of Health and Human Services Pain Management Best Practices Inter-Agency Task Force	2019 Pain Management Best Practices Report	https://www.hhs.gov/sites/default /files/pain-mgmt-best-practices -draft-final-report-05062019.pdf

Health Promotion Activity: Gratitude Practice

Gratitude practice has been shown to contribute to reduced pain (Yuan et al., 2021). For this activity, create a gratitude jar.

Gather the following: a fist-sized jar or container of any kind, colored pens or markers, blank paper, tape or glue.

1. Take a moment to consider things for which you are grateful. These can be personal or professional, tangible or intangible (e.g., hugs, a significant person in your life, trees, a supportive colleague, a hobby).
2. Write each item on a scrap of paper and fold the paper.
3. Next, take a piece of paper that will wrap around your jar. Label your jar (e.g., Joy Jar, Gratitude Jar, Love Jar). Glue or tape the label onto the jar.
4. Fill your jar with the slips of paper noting items you are grateful for.
5. Keep nearby and grab a slip of paper as needed.

Consider how this simple activity might benefit a patient who suffers from chronic pain.

with chronic pain include adopting the Mediterranean or an anti-inflammatory diet, developing a mindfulness practice, engaging in CBT, walking, having physical therapy, sleeping adequately, and reducing alcohol and nicotine use.

The long-standing nature of chronic pain will necessitate reassessment, modification of the plan, and ongoing support to increase functionality and QOL. Nevertheless, a holistic lifestyle management approach helps patients, families, and clinicians move beyond merely rating pain on a 0 to 10 scale to optimizing wellness in the face of chronic pain conditions.

Acronyms

APP: advanced practice provider

A-SMART: adopt healthy eating, stress less, move often, avoid alcohol, rest more, and treat tobacco use

AUDIT: Alcohol Use Disorder Identification Tool

BPI: Brief Pain Inventory

CBT: cognitive behavioral therapy

CDC: Centers for Disease Control and Prevention

CLBP: chronic low back pain

CWP: chronic widespread pain

HHS: U.S. Department of Health and Human Services

HPA axis: hypothalamic-pituitary-adrenal axis

HRQOL: health-related quality of life

IASP: International Association for the Study of Pain

iCBT: cognitive behavioral therapy for insomnia

ICD-11: International Classification of Diseases 11

IL: interleukin (IL-2, IL-4, IL-6, IL-10)

IPRCC: Interagency Pain Research Coordinating Committee

LBP: low back pain

NASS: North American Spine Society

NSAID: nonsteroidal anti-inflammatory drug

OA: osteoarthritis

QOL: quality of life

RA: rheumatoid arthritis

ROM: range of motion

TNF-α: tumor necrosis factor alpha

References

Aaron, R. V., Finan, P. H., Wegener, S. T., Keefe, F. J., & Lumley, M. A. (2020). Emotion regulation as a transdiagnostic factor underlying co-occurring chronic pain and problematic opioid use. *American Psychologist*, 75(6), 796–810. https://doi.org/10.1037/amp0000678

Alford, D. P., German, J. S., Samet, J. H., Cheng, D. M., Lloyd-Travaglini, C. A., & Saitz, R. (2016). Primary care patients with drug use report chronic pain and self-medicate with alcohol and other drugs. *Journal of General Internal Medicine*, 31(5), 486–491. https://doi.org/10.1007/s11606-016-3586-5

Allen, S. F., Gilbody, S., Atkin, K., & van der Feltz-Cornelis, C. (2020). The associations between loneliness, social exclusion and pain in the general population: A N=502,528 cross-sectional UK Biobank study. *Journal of Psychiatric Research*, 130, 68–74. https://doi.org/10.1016/j.jpsychires.2020.06.028

American Heart Association. (n.d.). *What is the Mediterranean diet?* Retrieved May 31, 2023, from https://www.heart.org/en/healthy-living/healthy-eating/eat-smart/nutrition-basics/mediterranean-diet

Ballantyne, J. C., & Sullivan, M. D. (2016). Intensity of chronic pain—The wrong metric? *New England Journal of Medicine*, 373(22), 2098–2099. https://doi.org/10.1056/NEJMp1507136

Barrett, K., & Chang, Y. P. (2016). Behavioral interventions targeting chronic pain, depression, and substance use disorder in primary care. *Journal of Nursing Scholarship*, 48(4), 345–353. https://doi.org/10.1111/jnu.12213

Bell, L., Cornish, P., Gauthier, R., Argus, C., Rash, J., Robbins, R., Ward, S., & Poulin, P. A. (2020). Implementation of the Ottawa Hospital Pain Clinic stepped care program: A preliminary report. *Canadian Journal of Pain*, 4(1), 168–178. http://doi.org/10.1080/24740527.2020.1768059

Berger, J. M., & Zelman, V. (2016). Pathophysiology of chronic pain. *Pain Medicine Journal*, 1(2), 29–49.

Bjørklund, G., Aaseth, J., Doşa, M. D., Pivina, L., Dadar, M., Pen, J. J., & Chirumbolo, S. (2019). Does diet play a role in reducing nociception related to inflammation and chronic pain? *Nutrition*, 66, 153–165. https://doi.org/10.1016/j.nut.2019.04.007

Boone, D., & Kim, S. Y. (2019). Family strain, depression, and somatic amplification in adults with chronic pain. *International Journal of Behavioral Medicine*, 26(4), 427–436. https://doi.org/10.1007/s12529-019-09799-y

Booth, J., Moseley, G. L., Schiltenwolf, M., Cashin, A., Davies, M., & Hübscher, M. (2017). Exercise for chronic musculoskeletal pain: A biopsychosocial approach. *Musculoskeletal Care*, 15(4), 413–421. https://doi.org/10.1002/msc.1191

Burchum, J. R., & Chung, H. S. (2020). Pharmacology of the gastrointestinal tract. In B. T. Smith (Ed.), *Pharmacology for nurses* (pp. 209–233). Jones & Bartlett Learning.

Calabrese, L. H. (2020). *Maintaining empathy in rheumatology.* Expert Perspectives in Rheumatology. https://expertperspectives.com/Rheumatology/Rheumatoid%20Arthritis/maintaining-empathy-in-rheumatology

Caniglia, E. C., Stevens, E. R., Khan, M., Young, K. E., Ban, K., Marshall, B. D., Chichetto, N. E., Gaither, J. R., Crystal, S., Edelman, E. J., Fielein, D. A., Gordon, A. J., Bryant, K. J., Tate, J., Justice, A. C., & Braithwaite, R. S. (2020). Does reducing drinking in patients with unhealthy alcohol use improve pain interference, use of other substances, and psychiatric symptoms? *Alcoholism: Clinical and Experimental Research, 44*(11), 2257–2265. https://doi.org/10.1111/acer.14455

Casale, R., Symeonidou, Z., Ferfeli, S., Micheli, F., Scarsella, P., & Paladini, A. (2021). Food for special medical purposes and nutraceuticals for pain: A narrative review. *Pain and Therapy, 10*, 225–242. https://doi.org/10.6084/M9.FIGSHARE.13664294

Centers for Disease Control and Prevention. (n.d.). *Pocket guide: Tapering opioids for chronic pain.* Retrieved May 31, 2023, from https://www.cdc.gov/drug overdose/pdf/clinical_pocket_guide_tapering-a.pdf

Centers for Disease Control and Prevention. (2020). *Health related quality of life.* https://www.cdc.gov/hrqol

Chang, K., Yang, S. M., Kim, S. H., Han, K. H., Park, S. J., & Shin, J. I. (2014). Smoking and rheumatoid arthritis. *International Journal of Molecular Science, 15*(12), 22279–22295. https://doi.org/10.3390/ijms151222279

Chen, J., Hu, F., Yang, B. X., Cai, Y., & Cong, X. (2020). Experience of living with pain among older adults with arthritis: A systematic review and meta-synthesis. *International Journal of Nursing Studies, 111*, 103756. https://doi.org/10.1016/j.ijnurstu.2020.103756

Choo, Y. T., Jiang, Y., Hong, J., & Wenru, W. (2020). Effectiveness of tai chi on quality of life, depressive symptoms and physical function among community-dwelling older adults with chronic disease: A systematic review and meta-analysis. *International Journal of Nursing Studies, 111*, 103737. https://doi.org/10.1016/j.ijnurstu.2020.103737

Cleeland, C. S., Nakamura, Y., Mendoza, T. R., Edwards, K. R., Douglas, J., & Serlin, R. C. (1996). Dimensions of the impact of cancer pain in a four-country sample: New information from multidimensional scaling. *Pain, 67*, 267–273.

Coffey, C. P., Ulbrich, T. R., Baughman, K., & Awad, M. H. (2019). Effect of an interprofessional pain service on nonmalignant pain control. *American Journal of Health-System Pharmacy, 76*, S49–S54. https://doi.org/10.1093/ajhp/zxy084

Comachio, J., Magalhães, M. O., Moura Campos Carvalho e Silva, A. P., & Marques, A. P. (2018). A cross-sectional study of associations between kinesiophobia, pain, disability, and quality of life in patients with chronic low back pain. *Advances in Rheumatology, 58*(1), 8–13. https://doi.org/10.1186/s42358-018-0011-2

Craner, J. R., Sperry, J. A., Koball, A. M., Morrison, E. J., & Gilliam, W. P. (2017). Unique contributions of acceptance and catastrophizing on chronic pain adaptation. *International Journal of Behavioral Medicine, 24*(4), 542–551. https://doi.org/10.1007/s12529-017-9646-3

Crawford, C., Lee, C., Bingham. J., & Active Self-Care Therapies for Pain Working Group. (2014). Sensory art therapies for the self-management of chronic pain symptoms. *Pain Medicine, 15*, S66–S75. https://doi.org/10.1111/pme.12409

Crouch, T. B., Wedin, S., Kilpatrick, R. L., Christon, L., Balliet, W., Borckardt, J., & Barth, K. (2020). Pain rehabilitation's dual power: Treatment for chronic pain and prevention of opioid-related risks. *American Psychologist, 75*, 825–839. http://doi.org/10.1037/amp0000663

Dahlhamer, J., Lucas, J., Zelaya, C., Nahin, R., Mackey, S., DeBar, L., Kerns, R., Von Korff, M., Porter, L., & Helmick, C. (2018). Prevalence of chronic pain and high-impact chronic pain among adults—United States, 2016. *MMWR Morbidity and Mortality Weekly Reports, 67*, 1001–1006. https://doi.org/10.15585/mmwr.mm6736a2

Deane, K. D., & Holers, V. M. (2021). Rheumatoid arthritis pathogenesis, prediction, and prevention: An emerging paradigm shift. *Arthritis & Rheumatology, 73*(2), 181–193. https://doi.org/10.1002/art.41417

Devan, H., Farmery, D., Peebles, L., & Grainger, R. (2019). Evaluation of self-management support functions in apps for people with persistent pain: Systematic review. *JMIR mHealth and uHealth, 7*(2), e13080. https://doi.org/10.2196/13080

Dlugasch, L., & Story, L. (2021). *Applied pathophysiology for the advanced practice nurse.* Jones & Bartlett Learning.

Dowell, D., Haegerich, T. M., & Chou, R. (2016). CDC guideline for prescribing opioids for chronic pain—United States, 2016. *MMWR Recommendations and Reports, 65*(1), 1–35. https://www.cdc.gov/mmwr/volumes/65/rr/pdfs/rr6501e1.pdf

Dowell, D., Haegerich, T. M., & Chou, R. (2019). No shortcuts to safer opioid prescribing. *New England Journal of Medicine, 380*(24), 2285–2287. https://doi.org/10.1056/NEJMp1904190

Estévez-López, F., Gray, C. M., Segura-Jiménez, V., Soriano-Maldonado, A., Álvarez-Gallardo, I. C., Arrayás-Grajera, M. J., Carbonell-Baeza, A., Aparicio, V. A., Delgado-Fernández, M., & Pulido-Martos, M. (2015). Independent and combined association of overall physical fitness and subjective well-being with fibromyalgia severity: The al-Ándalus project. *Quality of Life Research, 24*(8), 1865–1873. https://doi.org/10.1007/s11136-015-0917-7

Ewing, J. A. (1984). Detecting alcoholism: The CAGE Questionnaire. *JAMA, 252*(14), 1905–1907. https://doi.org/10.1001/jama.1984.03350140051025

Field, R., Pourkazemi, F., Turton, J., & Rooney, K. (2021). Dietary interventions are beneficial for patients with chronic pain: A systematic review with meta-analysis. *Pain Medicine*, 22(3), 694–714. https://doi.org/10.1093/pm/pnaa378

Finley, C. R., Chan, D. S., Garrison, S., Korownyk, C., Kolber, M. R., Campbell, S., Eurich, D. T., Lindblad, A. J., Vandermeer, B., & Allan, G. M. (2018). What are the most common conditions in primary care? Systematic review. *Canadian Family Physician*, 64(11), 832–840.

Flynn, D., Eaton, L. H., Langford, D. J., Ieronimakis, N., McQuinn, H., Burney, R. O., Holmes, S. L., & Doorenbos, A. Z. (2018). A SMART design to determine the optimal treatment of chronic pain among military personnel. *Contemporary Clinical Trials*, 73, 68–74. https://doi.org/10.1016/j.cct.2018.08.008

Generaal, E., Vogelzangs, N., Penninx, B. W. J. H., & Dekker, J. (2017). Insomnia, sleep duration, depressive symptoms, and the onset of chronic multisite musculoskeletal pain. *Sleep*, 40(1), zsw030. https://doi.org/10.1093/sleep/zsw030

Gokhale, A., Yap, T., Heaphy, N., & McCullough, M. J. (2020). Group pain education is as effective as individual education in patients with chronic temporomandibular disorders. *Journal of Oral Pathology & Medicine*, 49(6), 470–475. https://doi.org/10.1111/jop.13061

Grol-Prokopczyk, H. (2017). Sociodemographic disparities in chronic pain, based on 12-year longitudinal data. *Pain*, 158(2), 313–322. https://doi.org/10.1097/j.pain.0000000000000762

Gruß, I., Firemark, A., McMullen, C. K., Mayhew, M., & Debar, L. L. (2020). Satisfaction with primary care providers and health care services among patients with chronic pain: A mixed-methods study. *Journal of General Internal Medicine*, 35(1), 190–197. https://doi.org/10.1007/s11606-019-05339-2

Guyatt, G. H., Oxman, A. D., Vist, G. E., Kunz, R., Falck-Ytter, Y., Alonso-Coello, P., Schünemann, H. J., & GRADE Working Group (2008). GRADE: An emerging consensus on rating quality of evidence and strength of recommendations. *BMJ*, 336(7650), 924–926. https://doi.org/10.1136/bmj.39489.470347.AD

Haack, M., Simpson, N., Sethna, N., Kaur, S., & Mullington, J. (2020). Sleep deficiency and chronic pain: Potential underlying mechanisms and clinical implications. *Neuropsychopharmacology*, 45(1), 205–216. https://doi.org/10.1038/s41386-019-0439-z

Hadi, M. A., Alldred, D. P., Briggs, M., Marczewski, K., & Closs, S. J. (2017). "Treated as a number, not treated as a person": A qualitative exploration of the perceived barriers to effective pain management of patients with chronic pain. *BMJ Open*, 7(6), e016454. https://doi.org/10.1136/bmjopen-2017-016454

Häuser, W., Jung, E., Erbslöh-Möller, B., Gesmann, M., Kühn-Becker, H., Petermann, F., Langhorst, J., Weiss, T., Winkelmann, A., & Wolfe, F. (2012). Validation

of the fibromyalgia survey questionnaire within a cross-sectional survey. *PLoS One*, 7(5), e37504. https://doi.org/10.1371/journal.pone.0037504

Hilton, L., Hempel, S., Ewing, B., Apaydin, E., Zenakis, L., Newberry, S., Colaiaco, B., Maher, A., Shanman, R., Sorbero, M., Maglinone, M., Ewing, B. A., Maher, A. R., Shanman, R. M., Sobero, M. E., & Maglinone, M. A. (2017). Mindfulness meditation for chronic pain: Systematic review and meta-analysis. *Annals of Behavioral Medicine*, 5(2), 199–213. https://doi.org/10.1007/s12160-016-9844-2

Hirsch, J. K., Cukrowicz, K. C., & Walker, K. L. (2016). Pain and suicidal behavior in primary care patients: Mediating role of interpersonal needs. *International Journal of Mental Health and Addiction*, 14(5), 820–830. https://doi.org/10.1007/s11469-016-9642-x

Inkelis, S. M., Hasler, B. P., & Baker, F. C. (2020). Sleep and alcohol use in women. *Alcohol Research: Current Reviews*, 40(2), 13. https://doi.org/10.35946/arcr.v40.2.13

Innes, K. E., Selfe, T. K., Kandati, S., Wen, S., & Huysmans, Z. (2018). Effects of mantra meditation versus music listening on knee pain, function, and related outcomes in older adults with knee osteoarthritis: An exploratory randomized clinical trial (RCT). *Evidence-Based Complementary & Alternative Medicine*, 2018, 7683897. https://doi.org/10.1155/2018/7683897

Interagency Pain Research Coordinating Committee. (2016). *National pain strategy report*. https://www.iprcc.nih.gov/national-pain-strategy-overview/national-pain-strategy-report

International Association for the Study of Pain. (2021). *Definition of pain*. https://www.iasp-pain.org/resources/terminology/#pain

Kandaswamy, C., & Rengaramanujam, P. (2019). Evaluation of standard questionnaire to assess chronic alcoholism. *Journal of Evolution of Medical and Dental Sciences*, 8(24), 1896–1899. https://www.jemds.com/data_pdf/chelladurai-june-17--.pdf

Kawai, K., Kawai, A. T., Wollan, P., & Yawn, B. P. (2017). Adverse impacts of chronic pain on health-related quality of life, work productivity, depression and anxiety in a community-based study. *Family Practice*, 34(6), 656–661. https://doi.org/10.1093/fampra/cmx034

Khan, J. S., Hah, J. M., & Mackey, S. C. (2019). Effects of smoking on patients with chronic pain: A propensity-weighted analysis on the Collaborative Health Outcomes Information Registry. *Pain*, 160(10), 2374–2379. https://doi.org/10.1097/j.pain.0000000000001631

Kim, H. J., Chang, S. J., Park, H., Choi, S. J., Juon, H. S., Lee, K., & Ryu, H. R. (2020). Intra-ethnic differences in chronic pain and the associated factors: An exploratory, comparative design. *Journal of Nursing Scholarship*, 52(4), 389–396. https://doi.org/10.1111/jnu.12564

Koebner, I. J., Fishman, S. M., Paterniti, D., Sommer, D., Witt, C. M., Ward, D., & Joseph, J. G. (2019). The art of analgesia: A pilot study of art museum tours to decrease pain and social disconnection among individuals with chronic pain. *Pain Medicine, 20*(4), 681–691. https://doi.org/10.1093/pm/pny148

Koffel, E., McCurry, S. M., Smith, M. T., & Vitiello, M. V. (2019). Improving pain and sleep in middle-aged and older adults: The promise of behavioral sleep interventions. *Pain, 160*(3), 529–534. https://doi.org/10.1097/j.pain.0000000000001423

Kolasinski, S. L., Neogi, T., Hochberg, M. C., Oatis, C., Guyatt, G., Block, J., Callahan, L., Copenhaver, C., Dodge, C., Felson, D., Gellar, K., Harvey, W. F., Hawker, G., Herzig, E., Kwoh, C. K., Nelson, A. E., Samuels, J., Scanzello, C., White, D., . . . Reston, J. (2020). 2019 American College of Rheumatology/Arthritis Foundation guideline for the management of osteoarthritis of the hand, hip, and knee. *Arthritis Care & Research, 72*(2), 149–162. https://doi.org/10.1002/acr.24131

Koncz, A., Demetrovics, Z., & Takacs, Z. K. (2020). Meditation interventions efficiently reduce cortisol levels of at-risk samples: A meta-analysis. *Health Psychology Review, 15*(1), 56–84. https://doi.org/10.1080/17437199.2020.1760727

Krebs, E. E., Lorenz, K. A., Bair, M. J., Damush, T. M., Wu, J., Sutherland, J. M., Asch, S. M., & Kroenke, K. (2009). Development and initial validation of the PEG, a three-item scale assessing pain intensity and interference. *Journal of General Internal Medicine, 24*(6), 733–738. https://doi.org/10.1007/s11606-009-0981-1

Lawford, B. J., Walters, J., & Ferrar, K. (2016). Does walking improve disability status, function, or quality of life in adults with chronic low back pain? A systematic review. *Clinical Rehabilitation, 30*(6), 523–536. https://doi.org/10.1177/0269215515590487

Lee, S., Smith, M. L., Dahlke, D. V., Pardo, N., & Ory, M. G. (2020). A cross-sectional examination of patients' perspectives about their pain, pain management and satisfaction with pain treatment. *Pain Medicine, 21*(2), e164–e171. https://doi.org/10.1093/pm/pnz244

Lindell, M., & Grimby-Ekman, A. (2022). Stress, nonrestorative sleep, and physical inactivity as risk factors for chronic pain in young adults: A cohort study. *PLoS ONE, 17*(1), 1–16. https://doi.org/10.1371/journal.pone.0262601

Louw, A., Zimney, K., Puentedura, E. J., & Diener, I. (2016). The efficacy of pain neuroscience education on musculoskeletal pain: A systematic review of the literature. *Physiotherapy Theory and Practice, 32*(5), 332–355. https://doi.org/10.1080/09593985.2016.1194646

Low, M. Y., Lacson, C., Zhang, F., Kesslick, A., & Bradt, J. (2020). Vocal music therapy for chronic pain: A mixed methods feasibility study. *Journal of Alternative & Complementary Medicine, 26*(2), 113–122. https://doi.org/10.1089/acm.2019.0249

Majlesi, J. (2019). Patients with chronic musculoskeletal pain of 3-6-month duration already have low levels of health-related quality of life and physical activity. *Current Pain and Headache Reports, 23*(11), 81. https://doi.org/10.1007/s11916-019-0817-6

Mansfield, K. E., Sim, J., Jordan, J. L., & Jordan, K. P. (2016). A systematic review and meta-analysis of the prevalence of chronic widespread pain in the general population. *Pain, 157*(1), 55–64. https://doi.org/10.1097/j.pain.0000000000000314

Mayes-Burnett, D. (2020). Central nervous system drugs. In B. T. Smith (Ed.), *Pharmacology for nurses* (pp. 91–129). Jones & Bartlett Learning.

McMurtry, M., Viswanath, O., Cernich, M., Strand, N., Freeman, J., Townsend, C., Kaye, A. D., Cornett, E. M., & Wie, C. (2020). The impact of the quantity and quality of social support on patients with chronic pain. *Current Pain and Headache Reports, 24*(11), 72. https://doi.org/10.1007/s11916-020-00906-3

Mikolasek, M., Berg, J., Witt, C. M., & Barth, J. (2018). Effectiveness of mindfulness- and relaxation-based eHealth interventions for patients with medical conditions: A systematic review and synthesis. *International Journal of Behavioral Medicine, 25*(1), 1–16. https://doi.org/10.1007/s12529-017-9679-7

Morales, F. A., Jimenez, M. J. M., Morales, A. J. M., Vegara, R. M., Mora, B. A. M., Aranda, G. M., & Canca, S. J. C. (2021). Impact of a nurse-led intervention on quality of life in patients with chronic non-malignant pain: An open randomized controlled trial. *Journal of Advanced Nursing, 77*(1), 255–265. https://doi.org/10.1111/jan.14608

Mundal, I., Gråwe, R. W., Bjørngaard, J. H., Linaker, O. M., & Fors, E. A. (2014). Prevalence and long-term predictors of persistent chronic widespread pain in the general population in an 11-year prospective study: The HUNT study. *BMC Musculoskeletal Disorders, 15*(1). https://doi.org/10.1186/1471-2474-15-213

Murphy, J. L., Palyo, S. A., Schmidt, Z. S., Holrah, L. N., Banour, E., VanKeuren, C. P., & Strigo, I. A. (2021). The resurrection of interdisciplinary pain rehabilitation: Outcomes across a Veterans Affairs collaborative. *Pain Medicine, 22*(2), 430–443. https://doi.org/10.1093/pm/pnaa417

National Center for Complementary and Integrative Health. (2020). *Chronic pain: What you need to know.* https://www.nccih.nih.gov/health/chronic-pain-in-depth

Nguyen, N. P., Kim, S. Y., Daheim, J., & Neduvelil, A. (2020). Social contribution and psychological well-being among midlife adults with chronic pain: A longitudinal approach. *Journal of Aging and Health, 32*(10), 1591–1601. https://doi.org/10.1177/0898264320947293

Nijs, J., D'Hondt, E., Clarys, P., Deliens, T., Polli, A., Malfliet, A., Coppieters, I., Willaert, W., Yilmaz, S. T., Elma, O., & Ickmans, K. (2020). Lifestyle and chronic pain across the lifespan: An inconvenient truth? *PM&R*, *12*(4), 410–419. https://doi.org/10.1002/pmrj.12244

North American Spine Society. (2020). *Evidence-based clinical guidelines for multidisciplinary spine care: Diagnosis and treatment of low back pain.* https://www.spine.org/Portals/0/assets/downloads/ResearchClinicalCare/Guidelines/LowBackPain.pdf

Nyen, S., & Tveit, B. (2018). Symptoms without disease: Exploring experiences of non-Western immigrant women living with chronic pain. *Health Care for Women International*, *39*(3), 322–342. https://doi.org/10.1080/07399332.2017.1370470

Paice, J. A. (2016). Pain in advanced practice palliative nursing. In C. Dahlin, P. Coyne, & B. Ferrell (Eds.), *Advanced practice palliative nursing* (pp. 219–232). Oxford.

Palermo, T. M., & Kerns, R. D. (2020). Psychology's role in addressing the dual crises of chronic pain and opioid-related harms: Introduction to the special issue. *American Psychologist*, *75*(6), 741–747. https://doi.org/10.1037/amp0000711

Petrosky, E., Harpez, R., Fowler, K. A., Bohm, M. K., Helmick, C. G., Yuan, K., & Betz, C. J. (2018). Chronic pain among suicide decedents, 2003 to 2014: Findings from the national violent death reporting system. *Annals of Internal Medicine*, *169*, 448–455. doi:10.7326/M18-0830

Physical Activity Guidelines Advisory Committee. (2008). *Physical Activity Guidelines Advisory Committee report, 2008.* U.S. Department of Health and Human Services. https://health.gov/sites/default/files/2019-10/CommitteeReport_7.pdf

Puljak, L., & Chiara, A. (2019). Can physical activity and exercise alleviate chronic pain in adults? A Cochrane review summary with commentary. *American Journal of Physical Medicine and Rehabilitation*, *98*(6), 626–627. https://doi.org/10.1097/PHM.0000000000001179

Roelsgaard, I. K., Ikdahl, E., Rollefstad, S., Wibetoe, G., Esbensen, B. A., Kitas, G. D., van Riel, P., Bariel, S., Kvien, T. K., Douglas, K., Wållberg-Jonsson, S., Dahlqvist, S. R., Karpouzas, G., Dessein, P. H., Tsang, L., El-Galawy, H., Hithcon, C. A., Pascual-Ramos, V., Conteras-Yáñez, I., . . . Semb, A. G. (2020). Smoking cessation is associated with lower disease activity and predicts cardiovascular risk reduction in rheumatoid arthritis patients. *Rheumatology*, *59*(8), 1997–2004. https://doi.org/10.1093/rheumatology/kez557

Ross, E. L., Jamison, R. N., Nicholls, L., Perry, B. M., & Nolen, K. D. (2020). Clinical integration of a smartphone app for patients with chronic pain: Retrospective analysis of predictors of benefits and patient engagement between clinic visits. *Journal of Medical Internet Research*, *22*(4), e16939. https://doi.org/10.2196/16939

Rui, P., & Okeyode, T. (2016). *National ambulatory medical care survey: 2016 National summary tables.* https://www.cdc.gov/nchs/data/ahcd/namcs_summary/2016_namcs_web_tables.pdf

Schneiderhan, J., & Orizondo, C. (2017). Chronic pain: How to approach these 3 common conditions. *Journal of Family Practice*, *66*(3), 145–157.

Sharma, S., Abbott, J. H., & Jensen, M. P. (2018). Why clinicians should consider the role of culture in chronic pain. *Brazilian Journal of Physical Therapy*, *22*(5), 345–346. https://doi.org/10.1016/j.bjpt.2018.07.002

Smith, D., Wilkie, R., Uthman, O., Jordan, J. L., & McBeth, J. (2014). Chronic pain and mortality: A systematic review. *PLoS One*, *9*(6), e99048. https://doi.org/10.1371/journal.pone.0099048

Sommer, C., Leinders, M., & Uceyler, N. (2018). Inflammation in the pathophysiology of neuropathic pain. *Pain*, *159*(3), 595–602. https://doi.org/10.1097/j.pain.0000000000001122

Stevens, M., Cruwys, T., & Murray, K. (2020). Social support facilitates physical activity by reducing pain. *British Journal of Health Psychology*, *25*(3), 576–595. https://doi.org/10.1111/bjhp.12424

Szeto, C., Sugano, K., Wang, J., Fujimoto, K., Whittle, S., Modi, G. K., Chen, C., Park, J. B., Tam, L. S., Vareesangthip, K., Tsoi, K. F., & Chan, F. K. (2020). Non-steroidal anti-inflammatory drug (NSAID) therapy in patients with hypertension, cardiovascular, renal or gastrointestinal comorbidities: Joint APAGE/APLAR/APSDE/APSH/APSN/PoA recommendations. *Gut*, *69*(4), 617–629. http://dx.doi.org/10.1136/gutjnl-2019-319300

Treede, R.-D., Rief, W., Barke, A., Aziz, Q., Bennett, M., Benoliel, R., Cohen, M., Evers, S., Finnerup, N., First, M., Giamberardino, M. A., Kaasa, S., Kosek, E., Lavand'homme, P., Nicholas, M., Perrot, S., Scholz, J., Schug, S., Smith, B. H., . . . Wang, S. J. (2015). A classification of chronic pain for ICD-11. *Pain*, *156*(6), 1003–1007. https://doi.org/10.1097/j.pain.0000000000000160

Treede, R.-D., Rief, W., Barke, A., Aziz, Q., Bennett, M. I., Benoliel, R., Cohen, M., Evers, S., Finnerup, N. B., First, M. B., Giamberardino, M. A., Kaasa, S., Korwisi, B., Kosek, E., Lavand'homme, B., Nicholas, M., Perrot, S., Scholz, J., Schug, S., . . . Wang, S. (2019). Chronic pain as a symptom or a disease: The IASP Classification of Chronic Pain for the International Classification of Diseases (ICD-11). *Pain*, *160*(1), 19–27. https://doi.org/10.1097/j.pain.0000000000001384

Tribble, A. G., Summers, P., Chen, H., Quandt, S. A., & Arcury, T. A. (2016). Musculoskeletal pain, depression, and stress among Latino manual laborers in North Carolina. *Archives of Environmental & Occupational Health*, *71*(6), 309–316. http://dx.doi.org/10.1080/19338244.2015.1100104

U.S. Department of Agriculture. (2020). *Dietary Guidelines for Americans, 2020–2025* (9th ed.). https://www.dietaryguidelines.gov/sites/default/files/2021-03/Dietary_Guidelines_for_Americans-2020-2025.pdf

U.S. Department of Health and Human Services. (2019). *Pain Management Best Practices Inter-Agency Task Force report: Updates, gaps, inconsistencies, and recommendations.* https://www.hhs.gov/sites/default/files/pain-mgmt-best-practices-draft-final-report-05062019.pdf

Usui, C., Krinio, E., Tanaka, S., Inami, R., Nishioka, K., Hatta, K., Nakajima, T., & Inoue, R. (2020). Music intervention reduces persistent fibromyalgia pain and alters function connectivity between the insula and default mode network. *Pain Medicine, 21*(8), 1546–1552. https://doi.org/10.1093/pm/pnaa071

Vehof, J., Zavos, H. M. S., Lachance, G., Hammond, C. J., & Williams, F. M. K. (2014). Shared genetic factors underlie chronic pain syndromes. *Pain, 155*(8), 1562–1568. https://doi.org/10.1016/j.pain.2014.05.002

Wu, P., Chen, K., & Tsai, W. (2020). The Mediterranean dietary pattern and inflammation in older adults: A systematic review and meta-analysis. *Advances in Nutrition, 12*(2), 363–373. https://doi.org/10.1093/advances/nmaa116

Yuan, S. L. K., Couto, L. A., & Marques, A. P. (2021). Effects of a six-week mobile app versus paper book intervention on quality of life, symptoms, and self-care in patients with fibromyalgia: A randomized parallel trial. *Brazilian Journal of Physical Therapy, 25*(4), 428–436. https://doi.org/10.1016/j.bjpt.2020.10.003

Zhao, J., Salemohamed, N., Stinson, J., Carlin, L., Seto, E., Webster, F., & Furlan, A. D. (2020). Health care providers' experiences and perceptions participating in a chronic pain telementoring education program: A qualitative study. *Canadian Journal of Pain, 4*(1), 111–121. https://doi.org/10.1080/24740527.2020.1749003

CHAPTER 21

Healthy Lifestyle Promotion for the Cancer Continuum

Kara Mosesso, MSN, ANP-BC, AOCNP, DipACLM

If we could give every individual the right amount of nourishment and exercise, not too little and not too much, we would have found the safest way to health.

Hippocrates

OBJECTIVES

This chapter will enable the reader to:

1. Demonstrate an understanding of the economic and psychosocial burden of cancer.
2. Examine factors intertwined in cancer development and proliferation, such as infectious agents, environmental exposures, and lifestyle factors.
3. Identify the most prevalent cancer types for which lifestyle modification can mitigate risk.
4. Implement evidence-informed lifestyle strategies for cancer prevention and cancer survivorship.

Overview

Cancer was the second leading cause of death in the United States when the war on cancer was waged in 1971, and presently it remains the second leading cause of death (World Health Organization [WHO], 2022a). However, in countries like the United States, Canada, and Australia, where health systems are strong, survival rates of many types of cancers are improving thanks to accessible early detection, improvements in treatment, and a growing focus on survivorship care (Allemani et al., 2018; WHO, 2022a). These are important advancements, but while billions of research dollars have been poured into finding a cure, little attention has been paid to cancer prevention even though 30% to 50% of cancers are preventable (WHO, 2022a). Prevention offers the most cost-effective, long-term strategy for the control of cancer.

Nearly one-third of deaths from cancer are due to five leading behavioral and dietary risks: high body mass index, low fruit

© Kathleen Gail/Shutterstock; © StoryTime Studio/Shutterstock; © kali9/Getty Images

and vegetable intake, lack of physical activity, tobacco use, and alcohol use (WHO, 2021). The cancer process is multifactorial, and many causes, such as environmental exposures or certain genetic predispositions, may not be prevented by lifestyle changes. However, for most individuals, turning attention to lifestyle modification can significantly reduce the incidence of many types of cancer. Lifestyle modification can also strengthen the body and immune system to undergo and recover from cancer treatment, mitigate treatment-related side effects, and help prevent secondary cancers. This chapter provides an overview of the cancer process and modifiable cancer risk factors and outlines a plan to prevent cancer and improve cancer outcomes. The chapter focuses on the current evidence related to cancers that are modulated by lifestyle behaviors. It is not an exhaustive description of all types of cancers.

Effect of Cancer

The cancer burden continues to grow globally, inflicting tremendous physical, emotional, and financial strain on individuals, families, communities, and health systems. It was estimated that 1.8 million new cancer cases were diagnosed in the United States in 2020, equivalent to 4,950 new cases each day (Siegel et al., 2020). According to estimates from Siegel et al., an estimated 606,520 Americans died from cancer in 2020. Between 2020 and 2022, it is estimated that there will be as many as 19 million cancer survivors (Park & Look, 2019).

Economic Effect

The economic burden of cancer is high for both the individual faced with a diagnosis and for society. Healthcare expenditures on cancer treatment have increased significantly over the past two decades. The National Cancer Institute (NCI) estimates that cancer-related direct medical costs in the United States were $183 billion in 2015 and are projected to increase to $246 billion by 2030 (American Cancer Society [ACS], 2021).

Aside from direct costs, cancer deaths impose a significant economic burden because of productivity losses due to premature death. *Potential years of life lost* (PYLL), which incorporates age and residual life expectancy at death to represent the average number of years a person would have lived in the absence of cancer, is often used as a measure to assess this burden (Song et al., 2020). In 2015, there were 492,146 cancer deaths in persons aged 16 to 84 in the United States, translating to 8,739,939 PYLL, or 8.7 million years of life lost (Islami et al., 2019). Overall lost earnings were $94.4 billion. PYLL and lost earnings were high for many cancers associated with modifiable risk factors, such as lung cancer, which suggests that a large proportion of the mortality burden is avoidable.

Cancer patients have an estimated four times higher mean annual healthcare expenses than those without cancer (Park & Look, 2019). Several factors compound the out-of-pocket cost burden on the individual, including lack of health insurance, employment disability, and missed workdays, leading to reduced income, lost household productivity, medical debt, and even bankruptcy (Altice et al., 2017). Depending on the type and stage of cancer, the primary caretaker of the person with cancer may also require significant time off from work, potentially further reducing household income and productivity. Cancer survivors reporting financial hardship are more likely to delay, forgo, and have poorer adherence to cancer care (Kent et al., 2013).

Psychosocial Effect

In addition to an economic burden, cancer and its treatment can significantly affect the patients' roles and responsibilities and various other facets of their psychosocial life. Cancer survivors have a six-time higher risk for psychological disability than people without cancer (Martinez & Pasha, 2017). The incidence of psychological disorders such as depression and anxiety in survivors is between 30% and 60%, but it is estimated that less than 10% of patients are referred for psychological help (Anuk et al., 2019). The threat of recurrence causes significant anxiety. People often relive their initial fear and despair with each follow-up test, especially if left waiting for blood tests or imaging results. The economic and psychosocial burden of cancer are closely intertwined. Financial hardship before or as a result of cancer treatment can cause stress for the individuals and their families.

Cancer Process

Normal progression through the cell cycle has several checkpoints that sense damage and erroneous copying of sequences. These checkpoints stop the cell cycle, allowing cells to repair defects and prevent their transmission to daughter cells. If repair is unsuccessful, cells may undergo apoptosis, or death. This process protects the tissues from accumulating cells with damaged deoxyribonucleic acid (DNA). However, an optimal environment is required for the checkpoints to function as intended. According to the World Cancer Research Fund (WCRF) and the American Institute for Cancer Research (AICR), somatic mutations, viruses, aging, nutritional factors, physical activity, and body fatness are important determinants of the function of these protective processes (WCRF/AICR, 2018f). Cancer develops when the normal processes that regulate cell behavior fail. Cancer development and proliferation are complex processes generally induced by factors related to aging and exogenous (environmental) and endogenous (host) influences over the life span (WCRF/AICR, 2018f). Epidemiology has demonstrated that while genetic factors may contribute to cancer risk on the individual level, the patterns of cancer are determined mainly by modifiable factors (diet, lifestyle) at the population level (see **Figure 21.1**).

Host Factors

Host, or endogenous, factors in the cancer process arise within the body at a cellular level. These factors include genetics, epigenetics, hormones, inflammatory state and immune function, aging, oxidative stress, and other factors.

Genetics

DNA replication in the growth and maintenance phase of a cell cycle is complex, and errors in the copying sequence of nucleotides are inevitable. Each time a cell in the body divides into two new daughter cells, there is the potential for errors in the replication of DNA. Cells are constantly exposed to factors that can damage DNA. These include agents from the environment outside the body, such as radiation or chemicals in cigarette smoke, and agents generated by processes within the body, such as free radicals or other by-products of metabolism (WCRF/AICR, 2018f). Cells that have abnormal DNA may reproduce with permanent mutations. Though some mutations can be beneficial, others are harmful, such as cancer. Most mutations are a result of an accumulation of genetic damage in cells over time.

Familial cancers are uncommon at a population level and play a major role in less than 10% of all cancers (Morin et al., 2017). The relatively small number of individuals with inherited mutations are at high risk of developing cancer since they need to acquire fewer subsequent mutations over the life span (WCRF/AICR, 2018f). In people with an inherited genetic predisposition to cancer, the effect of other risk factors for cancer is at least as great as in people who do not have an inherited susceptibility. However, the inheritance of a cancer-linked germ-line mutation does not mean a person will ultimately develop cancer. Most people with a family history of cancer do not require genetic screening (ACS, 2017). As with many medical tests, genetic testing may provide false-negative or false-positive results. Therefore, the risks and benefits of genetic

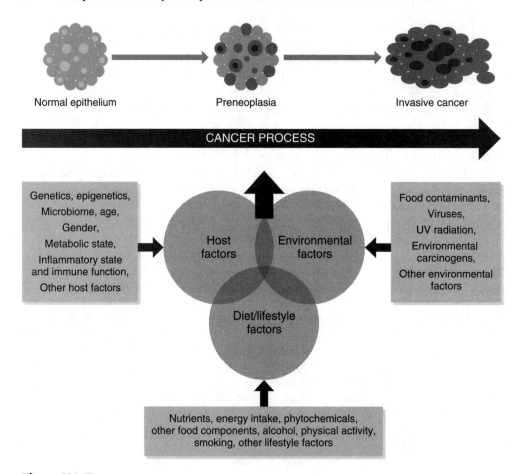

Figure 21.1 The cancer process.

This material has been reproduced from the World Cancer Research Fund and American Institute for Cancer Research. Diet, Nutrition, Physical Activity and Cancer: a Global Perspective. Continuous Update Project Expert Report 2018. Available at dietandcancerreport.org

Pros and Cons of Genetic Testing

A genetic counseling session to discuss the pros and cons of screening may be advised if:

- Someone has several first-degree relatives with cancer, especially if family members were diagnosed at a young age.
- A person has many relatives on one side of the family who have had the same type of cancer.
- Someone has a cluster of cancers in the family known to be linked to a single gene mutation (such as the BRCA 1 or 2 mutation linked to breast and ovarian cancers).
- There is a family member with rare cancer, such as breast cancer in a male.
- A person has known family members with an inherited gene mutation that increases risk.

testing must be weighed carefully. See the preceding box for the pros and cons of genetic testing.

Epigenetics

Epigenetics change as humans age, both as a normal part of development and aging and in response to behaviors, infections, and the environment (Centers for Disease Control and Prevention [CDC], 2020b). Lifestyle and environment are closely intertwined with epigenetics, helping to turn certain genes *on* or *off* and thus playing a major role in gene expression. The role of epigenetic control mechanisms in the development of human cancer is unclear, but together with the mutation of specific genes, these mechanisms may be crucial in the development of certain malignancies (Morin et al., 2017). For example, having a mutation in the breast cancer gene 1 (BRCA1) that prevents the gene from functioning properly increases the likelihood of breast, ovarian, pancreatic, and prostate cancers (CDC, 2020b). Similarly, an increase in the epigenetic mechanism involving direct chemical modification to the DNA, called DNA methylation, results in decreased BRCA1 gene expression and raises the risk for breast and other cancers (Tang et al., 2016).

Hormones

Imbalances in the homeostasis of various hormone pathways are also linked to the development and progression of hormone-dependent cancers (NCI, 2015b). Hormone receptor-positive breast, ovarian, endometrial, and prostate cancers depend on the respective male and female hormones for their growth and proliferation (Ulm et al., 2019). These types of cancers are often treated with therapy meant to block the hormone receptor or reduce the production of the causative hormone. For example, treatments that decrease androgen levels or block androgen activity can inhibit the growth of prostate cancer, so hormone depletion remains a mainstay of therapy (Ulm et al., 2019).

The insulin and insulin-like growth factor 1 (IGF-1) signaling pathways are also linked to cancer development (Knuppel et al., 2020). Not only do insulin and IGF-1 have metabolic effects for regulating glucose uptake, but they also have mitogenic and anti-apoptotic activity, which plays a role in organ development. Insulin and IGF-1 have been shown to stimulate cell proliferation in normal tissues and human cancer cell lines. The evidence further suggests that certain lifestyles, such as one involving a high-energy diet, may increase IGF-I levels, contributing to cancer risk (WCRF/AICR, 2018b).

Inflammatory State and Immune Function

Though acute inflammation is a normal physiological response to tissue injury, chronic inflammation is associated with DNA and tissue damage, including genetic and epigenetic changes that lead to cancer (WCRF/AICR, 2018f). A predisposition to chronic inflammation can be acquired through both single-gene inheritance (e.g., hemochromatosis) and multiple-gene inheritance (e.g., inflammatory bowel disease) and increase an individual's risk of cancer. Likewise, lifestyle choices can contribute to chronic inflammation. For example, the inflammatory response to acid reflux, which is more common with the standard American diet, is likely responsible for the increased incidence of esophageal carcinoma (Mayer, 2017).

Systemic immunity may also play a role in cancer risk (Song & Tworoger, 2020). Though direct evidence linking prediagnosis systemic immunity to cancer risk is limited, people who have human immunodeficiency virus (HIV) infection or take immunosuppressant medication have a higher cancer risk than the general population. This is because an immunocompromised system is less able to detect and destroy cancer cells or fight off infections that cause cancer, such as the Epstein-Barr virus (EBV) or hepatitis C virus (HCV) (NCI, 2015a).

Some hypothesize that an aging immune system is a primary reason cancer risk increases with age (Laconi et al., 2020; Palmer et al., 2018). The immunosurveillance hypothesis postulates that cancer cells continually arise in the body, but usually the immune system kills them before they can proliferate (Palmer et al., 2018). T cells generally scan for and destroy cancer cells, but as the thymus shrinks in size with age, the production of native T cells declines. This expected decline in T cell production is thought to be a significant component of the age-related deterioration of the immune system and thus the rise in cancer incidence with age.

Aging

For most cancers, increasing age is the most important risk factor (WCRF/AICR, 2018c). According to the National Institutes of Health (NIH), cancer of any site is most frequently diagnosed among people aged 65 to 74 (NCI, 2021a). Aging is characterized by a loss of reserve capacity and by the actual loss of function. As cells age, they become more likely to function abnormally. Biological aging includes an accumulation of DNA damage and mutations over time coupled with disruption of the DNA repair and cell growth regulation system (Laconi et al., 2020). Some of these mutations cause cancer, and the aging body is less able to purge dysfunctional cells. Though aging is a significant risk factor for cancer, it does not mean cancer is inevitable. It is also important to remember that the aging process can be accelerated by environmental and lifestyle influences, such as tobacco use and alcohol consumption (Bosnes et al., 2019).

Oxidative Stress

The normal process by which oxygen is used to make energy from carbohydrates can generate a type of unstable molecule, called reactive oxygen species, and unstable atoms, known as free radicals, that have the potential to cause extensive damage to a cell's proteins, DNA, and membrane lipids (Saha et al., 2017). Nutrition plays a major supportive role in combating oxidative stress. Antioxidants can extinguish reactive oxygen species and other free radicals. Vitamins C and E, for example, act as antioxidants, blocking the damage that free radicals cause. Other plant-derived compounds, such as phytochemicals, also show antioxidant activity in lab studies. However, the degree to which these components affect the damage of free radicals is still uncertain (WCRF/AICR, 2018g). On the other hand, overnutrition, inflammatory foods, alcohol, tobacco, and physical inactivity in the postprandial state can contribute to oxidative stress, increasing cellular damage, cellular age, and cancer risk (Saha et al., 2017).

Environmental Factors

In addition to host factors, several environmental factors influence the cancer process. These include environmental carcinogens, radiation, and infectious agents in air, water, soil, and food.

Environmental Carcinogens

The environment contains several natural and human-made chemicals that can cause DNA damage, disrupt cell function, and contribute to cancer, such as asbestos, benzene, formaldehyde, and arsenic (NCI, 2018a). To have carcinogenic potential, a compound must undergo metabolic activation to produce reactive intermediates that bind to and damage DNA (WCRF/AICR, 2018f). Activation of these carcinogens is generally catalyzed by the cytochrome P450 family of phase I enzymes through oxidative reactions. Humans have various physiological mechanisms for protecting against the adverse effects of some carcinogens. Still, these mechanisms can be overwhelmed by large exposures and may not work as well to protect against newer exposures throughout human development, such as with industrial pollution.

Solar and Other Radiation

Ionizing radiation, which carries sufficient energy to detach electrons from atoms or molecules, can damage DNA and cause cancer (WCRF/AICR, 2018f). This type of radiation comes from ultraviolet (UV) light, gamma rays, X-rays, cosmic radiation, natural radioactivity in rock and soil (e.g., radon), airplanes, and atomic radiation from weapons and nuclear accidents. Most notably, UV rays from the sun cause malignant melanoma and nonmelanoma skin cancers. UV light is categorized into three bands of varying wavelengths: UVA, UVB, and UVC. UVB has the highest energy and is absorbed by the bases in DNA, causing patterns of DNA damage. UVA damages DNA through the generation of reactive oxygen species. The other forms of ionizing radiation increase the risk of various cancers, including leukemia, breast, and thyroid cancers, by causing DNA damage.

Infectious Agents

Many infectious agents—viruses, bacteria, and parasites—can cause cancer by disrupting normal cell signaling (de Martel et al., 2020; NCI, 2019). This disruption causes dysregulation of cell growth and proliferation, inhibiting the expression of tumor suppressor genes or causing chronic inflammation. Overall, 2.2 million new cancer cases were attributable to infections in 2018, representing 13% of all cancer cases (excluding nonmelanoma skin cancers) (de Martel et al., 2020). The burden of infectious-born cancer disproportionately affects low- and middle-income countries.

Helicobacter pylori (H. pylori) is the most important infectious cause of cancer worldwide, responsible for 810,000 new cases of gastric-associated carcinoma in 2018 (de Martel et al., 2020). Human papillomavirus (HPV) was responsible for 690,000 new cases (80% cervical and oropharyngeal). Hepatitis B

virus (HBV) contributed 360,000 new cases, and HCV caused 160,000 new cases, mainly hepatocellular carcinoma. Other infectious pathogens, namely, EBV (which causes nasopharyngeal carcinoma and lymphoma), human T cell lymphotropic virus type 1, human herpesvirus type 8 (also known as Kaposi sarcoma herpesvirus), and parasitic infections (such as Opisthorchis viverrini from the consumption of raw or undercooked contaminated freshwater fish) were together responsible for the remaining 210,000 new cases. Vaccinations against certain viruses such as HPV, HBV, and HCV are important for cancer prevention (WHO, 2020, 2022b).

Lifestyle Factors

Fewer than 10% of all cancer cases are rooted only in hereditary factors (Morin et al., 2017). Most cancer cases (about 90%) are attributable to potentially modifiable environmental and lifestyle factors, including tobacco use, diet, alcohol, sun exposure, stress, obesity, and physical inactivity (Anand et al., 2008). Lifestyle factors may confer a direct cancer risk or increase cancer risk by creating a cancer conducive environment (see **Table 21.1**).

Diet

The significant variation in rates of specific cancers among countries and the dramatic changes in cancer incidence among populations emigrating to regions with different cancer rates indicate the importance of diet to prevent cancer (Willett, 2000). The extent to which diet contributes to cancer varies according to the type of cancer. For example, Willett (2000) found that diet contributes to 70% of colorectal cancer (CRC) and about 20% of lung cancers. Some links between diet and the cancer process are indirect. For example, the dietary pattern is a key component of weight management, and obesity is a risk factor for many cancers (see the section titled Weight).

Table 21.1 Effect of Lifestyle Factors on Susceptibility to Cancer

Exposure	Systemic Effect
Greater intake of red and processed meat	Elevated exposure to nitrites; endogenous N-nitroso compound formation
Greater body fatness	Hyperinsulinemia
	Increased estrogen
	Inflammation
Greater alcohol intake	Elevated acetaldehyde
	Increased estrogen
	Inflammation
Greater tobacco use	Systemic circulation of carcinogenic compounds
	Inflammation; weakened immune system

Data from World Cancer Research Fund and American Institute for Cancer Research. (2018). *The cancer process, table 1: Potential impact of diet, nutrition, physical activity and height in increasing susceptibility to cancer.* https://www.wcrf.org/wp-content/uploads/2021/02/The-cancer-process.pdf

Other links between diet and the cancer process are specific, such as the relationship between consumption of red and processed meat and CRC (Vieira et al., 2017; WCRF/AICR, 2018d). The more red and processed meats people consume, the higher the risk (Norat et al., 2005; Willett et al., 1990). Processed meats can include sausages, bratwursts, chorizo, frankfurters, and hot dogs, to which nitrites or other preservatives are added (WCRF/AICR, 2018d; WHO, 2015). Nitrite is used to preserve processed meats and gives cured meats their distinct color and flavor. Nitrite can react with the degradation products of amino acids to form exogenously derived N-nitrosodimethylamine (N-nitroso) compounds, which have carcinogenic potential (Han et al., 2019). These compounds may be included in meat during the curing process or formed in the body following dietary nitrate intake. Additionally, the high salt content of processed meats may damage the stomach's mucosal lining, leading to inflammation, atrophy, and H. pylori colonization.

Some biological mechanisms may underlie the association of red and processed meats with cancer. Cooking meats at high temperatures (up to 300°F), such as with grilling and frying, results in the formation of heterocyclic amines (HCAs) and polycyclic aromatic hydrocarbons (PAHs), which have mutagenic potential and have been linked to cancer development (Bouvard et al., 2015; Cross & Sinha, 2004). The longer meat is cooked, the more HCAs are produced. Heme iron, which is iron attached to a hemoprotein found only in food of animal origin, is present at high levels in red meat (WCRF/AICR, 2018d). This type of iron has also been shown to promote CRC growth by stimulating the formation of carcinogenic N-nitroso compounds (Fiorito et al., 2020).

Cantonese-style salted fish increases the risk for nasopharyngeal cancer (WCRF/AICR, 2018d). Salting is a traditional method of preserving raw fish throughout Asia, Africa, and parts of the Mediterranean. Other foods preserved by salting increase the risk of stomach cancer, including pickled vegetables and salted or dried fish as traditionally prepared in East Asia. With Cantonese-style salted fish and salt-preserved foods, the more people consume, the higher the risk.

On the other hand, high consumption of fruits and vegetables can reduce the risk of many cancers, but the constituents of these foods responsible for this risk reduction are not as clear (Willett, 2000). A pooled meta-analysis of four studies analyzing cancer incidence in those with a vegetarian or vegan diet found an 8% lower risk of cancer among vegetarians and a 15% lower risk among individuals following a completely plant-based diet (Dinu et al., 2017). There is also evidence that consumption of food rich in dietary fiber is associated with a reduced risk of total cancer and a reduced risk of total cancer mortality (Kaluza et al., 2020; Kyrø et al., 2018; Lohse et al., 2016).

Weight

Obesity has emerged as a major preventable cause of cancer (Ellulu et al., 2017). Aside from not smoking, maintaining a healthy weight is the most important thing individuals can do to protect themselves against cancer (AICR, 2020). Cancer risk likely increases as body mass index (BMI) rises above 25 kg/m^2 (Croswell et al., 2017). In general, the more excess weight someone carries, the higher the risk of certain cancers (WCRF/AICR, 2018b). It is estimated that in the United States, excess adiposity accounts for about 17% of the risk for postmenopausal breast cancer, 15% to 17% for CRC, 20% to 28% for renal cell cancer, and 17% to 20% for pancreatic cancer (WCRF/AICR, 2018b). Obesity is also associated with several other cancers, including liver, gallbladder, ovarian, esophageal, thyroid, meningioma, multiple myeloma, endometrial, and uterine (Lauby-Secretan et al., 2016).

The exact mechanism by which obesity causes cancer is unclear, but chronic inflammation associated with obesity may enhance cancer progression and any chronic comorbid conditions, such as diabetes. Adipose tissue, especially visceral fat, is metabolically active tissue. Excess adipose tissue leads to the elevated secretion of some pro-inflammatory cytokines, including interleukin-6, interleukin-8, and tumor necrosis factor-α (Stępień et al., 2014). Adipose cells also produce various proteins that cause high levels of circulating insulin and IGF-1, both of which signal inflammation (Yeh et al., 2020). Insulin and inflammatory pathways are all upregulated in obesity, preventing the process of apoptosis. These inflammatory proteins create a metabolic state conducive to accumulating the genetic and epigenetic alterations that may lead to cancer. Having a large amount of adipose tissue also affects sex hormone metabolism and causes the body to produce excess estrogen, which is linked to the development of several cancers (AICR, 2020) (see the section titled Hormones).

Epidemiological studies, such as the Nurses' Health Study, and observational studies, such as the Women's Health Initiative, have demonstrated a statistically significant reduction in cancer risk with weight loss (Eliassen et al., 2006; Morimoto et al., 2002; Yeh et al., 2020). This reduced risk is because weight loss may reduce central adiposity and levels of the endogenous insulin-sensitizing hormone adiponectin, which in turn improves insulin and pro-inflammatory cytokines and may lead to lower cell proliferation and a lower likelihood of developing cancers. Another study showed that intentional weight loss of 5% or greater significantly lowered endometrial cancer risk (Luo et al., 2017). However, this study is not generalizable to other cancer types. Though it is clear that weight loss reduces obesity-related cancer risk, more research is needed to determine how much weight needs to be lost to reduce risk, how much of the obesity-related cancer risk can be reduced with weight loss, and whether the benefits of weight loss can be offset by any subsequent regain (Luo et al., 2017; Yeh et al., 2020).

Exercise

There is strong evidence from WCRF/AICR (2018e) that leading a sedentary lifestyle increases the risk of many cancers. In contrast, moderate- and vigorous-intensity physical activity directly protects against cancers of the colon, breast, and endometrium (WCRF/AICR, 2018e). There is also limited evidence suggesting that physical activity decreases esophageal, lung, bladder, renal cell, stomach, and liver cancers.

Observational studies have shown that the most physically active people have the lowest risk of some cancers, including bladder (Keimling et al., 2014), breast (Pizot et al., 2016), colon (Liu et al., 2016), and endometrial (Schmid et al., 2015). Regular exercise may prevent excess weight; therefore, it might indirectly reduce the risk of obesity-related cancers through reductions in circulating estrogen, insulin, and IGF-1 levels (Winzer et al., 2011). Exercise reduces inflammation and has been shown to have immunomodulatory effects, improving both innate and acquired immunity (Krüger et al., 2016). It also decreases oxidative stress, prevents telomere shortening, and enhances DNA repair mechanisms.

Alcohol

Acetaldehyde, a human metabolite of ethanol formed by the metabolic activity of human cells, has been classified as a group 1 carcinogen by the International Agency for Cancer Research (IARC), meaning it is carcinogenic for humans (WCRF/AICR, 2018a). In addition to being a carcinogen, higher ethanol consumption can induce oxidative stress and genomic instability, interfere with DNA repair mechanisms, alter hormone metabolism (e.g., increase estrogen), and negatively affect the gut microbiome leading to inflammation and gut permeability (Bajaj, 2019; WCRF/AICR, 2018a).

Drinking alcohol increases the risk of several cancers, including cancers of the oral cavity, pharynx, larynx, esophagus, liver, colon, and breast (CDC, 2019; WCRF/AICR, 2018a). Two or more alcoholic drinks a day (about 30 grams or more of alcohol) increase the risk of CRC and three or more alcoholic drinks a day (about 45 grams or more) increase the risk of stomach and liver cancer (WCRF/AICR, 2018a). All alcoholic beverages, including red and white wine, beer, and liquor, are linked with cancer (CDC, 2019). The more alcohol consumed, the higher the cancer risk.

Tobacco

Tobacco use is the single most important risk factor for cancer (CDC, 2021a). Tobacco smoke contains at least 70 carcinogens that can damage DNA. Inhalation of tobacco smoke causes these carcinogenic compounds to enter the bloodstream and circulate through the body. For this reason, the use of tobacco can cause cancer almost anywhere in the body. Tobacco can alter cell-signaling pathways and likely contributes to systemic inflammation (Anand et al., 2008). Additionally, tobacco use weakens the immune system, making it harder to eliminate cancer cells (CDC, 2010). Secondhand smoke, smokeless tobacco products (e.g., snuff, chewing tobacco), and electronic cigarettes are also associated with cancer risk (CDC, 2021a).

Although typically associated with lung cancer, tobacco use increases the risk of developing at least 14 types of cancer, including acute myeloid leukemia and cancer of the mouth, bladder, liver, pancreas, larynx, cervix, colon, and rectum (Anand et al., 2008) (see **Figure 21.2**). Tobacco use is responsible for about 20% of all cancer-related deaths (ACS, 2020; NCI, 2017).

Types and Prevalence

Cancer is not one disease but a collection of related conditions that have one thing in common: division and abnormal proliferation of cells that can spread into surrounding tissues.

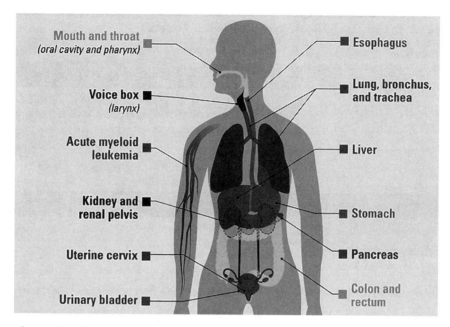

Figure 21.2 Cancers linked to tobacco use.

Source: Centers for Disease Control and Prevention. (2021). *Tobacco and Cancer*. https://www.cdc.gov/cancer/tobacco/index.htm

There are more than 100 types of cancer (WCRF/AICR, 2018f). Even tumors arising from the same tissue make up several different subtypes. It is estimated that 1.8 million new cancer cases were diagnosed in the United States in 2020, equivalent to nearly 5,000 new cases per day (Siegel et al., 2020). The lifetime probability of being diagnosed with an invasive cancer is about 40.1% for men and 38.7% for women. Lung, prostate, and CRC are the most common and are responsible for the most deaths in men while lung, breast, and CRC are the most common and responsible for the greatest number of deaths among women (CDC, 2021b).

Cancer occurrence and outcomes vary considerably among racial and ethnic groups. Survival rates are lower for Blacks than Whites for almost every cancer type, except cancers of the kidney and pancreas, for which they are the same (Siegel et al., 2020). The disparity is even larger for American Indians and Alaska Natives, among whom the risk of cancer death

is 51% higher than that for Whites. These disparities are partly due to systemic racism, reflecting differences in risk factor exposure, a later stage of disease at diagnosis due to less emphasis on or access to screening, and inconsistencies in recommended follow-up after diagnosis.

It is estimated that there are 26 cancer types attributable to potentially modifiable risk factors, including tobacco use; excess body weight; alcohol intake; consumption of red and processed meat; low consumption of fruits, vegetables, and dietary fiber; physical inactivity; UV radiation exposure; and infection with H. pylori, HBV, HCV, human herpesvirus type 8, HIV, or HPV (Islami et al., 2018) (see **Table 21.2**). The proportion of cases caused by potentially modifiable risk factors ranges from about 100% for cervical cancer to 4.3% for Kaposi sarcoma. However, of all cancers associated with modifiable risk factors, lung cancer has the highest number of attributable cases. Skin melanoma, colorectal,

Table 21.2 Cancers Associated with Modifiable Risk Factors

Risk Factor	Cancer Types
Substances	
Tobacco use (CDC, 2021a; NCI, 2017)	Oral cavity, pharynx; esophagus; stomach; colorectum; liver; pancreas; nasal cavity/paranasal sinus; larynx; lung, bronchus, trachea; cervix; kidney, renal pelvis, ureter; urinary bladder; acute myeloid leukemia
Alcohol intake (CDC, 2019)	Lip, oral cavity, pharynx; larynx; esophagus; female breast; liver; colorectum
Poor diet	
Red meat consumption (WCRF/AICR, 2018d)	Colorectum
Processed meat consumption (Rawla & Barsouk, 2019; WCRF/AICR, 2018d)	Stomach; colorectum
Low fruit/vegetable consumption (WCRF/AICR, 2018g)	Oral cavity, pharynx, larynx; lung, bronchus, trachea
Low dietary fiber consumption (WCRF/AICR, 2018g)	Colorectum
Physical inactivity and excess body weight	
Excess body weight (WCRF/AICR, 2018b)	Esophagus; stomach; colorectum; liver; gallbladder; pancreas; female breast; endometrium; ovary; kidney, renal pelvis; multiple myeloma
Physical inactivity (WCRF/AICR, 2018e)	Colon; female breast; endometrial
Environmental	
UV radiation (Sample & He, 2018)	Melanoma of the skin
Infections	
H. pylori (de Martel et al., 2020)	Stomach
HBV (de Martel et al., 2020)	Liver
HCV (de Martel et al., 2020)	Liver; non-Hodgkin lymphoma
Human herpes virus type 8 (de Martel et al., 2020)	Kaposi sarcoma
HIV (de Martel et al., 2020)	Anus; Kaposi sarcoma; cervix; Hodgkin lymphoma; non-Hodgkin lymphoma
HPV (de Martel et al., 2020)	Oral cavity; oropharynx, tonsils, base of tongue; anus; cervix; vulva; vagina; penis

Data from Islami, F., Goding Sauer, A., Miller, K. D., Siegel, R. L., Fedewa, S. A., Jacobs, E. J., McCullough, M. L., Patel, A. V., Ma, J., Soerjomataram, I., Flanders, W. D., Brawley, O. W., Gapstur, S. M., & Jemal, A. (2018). Proportion and number of cancer cases and deaths attributable to potentially modifiable risk factors in the United States. Table 1, p. 33. *CA: A Cancer Journal for Clinicians, 68*(1), 31–54. https://doi.org/10.3322/caac.21440

breast, and endometrial cancers follow lung cancer in the number of cases attributed to lifestyle factors (Islami et al., 2018). These five cancers most associated with modifiable factors are reviewed in the following sections.

Lung Cancer

Cancer of the lung was rare before 1900, but by the mid-20th century, it was established as the leading cause of cancer-related death in North America and Europe (Horn et al., 2017). Though the incidence has declined significantly in both men and women over the past few decades due to tobacco cessation, lung cancer is still responsible for the most cancer-related deaths (135,720 in 2020) (U.S. Preventive Services Task Force [USPSTF], 2021c). It is the second most prevalent cancer type, with over 235,000 cases diagnosed annually (NCI, 2020a).

About 8.9% of lung cancer cases are attributed to insufficient consumption of fruits and nonstarchy vegetables (Islami et al., 2018; WCRF/AICR, 2018g). However, most lung cancer cases (82%) are smoking related (Islami et al., 2018). Smokers have a 10-fold or greater risk of developing lung cancer than those who never smoked (Horn et al., 2017). According to the USPSTF (2021a), the risk for lung cancer increases with age and cumulative tobacco exposure and decreases with time after smoking cessation.

The average five-year survival rate for lung cancer is among the lowest (20.5%) of all types of cancer, but the prognosis is better when diagnosed at an early stage (USPSTF, 2021c). Low-dose computed tomography (LCDT) is the only screening test recommended for lung cancer (USPSTF, 2021b). The USPSTF recommends annual screening for lung cancer with LDCT in adults aged 50 to 80 who have a 20 pack-year smoking history and currently smoke or have quit within the past 15 years. Screening should be discontinued once a person has not smoked for 15 years or develops a health problem that significantly limits life expectancy or the ability or willingness to have curative lung surgery. LDCT screening should be done as part of a cancer screening program in which tobacco cessation counseling is also offered.

As with any cancer screening methodology, the decision to begin screening should result from a thorough discussion between the APP and the patient of the possible benefits, limitations, and known and uncertain harms. The most notable harm of lung cancer screening is the risk for false-positive results and incidental findings that lead to a cascade of testing, treatment, and the anxiety of living with a lesion that may be cancer (USPSTF, 2021a). The sensitivity of chest radiography for detecting lung cancer varies depending on the size and location of the lesion, the image quality of the scan, and the skill of the radiologist who interprets the scan. For this reason, it is best for screening to be performed at a medical center with expertise in lung cancer screening and treatment. To minimize the uncertainty and variation about the evaluation and management of lung nodules and to standardize the reporting of LDCT screening results, the American College of Radiology (2021) developed a classification system called the Lung Imaging Reporting and Data System (Lung-RADS) and endorses its use in lung cancer screening. Lung-RADS provides guidance to clinicians about which findings are suspicious for cancer and the suggested management of nodules detected with screening.

Skin Melanoma

In order of incidence, the three most common types of skin cancer are basal cell carcinoma, squamous cell carcinoma, and melanoma (Watson et al., 2016). Though melanoma is the least common of the three, it is the skin cancer responsible for the most deaths. It was estimated that more than 1.3 million Americans live with melanoma and that nearly 20 Americans die from melanoma daily (NCI, 2021b; Siegel et al., 2021). Invasive melanoma was projected to be the fifth most diagnosed cancer for both men and women in 2021 (Siegel et al., 2021).

Most melanoma cases worldwide are attributed to skin cell damage from UV radiation exposure (Arnold et al., 2018; Islami et al., 2018). An increasing number of sunburns throughout the life span, especially those with blisters or pain lasting two or more days, increases the risk of cutaneous melanoma (Dennis et al., 2008). Each tan also hastens skin aging and increases the risk for all types of skin cancer (American Academy of Dermatology [AAD], 2021). Exposure to tanning beds for more than 10 tanning sessions is strongly associated with cutaneous melanoma (Colantonio et al., 2014). The USPSTF has not found sufficient evidence to recommend standardized clinical screening for melanoma; however, the AAD (2021) recommends regular skin self-exams. A dermatologist can make individual recommendations about how often an individual with fair skin or a history of sun exposure requires a skin exam from a healthcare provider.

To prevent melanoma, the AAD (2021) recommends everyone use sunscreen that is:

- Broad-spectrum protection against UVA and UVB rays
- SPF 30 or higher
- Water resistant

In addition to wearing sunscreen, dermatologists recommend seeking shade when appropriate; wearing a wide-brimmed hat, sunglasses, and lightweight sleeved shirts and pants when appropriate; avoiding tanning beds; and using extra caution near water, snow, and sand (AAD, 2021).

Colorectal Cancer

CRC, which includes colon and rectal cancer, is the fourth most prevalent cancer type and the fourth top cause of cancer-related death (CDC, 2021b). CRC occurred in 36.3 per 100,000 people in 2019 and was responsible for 12.8 deaths per 100,000 people. The initial symptoms of CRC are vague and atypical, leading to a poor prognosis and high fatality rate (NCI, 2018b).

In the United States, more than half of all CRCs are attributable to lifestyle factors, including an unhealthy diet, insufficient physical activity, BMI $\geq$30 kg/m^2, high alcohol consumption (daily average >3 drinks), and tobacco use (Bagnardi et al., 2015; Islami et al., 2018; Xue et al., 2017). Dietary patterns likely influence risk both indirectly through excess calories and obesity and directly through specific dietary elements (Islami et al., 2018). For example, red meat consumption in excess of 100 grams/day and processed meat consumption are directly attributable to CRC, with a stronger association for colon cancer than rectal cancer and for processed meat than red meat (Chan et al., 2011; Vieira et al., 2017). On the other hand, numerous studies have shown that people with healthy lifestyle behaviors (such as high fiber intake and regular exercise) have a 27% to 52% lower risk of CRC compared to those without these behaviors (Kohler et al., 2016).

The USPSTF (2021b) found that CRC screening has a substantial net benefit for reducing CRC mortality in adults aged 50 to 75 and a moderate net benefit in adults aged 45 to 49. Screening can reduce CRC mortality by decreasing the incidence of disease and increasing the likelihood of survival. The benefit of early detection and intervention of CRC declines after age 75. Thus, the USPSTF recommends screening for CRC starting at age 45 for those with average risk and continuing until age 75. The decision to screen for CRC in adults 76 to 85 should consider the patient's overall health and prior screening history (USPSTF, 2021b). Screening is most appropriate in adults who are healthy enough to undergo treatment if CRC is detected and who do not have comorbid conditions that would significantly limit their life expectancy. The USPSTF does not recommend screening in adults 86 years and older because the competing causes of mortality preclude a mortality benefit that would outweigh the harms.

Many different screening options are available, such as stool-based, direct visualization, and serology tests (USPSTF, 2021b). The USPSTF's recommendations stress the evidence that CRC screening can help save lives instead of emphasizing specific screening tests. The risks and benefits of screening methods vary and are reviewed in **Table 21.3**. Patients should be given information about the benefits and limitations of each screening test to increase the likelihood of screening. When screening results in the diagnosis of colorectal adenomas or cancer, patients are followed with a surveillance regimen, and recommendations for screening no longer apply (USPSTF, 2021b).

Breast Cancer

Breast cancer includes a malignant proliferation of epithelial cells lining the ducts or lobules of the breast. In 2019, new breast cancer cases occurred in 129.7 of every 100,000 people (CDC, 2021b). Fewer than 10% of breast cancers are related to genetic mutations, whereas nearly 30% of breast cancer cases are attributable to modifiable lifestyle factors (Bagnardi et al., 2015; Islami et al., 2018; Lippman, 2017). A slight rise in breast cancer incidence rates (by approximately 0.3% per year) since 2004 has been attributed at least in part to persistent declines in the fertility rate as well as increased obesity (Pfeiffer et al., 2018). In addition to obesity, alcohol consumption and estrogen levels contribute to breast cancer risk.

Fortunately, there is a growing body of evidence that breast cancer incidence can be reduced with a lifestyle that includes minimal alcohol intake and a high-quality diet consisting of fruits, vegetables, whole grains, and legumes, including minimally processed soy (Anand et al., 2008; Bagnardi et al., 2015; Xiao et al., 2019). A predominantly plant-based dietary pattern may reduce the risk of breast cancer because it is associated with a lower BMI (Orman et al., 2020). Overweight and obesity are associated with an increased risk of breast cancer. Postmenopausal women with obesity have a 20% to 40% increased risk of developing breast cancer when compared with women of a healthy weight (Munsell et al., 2014; Renehan et al., 2008).

The mechanism by which alcohol consumption exerts its carcinogenic effect on the breast is not fully understood, though excess calories may contribute to weight gain (WCRF/AICR, 2018b). Additionally, alcohol can increase levels of estrogen. The risk of breast cancer does increase linearly with increasing doses of alcohol (Bagnardi et al., 2015).

Before menopause, estradiol, the primary estrogenic hormone involved in sexual development and reproduction, is the major estrogen secreted by the ovaries. Ovarian estrogen production ceases in postmenopausal women, and the peripheral tissues, such as adipose, liver, and kidney tissue, become the major source of estrogen (NCI, 2015b; WCRF/AICR, 2018b). At this stage, adipose tissue has higher concentrations of circulating estrogen; therefore, someone with obesity has a higher circulating estrogen concentration. Higher circulating levels of estrogen over time are consistently associated with an increased risk of breast cancer (WCRF/AICR, 2018b). Because breast cancer is a hormone-dependent disease, a longer menstrual life is a major component of the total risk of breast cancer (Lippman, 2017). Factors that increase the length of menstrual life include early menarche, late menopause, overweight and obesity, nulliparity, and never having breastfed.

Understanding the potential role of exogenous hormones in breast cancer and appropriately educating women is crucial for the APP due to the number of women who regularly use oral contraceptive pills (OCPs) and postmenopausal hormone replacement therapy (HRT). Women who have used OCPs have a

Table 21.3 Benefits and Limitations of Colorectal Cancer Screening Options

Type	Benefits	Limitations	Screening Interval
Visual examination			
Colonoscopy	■ Examines entire colon and rectum ■ Can biopsy and remove polyps ■ Can diagnose non-cancer–related diseases ■ Required for abnormal results from other CRC screening tests	■ Full bowel cleansing ■ Sedation usually needed ■ Patient may miss a day of work ■ Highest risk of bowel tears or infections	10 years
Computed tomography colonoscopy (CTC)	■ Examine entire colon ■ Quick ■ Few complications ■ No sedation needed ■ Noninvasive	■ Full bowel cleansing ■ Cannot remove polyps or perform biopsies ■ Exposure to low-dose radiation ■ Colonoscopy necessary if abnormal findings ■ Limited insurance coverage	5 years
Flexible sigmoidoscopy	■ Fairly quick ■ Few complications ■ Minimal bowel preparation ■ Does not require sedation	■ Partial bowel cleansing ■ Views only one-third of colon ■ Cannot remove large polyps ■ Small risk of infection or bowel tear ■ Slightly more effective when combined with annual fecal occult blood testing ■ Colonoscopy necessary if abnormal findings	5 years alone OR Every 10 years + FIT annually
Stool tests			
Fecal immunochemical test (FIT)	■ No bowel cleansing or sedation ■ Performed at home ■ Low cost ■ Noninvasive	■ Requires multiple stool samples ■ Will miss most polyps ■ May produce false-positive test results ■ Slightly more effective when combined with a flexible sigmoidoscopy every 5 years ■ Colonoscopy necessary if positive	Annual
High-sensitivity guaiac-based fecal occult blood test (gFOBT)	■ No bowel cleansing ■ Performed at home ■ Low cost ■ Noninvasive	■ Requires stool samples from 3 separate bowel movements ■ Will miss most polyps ■ May produce false-positive test results ■ Pretest dietary and medication limitations ■ Slightly more effective when combined with a flexible sigmoidoscopy every 5 years ■ Colonoscopy necessary if positive	Annual

Type	Benefits	Limitations	Screening Interval
Stool DNA fecal immunochemical test (sDNA FIT)	▪ No bowel cleansing ▪ Can be performed at home ▪ Requires only a single stool sample ▪ Noninvasive	▪ Will miss most polyps ▪ More false-positive results than other tests ▪ Higher cost than gFOBT and FIT ▪ Colonoscopy necessary if positive	Every 1–3 years

Data from Davidson, K. W., Barry, M. J., Mangione, C. M., Cabana, M., Caughey, A. B., Davis, E. M., Donahue, K. E., Doubeni, C. A., Krist, A. H., Kubik, M., Li, L., Ogedegbe, G., Owens, D. K., Pbert, L., Silverstein, M., Stevermer, J., Tseng, C.-W., & Wong, J. B. (2021). Screening for colorectal cancer: U.S. Preventive Services Task Force Recommendation Statement, Table 1, p. 1967. *JAMA, 325*(19). https://doi.org/10.1001/jama.2021.6238

7% increase in the relative risk of breast cancer compared with women who have never used OCPs (Bassuk & Manson, 2015). Women currently using OCPs have a 24% increased risk that does not increase with the duration of use. Risk declines after OCPs are discontinued. Similarly, six to seven years of HRT can double breast cancer risk (Lippman, 2017).

The USPSTF (2016) found adequate evidence that mammography screening reduces breast cancer mortality in women aged 40 to 74. Breast cancer is most frequently diagnosed among women aged 55 to 64. Therefore, the USPSTF recommends screening mammography every two years for women in the general population aged 50 to 74. There is a paucity of evidence demonstrating the benefits of screening mammography in women older than 75, so persistent screening after this age is not recommended (USPSTF, 2016).

The risk of breast cancer is high in women treated for childhood cancer with chest irradiation, especially survivors of childhood Hodgkin lymphoma. Survivorship guidelines from the Children's Oncology Group (2018) recommend clinical breast exams annually until age 25 and then every six months. Additionally, these women should have an annual mammogram beginning eight years after radiation or at age 25, whichever occurs first. Because mammography is limited in evaluating breasts before menopause due to breast density, an annual MRI is recommended as an adjunct to mammography.

Endometrial Cancer

Endometrial cancer is the most common type of cancer that affects the female reproductive organs (NCI, 2021c). In 2021, it was estimated that there were 66,570 new cases and 12,940 deaths (ACS, 2021). Risk factors for endometrial cancer include increasing age, hormone therapy with unopposed estrogen, early menarche, late menopause, nulliparity, never having breastfed, BMI >25 mg/m^2, metabolic syndrome, and diabetes (Beral et al., 2005; Brown & Hankinson, 2015; Dossus et al., 2010; Esposito et al., 2014; NCI, 2021c; Tsilidis et al., 2015). Bariatric surgery with sustained weight loss and physical activity, including walking, is associated with a decreased risk of endometrial cancer (Anveden et al., 2017; Schmid et al., 2015).

The endometrium has both functional and basal layers (NCI, 2021c). The functional layer is hormonally sensitive, so factors that lead to an excess of estrogen, including obesity and anovulation, lead to an increase in the deposition of the endometrial lining. These changes can lead to endometrial hyperplasia and, in some cases, cancer. A thickened lining leads to sloughing of endometrial tissue, so heavy menstrual bleeding or bleeding after menopause is often the initial sign of endometrial cancer. For this reason, most patients are diagnosed early. The USPSTF has not found strong evidence to support routine screening for endometrial cancer (CDC, 2020a).

Health Promotion Research Study

Adherence to WCRF/AICR Recommendations and Cancer

Background: In 2018, the WCRF and AICR issued revised recommendations for cancer prevention related to body fatness, physical activity, and diet. Researchers examined the relationship between adherence to these recommendations and the risk of total cancer in two population-based Swedish prospective cohorts (29,451 men and 25,349 women).

Methodology: Standardized WCRF/AICR 2018 and simplified WCRF/AICR 2018 adherence scores were constructed based on the WCRF/AICR recommendations for body weight, physical activity, diet, alcohol consumption, and dietary supplement use. Data were collected using a self-administered questionnaire.

Results: During the 15.4 years of follow-up, 12,693 incident cancers were ascertained. Statistically significant associations were observed between categories of the standardized WCRF/AICR 2018 score and total cancer incidence in the overall study population as well as in men and women when examined separately. Participants in the highest category of the standardized WCRF/AICR 2018 score (4.1–7) compared with those in the lowest category (0–2) had a lower risk of cancer, hazard ratio (HR) = 0.88 (95% CI = 0.82–0.95) with HRs of 0.86 (95% CI = 0.79–0.95) in men and 0.87 (95% CI = 0.77–0.99) in women. Examining the shape of the association between risk of cancer and adherence to the WCRF/AICR 2018 recommendations using the standardized score, researchers observed a linear dose–response relationship; each 1-point increment was associated with a 3% (95% CI = 1–5%; P-trend = 0.001) lower risk of cancer. Based on the simplified scoring, most participants (>90%) did not meet WCRF/AICR 2018 recommendations regarding consumption of plant foods, limited consumption of red/processed meat, and fast-food/processed food, and <50% of participants met the weight and physical activity recommendations. Adherence to the 2018 WCRF/AICR recommendations substantially reduced the risk of total cancer.

Implication for Advanced Practice: Lack of adherence to the WCRF/AICR 2018 recommendations by a high percentage of men and women in the study population strongly indicates a need for societal-level education for primary cancer prevention. The observed lack of compliance to specific recommendations provides information regarding which recommendations are critical for cancer prevention at a population level. APPs can play a role in education and helping patients to set small, progressive behavioral goals to meet recommended guidelines over time.

Reference: Kaluza, J., Harris, H. R., Håkansson, N., & Wolk, A. (2020). Adherence to the WCRF/AICR 2018 recommendations for cancer prevention and risk of cancer: Prospective cohort studies of men and women. *British Journal of Cancer, 122*(10), 1562–1570. doi:10.1038/s41416-020-0806-x

Starting the Conversation

Prevention

Though it's unequivocally clear that most cancers are lifestyle related, the healthcare system rarely approaches cancer from a place of prevention and risk reduction. The most practical approach is to look at living as a constant state of prevention and treatment rather than waiting until a disease has progressed to the point of showing signs. Ideally, cancer prevention should start in childhood, but it is never too late to modify lifestyle habits for prevention. Broaching a discussion about cancer risk and lifestyle modification is challenging, especially if the patient has seen a loved one suffer from cancer. It is hard to accept that such a difficult diagnosis may have been prevented. Still, it is the collective responsibility of APPs and other healthcare providers to discuss cancer

Table 21.4 Conversation Starters for Cancer Prevention

Question	Clinician Tips
What does a typical dinner look like for you and your family?	Patients need to start where they are and set specific, achievable, and progressive goals. Once a baseline of eating habits is established, the APP can suggest incremental evidence-informed dietary modifications.
What proportion of your meals are home cooked? Where does the rest of your food come from?	Determine how often patients are eating at home versus eating out. The APP can help set goals for cooking at home more often, packing a lunch, or increasing the nutritional quality of a restaurant meal.
What types of movement do you enjoy most?	Patients are more likely to develop an exercise routine if they find an activity they enjoy. Help patients identify enjoyable forms of movement and set goals around prioritizing these activities.
What have been some challenges you've encountered when making changes to your lifestyle in the past?	Discuss barriers and work with patients to identify reasonable work-arounds.
Think about a time in the past when you successfully made a significant lifestyle change. What helped you to be successful at that time?	Elicit character traits, strengths, or strategies patients utilized successfully in the past. Use these to empower patients and remind them they can accomplish difficult endeavors.

prevention with patients early and often. A list of evidence-informed resources or office pamphlets emphasizing the importance of lifestyle can serve as an adjunct to this conversation. **Table 21.4** provides questions that can be used to initiate a cancer prevention conversation.

One of the key things for patients to understand is that cancer is not an event but rather a process that occurs over time. Focus the conversation on the lifestyle behaviors that impede that process, including a nutritionally dense dietary pattern, routine physical activity, meaningful social connection, stress management, avoidance of risky substances, and adequate sleep. Each of these factors, along with avoidance of direct UV exposure and following vaccine guidelines, individually and collectively creates an environment that prevents cancer from developing and proliferating. It is important to discuss with patients and the parents of adolescents about the positive effect of following vaccination guidelines, especially for HBV and HPV, to offer long-term protection against hepatocellular and cervical cancer, respectively. Vaccination against these viruses could prevent 1 million cancer cases each year (de Martel et al., 2020).

Cancer Survivorship

The National Comprehensive Cancer Network (NCCN) defines survivorship as living with and beyond cancer (NCCN, 2020). This means that cancer survivorship starts at diagnosis and includes patients who receive treatment over a longer period. Once the diagnosis of cancer is made, the management of the patient is best undertaken as a multidisciplinary collaboration among the APP, medical oncologists, surgical oncologists, radiation oncologists, oncology nurse specialists, pharmacists, social workers, rehabilitation medicine specialists, dieticians, and several other consulting professionals working closely with each other and with the patients and their families (Longo, 2017). Though an oncologist serves

Table 21.5 Conversation Starters for Cancer Survivorship

Question	Clinician Tips
What are some of your favorite comfort foods?	People often turn to comfort foods when distressed by a new cancer diagnosis, but nutritional quality is essential. Help patients identify ways to optimize the nutrition of their favorite comfort foods so that they can get comfort *and* good nutrition.
Who in your life supports you during difficult times?	Assess patients' support system and help them to identify appropriate groups if they could benefit from additional support.
On a scale of 0 to 10, how would you rate your distress over the last month?	For those newly diagnosed with cancer, undergoing treatment, experiencing financial burdens of treatment, or awaiting the results of an annual surveillance scan, distress is common. Assess patients' level of distress and help them identify the source (emotional, practical, social, etc.). Referral to a mental health professional or social worker may be warranted if the distress score is 4 or greater.
Did your oncology treatment team provide you with a survivorship care plan?	Survivorship care plans provide evidence-informed guidance for primary care providers. If patients don't receive a care plan, ASCO and NCCN are great posttreatment resources for patients and providers alike.

as the primary treatment provider after a diagnosis is made and through the completion of treatment, the primary care provider can still play an active role in curative or palliative care, particularly when it comes to maintaining and improving functional status, assessing for treatment-related side effects, and providing psychosocial support. **Table 21.5** illustrates some questions that can be used to initiate a conversation with a cancer survivor.

Treatment starts with the development of a treatment plan. Though the focus of the treatment plan includes chemotherapeutic, radiation, and/or surgical treatment protocols, the plan optimally includes lifestyle modification prescriptions. A cancer diagnosis is a significant challenge, and providers may assume that it is unreasonable to discuss lifestyle modification with participants who were recently diagnosed with cancer or are undergoing cancer treatment. Many patients feel a loss of control following a cancer diagnosis, but they often welcome the opportunity to play a more active role in their cancer treatment and surveillance plan. Focusing on prevention

methods like increasing physical activity or modifying tobacco use can provide patients with a sense of agency. Appropriate lifestyle modifications will also strengthen patients' functional reserve and help them navigate treatment-related side effects.

As time passes, the likelihood of recurrence of primary cancer diminishes (Longo, 2017). For many types of cancer, survival for five years without recurrence is tantamount to cure. Though survivorship begins at diagnosis, the focus of survivorship care is to address the long-term needs of cancer survivors. At the end of curative treatment, a person has gradually less frequent contact with their oncology healthcare team. As the primary care provider resumes a more central role in a patient's care, there are unique medical and psychosocial needs to account for (ACS, 2016; Institute of Medicine and National Research Council, 2006).

High-quality survivorship care includes surveillance for recurrence; assessment and management of psychosocial and medical late effects; referrals for secondary cancer screening; referrals to specialists and resources as needed; and guidance about dietary patterns, exercise, and other health promotion activities (Institute of Medicine and National Research Council, 2006). It is important to ask patients whether their oncologist provided them with a survivorship care plan. A cancer survivorship care plan generally contains important information about cancer type and stage and applicable information about treatment, such as the chemotherapy regimen received, the number of treatment cycles, surgeries performed, radiation location and dose, and hormonal therapy (Fashoyin-Aje et al., 2012). Care plans also provide information about potential late effects of treatment, future screening recommendations, and health promotion opportunities. **Figure 21.3** demonstrates a standard survivorship care plan from the American Society of Clinical Oncology (ASCO).

A-SMART Prescriptions for the Cancer Continuum

The evidence for the effect of modifiable lifestyle factors on primary and secondary cancer risk is strong (Anand et al., 2008; Islami et al., 2018; Kaluza et al., 2020). Nutritious dietary choices, weight management, regular physical activity, and avoidance of alcohol and tobacco are interrelated and play a significant role (see **Figure 21.4**). Kaluza et al. (2020) found that the more WCRF/AICR 2018 cancer prevention recommendations were adhered to, the lower the cancer risk. Though there is no clear evidence that stress management, meaningful social connections, or restorative sleep directly reduce cancer risk, these lifestyle behaviors likely improve the environmental milieu, indirectly reducing cancer risk (Morey et al., 2015).

The effect of these lifestyle factors on survival after diagnosis is less clear (WCRF/AICR, 2018c). There is, however, growing evidence that lifestyle factors play an important role in determining rates of recurrence and prognosis among breast cancer survivors, and there is

evidence to suggest this may be true with other cancers as well (Farvid et al., 2020; Orman et al., 2020; WCRF/AICR, 2018c). Though the evidence is inadequate for organizations to generate guidelines for cancer survivors, cancer prevention guidelines are unlikely to be harmful to survivors who have completed the acute phase of treatment (WCRF/AICR, 2018c).

Adopt Healthy Eating
Cancer Prevention

For cancer prevention, the WCRF/AICR encourages people to follow a dietary pattern rich in whole grains, fruits, vegetables, and legumes and to limit consumption of sugar-sweetened drinks, fast foods, and other processed foods high in fat, refined starches, or added sugars (WCRF/AICR, 2018c). The recommendation for most adults is to consume one and a half to two cups of fruit and two to three cups of vegetables each day (U.S. Department of Agriculture and U.S. Department of Health and Human Services, 2020). One strategy to shift the composition of the plate and help patients adopt this more plant-based dietary pattern is to encourage patients to fill at least half of their lunch and dinner plates with a colorful variety of nonstarchy veggies each meal. Fresh, frozen, or canned vegetables (without added sodium, sugar, or fat) are acceptable. Eating these fiber and water-filled veggies before anything else on the plate may reduce the overall energy density of the meal for those who could benefit from weight loss. Additionally, eating at least three servings of whole grains per day (half a cup of cooked brown rice, oatmeal, or pasta is equivalent to one serving) can reduce CRC risk (WCRF/AICR, 2018g).

Survivorship

Traditionally, dietary advice for patients undergoing treatment focused on a high-calorie intake to maintain weight and energy needs and mitigate the effects of treatment-related nausea and gastrointestinal toxicity. However, as with

Patient Information	
Name:	DOB:
Phone:	Email:
Healthcare Providers (name and institution)	
Primary Care Provider:	
Surgeon:	
Radiation Oncologist:	
Medical Oncologist:	
Other Providers:	

Treatment Summary	
Cancer Type/Location/Stage:	Year of Diagnosis:
Surgery Procedure/Location (if applicable):	Surgery Date(s):
Radiation Dose/Areas treated (if applicable):	Radiation End Date:
Chemotherapy Agents used (if applicable):	Chemotherapy End Date:
Hormonal Therapy used (if applicable):	Hormonal Therapy End Date:
Persistent symptoms or side effects at completion of treatment (if applicable):	

Survivorship Care	
Primary/Secondary Cancer Surveillance and Other Tests	
Coordinating Provider:	Test And Frequency:
Possible late-and long-term treatment-related effects:	
Helpful Resources:	

Figure 21.3 Cancer survivorship care plan.

Data from American Society of Clinical Oncology. (2013). *ASCO treatment summary and survivorship care plan.* https://www.cancer.org/treatment/survivorship-during-and-after-treatment/long-term-health-concerns/survivorship-care-plans.html

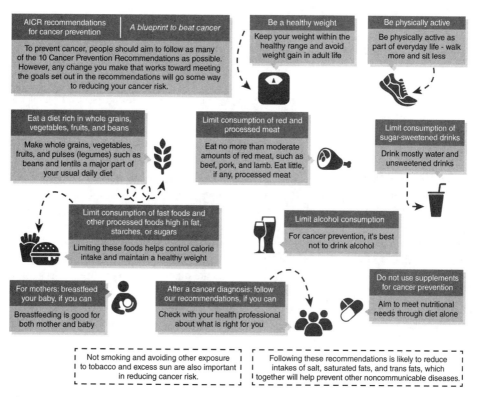

Figure 21.4 Lifestyle modifications for cancer prevention.

American Institute for Cancer Research. (2021). *10 cancer prevention recommendations.* https://www.aicr.org/resources/media-library/10-cancer-prevention-recommendations

the general population, obesity among cancer survivors is growing. Evidence suggests that elevated body fatness predicts poor outcomes in breast cancer survivors (WCRF/AICR, 2018b). For these reasons, ACS and ASCO recommend that cancer survivors be counseled to follow a dietary pattern high in vegetables, fruits, whole grains, and legumes and low in saturated fats (Rock et al., 2020). Consuming predominantly whole-plant foods can have an immediate positive effect on weight and health.

Though the use of supplements to help treat cancer is widespread, routine use of dietary supplements is not recommended by AICR or NCCN for cancer control (NCCN, 2020; WCRF/AICR, 2018c). Some supplements may interact with chemotherapeutic agents, leading to unexpected toxicities. The WCRF/AICR recommends patients meet

nutritional needs through diet alone because supplements do not offer the same benefit as eating whole food (WCRF/AICR, 2018c). Eating a variety of fruits and vegetables each day, plus whole grains and beans, helps patients ensure they are getting as many cancer-protective antioxidants, vitamins, minerals, fiber, and phytochemicals as possible. It is essential to maintain an open and nonjudgmental line of communication with patients so that they are more likely to discuss the use of supplements with their healthcare team.

There will be some patients for whom unintentional weight loss during treatment due to sarcopenia or cachexia is a problem. Unintentional weight loss is associated with poor outcomes in patients with cancer (WCRF/AICR, 2018c). Patients for whom unintentional weight loss is a problem can be guided to consume foods that are both energy and nutrient dense, such as nuts, nut butters, avocados, and potatoes rather than foods like ice cream commonly chosen by patients and recommended by providers. Referral to a lifestyle medicine certified dietician with expertise in cancer care is imperative for these patients.

Stress Less

Cancer Prevention

While short-term stress is beneficial to health, productivity, and survival, chronic stress has a detrimental effect on health. Though the evidence that stress causes cancer is weak, chronic stress does suppress or dysregulate innate and adaptive immune responses by altering cytokine balance, inducing low-grade chronic inflammation, and suppressing numbers and function of immunoprotective cells (Morey et al., 2015). Acceleration of immunosenescence is another mechanism by which chronic stress negatively affects immune function. These impedances to the immune response can leave people more susceptible to cancer. Additionally, those with prolonged psychosocial stressors may be more likely to smoke, drink alcohol, be sedentary, eat an unfavorable diet, and become obese—which are all risk factors for cancer and contribute to poorer outcomes (Anand et al., 2008; WCRF/AICR, 2018c).

As with chronic stress, those who feel lonely or are socially isolated may be more likely to smoke, drink alcohol, lead a sedentary lifestyle, eat foods detrimental to health, and gain weight (Lauder et al., 2006). Socially isolated individuals may suffer more stress than others due to a lack of social networks and support (Leigh-Hunt et al., 2017). Though social isolation and loneliness may not directly affect cancer risk, they may influence it indirectly through risky behaviors, downregulation of the immune system, and impaired immune function (Koh-Bell et al., 2021).

Patient's social connectedness and life stressors can be evaluated at each office visit. Marital status, frequency of church/temple attendance and club meetings/group activities, and the number of close friends/relatives can all provide information about their degree of social connectedness. Addressing social isolation by recommending exploration of volunteer opportunities, taking a class, or joining a group can help patients feel more socially connected and may help them develop a new sense of purpose or meaning. Assisting patients in identifying stressors, recognizing the signs of their body's response to stress, and creating personalized stress management strategies can reduce feelings of helplessness and return a sense of agency. Stress management is generally a multipronged approach, including adequate sleep, regular exercise, good nutrition, social support, cognitive behavioral therapy, mindfulness-based stress reduction, journaling, yoga, and breathing.

Survivorship

There is no evidence that successful management of psychological stress improves cancer survival. However, experimental laboratory evidence suggests that psychological stress can affect a tumor's ability to grow and metastasize (PDQ Supportive and Palliative Care Editorial Board, 2019). This is because the stress hormone norepinephrine may promote angiogenesis and metastasis. The recommendations to improve stress and social connection before and after a cancer diagnosis are similar, but the way patients experience stress and social isolation before and following a cancer diagnosis can be quite different. Patients with cancer often live under chronic stress resulting from the diagnosis itself, the threat of recurrence or mortality, and various difficulties associated with treatment, such as job discrimination, financial burden, and treatment-related symptoms. Juggling the demands of work and family with treatment demands can create an enormous amount of stress. Around a third of patients in treatment or long-term follow-up report levels of distress that warrant intervention (PDQ Supportive and Palliative Care Editorial Board, 2019). Those who have a baseline level of elevated stress or display stress soon after diagnosis are more vulnerable to longer-term distress (Cook et al., 2018). Similarly, experiencing treatment-related side effects such as alopecia or other physically disfiguring side effects can be emotionally isolating (NCI, 2021d). Following cancer, people may feel socially isolated because friends may not have stayed connected during treatment or because loved ones don't understand what the patient is going through. Some cancer survivors may attempt to manage their disease-related stress or isolation with risky behaviors such as drinking, smoking, or emotional eating (Cook et al., 2018). Others may develop a sense of helplessness or hopelessness, which may affect treatment adherence.

New stressors can arise for patients throughout the cancer treatment trajectory, including posttreatment remission, so ongoing assessment is vital. NCCN has developed a distress thermometer to help patients and providers assess distress in a nonjudgmental way (NCCN, 2022b). The thermometer allows patients to rate distress on a scale of 0 to 10, similar to a pain assessment. Those who rate their distress as a 4 or higher could benefit from additional emotional and social support to help cope with stress, reduce levels of depression and anxiety, and reduce fear of recurrence (Koch-Gallenkamp et al., 2016; NCCN, 2022a). Training in meditation, breathing, and other relaxation techniques; counseling; discussion with a religious or spiritual counselor; cognitive behavioral therapy; cancer education sessions; exercise; and social support groups can be helpful interventions at any point in the cancer continuum (NCCN, 2022a).

Move Often

Cancer Prevention

Regular physical activity helps support the immune system, maintain a healthy weight, reduce chronic inflammation, and regulate healthy levels of hormones such as insulin and estrogen (Orman et al., 2020). For cancer prevention, the AICR and WCRF recommend getting at least 150 minutes of moderate or 75 minutes of vigorous exercise per week (AICR, 2020). Though moderate to vigorous exercise is optimal, any amount of activity during the day, including walking, taking the stairs, and avoiding prolonged sedentary periods, is beneficial. The more someone moves, the greater the cancer-protective benefit (WCRF/AICR, 2018e). In addition to aerobic activity, patients should engage in muscle resistance and flexibility exercises at least two nonconsecutive days per week.

APPs should assess current physical activity regularly, counsel patients about the importance of physical activity, write activity prescriptions, help patients navigate exercising with physical limitations or other barriers, and provide local activity-related resources. Patients should be encouraged to start where they are, even if they only add a few minutes of physical activity to their routine each day or week initially. Most importantly, APPs should convey that moving matters and every little bit helps.

Survivorship

In addition to improving long-term outcomes and comorbidities in cancer survivors, exercise can lessen treatment-related toxicities and improve quality of life (WCRF/AICR, 2018e). Most of the available literature regarding exercise in people who have survived cancer is for the most common cancers, such as breast, prostate, and CRC (Ibrahim & Al-Homaidh, 2011; Meyerhardt, 2009; Meyerhardt et al., 2006; Newton et al., 2018). However, it is reasonable to assume that in the absence of any unique safety concerns for survivors of other types of cancer, the efficacy of exercise on various outcomes would be similar (Campbell et al., 2019). Combined aerobic and resistance training play a major role in addressing common problems experienced by cancer survivors, including anxiety, depression, fatigue, physical functioning, and health-related quality of life (WCRF/AICR, 2018c). Despite this, only about 23% of cancer survivors meet current physical activity guidelines (Webb et al., 2016).

In 2018, the American College of Sports Medicine (ACSM) distilled the literature on the safety and efficacy of exercise in cancer survivors and concluded that exercise training is safe during and after cancer treatment and can improve outcomes in breast, prostate, and colon cancer (Campbell et al., 2019; Patel et al., 2019). Similarly, the ACS advises cancer survivors to avoid inactivity, return to normal daily activities, and continue to follow the 2018 *Physical Activity Guidelines for Americans* as soon as possible following diagnosis (Rock et al., 2020).

A patient with a cancer diagnosis may have treatment-related side effects, such as chemo-induced peripheral neuropathy, bone metastases, cachexia, extreme fatigue, or lymphedema, that affect their ability to exercise. None of these symptoms are contraindications to exercise, though adjustments may be necessary to implement exercise safely (Patel et al., 2019). Patients with these symptoms may benefit from evaluation and guidance by outpatient rehabilitation therapy or by cancer-certified fitness professionals listed in the ACSM *Moving Through Cancer* registry. Additionally, Livestrong at the YMCA is a 12-week physical activity program that adheres to ACSM guidelines for survivors engaging in exercise and serves over 707 communities.

Avoid Alcohol

Cancer Prevention

Avoiding alcoholic beverages directly reduces cancer risk (Anand et al., 2008; WCRF/AICR, 2018a). The WCRF/AICR recommends that it is best to avoid alcohol altogether for cancer prevention (WCRF/AICR, 2018a). Those who choose to drink alcohol are encouraged to follow national guidelines. As part of alcohol risk reduction, APPs should regularly use a validated method, such as the Single Alcohol Screening

Question (SASQ) or Alcohol Use Disorders Identification Test–Consumption (AUDIT-C) (Curry et al., 2018), to screen for alcohol use and educate patients about the association between alcohol consumption and cancer risk. Screening is vital in younger patients and smokers who are more likely to report drinking in excess of the guidelines. Those who screen positively for a risky or an unhealthy use pattern should undergo a more thorough assessment.

Survivorship

In a large population-based study of alcohol consumption among adult cancer survivors, most participants with a history of cancer (56.5%) self-reported as current drinkers, including 34.9% who exceeded moderate drinking limits and 21% who engaged in binge drinking (Sanford et al., 2020). In those diagnosed with cancer, alcohol is associated with worsened cancer-related outcomes and can interfere with the metabolization of some chemotherapeutics (Sanford et al., 2020); therefore, screening for alcohol use disorder in the survivorship population is crucial. The ACS recommends that cancer survivors be counseled to limit or, better yet, avoid alcohol consumption (Rock et al., 2020).

Rest More
Cancer Prevention

There is no clear association between sleep quality and duration and cancer risk (Chen et al., 2018). Still, the cancer process is multifactorial, and it is unquestionable that adequate sleep is essential for proper immune function and stress management. Those who sleep poorly are also more likely to be obese, a risk factor for cancer (Fritschi et al., 2011; Markwald et al., 2013; WCRF/AICR, 2018b). Some studies have shown that disruption of the circadian rhythm may increase the risk of cancer (Jones et al., 2019; Konturek et al., 2011). Similarly, exposure to light while working overnight shifts for a prolonged time can reduce melatonin levels, which may interact with estrogen-signaling pathways and encourage cancer growth (Blask, 2009; Fritschi et al., 2011; Grandner et al., 2010), but data on these theories are mixed.

Patients can follow sleep guidelines from the American Academy of Sleep Medicine and the Sleep Research Society. It is important for the APP to regularly assess for sleep–wake disturbances by inquiring about subjective quantity and quality of sleep. For those who report insufficient sleep, perform a complete assessment of potential contributory factors to poor sleep, such as shift work, poor sleep hygiene, tobacco use, alcohol, pain, distress, or certain medications. Guide patients to optimize sleep hygiene and identify personalized sleep strategies, such as getting ample light during nonsleep hours, limiting caffeine, and creating a dark sleep environment (NCI, 2020b). Encouraging patients to keep a sleep journal may help them connect new behaviors to positive sleep outcomes, reinforcing the behaviors.

Survivorship

During and after a cancer diagnosis, anxiety, depression, fatigue, gastrointestinal upset, hot flashes, night sweats, nausea, and pain can all affect sleep quantity and quality (NCI, 2020b). Physical inactivity and frequent naps common during cancer treatment may further reduce sleep quality. Certain components of cancer treatment, such as anti-emetics, corticosteroids, and opioids, may disrupt circadian rhythm. It is estimated that up to 50% of people with cancer experience sleep disturbance (Berger et al., 2017). Chronic sleep disturbance resulting from cancer can significantly affect the quality of life and compound treatment-related fatigue and cognitive impairment. Relaxation techniques, mindfulness-based stress reduction, and cognitive behavioral therapy can benefit those suffering from significant anxiety and depression as a result of their cancer (Berger et al., 2017). If other strategies do not work, pharmacological intervention may be warranted.

Treat Tobacco Use
Cancer Prevention

No matter how long someone has used tobacco, quitting can reduce the risk of lung, mouth, throat, esophagus, and larynx cancers (CDC, 2021a). The level of cancer risk reduction increases with the length of time since the person has quit using tobacco. Within five years of quitting, the risk of mouth, throat, esophagus, and bladder cancers is reduced by half (CDC, 2010). Ten years after quitting, the risk of lung cancer is about half that of a person who is still smoking, and the risk of bladder, esophageal, and kidney cancers continues to decrease.

To aid cancer prevention, screen all adults for tobacco use according to general guidelines (Krist et al., 2021). Treat tobacco use as a vital sign, asking about and recording tobacco use status at every health visit (Agency for Healthcare Research and Quality, 2008). Tobacco use refers to the use of any tobacco product, including but not limited to cigarettes, cigars, hookahs, pipes, electronic nicotine delivery systems, and smokeless tobacco products (U.S. Food & Drug Administration, 2020). For those who use any amount of tobacco, provide behavioral interventions and pharmacotherapy for cessation (Krist et al., 2021).

Survivorship

Smoking cessation is equally important and beneficial in individuals with an established cancer diagnosis because it may halt the early stages of the cancer process (Croswell et al., 2017). However, cessation may not affect late-stage carcinomas, and it may not significantly decrease the cured cancer patient's risk of a second malignancy. Nonetheless, tobacco cessation is associated with improved survival, fewer side effects from treatment, and an overall improvement in quality of life (Longo, 2017). Tobacco use can alter the metabolism of many chemotherapy drugs, potentially causing unexpected toxicities and interfering with the therapeutic benefits of the agents. Assess for tobacco use in patients in any phase of the cancer continuum and offer referral for behavioral interventions. See **Table 21.6** for a summary of A-SMART prescriptions for the cancer continuum.

Table 21.6 A-SMART Prescriptions for the Cancer Continuum

Adopt healthy eating	■ Fill half of the plate at lunch and dinner with nonstarchy veggies and eat those first.
	■ Eat three servings of whole grains per day.
	■ Limit consumption of sugar-sweetened drinks.
	■ Reduce intake of fast food and processed foods.
	■ Limit red and processed meat consumption.
Stress less	■ Explore volunteer opportunities, take a class, or join a group.
	■ Learn to identify stressors and to recognize the body's response to stress.
	■ Develop personalized stress management strategies such as cognitive behavioral therapy, mindfulness-based stress reduction, journaling, exercise, or breathing.
Move often	■ Get at least 150 minutes of moderate or 75 minutes of vigorous exercise per week for cancer prevention.
	■ Engage in muscle resistance and flexibility exercises at least two nonconsecutive days/week.
	■ Cancer survivors continue to follow the 2018 *Physical Activity Guidelines for Americans* as soon as possible following diagnosis.
	■ For those with cancer-related symptoms, find a cancer-certified fitness professional using the ACSM *Moving Through Cancer* registry.
Avoid alcohol	■ If possible, avoid alcohol altogether for cancer prevention.
	■ Survivors should limit or avoid alcohol.
	■ For anyone who does drink alcohol, follow national guidelines.
Rest more	■ Identify personalized sleep strategies.
	■ Consider cognitive behavioral therapy or mindfulness-based stress reduction with a therapist or validated digital therapeutic tool.
	■ Keep a sleep journal to identify behaviors that help or interfere with sleep.
Treat tobacco use	■ Connect with a tobacco cessation program.
	■ Identify healthy behaviors to replace smoking.
	■ Remember that any reduction in tobacco use helps.

An Interprofessional Approach to Cancer Prevention and Survivorship

Cancer prevention will work best when a person-centered approach involving the APP, the family, a multidisciplinary team, and the wider community is taken. Interprofessional collaboration is important for optimizing widespread cancer prevention by means of health promotion, behavioral interventions, and cancer screening. Once patients establish care, the APP can thoroughly assess habits and behaviors associated with cancer risk and coordinate appropriate referrals based on each one's needs. The APP may develop relationships and a referral network with professionals such as certified health coaches or behavioral therapists, mental health specialists, chefs, dieticians, social workers, physical trainers, food pharmacies, teaching kitchens, community exercise programs, and individual public and community health advocates. A coordinated care effort incorporating any or all of these professions can play a role in influencing the modifiable risk factors related to cancer and improving cancer prevention at a systems level. Educational and hands-on events teaching actionable behavioral interventions, such as a cancer prevention cooking class, can effectively spread the prevention message at an individual and a community level. The prevention effort is more successful when an interprofessional team works together and learns from one another.

Summary

A nontoxic curative compound for cancer remains undiscovered; however, a greater focus on cancer prevention effectively reduces cancer morbidity and mortality. APPs with knowledge of lifestyle promotion play a vital role in educating and empowering patients of all ages and socioeconomic backgrounds to make lifestyle changes to prevent cancer and improve outcomes following a cancer diagnosis. Lifestyle modifications and behavioral interventions are crucial at any phase in the cancer trajectory, from prevention to improving cancer survivors' physical health and mental well-being to reducing the risk of recurrence and overall mortality from cancer and treatment-related side effects (see **Table 21.7**). Cancer takes a tremendous economic and psychosocial toll on individuals and society, but it does not have to.

Health Promotion Case Study: Addressing Cancer in a Postmenopausal Female

Case Description: C.K. is a 62-year-old postmenopausal female who presents to the clinic noting a large, nontender mass in her left breast. She admits not following through with recommended breast cancer screening. She appears distressed and tells you that her husband's first wife died of breast cancer.

- Past medical history: Unremarkable.
- Social history: Happily married. Works as a minister in a nondenominational Christian church.
- Vital signs: Normal.
- Physical exam: Fixed, nontender mass in the left breast approximately 3 x 4 cm in size. Dimpling of the left nipple is noted.
- Diagnostic tests: A diagnostic mammogram and ultrasound performed later that week reveal a 4.3 x 3.1 x 3.5 cm mass. She is referred for a biopsy, and pathology shows a T2 triple-negative invasive ductal carcinoma. There is no known lymphatic involvement.

(continues)

Health Promotion Case Study Addressing CVD in an Adult Male (*continued*)

Lifestyle Vital Signs

- Adopt healthy eating: Follows a predominantly plant-based dietary pattern.
- Stress less: Not assessed.
- Move often: Walks daily.
- Avoid alcohol: Consumes 1–2 glasses of wine nightly.
- Rest more: Not assessed.
- Treat tobacco use: Nonsmoker.
- BMI: 25 kg/m^2.

Assessment: T2 triple-negative invasive ductal carcinoma.

Plan: The APP offers emotional support and refers C.K. to a breast oncologist to discuss treatment options. From experience, the APP knows that the oncologist generally assumes most of the care during cancer treatment, but patients generally benefit when primary care providers play a regular supportive role.

Critical Thinking Questions

Though the oncology team is generally responsible for making treatment decisions following a cancer diagnosis, the APP can still play an important role in improving treatment outcomes, addressing treatment and diagnosis-related side effects, and enhancing the quality of life. Understanding health and treatment goals, assessing lifestyle habits, and implementing behavioral interventions are just as important in the cancer survivorship phase as they are for cancer prevention.

1. What lifestyle management strategies would you immediately consider optimizing for C.K.'s treatment outcomes?
2. What subjective data would you continue to assess throughout the treatment trajectory?

Health Promotion Activity: Addressing Lifestyle in Cancer Survivors

Review the "Exercise Guidelines for Cancer Survivors: Consensus Statement from International Multidisciplinary Roundtable" (Campbell et al., 2019). Then consider the 62-year-old female stage IIA breast cancer survivor from the chapter case study. She is now one-year status postcompletion of treatment, which included surgical resection of the tumor followed by chemotherapy. She has a BMI of 28 kg/m^2 and persistent chemotherapy-induced peripheral neuropathy. She is currently inactive but is motivated to start an exercise regimen. How would you advise her to begin?

TABLE 21.7 Evidence-Based Resources for Cancer Prevention and Survivorship

Resource	URL
Exercise Guidelines for Cancer Survivors: Consensus Statement from International Multidisciplinary Roundtable	https://journals.lww.com/acsm-msse/Fulltext/2019/11000/Exercise_Guidelines_for_Cancer_Survivors_.23.aspx
NCCN Guidelines	https://www.nccn.org/professionals/physician_gls/default.aspx

Resource	URL
Centers for Disease Control and Prevention, Let's Talk: Nutrition, Physical Activity and Cancer Survivors (An Interactive Training Simulation for Primary Healthcare Providers)	https://www.cdc.gov/cancer/survivors/health-care-providers/nutrition-pa-survivorship.htm
World Cancer Research Fund and American Institute for Cancer Research: Continuous Update Project, The Third Expert Report	https://www.wcrf.org/diet-activity-and-cancer/global-cancer-update-programme/about-the-third-expert-report
World Cancer Research Fund: Summary of Strong Evidence on Diet, Nutrition, Physical Activity and the Prevention of Cancer	https://www.wcrf.org/wp-content/uploads/2021/01/CUP-Strong-Evidence-Matrix.pdf
Anticancer Lifestyle Program	https://anticancerlifestyle.org
NCCN Guidelines for Patients for Survivorship Care for Healthy Living	https://www.nccn.org/patients/guidelines/content/PDF/survivorship-hl-patient.pdf
ACSM *Moving Through Cancer*	https://www.exerciseismedicine.org/support_page.php/moving-through-cancer
iTHRIVE	https://www.aicr.org/cancer-survival/ithrive

Acronyms

AAD: American Academy of Dermatology
ACS: American Cancer Society
ACSM: American College of Sports Medicine
AICR: American Institute for Cancer Research
ASCO: American Society of Clinical Oncology
AUDIT-C: Alcohol Use Disorders Identification Test–Consumption
BMI: body mass index
BRCA1: breast cancer gene 1
CDC: Centers for Disease Control and Prevention
CRC: colorectal cancer
CTC: computed tomography colonoscopy
DNA: deoxyribonucleic acid
EBV: Epstein-Barr virus
FIT: fecal immunochemical test
gFOBT: guaiac-based fecal occult blood test
HBV: hepatitis B virus
HCAs: heterocyclic amines
HCV: hepatitis C virus
HIV: human immunodeficiency virus
H. pylori: Helicobacter pylori

HPV: human papilloma virus
HRT: hormone replacement therapy
IARC: International Agency for Cancer Research
IFG-1: insulin-like growth factor 1
LDCT: Low-dose computed tomography
Lung-RADS: Lung Imaging Reporting and Data System
NCCN: National Comprehensive Cancer Network
NCI: National Cancer Institute
N-nitroso: N-nitrosodimethylamine
NIH: National Institutes of Health
OCPs: oral contraceptive pills
PAHs: polycyclic aromatic hydrocarbons
PYLL: potential years of life lost
SASQ: Single Alcohol Screening Question
sDNA FIT: stool DNA fecal immunochemical test
USPSTF: U.S. Preventive Services Task Force
UV: ultraviolet
WCRF: World Cancer Research Fund
WHO: World Health Organization

References

Agency for Healthcare Research and Quality. (2008). *Treating tobacco use and dependence: 2008 update*. https://www.ahrq.gov/prevention/guidelines/tobacco/index.html

Allemani, C., Matsuda, T., di Carlo, V., Harewood, R., Matz, M., Nikšić, M., Bonaventure, A., Valkov, M., Johnson, C. J., Estève, J., Ogunbiyi, O. J., Azevedo e Silva, G., Chen, W. Q., Eser, S., Engholm, G., Stiller, C. A., Monnereau, A., Woods, R. R., Visser, O., . . . Lewis, C. (2018). Global surveillance of trends in cancer survival 2000–14 (CONCORD-3): Analysis of individual records for 37 513 025 patients diagnosed with one of 18 cancers from 322 population-based registries in 71 countries. *The Lancet*, *391*(10125), 1023–1075. https://doi.org/10.1016/S0140-6736(17)33326-3

Altice, C. K., Banegas, M. P., Tucker-Seeley, R. D., & Yabroff, K. R. (2017). Financial hardships experienced by cancer survivors: A systematic review. *Journal of the National Cancer Institute*, *109*(2). doi: 10.1093/jnci/djw205

American Academy of Dermatology. (2021). *How to prevent skin cancer*. https://www.aad.org/public/diseases/skin-cancer/prevent/how

American Society of Clinical Oncology. (2013). *ASCO treatment summary and survivorship care plan*. https://www.cancer.org/treatment/survivorship-during-and-after-treatment/long-term-health-concerns/survivorship-care-plans.html

American Cancer Society. (2016). *Cancer treatment and survivorship facts and figures 2016–2017*. https://www.cancer.org/research/cancer-facts-statistics/survivor-facts-figures.html

American Cancer Society. (2017). *Understanding genetic testing for cancer*. https://www.cancer.org/cancer/cancer-causes/genetics/understanding-genetic-testing-for-cancer.html

American Cancer Society. (2020). *Health risks of smoking tobacco*. https://www.cancer.org/healthy/stay-away-from-tobacco/health-risks-of-tobacco/health-risks-of-smoking-tobacco.html

American Cancer Society. (2021). *Cancer facts and figures 2021*. https://www.cancer.org/content/dam/cancer-org/research/cancer-facts-and-statistics/annual-cancer-facts-and-figures/2021/cancer-facts-and-figures-2021.pdf

American College of Radiology. (2021). *Lung CT screening reporting and data system (Lung-RADS)*. https://www.acr.org/Clinical-Resources/Reporting-and-Data-Systems/Lung-Rads

American Institute for Cancer Research. (2020). *Be a healthy weight*. https://www.aicr.org/cancer-prevention/recommendations/be-a-healthy-weight

American Institute for Cancer Research. (2021). *10 cancer prevention recommendations*. https://www.aicr.org/resources/media-library/10-cancer-prevention-recommendations/

Anand, P., Kunnumakara, A. B., Sundaram, C., Harikumar, K. B., Tharakan, S. T., Lai, O. S., Sung, B., & Aggarwal, B. B. (2008). Cancer is a preventable disease that requires major lifestyle changes. *Pharmaceutical Research*, *25*(9), 2097–2116. https://doi.org/10.1007/s11095-008-9661-9

Anuk, D., Özkan, M., Kizir, A., & Özkan, S. (2019). The characteristics and risk factors for common psychiatric disorders in patients with cancer seeking help for mental health. *BMC Psychiatry*, *19*(1), 269. https://doi.org/10.1186/s12888-019-2251-z

Anveden, Å., Taube, M., Peltonen, M., Jacobson, P., Andersson-Assarsson, J. C., Sjöholm, K., Svensson, P.-A., & Carlsson, L. M. S. (2017). Long-term incidence of female-specific cancer after bariatric surgery or usual care in the Swedish Obese Subjects Study. *Gynecologic Oncology*, *145*(2), 224–229. https://doi.org/10.1016/j.ygyno.2017.02.036

Arnold, M., de Vries, E., Whiteman, D. C., Jemal, A., Bray, F., Parkin, D. M., & Soerjomataram, I. (2018). Global burden of cutaneous melanoma attributable to ultraviolet radiation in 2012. *International Journal of Cancer*, *143*(6), 1305–1314. https://doi.org/10.1002/ijc.31527

Bagnardi, V., Rota, M., Botteri, E., Tramacere, I., Islami, F., Fedirko, V., Scotti, L., Jenab, M., Turati, F., Pasquali, E., Pelucchi, C., Galeone, C., Bellocco, R., Negri, E., Corrao, G., Boffetta, P., & la Vecchia, C. (2015). Alcohol consumption and site-specific cancer risk: A comprehensive dose–response meta-analysis. *British Journal of Cancer*, *112*(3), 580–593. https://doi.org/10.1038/bjc.2014.579

Bajaj, J. S. (2019). Alcohol, liver disease and the gut microbiota. *Nature Reviews Gastroenterology & Hepatology*, *16*(4), 235–246. https://doi.org/10.1038/s41575-018-0099-1

Bassuk, S. S., & Manson, J. E. (2015). Oral contraceptives and menopausal hormone therapy: Relative and attributable risks of cardiovascular disease, cancer, and other health outcomes. *Annals of Epidemiology*, *25*(3), 193–200. https://doi.org/10.1016/j.annepidem.2014.11.004

Beral, V., Bull, D., & Reeves, G. (2005). Endometrial cancer and hormone-replacement therapy in the Million Women Study. *The Lancet*, *365*(9470), 1543–1551. https://doi.org/10.1016/S0140-6736(05)66455-0

Berger, A. M., Matthews, E. E., & Kenkel, A. M. (2017). Management of sleep-wake disturbances comorbid with cancer. *Cancer Network*, 610–617.

Blask, D. E. (2009). Melatonin, sleep disturbance and cancer risk. *Sleep Medicine Reviews*, *13*(4), 257–264. https://doi.org/10.1016/j.smrv.2008.07.007

Bosnes, I., Nordahl, H. M., Stordal, E., Bosnes, O., Myklebust, T. Å., & Almkvist, O. (2019). Lifestyle predictors of successful aging: A 20-year prospective

HUNT study. *PLoS ONE, 14*(7), e0219200. https://doi.org/10.1371/journal.pone.0219200

Bouvard, V., Loomis, D., Guyton, K. Z., Grosse, Y., El Ghissassi, F., Benbrahim-Tallaa, L., Guha, N., Mattock, H., & Straif, K. (2015). Carcinogenicity of consumption of red and processed meat. *The Lancet Oncology, 16*(16), 1599–1600. https://doi.org/10.1016/S1470-2045(15)00444-1

Brown, S. B., & Hankinson, S. E. (2015). Endogenous estrogens and the risk of breast, endometrial, and ovarian cancers. *Steroids, 99*, 8–10. https://doi.org/10.1016/j.steroids.2014.12.013

Campbell, K. L., Winters-Stone, K. M., Wiskemann, J., May, A. M., Schwartz, A. L., Courneya, K. S., Zucker, D. S., Matthews, C. E., Ligibel, J. A., Gerber, L. H., Morris, G. S., Patel, A. V., Hue, T. F., Perna, F. M., & Schmitz, K. H. (2019). Exercise guidelines for cancer survivors: Consensus statement from International Multidisciplinary Roundtable. *Medicine & Science in Sports & Exercise, 51*(11), 2375–2390. https://doi.org/10.1249/MSS.0000000000002116

Centers for Disease Control and Prevention. (2010). *How tobacco smoke causes disease: The biology and behavioral basis for smoking-attributable disease: A report of the Surgeon General.* https://www.ncbi.nlm.nih.gov/books/NBK53017

Centers for Disease Control and Prevention. (2019). *Alcohol and cancer.* https://www.cdc.gov/cancer/alcohol/index.htm

Centers for Disease Control and Prevention. (2020a). *Cancer screening tests.* https://www.cdc.gov/cancer/dcpc/prevention/screening.htm

Centers for Disease Control and Prevention. (2020b). *What is epigenetics?* https://www.cdc.gov/genomics/disease/epigenetics.htm

Centers for Disease Control and Prevention. (2021a). *Tobacco and cancer.* https://www.cdc.gov/cancer/tobacco/index.htm

Centers for Disease Control and Prevention. (2021b). *United States cancer statistics: Data visualizations.* https://gis.cdc.gov/Cancer/USCS/DataViz.html

Chan, D. S. M., Lau, R., Aune, D., Vieira, R., Greenwood, D. C., Kampman, E., & Norat, T. (2011). Red and processed meat and colorectal cancer incidence: Meta-analysis of prospective studies. *PLoS ONE, 6*(6), e20456. https://doi.org/10.1371/journal.pone.0020456

Chen, Y., Tan, F., Wei, L., Li, X., Lyu, Z., Feng, X., Wen, Y., Guo, L., He, J., Dai, M., & Li, N. (2018). Sleep duration and the risk of cancer: A systematic review and meta-analysis including dose-response relationship. *BMC Cancer, 18*. https://doi.org/10.1186/s12885-018-5025-y

Children's Oncology Group. (2018). *Long-term follow-up guidelines for survivors of childhood, adolescent, and young adult cancers, version 5.0.* http://www.survivorshipguidelines.org/pdf/2018/COG_LTFU_Guidelines_v5.pdf

Colantonio, S., Bracken, M. B., & Beecker, J. (2014). The association of indoor tanning and melanoma in adults: Systematic review and meta-analysis. *Journal of the American Academy of Dermatology, 70*(5), 847–857, e18. https://doi.org/10.1016/j.jaad.2013.11.050

Cook, S. A., Salmon, P., Hayes, G., Byrne, A., & Fisher, P. L. (2018). Predictors of emotional distress a year or more after diagnosis of cancer: A systematic review of the literature. *Psycho-Oncology, 27*(3), 791–801. https://doi.org/10.1002/pon.4601

Cross, A. J., & Sinha, R. (2004). Meat-related mutagens/carcinogens in the etiology of colorectal cancer. *Environmental and Molecular Mutagenesis, 44*(1), 44–55. https://doi.org/10.1002/em.20030

Croswell, J. M., Brawley, O. W., & Kramer, B. S. (2017). Prevention and early detection of cancer. In D. L. Longo (Ed.), *Harrison's hematology and oncology* (3rd ed., pp. 373–385). McGraw-Hill Medical.

Curry, S. J., Krist, A. H., Owens, D. K., Barry, M. J., Caughey, A. B., Davidson, K. W., Doubeni, C. A., Epling, J. W., Kemper, A. R., Kubik, M., Landefeld, C. S., Mangione, C. M., Silverstein, M., Simon, M. A., Tseng, C.-W., & Wong, J. B. (2018). Screening and behavioral counseling interventions to reduce unhealthy alcohol use in adolescents and adults. *JAMA, 320*(18), 1899. https://doi.org/10.1001/jama.2018.16789

Davidson, K. W., Barry, M. J., Mangione, C. M., Cabana, M., Caughey, A. B., Davis, E. M., Donahue, K. E., Doubeni, C. A., Krist, A. H., Kubik, M., Li, L., Ogedegbe, G., Owens, D. K., Pbert, L., Silverstein, M., Stevermer, J., Tseng, C.-W., & Wong, J. B. (2021). Screening for colorectal cancer: U.S. Preventive Services Task Force Recommendation Statement, Table 1, p. 1967. *JAMA, 325*(19). https://doi.org/10.1001/jama.2021.6238

de Martel, C., Georges, D., Bray, F., Ferlay, J., & Clifford, G. M. (2020). Global burden of cancer attributable to infections in 2018: A worldwide incidence analysis. *The Lancet Global Health, 8*(2), e180–e190. https://doi.org/10.1016/S2214-109X(19)30488-7

Dennis, L. K., Vanbeek, M. J., Beane Freeman, L. E., Smith, B. J., Dawson, D. V., & Coughlin, J. A. (2008). Sunburns and risk of cutaneous melanoma: Does age matter? A comprehensive meta-analysis. *Annals of Epidemiology, 18*(8), 614–627. https://doi.org/10.1016/j.annepidem.2008.04.006

Dinu, M., Abbate, R., Gensini, G. F., Casini, A., & Sofi, F. (2017). Vegetarian, vegan diets and multiple health outcomes: A systematic review with meta-analysis of observational studies. *Critical Reviews in Food Science and Nutrition, 57*(17), 3640–3649. https://doi.org/10.1080/10408398.2016.1138447

Dossus, L., Allen, N., Kaaks, R., Bakken, K., Lund, E., Tjonneland, A., Olsen, A., Overvad, K., Clavel-Chapelon, F., Fournier, A., Chabbert-Buffet, N., Boeing, H., Schütze, M., Trichopoulou, A., Trichopoulos, D., Lagiou, P., Palli, D.,

Krogh, V., Tumino, R., . . . Riboli, E. (2010). Reproductive risk factors and endometrial cancer: The European Prospective Investigation into Cancer and Nutrition. *International Journal of Cancer*, *127*, 442–451. https://doi.org/10.1002/ijc.25050

Eliassen, A. H., Colditz, G. A., Rosner, B., Willett, W. C., & Hankinson, S. E. (2006). Adult weight change and risk of postmenopausal breast cancer. *JAMA*, *296*(2), 193. https://doi.org/10.1001/jama.296.2.193

Ellulu, M. S., Patimah, I., Khaza'ai, H., Rahmat, A., & Abed, Y. (2017). Obesity and inflammation: The linking mechanism and the complications. *Archives of Medical Science*, *4*, 851–863. https://doi.org/10.5114/aoms.2016.58928

Esposito, K., Chiodini, P., Capuano, A., Bellastella, G., Maiorino, M. I., & Giugliano, D. (2014). Metabolic syndrome and endometrial cancer: A meta-analysis. *Endocrine*, *45*(1), 28–36. https://doi.org/10.1007/s12020-013-9973-3

Farvid, M. S., Holmes, M. D., Chen, W. Y., Rosner, B. A., Tamimi, R. M., Willett, W. C., & Eliassen, A. H. (2020). Postdiagnostic fruit and vegetable consumption and breast cancer survival: Prospective analyses in the Nurses' Health Studies. *Cancer Research*, *80*(22), 5134–5143. https://doi.org/10.1158/0008-5472.CAN-18-3515

Fashoyin-Aje, L. A., Martinez, K. A., & Dy, S. M. (2012). New patient-centered care standards from the Commission on Cancer: Opportunities and challenges. *Journal of Supportive Oncology*, *10*(3), 107–111. https://doi.org/10.1016/j.suponc.2011.12.002

Fiorito, V., Chiabrando, D., Petrillo, S., Bertino, F., & Tolosano, E. (2020). The multifaceted role of heme in cancer. *Frontiers in Oncology*, *9*(1540). https://doi.org/10.3389/fonc.2019.01540

Fritschi, L., Glass, D. C., Heyworth, J. S., Aronson, K., Girschik, J., Boyle, T., Grundy, A., & Erren, T. C. (2011). Hypotheses for mechanisms linking shiftwork and cancer. *Medical Hypotheses*, *77*(3), 430–436. https://doi.org/10.1016/j.mehy.2011.06.002

Grandner, M. A., Patel, N. P., Gehrman, P. R., Perlis, M. L., & Pack, A. I. (2010). Problems associated with short sleep: Bridging the gap between laboratory and epidemiological studies. *Sleep Medicine Reviews*, *14*(4), 239–247. https://doi.org/10.1016/j.smrv.2009.08.001

Han, M. A., Zeraatkar, D., Guyatt, G. H., Vernooij, R. W. M., El Dib, R., Zhang, Y., Algarni, A., Leung, G., Storman, D., Valli, C., Rabassa, M., Rehman, N., Parvizian, M. K., Zworth, M., Bartoszko, J. J., Lopes, L. C., Sit, D., Bala, M. M., Alonso-Coello, P., & Johnston, B. C. (2019). Reduction of red and processed meat intake and cancer mortality and incidence. *Annals of Internal Medicine*, *171*(10), 711. https://doi.org/10.7326/M19-0699

Horn, L., Lovly, C. M., & Johnson D. H. (2017). Neoplasms of the lung. In D. L. Longo (Ed.), *Harrison's hematology and oncology* (3rd ed., pp. 500–525). McGraw-Hill Medical.

Ibrahim, E. M., & Al-Homaidh, A. (2011). Physical activity and survival after breast cancer diagnosis: Meta-analysis of published studies. *Medical Oncology*, *28*(3), 753–765. https://doi.org/10.1007/s12032-010-9536-x

Institute of Medicine and National Research Council. (2006). *From cancer patient to cancer survivor: Lost in transition*. The National Academies Press. https://doi.org/10.17226/11468

Islami, F., Goding Sauer, A., Miller, K. D., Siegel, R. L., Fedewa, S. A. Jacobs, E. J., McCullough, M. L., Patel, A. V., Ma, J., Soerjomataram, I., Flanders, W. D., Brawley, O. W., Gapstur, S. M., & Jemal, A. (2018). Proportion and number of cancer cases and deaths attributable to potentially modifiable risk factors in the United States. *CA: A Cancer Journal for Clinicians*, *68*(1), 31–54. https://doi.org/10.3322/caac.21440

Islami, F., Miller, K. D., Siegel, R. L., Zheng, Z., Zhao, J., Han, X., Ma, J., Jemal, A., & Yabroff, K. R. (2019). National and state estimates of lost earnings from cancer deaths in the United States. *JAMA Oncology*, *5*(9). https://doi.org/10.1001/jamaoncol.2019.1460

Jones, M. E., Schoemaker, M. J., Mcfadden, E. C., Wright, L. B., Johns, L. E., & Swerdlow, A. J. (2019). Epidemiology night shift work and risk of breast cancer in women: The Generations Study cohort. *British Journal of Cancer*, *121*, 172–179. https://doi.org/10.1038/s41416-019-0485-7

Kaluza, J., Harris, H. R., Håkansson, N., & Wolk, A. (2020). Adherence to the WCRF/AICR 2018 recommendations for cancer prevention and risk of cancer: Prospective cohort studies of men and women. *British Journal of Cancer*, *122*(10), 1562–1570. https://doi.org/10.1038/s41416-020-0806-x

Keimling, M., Behrens, G., Schmid, D., Jochem, C., & Leitzmann, M. F. (2014). The association between physical activity and bladder cancer: Systematic review and meta-analysis. *British Journal of Cancer*, *110*(7), 1862–1870. https://doi.org/10.1038/bjc.2014.77

Kent, E. E., Forsythe, L. P., Yabroff, K. R., Weaver, K. E., de Moor, J. S., Rodriguez, J. L., & Rowland, J. H. (2013). Are survivors who report cancer-related financial problems more likely to forgo or delay medical care? *Cancer*, *119*(20), 3710–3717. https://doi.org/10.1002/cncr.28262

Knuppel, A., Fensom, G. K., Watts, E. L., Gunter, M. J., Murphy, N., Papier, K., Perez-Cornago, A., Schmidt, J. A., Smith Byrne, K., Travis, R. C., & Key, T. J. (2020). Circulating insulin-like growth factor-I concentrations and risk of 30 cancers: Prospective analyses in UK Biobank. *Cancer Research*, *80*(18), 4014–4021. https://doi.org/10.1158/0008-5472.CAN-20-1281

Koch-Gallenkamp, L., Bertram, H., Eberle, A., Holleczek, B., Schmid-Höpfner, S., Waldmann, A., Zeissig, S. R.,

Brenner, H., & Arndt, V. (2016). Fear of recurrence in long-term cancer survivors—Do cancer type, sex, time since diagnosis, and social support matter? *Health Psychology, 35*(12), 1329–1333. https://doi.org/10.1037/hea0000374

Koh-Bell, A., Chan, J., Mann, A. K., & Kapp, D. S. (2021). Social isolation, inflammation, and cancer mortality from the National Health and Nutrition Examination Survey: A study of 3,360 women. *BMC Public Health, 21*(1), 1289. https://doi.org/10.1186/s12889-021-11352-0

Kohler, L. N., Garcia, D. O., Harris, R. B., Oren, E., Roe, D. J., & Jacobs, E. T. (2016). Adherence to diet and physical activity cancer prevention guidelines and cancer outcomes: A systematic review. *Cancer Epidemiology Biomarkers & Prevention, 25*(7), 1018–1028. https://doi.org/10.1158/1055-9965.EPI-16-0121

Konturek, P. C., Brzozowski, T., & Konturek, S. J. (2011). Gut clock: Implication of circadian rhythms in the gastrointestinal tract. *Journal of Physiology and Pharmacology, 62*(2), 139–150. https://pubmed.ncbi.nlm.nih.gov/21673361/

Krist, A. H., Davidson, K. W., Mangione, C. M., Barry, M. J., Cabana, M., Caughey, A. B., Donahue, K., Doubeni, C. A., Epling, J. W., Kubik, M., Ogedegbe, G., Pbert, L., Silverstein, M., Simon, M. A., Tseng, C.-W., & Wong, J. B. (2021). Interventions for tobacco smoking cessation in adults, including pregnant persons. *JAMA, 325*(3), 265. https://doi.org/10.1001/jama.2020.25019

Krüger, K., Mooren, F.-C., & Pilat, C. (2016). The immunomodulatory effects of physical activity. *Current Pharmaceutical Design, 22*(24), 3730–3748. https://doi.org/10.2174/1381612822666160322145107

Kyrø, C., Tjønneland, A., Overvad, K., Olsen, A., & Landberg, R. (2018). Higher whole-grain intake is associated with lower risk of type 2 diabetes among middle-aged men and women: The Danish Diet, Cancer, and Health Cohort. *Journal of Nutrition, 148*(9), 1434–1444. https://doi.org/10.1093/jn/nxy112

Laconi, E., Marongiu, F., & DeGregori, J. (2020). Cancer as a disease of old age: Changing mutational and microenvironmental landscapes. *British Journal of Cancer, 122*(7), 943–952. https://doi.org/10.1038/s41416-019-0721-1

Lauby-Secretan, B., Scoccianti, C., Loomis, D., Grosse, Y., Bianchini, F., & Straif, K. (2016). Body fatness and cancer—Viewpoint of the IARC Working Group. *New England Journal of Medicine, 375*(8), 794–798. https://doi.org/10.1056/nejmsr1606602

Lauder, W., Mummery, K., Jones, M., & Caperchione, C. (2006). A comparison of health behaviours in lonely and non-lonely populations. *Psychology, Health & Medicine, 11*(2), 233–245. https://doi.org/10.1080/13548500500266607

Leigh-Hunt, N., Bagguley, D., Bash, K., Turner, V., Turnbull, S., Valtorta, N., & Caan, W. (2017). An overview of systematic reviews on the public health consequences of social isolation and loneliness. *Public Health, 152*, 157–171. https://doi.org/10.1016/j.puhe.2017.07.035

Lippman, M. E. (2017). Breast cancer. In D. L. Longo (Ed.), *Harrison's hematology and oncology* (3rd ed., pp. 529–541). McGraw-Hill Medical.

Liu, L., Shi, Y., Li, T., Qin, Q., Yin, J., Pang, S., Nie, S., & Wei, S. (2016). Leisure time physical activity and cancer risk: Evaluation of the WHO's recommendation based on 126 high-quality epidemiological studies. *British Journal of Sports Medicine, 50*(6), 372–378. https://doi.org/10.1136/bjsports-2015-094728

Lohse, T., Faeh, D., Bopp, M., & Rohrmann, S. (2016). Adherence to the cancer prevention recommendations of the World Cancer Research Fund/American Institute for Cancer Research and Mortality: A census-linked cohort. *American Journal of Clinical Nutrition, 104*(3), 678–685. https://doi.org/10.3945/ajcn.116.135020

Longo, D. L. (2017). Approach to the patient with cancer. In D. L. Longo (Ed.), *Harrison's hematology and oncology* (3rd ed., pp. 360–372). McGraw-Hill Medical.

Luo, J., Hendryx, M., & Chlebowski, R. T. (2017). Intentional weight loss and cancer risk. *Oncotarget, 8*(47), 81719–81720. https://doi.org/10.18632/oncotarget.20671

Markwald, R. R., Melanson, E. L., Smith, M. R., Higgins, J., Perreault, L., Eckel, R. H., & Wright, K. P. (2013). Impact of insufficient sleep on total daily energy expenditure, food intake, and weight gain. *Proceedings of the National Academy of Sciences of the United States of America, 110*(14), 5695–5700. https://doi.org/10.1073/pnas.1216951110

Martinez, M. R., & Pasha, A. (2017). Prioritizing mental health research in cancer patients and survivors. *AMA Journal of Ethics, 19*(5), 486–492. https://doi.org/10.1001/journalofethics.2017.19.5.msoc2-1705

Mayer, R. J. (2017). Upper gastrointestinal tract cancers. In D. L. Longo (Ed.), *Harrison's hematology and oncology* (3rd ed., pp. 542–550). McGraw-Hill Medical.

Meyerhardt, J. A. (2009). Physical activity and male colorectal cancer survival. *Archives of Internal Medicine, 169*(22), 2102. https://doi.org/10.1001/archinternmed.2009.412

Meyerhardt, J. A., Giovannucci, E. L., Holmes, M. D., Chan, A. T., Chan, J. A., Colditz, G. A., & Fuchs, C. S. (2006). Physical activity and survival after colorectal cancer diagnosis. *Journal of Clinical Oncology, 24*(22), 3527–3534. https://doi.org/10.1200/JCO.2006.06.0855

Morey, J. N., Boggero, I. A., Scott, A. B., & Segerstrom, S. C. (2015). Current directions in stress and human immune function. *Current Opinion in Psychology, 5*, 13–17. https://doi.org/10.1016/j.copsyc.2015.03.007

Morimoto, L. M., White, E., Chen, Z., Chlebowski, R. T., Hays, J., Kuller, L., Lopez, A. M., Manson, J., Margolis,

K. L., Muti, P. C., Stefanick, M. L., & McTiernan, A. (2002). Obesity, body size, and risk of postmenopausal breast cancer: The Women's Health Initiative (United States). *Cancer Causes and Control*, *13*(8), 741–751. https://doi.org/10.1023/A:1020239211145

Morin, P. J., Trent, J. M., Collins, F. S., & Vogelstein, B. (2017). Cancer genetics. In D. L. Longo (Ed.), *Harrison's hematology and oncology* (3rd ed., pp. 320–332). McGraw-Hill Medical.

Munsell, M. F., Sprague, B. L., Berry, D. A., Chisholm, G., & Trentham-Dietz, A. (2014). Body mass index and breast cancer risk according to postmenopausal estrogen-progestin use and hormone receptor status. *Epidemiologic Reviews*, *36*(1), 114–136. https://doi.org/10.1093/epirev/mxt010

National Cancer Institute. (2015a). *Immunosuppression*. https://www.cancer.gov/about-cancer/causes-prevention/risk/immunosuppression

National Cancer Institute. (2015b). *Risk factors: Hormones*. https://www.cancer.gov/about-cancer/causes-prevention/risk/hormones

National Cancer Institute. (2017). *Tobacco*. https://www.cancer.gov/about-cancer/causes-prevention/risk/tobacco

National Cancer Institute. (2018b). *Cancer-causing substances in the environment*. https://www.cancer.gov/about-cancer/causes-prevention/risk/substances

National Cancer Institute. (2018a). *Cancer stat facts: Colorectal cancer*. https://seer.cancer.gov/statfacts/html/colorect.html

National Cancer Institute. (2019). *Infectious agents*. https://www.cancer.gov/about-cancer/causes-prevention/risk/infectious-agents

National Cancer Institute. (2020a). *Cancer statistics*. https://www.cancer.gov/about-cancer/understanding/statistics

National Cancer Institute. (2020b). *Sleep disorders (PDQ®)—Health professional version*. https://www.cancer.gov/about-cancer/treatment/side-effects/sleep-disorders-hp-pdq

National Cancer Institute. (2021a). *Cancer stat facts: Cancer of any site*. https://seer.cancer.gov/statfacts/html/all.html

National Cancer Institute. (2021b). *Cancer stat facts: Melanoma of the skin*. https://seer.cancer.gov/statfacts/html/melan.html

National Cancer Institute. (2021c). *Endometrial cancer treatment (PDQ®)—Health professional version*. https://www.cancer.gov/types/uterine/hp/endometrial-treatment-pdq

National Cancer Institute. (2021d). *Emotions and cancer*. https://www.cancer.gov/about-cancer/coping/feelings

National Comprehensive Cancer Network. (2020). *NCCN guidelines for patients: Survivorship care for healthy living*. https://www.nccn.org/patients/guidelines/content/PDF/survivorship-hl-patient.pdf

National Comprehensive Cancer Network. (2022a). *NCCN clinical practice guidelines in oncology: Distress management*. https://www.nccn.org/professionals/physician_gls/pdf/distress.pdf

National Comprehensive Cancer Network. (2022b). *NCCN distress thermometer*. https://www.nccn.org/docs/default-source/patient-resources/nccn_distress_thermometer.p

Newton, R. U., Kenfield, S. A., Hart, N. H., Chan, J. M., Courneya, K. S., Catto, J., Finn, S. P., Greenwood, R., Hughes, D. C., Mucci, L., Plymate, S. R., Praet, S. F. E., Guinan, E. M., van Blarigan, E. L., Casey, O., Buzza, M., Gledhill, S., Zhang, L., Galvão, D. A., . . . Saad, F. (2018). Intense exercise for survival among men with metastatic castrate-resistant prostate cancer (INTERVAL-GAP4): A multicentre, randomised, controlled phase III study protocol. *BMJ Open*, *8*(5), e022899. https://doi.org/10.1136/bmjopen-2018-022899

Norat, T., Bingham, S., Ferrari, P., Slimani, N., Jenab, M., Mazuir, M., Overvad, K., Olsen, A., Tjønneland, A., Clavel, F., Boutron-Ruault, M.-C., Kesse, E., Boeing, H., Bergmann, M. M., Nieters, A., Linseisen, J., Trichopoulou, A., Trichopoulos, D., Tountas, Y., . . . Riboli, E. (2005). Meat, fish, and colorectal cancer risk: The European Prospective Investigation into Cancer and Nutrition. *Journal of the National Cancer Institute*, *97*(12), 906–916. https://doi.org/10.1093/jnci/dji164

Orman, A., Johnson, D. L., Comander, A., & Brockton, N. (2020). Breast cancer: A lifestyle medicine approach. *American Journal of Lifestyle Medicine*, *14*(5), 483–494. https://doi.org/10.1177/1559827620913263

Palmer, S., Albergante, L., Blackburn, C. C., & Newman, T. J. (2018). Thymic involution and rising disease incidence with age. *Proceedings of the National Academy of Sciences of the United States of America*, *115*(8), 1883–1888. https://doi.org/10.1073/pnas.1714478115

Park, J., & Look, K. A. (2019). Health care expenditure burden of cancer care in the United States. *INQUIRY: The Journal of Health Care Organization, Provision, and Financing*, *56*. https://doi.org/10.1177/0046958019880696

Patel, A. V., Friedenreich, C. M., Moore, S. C., Hayes, S. C., Silver, J. K., Campbell, K. L., Winters-Stone, K., Gerber, L. H., George, S. M., Fulton, J. E., Denlinger, C., Morris, G. S., Hue, T., Schmitz, K. H., & Matthews, C. E. (2019). American College of Sports Medicine roundtable report on physical activity, sedentary behavior, and cancer prevention and control. *Medicine & Science in Sports & Exercise*, *51*(11), 2391–2402. https://doi.org/10.1249/MSS.0000000000002117

PDQ Supportive and Palliative Care Editorial Board. (2019). Adjustment to cancer: Anxiety and distress (PDQ®): Health professional version. In *PDQ Cancer Information Summaries*. https://www.ncbi.nlm.nih.gov/books/NBK65960

Pfeiffer, R. M., Webb-Vargas, Y., Wheeler, W., & Gail, M. H. (2018). Proportion of U.S. trends in breast cancer incidence attributable to long-term changes in risk factor distributions. *Cancer Epidemiology Biomarkers and Prevention*, 27(10), 1214–1222. https://doi.org/10.1158/1055-9965.EPI-18-0098

Pizot, C., Boniol, M., Mullie, P., Koechlin, A., Boniol, M., Boyle, P., & Autier, P. (2016). Physical activity, hormone replacement therapy and breast cancer risk: A meta-analysis of prospective studies. *European Journal of Cancer*, 52, 138–154. https://doi.org/10.1016/j.ejca.2015.10.063

Rawla, P., & Barsouk, A. (2019). Epidemiology of gastric cancer: Global trends, risk factors and prevention. *Gastroenterology Review*, 14(1), 26–38. https://doi.org/10.5114/pg.2018.80001

Renehan, A. G., Tyson, M., Egger, M., Heller, R. F., & Zwahlen, M. (2008). Body-mass index and incidence of cancer: A systematic review and meta-analysis of prospective observational studies. *The Lancet*, 371(9612), 569–578. https://doi.org/10.1016/S0140-6736(08)60269-X

Rock, C. L., Thomson, C., Gansler, T., Gapstur, S. M., McCullough, M. L., Patel, A. V., Andrews, K. S., Bandera, E. V., Spees, C. K., Robien, K., Hartman, S., Sullivan, K., Grant, B. L., Hamilton, K. K., Kushi, L. H., Caan, B. J., Kibbe, D., Black, J. D., Wiedt, T. L., . . . Doyle, C. (2020). American Cancer Society guideline for diet and physical activity for cancer prevention. *CA: A Cancer Journal for Clinicians*, 70(4), 245–271. https://doi.org/10.3322/caac.21591

Saha, S. K., Lee, S. B., Won, J., Choi, H. Y., Kim, K., Yang, G. M., Dayem, A. A., & Cho, S. G. (2017). Correlation between oxidative stress, nutrition, and cancer initiation. *International Journal of Molecular Sciences*, 18(7). https://doi.org/10.3390/ijms18071544

Sample, A., & He, Y.-Y. (2018). Mechanisms and prevention of UV-induced melanoma. *Photodermatology, Photoimmunology & Photomedicine*, 34(1), 13–24. https://doi.org/10.1111/phpp.12329

Sanford, N. N., Sher, D. J., Xu, X., Ahn, C., D'Amico, A. V., Aizer, A. A., & Mahal, B. A. (2020). Alcohol use among patients with cancer and survivors in the United States, 2000–2017. *Journal of the National Comprehensive Cancer Network*, 18(1), 69–79. https://doi.org/10.6004/jnccn.2019.7341

Schmid, D., Behrens, G., Keimling, M., Jochem, C., Ricci, C., & Leitzmann, M. (2015). A systematic review and meta-analysis of physical activity and endometrial cancer risk. *European Journal of Epidemiology*, 30(5), 397–412. https://doi.org/10.1007/s10654-015-0017-6

Siegel, R. L., Miller, K. D., Fuchs, H. E., & Jemal, A. (2021). Cancer statistics, 2021. *CA: A Cancer Journal for Clinicians*, 71(1), 7–33. https://doi.org/10.3322/caac.21654

Siegel, R. L., Miller, K. D., & Jemal, A. (2020). Cancer statistics, 2020. *CA: A Cancer Journal for Clinicians*, 70(1), 7–30. https://doi.org/10.3322/caac.21590

Song, M., Hildesheim, A., & Shiels, M. S. (2020). Premature years of life lost due to cancer in the United States in 2017. *Cancer Epidemiology Biomarkers & Prevention*, 29(12), 2591–2598. https://doi.org/10.1158/1055-9965.EPI-20-0782

Song, M., & Tworoger, S. S. (2020). Systemic immune response and cancer risk: Filling the missing piece of immuno-oncology. *Cancer Research*, 80(9), 1801–1803. https://doi.org/10.1158/0008-5472.can-20-0730

Stępień, M., Stępień, A., Wlazeł, R. N., Paradowski, M., Banach, M., & Rysz, J. (2014). Obesity indices and inflammatory markers in obese non-diabetic normo- and hypertensive patients: A comparative pilot study. *Lipids in Health and Disease*, 13(1), 29. https://doi.org/10.1186/1476-511X-13-29

Tang, Q., Cheng, J., Cao, X., Surowy, H., & Burwinkel, B. (2016). Blood-based DNA methylation as biomarker for breast cancer: A systematic review. *Clinical Epigenetics*, 8(1), 115. https://doi.org/10.1186/s13148-016-0282-6

Tsilidis, K. K., Kasimis, J. C., Lopez, D. S., Ntzani, E. E., & Ioannidis, J. P. A. (2015). Type 2 diabetes and cancer: Umbrella review of meta-analyses of observational studies. *BMJ*, 350, g7607. https://doi.org/10.1136/bmj.g7607

Ulm, M., Ramesh, A. V., McNamara, K. M., Ponnusamy, S., Sasano, H., & Narayanan, R. (2019). Therapeutic advances in hormone-dependent cancers: Focus on prostate, breast and ovarian cancers. *Endocrine Connections*, 8(2), R10–R26. https://doi.org/10.1530/EC-18-0425

U.S. Department of Agriculture and U.S. Department of Health and Human Services. (2020). *Dietary guidelines for Americans: 2020–2025*. https://www.dietaryguidelines.gov/sites/default/files/2021-03/Dietary_Guidelines_for_Americans-2020-2025.pdf

U.S. Food & Drug Administration. (2020, May 28). *Tobacco products: Products, ingredients and components*. https://www.fda.gov/tobacco-products/products-guidance-regulations/products-ingredients-components

U.S. Preventive Services Task Force. (2016). *Final recommendation statement: Breast cancer screening*. https://www.uspreventiveservicestaskforce.org/uspstf/recommendation/breast-cancer-screening

U.S. Preventive Services Task Force. (2021a). *Final recommendation statement: Lung cancer screening*. https://www.uspreventiveservicestaskforce.org/uspstf/recommendation/lung-cancer-screening

U.S. Preventive Services Task Force. (2021b). Screening for colorectal cancer: U.S. Preventive Services Task Force Recommendation Statement. *JAMA*, 325(19), 1965–1977. https://doi.org/10.1001/jama.2021.6238

U.S. Preventive Services Task Force. (2021c). Screening for lung cancer: U.S. Preventive Services Task Force Recommendation Statement. *JAMA*, *325*(10), 962–970. https://doi.org/10.1001/jama.2021.1117

Vieira, A. R., Abar, L., Chan, D. S. M., Vingeliene, S., Polemiti, E., Stevens, C., Greenwood, D., & Norat, T. (2017). Foods and beverages and colorectal cancer risk: A systematic review and meta-analysis of cohort studies, an update of the evidence of the WCRF-AICR Continuous Update Project. *Annals of Oncology*, *28*(8), 1788–1802. https://doi.org/10.1093/annonc/mdx171

Watson, M., Holman, D. M., & Maguire-Eisen, M. (2016). Ultraviolet radiation exposure and its impact on skin cancer risk. *Seminars in Oncology Nursing*, *32*(3), 241–254. https://doi.org/10.1016/j.soncn.2016.05.005

Webb, J., Foster, J., & Poulter, E. (2016). Increasing the frequency of physical activity very brief advice for cancer patients. Development of an intervention using the behaviour change wheel. *Public Health*, *133*, 45–56. https://doi.org/10.1016/j.puhe.2015.12.009

Willett, W. C. (2000). Diet and cancer. *The Oncologist*, *5*(5), 393–404. https://doi.org/10.1634/theoncologist.5-5-393

Willett, W. C., Stampfer, M. J., Colditz, G. A., Rosner, B. A., & Speizer, F. E. (1990). Relation of meat, fat, and fiber intake to the risk of colon cancer in a prospective study among women. *New England Journal of Medicine*, *323*(24), 1664–1672. https://doi.org/10.1056/NEJM199012133232404

Winzer, B. M., Whiteman, D. C., Reeves, M. M., & Paratz, J. D. (2011). Physical activity and cancer prevention: A systematic review of clinical trials. *Cancer Causes & Control*, *22*(6), 811–826. https://doi.org/10.1007/s10552-011-9761-4

World Cancer Research Fund and American Institute for Cancer Research. (2018a). *Alcoholic drinks and cancer risk*. Continuous Update Project Expert Report 2018. https://www.wcrf.org/dietandcancer/exposures/alcoholic-drinks

World Cancer Research Fund and American Institute for Cancer Research. (2018b). *Obesity, weight gain, and cancer risk*. Continuous Update Project Expert Report 2018. https://www.wcrf.org/dietandcancer/exposures/body-fatness

World Cancer Research Fund and American Institute for Cancer Research. (2018c). *Continuous Update Project recommendations and public health and policy implications*. https://www.wcrf.org/wp-content/uploads/2021/01/Recommendations.pdf

World Cancer Research Fund and American Institute for Cancer Research. (2018d). *Meat, fish, dairy & cancer risk*. Continuous Update Project Expert Report 2018. https://www.wcrf.org/dietandcancer/exposures/meat-fish-dairy

World Cancer Research Fund and American Institute for Cancer Research. (2018e). *Physical activity and cancer risk*. Continuous Update Project Expert Report 2018. https://www.wcrf.org/dietandcancer/exposures/physical-activity

World Cancer Research Fund and American Institute for Cancer Research. (2018f). *The cancer process*. https://www.wcrf.org/wp-content/uploads/2021/02/The-cancer-process.pdf

World Cancer Research Fund and American Institute for Cancer Research. (2018g). *Wholegrains, vegetables, fruit, and cancer risk*. Continuous Update Project Expert Report 2018. https://www.wcrf.org/dietandcancer/exposures/wholegrains-veg-fruit

World Health Organization. (2015). *Cancer: Carcinogenicity of the consumption of red and processed meat*. https://www.who.int/news-room/questions-and-answers/item/cancer-carcinogenicity-of-the-consumption-of-red-meat-and-processed-meat

World Health Organization. (2020). *World Health Assembly adopts global strategy to accelerate cervical cancer elimination*. https://www.who.int/news/item/19-08-2020-world-health-assembly-adopts-global-strategy-to-accelerate-cervical-cancer-elimination

World Health Organization. (2021). *Cancer key facts*. https://www.who.int/news-room/fact-sheets/detail/cancer

World Health Organization. (2022a). *Cancer overview*. https://www.who.int/health-topics/cancer#tab=tab_1

World Health Organization. (2022b). *Preventing cancer*. https://www.who.int/activities/preventing-cancer

Xiao, Y., Xia, J., Li, L., Ke, Y., Cheng, J., Xie, Y., Chu, W., Cheung, P., Kim, J. H., Colditz, G. A., Tamimi, R. M., & Su, X. (2019). Associations between dietary patterns and the risk of breast cancer: A systematic review and meta-analysis of observational studies. *Breast Cancer Research*, *21*(1), 16. https://doi.org/10.1186/s13058-019-1096-1

Xue, K., Li, F.-F., Chen, Y.-W., Zhou, Y.-H., & He, J. (2017). Body mass index and the risk of cancer in women compared with men: A meta-analysis of prospective cohort studies. *European Journal of Cancer Prevention*, *26*(1), 94–105. https://doi.org/10.1097/CEJ.0000000000000231

Yeh, H., Bantle, J. P., Cassidy-Begay, M., Blackburn, G., Bray, G. A., Byers, T., Clark, J. M., Coday, M., Egan, C., Espeland, M. A., Foreyt, J. P., Garcia, K., Goldman, V., Gregg, E. W., Hazuda, H. P., Hesson, L., Hill, J. O., Horton, E. S., Jakicic, J. M., . . . Yanovski, S. Z. (2020). Intensive weight loss intervention and cancer risk in adults with type 2 diabetes: Analysis of the Look AHEAD randomized clinical trial. *Obesity*, *28*(9), 1678–1686. https://doi.org/10.1002/oby.22936

CHAPTER 22

Health Promotion Interventions for Alzheimer's Disease and Dementia

Alicia Craig-Rodriguez, DNP, MBA, APRN, FNP-BC, DipACLM
Carli A. Carnish, DNP, APRN-CNP

A healthy body is the guest-chamber of the soul; a sick body, its prison.

Francis Bacon, 1561–1626

OBJECTIVES

This chapter will enable the reader to:

1. Describe the prevalence and pathophysiology of dementia and Alzheimer's disease.
2. Summarize early biomarkers predictive of cognitive decline.
3. Distinguish between the different types of dementia.
4. Integrate evidence-informed guidelines for screening and management of dementia and Alzheimer's disease into advanced practice.
5. Appraise the different lifestyle approaches to prevent and reverse cognitive decline.
6. Discuss current interprofessional approaches to dementia management.
7. Apply key principles of lifestyle medicine in dementia prevention.

Overview

Alzheimer's disease (AD) is a diagnosis that many fear above all others, even cancer, heart attack, stroke, and COVID-19 (Edward Jones et al., 2021). It is the affliction that robs individuals of their identities; it decimates families, friends, and caregivers; and it is a disease that continues to baffle researchers and scientists because there has been no approved medication or treatment that has been able to slow or halt the progression of the disease.

© Kathleen Gail/Shutterstock; © StoryTime Studio/Shutterstock; © kali9/Getty Images

By the time AD is diagnosed, the destructive process has likely been underway for as long as 20 years (Alzheimer's Association, 2022). Failure to identify early markers of AD and to intervene early has resulted in unnecessary physical, emotional, and financial trauma in patients and their family members. Traditional treatment of AD, which comprises a symptom management approach, has yielded minimal results. Ongoing research, however, continues to provide clarity and hope because there is now substantial evidence that indicates an opportunity to reverse and prevent the cognitive decline using lifestyle interventions. This chapter explores the pathophysiology and prevalence of AD and other dementias and provides evidence-informed tools for advanced practice providers (APPs) to support patients and their families in the prevention and reversal of cognitive decline.

Description and Prevalence

Dementia is the general term used to describe a constellation of symptoms that include difficulties with language, memory, and other cognitive abilities that adversely affect a person's ability to perform the normal activities of daily living (Alzheimer's Association, 2021). Common causes of dementia and associated characteristics are found in **Table 22.1**. AD is the most common cause of dementia, comprising between 60% and 80% of all cases of dementia, and it is the sixth leading cause of death in the United States and the fifth leading cause of death in individuals 65 and older (Tobore, 2019).

More than 5 million Americans currently live with AD, and the number of cases continues to rise due to the aging of the U.S. population (see **Figure 22.1**). A large segment of the American population—the baby boomer generation—has started reaching age 65 and older, when the risk for AD and other dementias increases. By 2060, the number of people aged 65 and older with AD is projected to reach 13.8 million, barring the development of a solution to prevent, slow, or cure AD.

The number of deaths attributed to AD increased by 146% between 2000 and 2018; this rise in AD deaths is in stark contrast to heart disease (the number one cause of death), which decreased by 7.8% during that same period (Alzheimer's Association, 2020). It is sobering to note that of the top 10 leading causes of death, AD is the only condition for which there is no effective treatment (Bredesen, 2017; Tobore, 2019). Despite decades of research and billions of dollars spent by government agencies and pharmaceutical and biotech companies, successful treatment of AD remains an elusive target because not a single drug treatment developed in the past 25 years has yielded promising results in preventing or slowing the progression of the disease (Bredesen, 2017; Cummings et al., 2018).

Pathophysiology

AD is a progressive disorder in which pathological changes in the brain begin decades before the appearance of any symptoms (Oxford et al., 2020). There are several mechanisms at play in the neuropathology of AD, including brain inflammation, shrinkage with cortical thinning and atrophy, an accumulation and deposition of amyloid-beta plaques, and an abnormal protein tau, the primary component of neurofibrillary tangles (Chen & Mobley, 2019; Tobore, 2019).

While aging is the most significant risk factor for developing AD, there is ample evidence to suggest that AD is not a single disease but rather a confluence of numerous other influences, all of which contribute to the pathogenesis and progression of AD. Bredesen (2017) posits that there are 36 factors that affect the pathogenesis of AD and suggests that the current approach of targeting AD with a single drug candidate is analogous to patching a single hole of a leaky roof that has 36 holes.

Table 22.1 Dementia: Types of Dementia and Associated Characteristics

Type	Pathology	Common Symptoms
Alzheimer's disease (AD) AD is a slowly progressive brain disease that begins many years before the symptoms emerge. Alzheimer's disease is the most common cause of dementia, accounting for an estimated 60–80% of cases.	The hallmark pathologies of AD are an accumulation of the protein fragment amyloid-beta (plaques) outside neurons in the brain and twisted strands of the protein tau (tangles) inside neurons. These changes are accompanied by the death of neurons and damage to brain tissue.	Symptoms include difficulty remembering recent conversations, names, or events. Apathy and depression are also often early symptoms. Later symptoms include impaired communication; disorientation; confusion; poor judgment; behavior changes; and difficulty speaking, swallowing, and walking.
Cerebrovascular disease (vascular dementia) Cerebrovascular disease refers to the process by which blood vessels in the brain are blocked or damaged, leading to brain tissue injury from insufficient blood, oxygen, or nutrients.	Vascular dementia is more common as a mixed pathology, with most people living with dementia showing the brain changes of cerebrovascular disease and AD.	Initial symptoms include impaired judgment and ability to make decisions, plan, or organize; memory may also be affected, especially when the brain changes of other causes of dementia are present. Other symptoms include difficulty with motor function, such as a slow gait, and poor balance.
Lewy body dementia (LBD) About 5% of individuals with dementia show evidence of LBD alone, but most people with LBD also have AD pathology.	Lewy bodies are abnormal aggregations (or clumps) of the protein alpha-synuclein in neurons that develop in the cortex of the brain.	Symptoms are similar to those with AD but are more likely to have initial or early symptoms of sleep disturbances, well-formed visual hallucinations, and visuospatial impairment. These may occur in the absence of significant memory impairment, but memory loss often occurs, especially when the brain changes of other causes of dementia are present.
Frontotemporal lobar degeneration (FTLD) FTLD includes dementias such as behavioral-variant FTLD, primary progressive aphasia, Pick's disease, corticobasal degeneration, and progressive supranuclear palsy.	Nerve cells in the frontal and temporal lobes of the brain are especially affected, and these regions become markedly atrophied. In addition, the upper layers of the cortex typically become soft and spongy and have abnormal protein inclusions (usually tau protein or the transactive response DNA-binding protein, TDP-43).	Typical early symptoms include marked changes in personality and behavior and difficulty producing or comprehending language. Unlike AD, memory is typically spared in the early stages of the disease. Symptoms may occur in people 65 years and older; however, most develop symptoms at a younger age. About 60% of those with FTLD are 45–60 years old.

(continues)

Table 22.1 Dementia: Types of Dementia and Associated Characteristics   *(continued)*

Type	Pathology	Common Symptoms
Parkinson's disease (PD), or Parkinson's disease dementia	Alpha-synuclein aggregates appear in an area deep in the brain called the substantia nigra. The aggregates are thought to cause degeneration of the nerve cells that produce dopamine. As PD progresses, it often results in dementia secondary to the accumulation of alpha-synuclein in the cortex (similar to LBD).	Problems with movement (slowness, rigidity, tremor, and changes in gait) are common symptoms of PD. Cognitive symptoms develop either just before movement symptoms or later in the disease.
Hippocampal sclerosis (HS) **(HS dementia)** HS is a common cause of dementia in the *oldest-old*, individuals aged 85 or older.	HS is the hardening of tissue in the hippocampus of the brain. The hippocampus plays a key role in forming memories. HS brain changes are often accompanied by accumulations of a misfolded form of a protein called TDP-43.	The most pronounced symptom of HS is memory loss, and individuals may be misdiagnosed as having AD.
Mixed pathologies (mixed dementia) Studies suggest that mixed dementia is more common than previously recognized, with more than 50% of people with dementia who were studied at Alzheimer's Disease Research Centers having pathological evidence of more than one cause of dementia.	The likelihood of having mixed dementia increases with age and is highest in people aged 85 or older.	Symptoms are consistent with impairments associated with the associated form of dementia noted above.

Data from Alzheimer's Association. (2021). *Alzheimer's disease facts and figures.* https://www.alz.org/media/Documents/alzheimers-facts-and-figures.pdf

Risk Factors for Dementia

The development of dementia is a complex multifactorial process resulting from environmental, genetic, and lifestyle factors. Genetic predisposition (Armstrong, 2019; Bredesen, 2017; Chen & Mobley, 2019; Prendecki et al., 2020; Tobore, 2019), metabolic dysfunction (Armstrong, 2019; Tobore, 2019; Zheng et al., 2018), blood–brain barrier dysfunction (Huang et al., 2020), inflammation and oxidative stress (Tobore, 2019; Walker et al., 2017),

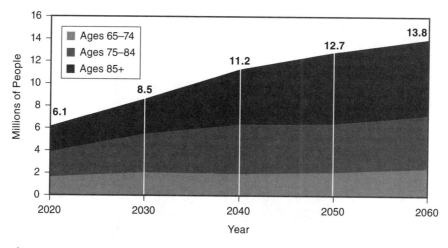

Figure 22.1 Alzheimer's disease projections in U.S. population through 2060.

Courtesy of the Centers for Disease Control and Prevention. Reference to specific commercial products, manufacturers, companies, or trademarks does not constitute its endorsement or recommendation by the U.S. Government, Department of Health and Human Services, or Centers for Disease Control and Prevention. Available free of charge at https://www.cdc.gov/hai/pdfs/ppe/PPE-Sequence.pdf

hormonal depletion (Huang et al., 2020; Tobore, 2019), infections (Armstrong, 2019), and environmental toxins (Armstrong, 2019) are all contributing influences that evoke ongoing damage to the body and the brain, making dementia prevention and treatment an extremely challenging endeavor. This multifactorial process is evidenced by the numerous drug targets that have failed to slow or halt the progression of the disease.

Tobore (2019) underscores the importance of addressing all of these influences in the treatment of AD dementia. He describes a new hypothesis that encompasses most, if not all, the recognized risk factors involved with the pathophysiology and etiopathogenesis of AD: mitochondrial dysfunction and oxidative stress, vitamin D deficiency, melatonin deficiency, thyroid hormone dysfunction, and sex hormone dysfunction. He recommends addressing this quintuple framework (shown in **Figure 22.2**) to help slow the progression of AD dementia and improve future treatment options.

In 2017, the Lancet Commission published the report *Dementia Prevention, Intervention, and Care*, which identified nine modifiable risk factors for dementia: less education, hypertension, hearing impairment, smoking, obesity, depression, physical inactivity, diabetes, and infrequent social contact. In 2020, this report was updated, presenting newer, more compelling evidence that confirmed these previously identified risk factors and added three additional modifiable risks for dementia: excessive alcohol consumption, head injury, and air pollution. These 12 risk factors combined account for 40% of all dementias worldwide, and thus modifying these risk factors has the potential to delay up to 40% of all dementia diagnoses (Livingston et al., 2020). **Figure 22.3** captures the possible risk reduction strategies that may help to prevent or delay the onset of dementia. These strategies emphasize the importance of reducing inflammatory insults to the body and brain to maintain cognitive reserve and reduce neuropathological damage.

Prevention and Management

The World Health Organization (WHO, 2017) has identified dementia as an international public health priority. In 2017, the World Health Assembly released a global action plan to reduce the risk of dementia and improve the lives of people living with dementia and

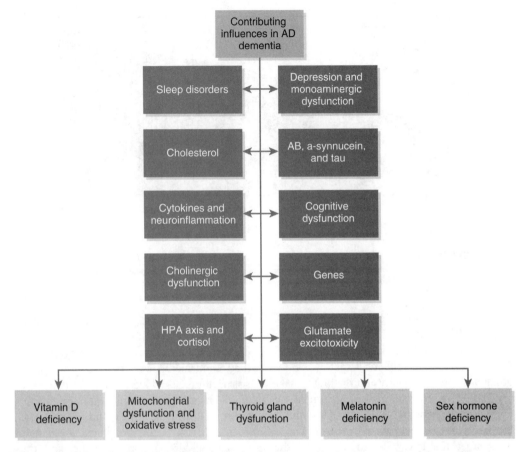

Figure 22.2 Contributing influences in the pathophysiology and etiopathogenesis of dementia.

There are multiple contributing influences involved with the pathophysiology and etiopathogenesis of AD. The authors hypothesize that among these influences, there are five areas of dysfunction that if addressed and corrected, may help slow the progression of AD and improve future treatment options.

Based on Tobore, O. T. (2019). On the etiopathogenesis and pathophysiology of Alzheimer's disease: A comprehensive theoretical review. *Journal of Alzheimer's Disease, 68*, 417–437. https://doi.org/10.3233/JAD-181052

their caregivers (WHO, 2017). Included in their global action plan were seven specific areas for improvement, including the following:

- Recognition of dementia as a public health priority
- Improved dementia awareness and friendliness to reduce stigmatization
- Dementia risk reduction
- Increased dementia diagnosis, treatment, care, and support
- Improved support for dementia caregivers
- Access to information systems
- Dementia research and innovation

Currently, there is not one specific cure for dementia. Treatment has traditionally focused on symptom management rather than on the reversal of cognitive decline. Clinical practice guidelines for dementia are limited to those related to screening recommendations.

Lifestyle Interventions for Dementia

There is a growing body of evidence on lifestyle interventions that show great promise for risk reduction and prevention of AD

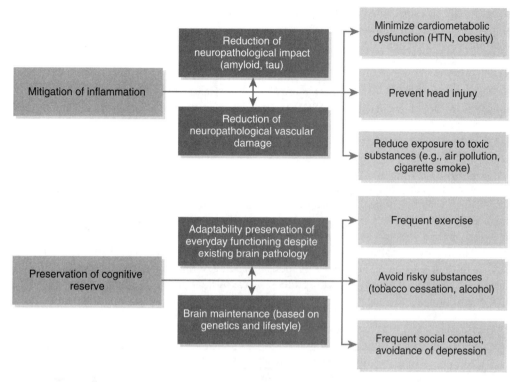

Figure 22.3 Risk reduction strategies for AD.

Possible brain mechanisms for dementia protection include enhancing or maintaining cognitive reserve and modifying behaviors to reduce risk factors of dementia.

Data from Livingston, G., Huntley, J., Sommerlad, A., Ames, D., Ballard, C., Banerjee, S., Brayne, C., Burns, A., Cohen-Mansfield, J., Cooper, C., Costafreda, S. G., Dias, A., Fox, N., Gitlin, L. N., Howard, R., Kales, H. C., Kivimäki, M., Larson, E. B., Ogunniyi, A., ... Mukadam, N. (2020). Dementia prevention, intervention, and care: 2020 report of the Lancet Commission. *The Lancet, 396*(10248), 413–446. https://doi.org/10.1016/S0140-6736(20)30367-6

and other types of dementia, including the following:

- Diet (Blumenthal et al., 2019; Bredesen, 2020; Loughrey et al., 2017; McEvoy et al., 2017; McGrattan et al., 2019; Morris et al., 2015; Pistollato et al., 2018; Poulose et al., 2017; Sherzai & Sherzai, 2019)
- Exercise (Blumenthal et al., 2019; Bredesen, 2020; Erickson et al., 2019; Groot et al., 2016; Jia et al., 2019; Northey et al., 2018; Santos-Lozano et al., 2016; Sherzai & Sherzai, 2019)
- Sleep (Mander et al., 2016; Sabia et al., 2021; Sherzai & Sherzai, 2019)
- Social networks (Kelly et al., 2017; Small et al., 2012)

- Optimization of metabolic parameters (Bredesen, 2017, 2020; Isaacson et al., 2018; Shetty & Youngberg, 2018; Walker et al., 2017; Zheng et al., 2018).

These lifestyle interventions correspond with select A-SMART (adopt healthy eating, stress less, move often, avoid alcohol, rest more, and treat tobacco use) lifestyle prescriptions to adopt healthy eating, move often, and rest more.

Adopt Healthy Eating

The standard American diet is a significant contributor to the chronic inflammatory process that promotes neurodegeneration and increases the risk for dementia later in life. A summary of the nutritional patterns associated with dementia and AD risk is displayed in **Figure 22.4**. Several dietary patterns have been found to improve neurocognition and decrease AD risk, including the Dietary Approaches to Stop Hypertension (DASH), the Mediterranean diet, and the Mediterranean–DASH Diet Intervention for Neurogenerative Delay (MIND).

The DASH and Mediterranean diets contain neuroprotective components that may inhibit the development or progression of dementia. Regular adherence to a plant-focused diet high in antioxidants and elimination of pro-inflammatory foods (high in saturated fats and sodium and artificial or processed food products) has been shown to be neuroprotective in addition to inducing neurogenesis and

improving concentration, processing speed, and memory (McGrattan et al., 2019; Pistollato et al., 2018; Poulose et al., 2017).

The MIND diet is a modified version of the Mediterranean, DASH, and American Heart Association diets. The MIND diet was developed and studied among 960 community-dwelling older adults with no dementia or mild cognitive impairment. This diet specifically recommends eating foods that, based on prospective studies, have the highest potential to reduce the risk of or slow cognitive decline in at-risk older adults. The diet includes green leafy vegetables, other raw and cooked vegetables, berries, nuts, beans, whole grains, poultry, and fish. The MIND diet discourages intake of cheese, oils (other than olive oil), red meat, fast foods, and sweets. This research study found a positive relationship

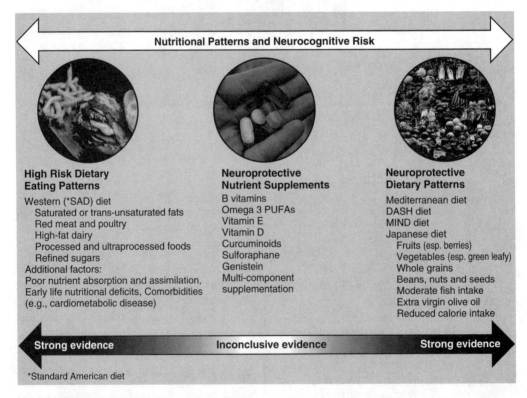

Nutritional Patterns and Neurocognitive Risk

High Risk Dietary Eating Patterns

Western (*SAD) diet
    Saturated or trans-unsaturated fats
    Red meat and poultry
    High-fat dairy
    Processed and ultraprocessed foods
    Refined sugars
Additional factors:
Poor nutrient absorption and assimilation,
Early life nutritional deficits, Comorbidities
(e.g., cardiometabolic disease)

Neuroprotective Nutrient Supplements

B vitamins
Omega 3 PUFAs
Vitamin E
Vitamin D
Curcuminoids
Sulforaphane
Genistein
Multi-component
supplementation

Neuroprotective Dietary Patterns

Mediterranean diet
DASH diet
MIND diet
Japanese diet
    Fruits (esp. berries)
    Vegetables (esp. green leafy)
    Whole grains
    Beans, nuts and seeds
    Moderate fish intake
    Extra virgin olive oil
    Reduced calorie intake

Strong evidence   Inconclusive evidence   **Strong evidence**

*Standard American diet

Figure 22.4 Nutrients and nutritional patterns in neurocognition and AD risk.

Source: Pistollato, F., Iglesias, R. C., Ruiz, R., Aparicio, S., Crespo, J., Lopez, L. D., Manna, P. P., Giampieri, F., & Battino, M. (2018). Nutritional patterns associated with the maintenance of neurocognitive functions and the risk of dementia and Alzheimer's disease: A focus on human studies. *Pharmacological Research*, 131, 32–43. https://doi.org/10.1016/j.phrs.2018.03.012

between higher scores among multiple cognitive domains and the prescribed diet servings and scores (Morris et al., 2015).

Move Often

The U.S. Department of Health and Human Services published the second edition of *Physical Activity Guidelines for Americans* in 2018. New to this edition is an emphasis on the relationship between physical activity and overall health, including mood and cognition. There is strong evidence to support the role of physical inactivity in the development and progression of dementia (Erickson et al., 2019; Jia et al., 2019). Replacing sedentary activities, such as sitting, with regular exercise, such as walking, dancing, and weight training, has been shown to be beneficial in reducing insulin resistance and improving vascular function, stress reduction, and mood—all significant contributors to optimal cognitive health (Bredesen, 2017).

A multicomponent exercise prescription should be given to all adults and tailored to their interests, abilities, and availability. Exercise programs that include aerobic, muscle strengthening, and stretching are effective in improving cognitive function for adults regardless of their cognitive status prior to engaging in the activity (Groot et al., 2016; Northey et al., 2018). Numerous studies have demonstrated the relationship between regular physical activity and dementia risk reduction, especially in apolipoprotein E gene (APOE4) carriers (Groot et al., 2016; Santos-Lozano et al., 2016).

In addition to the neuroprotective effects of physical activity, it has been demonstrated that exercise can improve both cognitive function and function in patients with dementia, regardless of subtype. It is important to note that cognitive performance improved in dementia patients with engagement in physical activity interventions, regardless of program intensity or disease severity. This finding underscores the value of incorporating physical activity into the plan of care for all older adults diagnosed with dementia (Groot et al., 2016; Jia et al., 2019).

Rest More

The effect of sleep disturbances on cognitive function is widespread, interfering with processing speed, concentration, memory, and mood (Considine et al., 2018; Dufort-Gervais et al., 2019). Sleep disturbances occur in over 60% of those diagnosed with mild cognitive impairment and AD (Wennberg et al., 2017). Evidence supports that not only do sleep disorders often precede diagnoses of mild cognitive impairment and AD but also that patients with sleep disturbances are more likely to have a diagnosis of mild cognitive impairment or AD earlier in life (Mander et al., 2016). Furthermore, patients with dementia and comorbid sleep disorders have poorer prognosis and clinical outcomes. Promoting healthy sleep patterns is increasingly important in older adults with dementia diagnoses because it contributes to functional impairment and behavior disturbances (Wennberg et al., 2017).

It is important to determine how many hours of uninterrupted sleep patients get each night. Excess sleep can be equally as harmful as a sleep deficit. Adults who exceed the recommended number of sleep hours each night are at increased risk for metabolic syndrome or one of its components, each of which is an AD risk factor (Xu et al., 2020). Evidence supports that the relationship between sleep and cognitive impairment is bidirectional and the neuroprotective effect of good sleep hygiene is of growing interest (Blackman et al., 2021; Dufort-Gervais et al., 2019).

Cognitive impairment spurred by poor sleep quality occurs via multiple trajectories. Cortical thinning has been associated with both shortened and extended sleep duration of less than six or more than eight hours, respectively. Cortical thinning has also been linked to fragmented sleep patterns and self-reported daytime sleepiness. Ventricular enlargement, reflective of brain volume loss, is commonly found among patients reporting shortened sleep duration (Wennberg et al., 2017).

The APOE4 gene linked to AD has also been associated with an increased risk for obstructive sleep apnea (Mander et al., 2016). It is estimated that up to 80% of people diagnosed with dementia have sleep apnea. Sleep apnea severity also appears to correlate with dementia severity (Mander et al., 2016). History of sleep apnea has been linked to earlier onset of cognitive impairment and dementia risk (Bredesen, 2020; Considine et al., 2018). Obstructive sleep apnea treatment with continuous positive airway pressure could delay the onset of cognitive impairment, suggesting that hypoxia plays a key role in dementia development and progression (Considine et al., 2018).

Good sleep hygiene is also associated with improved concentration and memory. Although there are expected alterations in sleep architecture as a person ages, not all are a normal part of the aging process. Daytime drowsiness and napping may result from the change in circadian rhythms, causing further sleep pattern disruptions. Insomnia, which is highly prevalent among older adults, is often treated with anxiolytic, antidepressant, hypnotic, or antipsychotic drugs. Most of these medications carry a significant risk for older adults, especially those diagnosed with AD or other dementia (Blackman et al., 2021).

While a reduced amount of time spent in slow-wave sleep per night is an expected part of aging, the degree to which this occurs is also related to cognitive function. In other words, older adults with the least amount of slow-wave sleep per night are more likely to have a diagnosis of AD (Mander et al., 2016). There is also a correlation between middle-aged adults with poor self-reported sleep quality and increased amyloid-beta plaque burden found on positron emission tomography scans. These findings suggest a bidirectional relationship between poor sleep hygiene and cognitive impairment rather than one occurring only because of the other (Dufort-Gervais et al., 2019; Mander et al., 2016).

Multicomponent Lifestyle Interventions

Growing evidence supports the value of multicomponent interventions in improving cognitive health. The Exercise and Nutritional Interventions for Neurocognitive Health Enhancement (ENLIGHTEN) trial, initiated in 2013, was the first to compare the effects of diet and exercise and their combination on neurocognitive performance (Blumenthal et al., 2019). The 160-person sample for the randomized controlled trial included sedentary adults at least 55 years of age, with either cardiovascular disease risk factors or cognitive impairment without a diagnosis of dementia. Participants were randomized to a control group receiving health education alone or an intervention group of either DASH diet, exercise, or a combination (DASH diet plus exercise). Interventions were given and monitored for six months. The study findings demonstrated significant improvements in executive function among the exercise intervention group and even greater improvements among the combination group (Blumenthal et al., 2019). A one-year follow-up study on the ENLIGHTEN trial found that participants sustained the improvements in cognitive function, even among those who discontinued the lifestyle changes implemented during the original trial.

Similarly, the Finnish Geriatric Intervention Study to Prevent Cognitive Impairment and Disability (FINGER) trial, a two-year, intensive intervention that included aerobic exercise, dietary modification, vascular risk management, and cognitive training, was associated with improved cognitive performance among older adults at risk for dementia (Rosenberg et al., 2018). Since it appears that there may be combined effects of multicomponent lifestyle interventions on neurocognitive function, APPs should consider several or all

A-SMART lifestyle interventions when discussing strategies for improved cognition.

Alzheimer's Dementia Screening and Assessment

Given that the pathogenesis of AD occurs years before showing any symptoms, it is imperative to begin the screening process early. Obtaining baseline function should be established in the same way that one undergoes other preventive screenings, such as a colonoscopy or a mammogram. Several validated cognitive screening tools are available, including the General Practitioner Assessment of Cognition (GPCOG), the Mini-Mental State Examination (MMSE) (a.k.a. the Folstein test), Mini-Cog, the Saint Louis University Mental Status (SLUMS), and the Eight-Item Interview to Differentiate Aging and Dementia (AD8) (see **Table 22.2**). A positive screen requires further assessment, including history, physical examination, additional cognitive assessment instruments, laboratory testing, and brain imaging to establish a dementia diagnosis. A geriatrician or neurologist may also be consulted as necessary.

Along with cognitive screening interviews, specific laboratory biomarkers routinely used to detect cardiometabolic conditions, such as diabetes and heart disease, can also be utilized in the early screening of mild cognitive impairment (Bredesen, 2020). In addition to standard routine laboratory tests, such as a comprehensive metabolic panel that includes blood urea nitrogen (BUN), creatinine, estimated glomerular filtration rate (eGFR), albumin, globulin, calcium, and potassium, additional metabolic markers, such as fasting insulin, and inflammatory markers, such as homocysteine, C-reactive protein (CRP), and interleukin 6 (IL-6) should be tested because they are implicated in the earliest stages of cognitive decline (Bredesen, 2017). Early testing using key biomarkers provides a vital window of opportunity to identify, prevent, and reverse cognitive decline much earlier before symptoms begin (Bredesen, 2020). A list of inflammatory biomarkers and target values can be found in **Table 22.3**.

Starting the Conversation

The body of evidence supports that the physiological changes leading to dementia begin decades before the onset of symptoms. Therefore, APPs should point out the prevention of cognitive decline as a motivating factor to engage patients in healthy behaviors. Healthy diet, exercise, sleep patterns, and psychological well-being each play an important role in the prevention and progression of cognitive deterioration. APPs must seize every opportunity to address health behaviors early in life when the greatest opportunity exists to improve the patient's quality and length of life. Once the patient has become symptomatic, experiencing moderate or advanced disease, options become more limited, resulting in a symptom management approach rather than an attempt to solve the underlying problem.

In addition to assessing A-SMART lifestyle vital signs, examples of questions the APP should ask when assessing lifestyle behaviors that promote or reduce the risk of dementia are included in **Table 22.4**. These questions can identify knowledge gaps and opportunities for patient education related to dementia prevention. They can also be used to explore patients' perceived barriers and social determinants that may interfere with their ability to make proposed lifestyle changes.

Planning Lifestyle Interventions for Addressing Cognitive Health

Healthy lifestyle modifications have been shown to significantly decrease the risk for cognitive decline in later life (Rosenberg et al.,

Table 22.2 Screening Instruments for Cognitive Impairment

Tool	Description	Interpretation	URL
General Practitioner Assessment of Cognition (GPCOG)	A brief cognitive screening tool specifically designed for use in the primary care setting. The GPCOG consists of both a cognitive test of the patient (9 questions) and an informant interview (5 questions) to increase the predictive power. Both parts can be scored separately or together. Printed and web-based versions are available.	A score of 9 (out of 9) indicates normal cognition; 5–8 indicates some impairment, and the informant interview is recommended; a score of ≤4 is very likely to indicate cognitive impairment.	http://gpcog.com.au
Mini-Mental State Examination (MMSE) Also called the Folstein test.	An 11-question measure that tests five areas of cognitive function: orientation, registration, attention and calculation, recall, and language. It has both validity and reliability for the diagnosis and longitudinal assessment of AD. The MMSE relies heavily on verbal response and reading and writing ability. Not to be confused with the Mental Status Examination (MSE).	A score of ≥24 (out of 30) indicates a normal cognition. Below this, scores can indicate severe (≤9), moderate (10–18), or mild (19–23) cognitive impairment.	https://www.dementiacarecentral.com/mini-mental-state-exam
Mini-Cog	A 3-minute instrument consisting of a 3-item recall and clock drawing. The results do not diagnose dementia but permit the APP to know if further action is necessary.	A total score of 3–5 (out of 5) indicates a lower likelihood of dementia but does not rule out some degree of cognitive impairment.	https://mini-cog.com

Test	Description	Scoring	Reference
Saint Louis University Mental Status (SLUMS)	Consists of 11 questions assessing attention, immediate recall, immediate recall with interference, delayed recall with interference, numerical calculation, registration, digit span, visual spatial, executive function, extrapolation, and orientation. Sensitive to mild impairment.	Scoring is adjusted based on educational level. For patients with a high school education, a score of 27–30 indicates normal cognition; 21–26 mild neurocognitive disorder; and 1–20 dementia. For patients with less than a high school education, 25–30 indicates normal cognition; 20–24 mild neurocognitive disorder; and 1–19 dementia.	https://www.slu.edu/medicine/internal-medicine/geriatric-medicine/aging-successfully/assessment-tools/mental-status-exam.php
Eight-Item Interview to Differentiate Aging and Dementia (AD8) Also called he Washington University Dementia Screening Test.	Developed as a brief instrument to help discriminate between signs of normal aging and mild dementia. It contains eight items that test for memory, orientation, judgment, and function. Sensitive to early signs of dementia regardless of etiology. Validated as a direct questionnaire for the patient and as an informant-based interview.	0–1: Normal cognition $\geq$2: Impairment in cognition	https://hign.org/sites/default/files/2020-06/Try_This_Dementia_14.pdf

Table 22.3 Early Laboratory Markers Used to Screen for Cognitive Decline

Laboratory Markers	Optimal Ranges	Key Considerations
Fasting insulin	3.0–5.0 μIU/mL	Measures of insulin resistance, glycotoxicity
Fasting glucose	70–90 mg/dL	
Hemoglobin A1C	4.0–5.3%	
Homeostatic Model Assessment for Insulin Resistance (HOMA-IR)	<1.2	
High-sensitivity C-reactive protein (hs-CRP)	<0.9 mg/dL	Measure of systemic inflammation
Homocysteine	>7 μmol/L	Reflects methylation, inflammation, and the body's ability to handle detoxification
Vitamin B6	25–50 mcg/L	Improves methylation, reduces homocysteine
Vitamin B9 (folate)	10–25 ng/mL	
Vitamin B12	500–1,500 pg/mL	

Data from Bredesen, D. E. (2020). *The end of Alzheimer's program: The first program to prevent and reverse cognitive decline*, pp. 21–24. Avery.

Table 22.4 Sample Screening Questions for Dementia Risk and Primary Prevention Strategies

Lifestyle Vital Sign	Screening Questions
Adopt healthy eating	■ How many days per week do you eat fresh fruits and vegetables? ■ How many days per week do you eat whole grains?
Stress less	■ Do you participate in any social groups or volunteer organizations? ■ Do you have family members or close friends with whom you communicate regularly? ■ Do you feel safe at home?
Move often	■ Have you fallen within the past month? ■ Do you have pain that would limit you from participating in a regular exercise program?
Avoid alcohol	■ About how many days have you had an alcoholic beverage within the past month?
Rest more	■ Do you feel well rested in the morning? ■ How many hours do you sleep uninterrupted on a typical night?
Treat tobacco use	■ Have you used tobacco products within the past month? ■ Do any members of your household use tobacco products daily?

Health Promotion Research Study

Association Between Diabetes and Cognitive Decline

Background: The association between diabetes and dementia has been well documented; however, the association between diabetes and cognitive decline is less well studied.

Methodology: A study was conducted to evaluate longitudinal associations among HbA1c levels, diabetes status, and subsequent cognitive decline. A total of 5,189 participants (55.1% women, mean age 65.6 ± 9.4 years) with baseline HbA1c levels ranging from 15.9 to 126.3 mmol/mol (3.6–13.7%) were studied over a 10-year follow-up period.

Results: There were significant longitudinal associations among HbA1c levels, diabetes status, and long-term cognitive decline. Future studies are required to determine the effects of maintaining optimal glucose control on the rate of cognitive decline in people with diabetes.

Implications for Advanced Practice: Findings suggest that interventions that delay diabetes onset, as well as management strategies for glucose control, may help to alleviate the progression of subsequent cognitive decline over the long term. Although more research is needed, diabetes has been associated with microvascular complications that affect the central nervous system and is thus a strong risk factor for cognitive decline. Early intervention to address the risk factors for diabetes may offer significant promise in preventing the decline in cognitive function.

Reference: Zheng, F., Yan, L., Zhong, B., & Xie, W. (2018). HbA1c, diabetes and cognitive decline: The English Longitudinal Study of Ageing. *Diabetologia, 61*(4), 839–848. https://doi.org/10.1007/s00125-017-4541-7

Data from Zheng, F., Yan, L., Zhong, B., & Xie, W. (2018). HbA1c, diabetes and cognitive decline: The English Longitudinal Study of Ageing. *Diabetologia, 61*(4), 839–848. https://doi.org/10.1007/s00125-017-4541-7

2018; Shetty & Youngberg, 2018; Zheng et al., 2018). However, even rigorous evidence is not always enough to galvanize behavioral change. Individuals may have a genuine desire to improve their health yet are unable to turn those intentions into actions unless they are willing to commit to setting well-defined, measurable goals to address maladaptive health behaviors (Bailey, 2019). Implementing lifestyle interventions such as exercise and diet can be particularly challenging to older adults and their providers, especially if there are ongoing chronic comorbid conditions (Murdoch et al., 2020). APPs have a unique opportunity to influence positive behavior change with each patient encounter. However, most are not routinely providing adequate counseling and coaching often due to time constraints (Lacagnina et al., 2018) or a perceived lack of knowledge on the clinician's part to provide adequate nutrition counseling (Crowley et al., 2019; Frates, 2015).

Moreover, traditional medical training typically uses a problem-based approach, which prepares APPs to be experts in assessing problems and implementing treatment but does not adequately prepare them to serve in the roles of mentor, partner, and health coach (Frates & Bonnet, 2016). The partnering approach, as described by Frates and Bonnet, necessitates that the provider transition their role from *expert* to *collaborator*, shifting the responsibility for behavior change away from the provider and toward the patient. In this way, the authors emphasize, (a) patients are intricately involved in the planning and evaluating process and thus become accountable for their own health actions and behaviors, and (b) both the provider and the patients can achieve more collaboratively than they could have achieved on their own.

SMART Goals

"The best goal is the one that the patient feels is important, the one the patient feels confident that he or she can complete, and the one that is SMART" (Frates, 2021, p. 10). Once patients express their desire to embrace lifestyle approaches to improve their health, the APP needs to tailor goals specific to them; in other words, the APP will meet the patients where they are. SMART goals, which originated in the 1960s in the business and engineering realm, are routinely used to achieve objectives by setting *specific*, *measurable*, *achievable*, *relevant*, and *time-bound* goals. SMART goals were further developed into SMART-EST to include the characteristics of *evidence-informed*, *strategic*, and *tailored* to the patient (White et al., 2020).

A-SMART Lifestyle Prescriptions

The SMART-EST approach to goal setting includes a written prescription with actionable steps for lifestyle change. However, unlike a traditional directive prescription where the APP provides instructions on what to do and how to do it, the SMART-EST goals are person centered and involve a collaborative effort

---

Example of an Individualized A-SMART Prescription for Addressing Cognitive Health

For the next four weeks, do the following:

- Eat one serving of leafy vegetables like kale, spinach, and collard greens daily.
- Walk 15 minutes after dinner each day.
- Turn off TV and devices one hour before bedtime.

---

between the patients and the providers after using a motivational interviewing approach to determine which lifestyle strategies the patients are able, willing, and ready to implement. The following box provides an example of an individualized A-SMART prescription that could be given to patients with identified risk factors for dementia and a desire to implement lifestyle change to promote optimal cognitive health.

Interprofessional Approach to Dementia

Worldwide, dementia management programs are striving to develop and foster holistic, person-centered interprofessional approaches that provide educational support for patients and their caregivers regarding medical care content, prevention of disease progression, symptom management, coping skills, and social support services (Rodriguez et al., 2020; Seike et al., 2014). One such integrated care model that incorporates interprofessional approaches to dementia care was described by Richter (2016), who evaluated an established care model in northeast Germany to determine whether this successful model could be replicated in other countries and healthcare systems. The model, known as the Dementia Care Centre, is patient and family centered and led by a geriatric psychiatrist who serves as a gatekeeper and includes nurses, physical and occupational therapists, rehabilitation specialists, counselors, occupational therapists, and other specialists. These services are provided in a single dementia-friendly building that promotes and nurtures independent and assisted living within an enclosed community setting. In the United States, similar models have emerged, such as the Continuing Care Communities (continuingcarecommunities .org), which provide a continuum of care for the aging population. However, these communities are not affordable to much of the population.

Summary

The goals of this chapter were to provide a robust understanding of the prevalence and pathophysiology of AD and other types of dementia; to recognize early biomarkers that can identify risks of cognitive decline; and to introduce evidence-informed lifestyle approaches that can prevent, treat, and, in some cases, reverse cognitive decline (Bredesen et al., 2016; Bredesen, 2020; Sherzai & Sherzai, 2019). The etiology of AD and, other dementias is multifactorial, involving many environmental, genetic, and lifestyle influences. For this reason, no stand-alone intervention is effective. Strategies to mitigate cognitive decline must include behavioral approaches that reduce and eliminate modifiable risk factors contributing to cognitive decline, such as chronic inflammation, insulin resistance, poor sleep, suboptimal nutrition, and lack of physical exercise. See **Table 22.5** for additional resources. APPs well versed in health promotion and lifestyle medicine are uniquely positioned to educate and empower patients to make evidence-informed lifestyle choices that include adopting healthy eating, becoming and remaining physically active, and getting restorative sleep.

Health Promotion Case Study: Addressing Cognitive Changes in an Adult Female

Case description: M.J. is a 63-year-old female who presented to her APP with a chief complaint of difficulty concentrating and forgetfulness over the last year. She has noticed that these changes have been much more frequent over the past month.

- Past medical history: Depression, hypertension, hypothyroidism, and osteoarthritis.
- Medications: Naproxen 220 mg one to two times daily as needed for knee pain; amlodipine 5 mg tablet daily.
- Social history: She works as a cashier at the local drugstore. She is divorced, lives alone, and has two healthy sons.
- Vital signs: Height 61 inches, weight 160 pounds, blood pressure 144/90 mmHg, heart rate 82, respiratory rate 17, temperature 97.0°F.
- Physical exam: Well-nourished, well-hydrated female. Slow but steady gait. SLUMS: 27/30, had difficulty with word recall but otherwise neurological exam essentially unremarkable. Physical exam otherwise notable only for bilateral knee crepitation and healing skin tear left calf (due to reported fall earlier in the week).
- Laboratory tests: Most recent laboratory tests (six months ago from primary care provider) were notable for HbA1c 6.6%, total cholesterol 170 mg/dL, low-density lipoproteins (LDL) 125 mg/dL, high-density lipoprotein (HDL) 40 mg/dL, and fasting blood glucose (FBG) 121 mg/dL. Basic metabolic panel (BMP) and complete blood count (CBC) were otherwise unremarkable. No other labs were drawn at that visit. At that time, she was instructed to modify her diet and exercise more.

Lifestyle Vital Signs

- Adopt healthy eating: 24-hour diet recall includes skipped breakfast; midmorning coffee; packed lunch of ham and cheese sandwich, apple, and cookies; afternoon snack of candy bar; takeout dinner on the way home from work; sips colas throughout the day.
- Stress less: Notes stressful job due to decreased staffing. Admits loneliness on weekends.
- Move often: Denies due to fear of falling.

(continues)

Health Promotion Case Study: Addressing Cognitive Changes in
an Adult Female   (*continued*)

- Avoid alcohol: Denies alcohol and substance use.
- Rest more: 9:00 p.m. bedtime; falls asleep without difficulty; 1–2 awakenings during the night (to urinate); returns to sleep without difficulty; awakens with alarm at 7:00 a.m.; 5/10 refreshed; unaware of snoring.
- Treat tobacco use: Denies current tobacco use; history of 100 pack-years of cigarette smoking.
- BMI: 30.2 kg/m^2.

Critical Thinking Questions

- What additional history would you be interested in gathering from M.J. for your subjective data?
- What additional lifestyle factors would you assess and why?
- What diagnostic tests would you run and why?
- What lifestyle management strategies would you recommend for improving M.J.'s outcomes?
- Find research evidence to support lifestyle management of M.J.'s symptoms.

Health Promotion Activity: Special Considerations in Exercise Prescription for Older Adults

Review and discuss the recommended screening guidelines in the article below. Pay particular attention to the framework that APPs can follow when modifying these guidelines for older adults with the most common age-associated comorbidities. Also, note the barriers and motivation for exercise adherence in this population. Role-play with a classmate or colleague how you might address these barriers.

Zaleski, A. L., Taylor, B. A., Panza, G. A., Wu, Y., Pescatello, L. S., Thompson, P. D., & Fernandez, A. B. (2016). Coming of age: Considerations in the prescription of exercise for older adults. *Methodist DeBakey Cardiovascular Journal, 12*(2), 98. https://doi.org/10.14797/mdcj-12-2-98

TABLE 22.5	Evidence-Based Resources for Alzheimer's Disease and Dementia

Organization	Resource	URL
Alzheimer's Association	Provider resources include AD statistics, diagnostic criteria, cognitive assessment tool kit, guidelines, Medicare Annual Wellness Visit Algorithm for Assessment of Cognition, and other resources. Patient and caregiver resources include educational material, support programs, a 24/7 helpline, and a resource finder.	https://www.alz.org

Organization	Resource	URL
Alzheimer's Impact Movement	Fiscal Year 2021 Alzheimer's Research Funding	https://act.alz.org /site/DocServer/2015 _Appropriations_Fact_Sheet __FY16_.pdf?docID=3641
Alzheimer's Disease International	World Alzheimer Report 2020	https://www.alz.co.uk /research/world-report-2020
Apollo Health	AD research, education, and protocols for prevention and reversal of cognitive decline	https://www.apollohealthco .com/bredesen-protocol
Dementia Care Central	Resources for dementia caregivers	https://www .dementiacarecentral.com
Physicians Committee for Responsible Medicine	News and resources related to AD	https://www.pcrm.org /search?keys=Alzheimers
Sherzai MD	*The Alzheimer's Solution* book and the NEURO Plan (nutrition, exercise, restorative sleep, unwinding, and optimization) brain health program for the prevention of Alzheimer's and other neurodegenerative diseases	https://www.theneuroplan .com
U.S. Department of Health and Human Services	*Physical Activity Guidelines for Americans*, 2nd edition	https://health.gov/sites /default/files/2019-09 /Physical_Activity _Guidelines_2nd_edition.pdf

Acronyms

AD: Alzheimer's disease

AD8: Eight-Item Interview to Differentiate Aging and Dementia

APP: advanced practice provider

A-SMART: adopt healthy eating, stress less, move often, avoid alcohol, rest more, and treat tobacco use

DASH: Dietary Approaches to Stop Hypertension

ENLIGHTEN: Exercise and Nutritional Interventions for Neurocognitive Health Enhancement

FINGER: Finnish Geriatric Intervention Study to Prevent Cognitive Impairment and Disability

FTLD: frontotemporal lobar degeneration

GPCOG: General Practitioner Assessment of Cognition

HS: hippocampal sclerosis

LBD: Lewy body dementia

MIND: Mediterranean–DASH Diet Intervention for Neurogenerative Delay

MMSE: Mini-Mental State Examination

PD: Parkinson's disease

SLUMS: Saint Louis University Mental Status
SMART: specific, measurable, achievable, relevant, and time-bound

SMART-EST: specific, measurable, achievable, relevant, time-bound, evidence-informed, strategic, and tailored

References

Alzheimer's Association. (2020). 2020 Alzheimer's disease facts and figures. *Alzheimer's & Dementia, 16*(3), 391–460. https://doi.org/10.1002/alz.12068

Alzheimer's Association. (2021). 2021 Alzheimer's disease facts and figures. *Alzheimer's & Dementia, 17*(3), 327–406. https://doi.org/ 10.1002/alz.12328

Alzheimer's Association. (2022). 2022 Alzheimer's disease facts and figures. *Alzheimer's & Dementia, 18,* 700–789. https://doi.org/10.1002/alz.12638

Armstrong, R. (2019). Risk factors for Alzheimer's disease. *Folia Neuropathologica, 57*(2), 87–105. https://doi.org/10.5114/fn.2019.85929

Bailey, R. R. (2019). Goal setting and action planning for health behavior change. *American Journal of Lifestyle Medicine, 13*(6), 615–618. https://doi.org/10.1177/1559827617729634

Blackman, J., Swirski, M., Clynes, J., Harding, S., Leng, Y., & Coulthard, E. (2021). Pharmacological and non-pharmacological interventions to enhance sleep in mild cognitive impairment and mild Alzheimer's disease: A systematic review. *Journal of Sleep Research, 30*(4), e13229. https://doi.org/10.1111/jsr.13229

Blumenthal, J. A., Smith, P. J., Mabe, S., Hinderliter, A., Lin, P.-H., Liao, L., Welsh-Bohmer, K. A., Browndyke, J. N., Kraus, W. E., Doraiswamy, P. M., Burke, J. R., & Sherwood, A. (2019). Lifestyle and neurocognition in older adults with cognitive impairments: A randomized trial. *Neurology, 92*(3), e212–e223. https://doi.org/10.1212/WNL.0000000000006784

Bredesen, D. E. (2017). *The end of Alzheimer's: The first program to prevent and reverse cognitive decline.* Penguin Random House.

Bredesen, D. E. (2020). *The end of Alzheimer's program: The first program to enhance cognition and reverse decline at any age.* Avery.

Bredesen, D. E. E., Amos, E. C. C., Canick, J., Ackerley, M., Raji, C., Fiala, M., & Ahdidan, J. (2016). Reversal of cognitive decline in Alzheimer's disease. *Aging, 8*(6), 1250–1258. https://doi.org/10.18632/aging.100981

Chen, X.-Q., & Mobley, W. C. (2019). Alzheimer disease pathogenesis: Insights from molecular and cellular biology studies of oligomeric Aβ and tau species. *Frontiers in Neuroscience, 13,* 659. https://doi.org/10.3389/fnins.2019.00659

Considine, C. M., Parker, H. A., Briggs, J., Quasney, E. E., Larson, E. R., Smith, H., Shollenbarger, S. G., & Abeare, C. A. (2018). Sleep biomarkers, health comorbidities, and neurocognition in obstructive sleep apnea. *Journal of the International Neuropsychological Society, 24*(8), 864–875. https://doi.org/10.1017/S1355617718000449

Crowley, J., Ball, L., & Hiddink, G. J. (2019). Nutrition in medical education: A systematic review. *The Lancet Planetary Health, 3*(9), e379–e389. https://doi.org/10.1016/S2542-5196(19)30171-8

Cummings, J., Reiber, C., & Kumar, P. (2018). The price of progress: Funding and financing Alzheimer's disease drug development. *Alzheimer's & Dementia: Translational Research & Clinical Interventions, 4*(1), 330–343. https://doi.org/10.1016/j.trci.2018.04.008

Dufort-Gervais, J., Mongrain, V., & Brouillette, J. (2019). Bidirectional relationships between sleep and amyloid-beta in the hippocampus. *Neurobiology of Learning and Memory, 160,* 108–117. https://doi.org/10.1016/j.nlm.2018.06.009

Edward Jones, Age Wave, & the Harris Poll. (2021). *The four pillars of the new retirement: An Edward Jones and Age Wave Study.* https://www.edwardjones.com/sites/default/files/acquiadam/2021-01/Edward-Jones-4-Pillars-US-report.pdf

Erickson, K. I., Hillman, C., Stillman, C. M., Ballard, R. M., Bloodgood, B., Conroy, D. E., Macko, R., Marquez, D. X., Petruzzello, S. J., Powell, K. E., & the 2018 Physical Activity Guidelines Advisory Committee. (2019). Physical activity, cognition, and brain outcomes: A review of the 2018 physical activity guidelines. *Medicine & Science in Sports & Exercise, 51*(6), 1242–1251. https://doi.org/10.1249/MSS.0000000000001936

Frates, E. P. (2015). The five step collaboration cycle: A tool for the doctors office. *International Journal of School and Cognitive Psychology, 2*(3). https://doi.org/10.4172/2469-9837.1000144

Frates, E. P. (2021). *Lifestyle medicine course syllabus.* American College of Lifestyle Medicine.

Frates, E. P., & Bonnet, J. (2016). Collaboration and negotiation: The key to therapeutic lifestyle change. *American Journal of Lifestyle Medicine, 10*(5), 302–312. https://doi.org/10.1177/1559827616638013

Groot, C., Hooghiemstra, A. M., Raijmakers, P. G. H. M., van Berckel, B. N. M., Scheltens, P., Scherder, E. J. A., van der Flier, W. M., & Ossenkoppele, R. (2016). The effect of physical activity on cognitive function in patients with dementia: A meta-analysis of randomized control trials. *Ageing Research Reviews, 25,* 13–23. https://doi.org/10.1016/j.arr.2015.11.005

Huang, Z., Wong, L.-W., Su, Y., Huang, X., Wang, N., Chen, H., & Yi, C. (2020). Blood-brain barrier integrity in the pathogenesis of Alzheimer's disease. *Frontiers in Neuroendocrinology*, *59*, 100857. https://doi.org/10.1016/j.yfrne.2020.100857

Isaacson, R. S., Ganzer, C. A., Hristov, H., Hackett, K., Caesar, E., Cohen, R., Kachko, R., Meléndez-Cabrero, J., Rahman, A., Scheyer, O., Hwang, M. J., Berkowitz, C., Hendrix, S., Mureb, M., Schelke, M. W., Mosconi, L., Seifan, A., & Krikorian, R. (2018). The clinical practice of risk reduction for Alzheimer's disease: A precision medicine approach. *Alzheimer's & Dementia*, *14*(12), 1663–1673. https://doi.org/10.1016/j.jalz.2018.08.004

Jia, R.-X., Liang, J.-H., Xu, Y., & Wang, Y.-Q. (2019). Effects of physical activity and exercise on the cognitive function of patients with Alzheimer disease: A meta-analysis. *BMC Geriatrics*, *19*(1), 181. https://doi.org/10.1186/s12877-019-1175-2

Kelly, M. E., Duff, H., Kelly, S., McHugh Power, J. E., Brennan, S., Lawlor, B. A., & Loughrey, D. G. (2017). The impact of social activities, social networks, social support and social relationships on the cognitive functioning of healthy older adults: A systematic review. *Systematic Reviews*, *6*(1), 259. https://doi.org/10.1186/s13643-017-0632-2

Lacagnina, S., Moore, M., & Mitchell, S. (2018). The lifestyle medicine team: Health care that delivers value. *American Journal of Lifestyle Medicine*, *12*(6), 479–483. https://doi.org/10.1177/1559827618792493

Livingston, G., Huntley, J., Sommerlad, A., Ames, D., Ballard, C., Banerjee, S., Brayne, C., Burns, A., Cohen-Mansfield, J., Cooper, C., Costafreda, S. G., Dias, A., Fox, N., Gitlin, L. N., Howard, R., Kales, H. C., Kivimäki, M., Larson, E. B., Ogunniyi, A., . . . Mukadam, N. (2020). Dementia prevention, intervention, and care: 2020 report of the Lancet Commission. *The Lancet*, *396*(10248), 413–446. https://doi.org/10.1016/S0140-6736(20)30367-6

Loughrey, D. G., Levecchia, S., Brennan, S., Lawlor, B. A., & Kelly, M. E. (2017). The impact of the Mediterranean diet on the cognitive functioning of healthy older adults: A systematic review and meta-analysis. *Advances in Nutrition*, *8*(4), 571–586. https://doi.org/10.3945/an.117.015495

Mander, B. A., Winer, J. R., Jagust, W. J., & Walker, M. P. (2016). Sleep: A novel mechanistic pathway, biomarker, and treatment target in the pathology of Alzheimer's disease? *Trends in Neurosciences*, *39*(8), 552–566. https://doi.org/10.1016/j.tins.2016.05.002

McEvoy, C. T., Guyer, H., Langa, K. M., & Yaffe, K. (2017). Neuroprotective diets are associated with better cognitive function: The health and retirement study. *American Geriatrics Society*, *65*(8), 1857–1862. https://doi.org/10.1111/jgs.14922

McGrattan, A. M., McGuinness, B., McKinley, M. C., Kee, F., Passmore, P., Woodside, J. V., & McEvoy, C. T. (2019). Diet and inflammation in cognitive ageing and Alzheimer's disease. *Current Nutrition Reports*, *8*(2), 53–65. https://doi.org/10.1007/s13668-019-0271-4

Morris, M. C., Tangney, C. C., Wang, Y., Sacks, F. M., Barnes, L. L., Bennett, D. A., & Aggarwal, N. T. (2015). MIND diet slows cognitive decline with aging. *Alzheimer's & Dementia*, *11*(9), 1015–1022. https://doi.org/10.1016/j.jalz.2015.04.011

Murdoch, J., Salter, C., Ford, J., Lenaghan, E., Shiner, A., & Steel, N. (2020). The "unknown territory" of goal-setting: Negotiating a novel interactional activity within primary care doctor-patient consultations for patients with multiple chronic conditions. *Social Science & Medicine*, *256*, 113040. https://doi.org/10.1016/j.socscimed.2020.113040

Northey, J. M., Cherbuin, N., Pumpa, K. L., Smee, D. J., & Rattray, B. (2018). Exercise interventions for cognitive function in adults older than 50: A systematic review with meta-analysis. *British Journal of Sports Medicine*, *52*(3), 154–160. https://doi.org/10.1136/bjsports-2016-096587

Oxford, A. E., Stewart, E. S., & Rohn, T. T. (2020). Clinical trials in Alzheimer's disease: A hurdle in the path of remedy. *International Journal of Alzheimer's Disease*, *2020*, 5380346. https://doi.org/10.1155/2020/5380346

Pistollato, F., Iglesias, R. C., Ruiz, R., Aparicio, S., Crespo, J., Lopez, L. D., Manna, P. P., Giampieri, F., & Battino, M. (2018). Nutritional patterns associated with the maintenance of neurocognitive functions and the risk of dementia and Alzheimer's disease: A focus on human studies. *Pharmacological Research*, *131*, 32–43. https://doi.org/10.1016/j.phrs.2018.03.012

Poulose, S. M., Miller, M. G., Scott, T., & Shukitt-Hale, B. (2017). Nutritional factors affecting adult neurogenesis and cognitive function. *Advances in Nutrition*, *8*(6), 804–811. https://doi.org/10.3945/an.117.016261

Prendecki, M., Kowalska, M., Lagan-Jedrzejczyk, U., Piekut, T., Krokos, A., Kozubski, W., & Dorszewska, J. (2020). Genetic factors related to the immune system in subjects at risk of developing Alzheimer's disease. *Journal of Integrative Neuroscience*, *19*(2), 359–371. https://doi.org/10.31083/j.jin.2020.02.110

Richter, S. (2016). Integrated care for people with dementia—Results of a social-scientific evaluation of an established dementia care model. *Geriatrics*, *2*(1), 1. https://doi.org/10.3390/geriatrics2010001

Rodriguez, F. S., Jackson, J., Ware, C., Churchyard, R., & Hanseeuw, B. (2020). Interdisciplinary and transdisciplinary perspectives: On the road to a holistic approach to dementia prevention and care. *Journal of Alzheimer's Disease Reports*, *4*(1), 39–48. https://doi.org/10.3233/ADR-180070

Rosenberg, A., Ngandu, T., Rusanen, M., Antikainen, R., Backman, L., Havulinna, S., Hanninen, T.,

Laatikainen, T., Lehtisalo, J., Levalahti, E., Lindstrom, J., Paajanen, T., Peltonen, M., Soininen, H., Stigsdotter-Neely, A., Strandberg, T., Tuomilehto, J., Solomon, A., & Kivipelto, M. (2018). Multidomain lifestyle intervention benefits a largely elderly population at risk for cognitive decline and dementia regardless of baseline characteristics: The FINGER trial. *Alzheimer's & Dementia*, *14*(3), 263–270. https://doi.org/10.1016/j.jalz.2017.09.006

Sabia, S., Fayosse, A., Dumurgier, J., van Hees, V. T., Paquet, C., Sommerlad, A., Kivimäki, M., Dugravot, A., & Singh-Manoux, A. (2021). Association of sleep duration in middle and old age with incidence of dementia. *Nature Communications*, *12*(1), 2289. https://doi.org/10.1038/s41467-021-22354-2

Santos-Lozano, A., Pareja-Galeano, H., Sanchis-Gomar, F., Quindós-Rubial, M., Fiuza-Luces, C., Cristi-Montero, C., Emanuele, E., Garatachea, N., & Lucia, A. (2016). Physical activity and Alzheimer disease: A protective association. *Mayo Clinic Proceedings*, *91*(8), 999–1020. https://doi.org/10.1016/j.mayocp.2016.04.024

Seike, A., Sumigaki, C., Takeda, A., Endo, H., Sakurai, T., & Toba, K. (2014). Developing an interdisciplinary program of educational support for early-stage dementia patients and their family members: An investigation based on learning needs and attitude changes: Interdisciplinary educational support. *Geriatrics & Gerontology International*, *14*, 28–34. https://doi.org/10.1111/ggi.12263

Sherzai, D., & Sherzai, A. (2019). *The Alzheimer's solution: A breakthrough program to prevent and reverse the symptoms of cognitive decline at every age*. HarperOne.

Shetty, P., & Youngberg, W. (2018). Clinical lifestyle medicine strategies for preventing and reversing memory loss in Alzheimer's. *American Journal of Lifestyle Medicine*, *12*(5), 391–395. https://doi.org/10.1177/1559827618766468

Small, B. A., Dixon, R. A., McArdle, J. J., & Grimm, K. J. (2012). Do changes in lifestyle engagement moderate cognitive decline in normal aging? Evidence from the Victoria Longitudinal Study. *Neuropsychology*, *26*(2), 144–155. https://doi.org/10.1037/a0026579

Tobore, O. T. (2019). On the etiopathogenesis and pathophysiology of Alzheimer's disease: A comprehensive theoretical review. *Journal of Alzheimer's Disease*, *68*, 417–437. https://doi.org/10.3233/JAD-181052

Walker, K. A., Hoogeveen, R. C., Folsom, A. R., Ballantyne, C. M., Knopman, D. S., Windham, B. G., Jack, C. R., & Gottesman, R. F. (2017). Midlife systemic inflammatory markers are associated with late-life brain volume: The ARIC Study. *Neurology*, *89*(22), 2262–2270. https://doi.org/10.1212/WNL.0000000000004688

Wennberg, A. M. V., Wu, M. N., Rosenberg, P. B., & Spira, A. P. (2017). Sleep disturbance, cognitive decline, and dementia: A review. *Seminars in Neurology*, *37*(4), 395–406. https://doi.org/10.1055/s-0037-1604351

White, N. D., Bautista, V., Lenz, T., & Cosimano, A. (2020). Using the SMART-EST goals in lifestyle medicine prescription. *American Journal of Lifestyle Medicine*, *14*(3), 271–273. https://doi.org/10.1177/1559827620905775

World Health Organization. (2017). *Global action plan on the public health response to dementia 2017–2025*. https://apps.who.int/iris/bitstream/handle/10665/259615/9789241513487-eng.pdf?sequence=1

Xu, W., Tan, C.-C., Zou, J.-J., Cao, X.-P., & Tan, L. (2020). Sleep problems and risk of all-cause cognitive decline or dementia: An updated systematic review and meta-analysis. *Journal of Neurology, Neurosurgery & Psychiatry*, *91*(3), 236–244. https://doi.org/10.1136/jnnp-2019-321896

Zaleski, A. L., Taylor, B. A., Panza, G. A., Wu, Y., Pescatello, L. S., Thompson, P. D., & Fernandez, A. B. (2016). Coming of age: Considerations in the prescription of exercise for older adults. *Methodist DeBakey Cardiovascular Journal*, *12*(2), 98. https://doi.org/10.14797/mdcj-12-2-98

Zheng, F., Yang, Z., & Xie, W. (2018). HbA$_{1c}$, diabetes and cognitive decline: The English longitudinal study of ageing. *Diabetologia*, *61*, 839–848. https://doi.org/10.1007/s00125-017-4541-7

CHAPTER 23

The Role of Healthy Lifestyles in Mental Health Promotion

Carol Essenmacher, DNP, RN, PMHCNS-BC
Joanne Evans, MEd, RN, PMHCNS-BC
Kelly Freeman, MSN, RN, AGPCNP-BC, DipACLM
Elizabeth Winings, DNP, APRN, PMHNP-BC

"If you are in a bad mood, go for a walk. If you are still in a bad mood, go for another walk."

Hippocrates

OBJECTIVES

This chapter will enable the reader to:

1. Identify the reciprocal nature of mental and physical health.
2. Review co-occurring mental health disorders and chronic diseases.
3. Explain the significance of the gut–brain axis in mental health.
4. Conceptualize the relationship between inflammation and mental health.
5. Discuss the impact of lifestyle choices on mental health.
6. Analyze lifestyle characteristics conducive to optimal mental health.
7. Identify ways to screen and assess for mental illness.
8. Formulate prescriptive lifestyle interventions to optimize mental health outcomes.

Overview

The co-occurrence of mental health disorders and chronic health problems merely hints at the complexities and connectedness between the mind and body. Implications of social determinants of health only add to the challenges of treating mental and physical diseases. Historically, providers have identified themselves as either physical or mental healthcare providers (Kalmakis, 2021). Patients have reported experiencing frustration

© Kathleen Gail/Shutterstock; © StoryTime Studio/Shutterstock; © kali9/Getty Images

and stress at their inability to find a provider who understood or was interested in the mind–body connection (Ramanuj et al., 2019). As a result, greater emphasis is being placed on treating the whole person—body and mind—because health problems in one affect the other.

Today's advanced practice providers (APPs) are tasked with offering holistic care regardless of their setting (Nazarko & Thorne, 2020). However, it can be challenging to fully appreciate the interplay between the mind and the body while managing the day-to-day tasks of advanced practice. Busy clinicians often do not have time to assess the impact that patients' choices have on their mental and physical health or to empower patients with chronic illnesses to learn new skills to improve their health outcomes. Furthermore, while demographic data and statistical trends for mental illness are essential to providing evidence-informed care, this information does not convey the lived experience of the patients, which is essential for establishing therapeutic rapport and developing effective person-centered strategies.

Patient adherence to prescribed healthy lifestyle interventions for optimal mental health depends on an accurate evaluation of their current needs and the implementation of a plan that is meaningful to them. This chapter discusses the common mental health issues seen in primary care settings and applicable assessments and screening tools. Resources are provided for effective communication strategies to support health behavior change, suggestions on starting conversations about mental health, and practical approaches to patient–provider collaboration. The chapter also provides evidence-informed lifestyle interventions to improve mental health outcomes and guides APPs in developing A-SMART (adopt healthy eating, stress less, move often, avoid alcohol, rest more, and treat tobacco use) prescriptions that support the pillars of a healthy lifestyle.

Complexity of Mental Health

Descriptions of mental health are complex and include several factors. The World Health Organization (WHO, 2022) defines mental health as "a state of mental well-being that enables people to cope with the stresses of life, realize their abilities, learn well and work well, and contribute to their community" (para. 1). What constitutes mental health is complex, highly subjective, and dependent on multiple determinants and personal perspectives and values. Fusar-Poli et al. (2020), in a scoping review of the literature, described 14 domains that define mental health: mental health literacy, attitude toward mental disorder, self-perceptions and values, cognitive skills, academic/occupational performance, emotions, behaviors, self-management strategies, social skills, family and significant relationships, physical health, sexual health, meaning of life, and quality of life. The context of optimal mental health and the lifestyle activities that support the best possible outcomes should be kept in mind as attention is turned toward possible threats to achieving and sustaining mental and physical health.

Co-Occurring Mental and Physical Health Issues

The reciprocal nature of mental and physical health is well documented and "inextricably linked" (Office of Disease Prevention and Health Promotion [ODPHP], n.d.-d, para. 5). Evidence of the mental–physical health relationship reveals that individuals experiencing chronic physical diseases also experience mental health issues (Conversano, 2019; McCarron et al., 2019) and vice versa. People with depression have a 40% higher risk of cardiovascular and metabolic diseases than the general public (National Alliance on Mental Illness, n.d.). Anxiety and substance use disorders (SUDs) can develop into chronic physical health issues (McCarron et al., 2019). Anxiety-like symptoms accompany many medical conditions, such as pneumonia, chronic obstructive pulmonary disease, cardiovascular conditions (e.g., coronary artery disease, heart failure, and pulmonary embolism), thyroid dysfunction, hyperparathyroidism, hypoglycemia, menopause, seizure disorders, and SUDs (McCarron et al., 2019). Persons experiencing mental health issues also struggle with treatment and medication adherence, which worsens the effects and outcomes of chronic diseases (Allegrante et al., 2019). These comorbidities occur across the life span. In the pediatric population, the Centers for Disease Control and Prevention (CDC) reports that 73.8% of children aged 3 to 17 years with depression also have anxiety and that almost one out of two (47.2%) also have behavior problems (National Center on Birth Defects and Developmental Disabilities [NCBDDD], n.d.-b).

Mental and physical health issues are widely noted as unintended side effects of the COVID-19 pandemic due to a substantial period of restrictions on lifestyle options and choices (Caroppo et al., 2021). Studies show a significant decline in physical activity, the impact of which is emerging as this chapter is being written (Caroppo et al., 2021; Giuntella et al., 2021). Social isolation also has led to adverse changes in sleep habits and eating patterns, both of which have long-term consequences yet to be fully understood.

Mental health conditions, such as anxiety and depression, can also impact physical health by interfering with healthy coping skills. The *Healthy People 2030* report describes symptoms of depression as a vicious cycle of people becoming less motivated and participating in activities that do not support mental and physical health (ODPHP, n.d.-c). When experiencing distress, people often indulge in unhealthy behaviors to self-soothe (Protogerou et al., 2020). Consequently, unhealthy dietary patterns, lack of regular exercise, and substance use can lead to hypertension, type 2 diabetes, and other chronic health problems.

Another consideration in the reciprocal nature of chronic disease treatment and prevention is the role of medications used to treat mental health issues. There are classes of psychotropic medications, including antipsychotics and mood stabilizers, that are implicated in the development of metabolic problems (Dikec et al., 2021; Penninx & Lange, 2018). Thus, medications to help treat mental illness can contribute to weight gain, elevated cholesterol, and increased risk for the development of type 2 diabetes (Dikec et al., 2021; Penninx & Lange, 2018). Further exacerbating the vicious cycle, people who struggle with their weight and type 2 diabetes often become depressed. Knowing this cycle can help prepare APPs to screen for metabolic changes and depression. If APPs identify areas of concern, they can collaborate with patients to create an individualized treatment plan for addressing the issues.

Common Mental Health Conditions in Primary Care Settings

Of note, the symptomology of depression, anxiety, loneliness due to isolation, and trauma-related mental illness occurs across a continuum of severity. Symptoms can range from mildly disrupting to clinically impairing and other debilitating effects. APPs can improve their skills in working with persons with mental illnesses by increasing their awareness of the risk factors and symptoms linked to negative mental health outcomes. It is also important to be familiar with the mental health conditions that are most prevalent in the primary care setting.

Depression

Widespread use of the term *depression* can be misleading. There are many types of depression, including major depressive disorder, persistent depressive disorder, perinatal depression, seasonal affective disorder, bipolar disorder, situational depression, psychotic depression, premenstrual dysphoric disorder, and atypical depression (National Institute of Mental Health [NIMH], n.d.-b). Patients with severe forms of depression, including psychotic features, suicidality, and a history of treatment resistance, should be referred to a provider specifically credentialed and specialized in psychiatric mental health services. In this chapter, the term depression will be used to describe a person who experiences common symptoms of depression (e.g., sadness, hopelessness, irritability, worthlessness, loss of interest in previously enjoyed activities, and sleep disturbances) (NIMH, n.d.-b).

Depression is one of the leading causes of disability in the United States (Anxiety and Depression Association of America [ADAA], n.d.-b). In the National Health Interview Study, the percentage of adults who experienced any symptoms of depression in 2019 was 21.0% of those aged 18 to 29, 16.8% of those aged 30 to 44, 18.4% of those aged 45 to 64, and 18.4% of those aged 65 and over (Villarroel & Terlizzi, 2020). Of those, in the past two weeks, 11.5% experienced mild symptoms of depression; 4.2%, moderate symptoms; and 2.8%, severe symptoms. A major depressive disorder affects about 6.7% of the population aged 18 and older each year, with a median age of onset at 32.5 years old (ADAA, n.d.-b). It is more prevalent in women than in men (Villarroel & Terlizzi, 2020).

People with depression have a higher risk for other medical conditions, such as cardiovascular disease, diabetes, stroke, pain, Alzheimer's disease, and osteoporosis; at the same time, people with chronic illness are more likely to experience depression (NIMH,

n.d.-a). The magnitude of depression's effects on the U.S. population is further reflected in data about treatment settings. Ballou et al. (2019) reported that emergency department visits specifically for treating severe, urgent cases of depression rose 25.9% from 2006 to 2014. Over half of these visits resulted in inpatient stays averaging six days. The CDC reports that a mental disorder was the primary diagnosis for 55.7 million physician visits in 2018 (National Center for Health Statistics, n.d.-b) and that over 10% of patients treated in physician office visits have depression listed as a chronic condition in their medical record (National Center for Health Statistics, n.d.-a). This data underscores a significant need for APPs in all clinical settings to have adequate education and training in assessing and addressing mental health.

Demographic data also show that in 2019, 13.6% of U.S. children received mental health care, with boys being more likely to receive treatment than girls (Zablotsky & Terlizzi, 2020). In children, depression may be exhibited by difficulty sleeping, frequent absences from school, frequent sadness, crying or tears, physical symptoms without a medical cause, difficulty in social situations, or a lack of interest in activities (NCBDDD, n.d.-a). Children with depression also may be susceptible to rejection or failure.

It is not always easy to recognize depression because symptoms can range in severity and may include puzzling symptoms that appear at odds with the diagnosis (Hunter et al., 2017; McCarron et al., 2019; Zimmerman et al., 2018). In some patients, depression may be exhibited by angry outbursts, frustration, or irritability. Others may find humor in sad situations. Some patients with depression complain about sleep problems, including difficulty falling asleep, waking in the middle of the night, or sleeping too much (Hunter et al., 2017; McCarron et al., 2019). Reports of lack of energy, constant fatigue, and somatic symptoms (especially pain) are common. Changes in appetite, significant fluctuations in weight, and food cravings (especially sugar) can indicate depression (Francis et al., 2019). Cognitive symptoms include trouble concentrating, diminished clarity of thought, and difficulty making important decisions. Further exploration may reveal recurring or present thoughts of death and attempts of self-harm (Melham et al., 2019).

Social Isolation and Loneliness

Research studies surrounding social connectivity and loneliness have been impactful, demonstrating the importance of social connectivity for mental health and the devastating effects of loneliness (Lam et al., 2021; Terziev, 2019). Loneliness predicted general anxiety, depression, and suicidal ideation (Beutel et al., 2017). Other studies also have demonstrated links between suboptimal social connectivity and mental health (Cacioppo & Cacioppo, 2018). After adjusting for chronic mental health disease–attenuated associations, Stickley and Koyanagi (2016) found that loneliness was still significantly associated with severe symptoms of depression, including hopelessness and thoughts of self-harm.

Episodes of social isolation and loneliness can be experienced by anyone. A community-based, prospective, observational cohort study of over 15,000 adults showed that 10.7% had some degree of loneliness (Beutel et al., 2017). Those most affected by loneliness tended to be female, single, without a partner, and without children. Loneliness tends to peak in adolescence, gradually decrease over the adult years, then increase again in later life (Lam et al., 2021; Luhmann & Hawkley, 2016). Subtle symptoms of depression may be noted in older adults who exhibit increasingly isolative behaviors due to age-related issues.

Humans are social beings. It is human nature to want to be a part of a larger group and purpose. Essential components of the human experience include conversations, sharing, coming together when there is a challenge or cause, and human touch (Cacioppo & Cacioppo, 2018; Terziev, 2019). The opposite of these experiences—isolation, withdrawal, change in the ability to show up for others, and divisiveness—are concerning symptoms of poor mental health. Given the influences of the COVID-19 pandemic, the APP needs to ask about social connectivity when assessing mental health.

Anxiety

Anxiety and stress are conceptually connected. Human beings experience stress and anxiety throughout their lives as a part of having a healthy nervous system. The difference is that a person experiences healthy stress or anxiety when encountering a real threat while clinical anxiety is a persistent and excessive worry about a perceived threat (ADAA, n.d.-a). Anxiety disorders are one of the most common mental illnesses and can interfere with all aspects of a person's life, including interpersonal relationships, work, school, and home.

According to the ADAA (n.d.-a), 40 million adults in the United States aged 18 and over (19.1% of the population) experience anxiety disorders every year. However, only a little over one-third (36.9%) receive treatment. Anxiety tends to be more prevalent in women than men (ADAA, n.d.-a). Symptoms vary widely and can include excessive worry with little or no justification. People who experience anxiety report feeling on edge, being unable to relax, nausea, trouble getting to and staying asleep, and feeling a sense of impending doom (ADAA, n.d.-c).

There are many forms of anxiety, including social anxiety disorder, panic disorder, obsessive–compulsive disorder (OCD), agoraphobia, separation anxiety, generalized anxiety disorder, and post-traumatic stress disorder (PTSD) (ADAA, n.d.-a). Each year, about 6.8 million U.S. adults, or 3.1% of the population, experience generalized anxiety disorder, and approximately 2.7% of adults experience panic attacks. Panic attacks usually begin in young adulthood but can occur in children. They are more prevalent in females (ADAA, n.d.-c).

Another type of severe anxiety is OCD, which manifests as intrusive thoughts called obsessions and behavioral responses known as compulsions. Some commonly known presentations of OCD include obsessive thoughts about contamination and cleanliness or a need for symmetry. Common compulsions include checking behaviors, washing, cleaning, and organizing or arranging (ADAA, n.d.-e). To the onlooker, there may not seem to be a logical reason for these behaviors. For individuals with OCD, intense internal experiences are driving their behaviors. Children and adolescents do not always have insight into their behaviors while adults with OCD typically do. Current evidence shows that OCD occurs in 1 in 40 adults and 1 in 100 children (ADAA, n.d.-e).

APPs should be mindful that some medical conditions, such as cardiovascular, pulmonary, endocrine, hematologic, neurologic, infections, or SUDs, may mimic psychiatric illnesses (Hunter et al., 2017; McCarron et al., 2019). Ruling out physical causes for anxiety and depression is crucial in assessing patients presenting with symptoms. These include thyroid imbalances, poorly controlled or undiagnosed diabetes, cardiac arrhythmias, cerebral issues, and somatic disorders (Hunter et al., 2017; McCarron et al., 2019).

Post-Traumatic Stress Disorder

In adults, recent data indicates that about 7 or 8 of every 100 people will experience PTSD in their lifetime (NIMH, n.d.-b), with women more likely to develop it than men. Currently, about 8 million people in the United States live with PTSD (ADAA, n.d.-d). Symptoms of PTSD are categorized into distinct areas: re-experiencing (flashbacks), avoidance, arousal and reactivity, and cognitive and mood symptoms (NIMH, n.d.-d). One hallmark symptom

of PTSD is irritability, which may result from a lack of trust in others after abuse or a lack of restorative sleep. Poor quality of sleep has impacts beyond the scope of this chapter but is important for APPs to assess in patients presenting with and without symptoms of trauma.

The causes of PTSD are vast, including bullying, war, physical abuse, emotional abuse, sexual assaults, natural disasters, and other life-threatening experiences. About 67% of people who experience a violent or life-threatening event, as well as individuals who have experienced previous traumatic events, are at a higher risk of developing PTSD (ADAA, n.d.-d). Not everyone who experiences trauma will develop PTSD.

PTSD occurs in both children and adults. In children, it can result from bullying; physical, sexual, or emotional abuse; witnessing a violent crime; natural disasters; severe car crashes; or the death of a loved one. Children with PTSD display symptoms such as lacking positive emotions; acting helpless, hopeless, or withdrawn; having intense fear or sadness; and denying the trauma ever happened (NCBDDD, n.d.-c). One practical, empirically validated tool for assessing trauma is the Adverse Childhood Events Questionnaire, which helps determine the severity of trauma exposure (see **Table 23.1**). A significant contributor to the vicious cycle of physical and mental health issues is undertreatment or inadequate trauma treatment (Grabbe, 2022). Inadequate treatment is especially true for childhood trauma and adverse childhood events.

Alcohol Use Disorder

The use of alcohol presents a unique conundrum in relation to mental health and healthy lifestyle maintenance. The link between alcohol and mental health is bidirectional. On the one hand, drinking alcohol can contribute to or exacerbate mental health problems. On the other hand, a patient may turn to alcohol

Table 23.1 Mental Health Screening and Assessment Tools

Tool	Population	Use	URL
Adverse Childhood Experience (ACE) Questionnaire	Life span	Assesses childhood trauma	http://www.odmhsas.org/picis/TraningInfo/ACE.pdf
CAGE Alcohol Questionnaire	Adults	Screens for alcohol use disorder	https://psychology-tools.com/test/cage-alcohol-questionnaire
Clinical Institute Withdrawal Assessment for Alcohol Scale, Revised (CIWA-Ar)	Adults	Assesses for alcohol withdrawal symptoms	https://umem.org/files/uploads/1104212257_CIWA-Ar.pdf
Clinical Opiate Withdrawal Scale (COWS) Subjective Opiate Withdrawal Scale (SOWS)	Adults	Measures opiate withdrawal symptoms. COWS is completed by the *clinician*. SOWS is completed by the *patient*.	https://www.drugabuse.gov/sites/default/files/ClinicalOpiateWithdrawalScale.pdf https://www.asam.org/docs/default-source/education-docs/sows_8-28-2017.pdf
Columbia-Suicide Severity Rating Scale (C-SSRS)	Adults	Identifies people at risk for suicide	https://cssrs.columbia.edu
General Anxiety Disorder-7 (GAD-7)	Adults	Measures severity of anxiety	https://adaa.org/sites/default/files/GAD-7_Anxiety-updated_0.pdf
Mental status examination (MSE) Mini Mental State Examination (MMSE)	Life span	Determines mental functioning	https://www.aafp.org/pubs/afp/issues/2016/1015/p635.html https://cgatoolkit.ca/Uploads/ContentDocuments/MMSE.pdf
Minnesota Multiphasic Personality Inventory-A (MMPI-A) Minnesota Multiphasic Personality Inventory (MMPI)	Adolescents Adults	Psychological testing. Typically completed by a psychologist with other mental health testing.	https://www.mentalhelp.net/psychological-testing/minnesota-multiphasic-personality-inventory
Mini-Cog	Older adult	Screens for dementia	https://mini-cog.com
Patient Health Questionnaire-9 (PHQ-9)	Adults	Screens for mental health	https://www.apa.org/depression-guideline/patient-health-questionnaire.pdf

because of mental illness, such as anxiety and depression, as a way of self-medicating to modify mood or improve sleep (Rani & Hemavathy, 2021).

Another critical understanding for APPs is the implication of the emerging literature on the effects of the chemical alcohol. According to Woodward (2020), the most accurate description of alcohol is that it is not just one chemical; it is several related compound groups, one of which is ethanol. Long-term and heavy intake of ethanol can lead to devastating gastrointestinal damage and cancers (National Center for Chronic Disease Prevention and Health Promotion, n.d.; Woodward, 2020) and chronic diseases, such as high blood pressure, heart disease, stroke, increasing memory difficulties, and mental health disorders such as depression (National Center for Chronic Disease Prevention and Health Promotion, n.d.; Stahl, 2021). Even low and moderate use of alcohol are implicated in coronary artery disease. Herron and Brennan (2020) provide information about the mental health implications of chronic physical health problems and the effects of excessive, moderate, and light use of alcohol.

The recent COVID-19 pandemic triggered an increase in the amount and frequency of alcohol consumption in U.S. adults (Grossman et al., 2020). Currently, more than half of U.S. adults report drinking alcohol in the past 30 days (Division of Population Health, n.d.-a) and two in three adult drinkers report drinking above moderate levels at least monthly (Division of Population Health, n.d.-b). One aspect of alcohol use that often evades medical attention is related to current research findings of the risks associated with low-level, or "light," use of alcohol. In a summary opinion article, Watson (2021) presented information from several studies and observed a phenomenon—people who use alcohol at low rates often do not see their use as problematic. People who follow the guidelines and embrace the purported health benefits of low alcohol intake may not be fully informed of the mental and physical health risks associated with low levels of alcohol use. Health risks associated with low levels of alcohol use can vary depending on one's genetics and co-occurring lifestyle factors (e.g., a sedentary lifestyle if accompanied by a regular diet of highly processed foods) (Watson, 2021). These risks are often misperceived or minimized by patients.

Tobacco Use Disorder

Healthcare workers, including APPs, may have become numb to the never-ending grim statistics about the mortality related to tobacco use. What may be missed are the implications of the surprisingly large number (16 million) of people living with serious medical issues due to tobacco use (Office on Smoking and Health, n.d.). Many people living with tobacco use–related illnesses also experience mental health issues. In 2019, 35% of people diagnosed with mental illnesses also used tobacco (Office on Smoking and Health, n.d.). Furthermore, people who experience mental health illnesses and use tobacco are more likely to die an average of 10 or more years earlier than those who do not use tobacco and who do not experience mental illness (Colton & Manderscheid, 2006).

This issue is further compounded due to the chemical effects of tobacco use. The human body metabolizes nicotine using some of the same metabolism cycles involved in breaking down and excreting many medications, such as some psychiatric medications (e.g., alprazolam, clozapine, olanzapine, tricyclic antidepressants, and benzodiazepines), and other medications that can influence mental health (e.g., insulin, beta blockers, and birth control pills) (Smoking Cessation Leadership Center, 2022; Stahl, 2021). Subsequently, dosages for these medications must be adjusted to accommodate this effect.

Additional problems related to treating patients with tobacco use disorder are the stubborn myths that have been debunked for over a decade. These myths include "it is their choice to smoke" or "it is the only thing they have left" (Prochaska, 2011). Successful tobacco abstinence is further sabotaged by misinformation about the risks of quitting during addiction treatment or during stabilization for severe mental illnesses (Prochaska, 2011; Schroeder et al., 2017). Other myths are "only quit one thing at a time" or "quitting smoking will destabilize their progress," both of which are false statements. On the contrary, evidence shows that supporting tobacco abstinence during mental health or addiction treatment *increases the odds that both efforts will be successful* (Prochaska, 2011; Schroeder et al., 2017).

Nevertheless, tobacco use disorders remain poorly understood and inadequately treated. Successful interventions to treat tobacco dependence have been available for decades. However, this information has been inconsistently translated into practice.

Other Substances

It is regularly noted in extant literature that SUDs are highly associated with impaired mental health (e.g., depression and anxiety) (Substance Abuse and Mental Health Services Administration, 2020). APPs must be aware that their patients may use other risky substances. Evidence shows that U.S. citizens regularly use marijuana. The CDC reports that marijuana was used by 48.2 million people in 2019 and that about 3 in 10 people who use it meet diagnostic criteria for marijuana use disorder (National Center for Injury Prevention and Control, n.d.-a). The legal issues about the medicinal and recreational use of marijuana and cannabis vary widely from state to state and defy concise instruction. When in doubt, it is best practice to inquire about the possibility of marijuana use in a nonjudgmental approach.

Current events also reveal the ongoing devastating opiate use epidemic. The CDC reports that almost 500,000 people died of an overdose from 1999 to 2019 (National Center for Injury Prevention and Control, n.d.-b). This problem is compounded by the increasing lethal concentrations of emerging formulations of opiates.

Access to Mental Health Care

APPs should be aware of a critical factor related to mental health care because it will affect them in clinical practice: limited access to mental health care. The 2018 America's Mental Health survey found that 53 million American adults (21%) sought mental health treatment at some point but were unable to do so for reasons outside of their control (Cohen Veterans Network and the National Council for Behavioral Health, 2018). Research estimates that only half of those with mental illnesses in the United States receive treatment (NIMH, n.d.-c). One significant factor is a shortage of healthcare professionals who are adequately educated, trained, and credentialed in mental health. This shortage is due to many complex issues, including insufficient funding for programs, the need for more educators, a lack of clinical sites, and few clinicians seeking training in this specialty. Social determinants of health, such as low income or lack of health insurance coverage, create other disparities that influence access to care.

The *Healthy People 2030* report illuminates the challenges associated with connecting people to mental health care and improving access to care (ODPHP, n.d.-a). In 2018, only 3.4% of adults aged 18 years and older with co-occurring SUDs and mental health disorders were able to receive treatment by providers specializing in those conditions (ODPHP, n.d.-b). A small but steady improvement to 8.2% has been set as the target goal (ODPHP, n.d.-b). Of the 3.4% of people who received care, 8.5% were seen in primary care office visits, which included screening for depression (ODPHP, n.d.-c).

The current challenges in access to care support the need for APPs in all settings to receive education and training in mental health strategies for facilitating optimal healthy lifestyles. It is also important that APPs of all backgrounds and training keep in mind the opportunity and necessity for providing a level of mental health care to the patients they treat while staying within their scope and standards of practice and licensing. The bottom line is that APPs must care for the *whole* person.

Health Promotion Research Study

Association Between Physical Activity and Depression

Background: Depression is the leading cause of mental health–related disease burden, a major cause of disability, and associated with premature mortality from suicide and other causes. Although the risk of depression may be reduced by physical activity, the dose-response relationship between activity and depression is uncertain. Previous meta-analyses have shown lower risks of depression among adults reporting high versus low physical activity and suggested a dose-response association using meta-regression without quantifying the association.

Methodology: A systematic review and meta-analysis were conducted to determine the dose-response association between physical activity and incident depression from published prospective studies of adults. Fifteen studies comprising 191,130 participants and 2,110,588 person-years were included. The samples used were adults who reported an element of physical activity and risk factors for depression. Data were extracted from the studies, including volume of physical activity, depression cases, participant number, and follow-up.

Results: An inverse and curvilinear dose-response association between physical activity and depression was observed, with the greatest differences in risk observed between low doses of physical activity, suggesting most benefits are realized when moving from no activity to at least some. Accumulating an activity volume equivalent to 2.5 hours of brisk walking per week was associated with a 25% lower risk of depression. At half that dose, the risk was 18% lower compared with no activity. Only minor additional benefits were observed at higher activity levels.

Implications for Advanced Practice: Results showed that the biggest benefit in participants' depression was moving from no physical activity to some physical activity. This suggests that substantial mental health benefits can be achieved at physical activity levels even below the public health recommendations. APPs can relate the mental health benefits of low doses of physical activity when making lifestyle recommendations, especially to inactive individuals who may perceive the currently recommended target as unrealistic.

Reference: Data from Pearce, M., Garcia, L., Abbas, A., Strain, T., Schuch, F. B., Golubic, R., Kelly, P., Khan, S., Utukuri, M., Laird, Y., Mok, A., Smith, A., Tainio, M., Brage, S., & Woodcock, J. (2022). Association between physical activity and risk of depression: A systematic review and meta-analysis. *JAMA Psychiatry, 79*(6), 550–559. https://doi.org/10.1001/jamapsychiatry.2022.0609

Mental Health Screening and Assessment

As APPs become more skilled in assisting the *whole* person to gain optimal mental health and avoid chronic diseases, an initial assessment helps direct the course of care. As noted previously, mental and physical health are highly intertwined. Therefore, it is essential to assess both.

Many screening tools and assessment scales are available to APPs to focus on what may or may not be affecting a person's mental health, including symptoms of anxiety, mood, psychosis, or substance use (McCarron et al., 2019). Table 23.1 lists empirically valid, commonly used tools that screen, assess, and support mental health. The mental status examination (MSE) is a standardized, efficient evaluation of a mental health review of systems. Carlat (2017) described the MSE as an evaluation of the "patient's current state of cognitive and emotional functioning" (p. 137). While some clinicians mistakenly think the MSE is a point-in-time snapshot of functioning, it is actually an ongoing assessment throughout the initial interview.

Certain mental health screenings, such as those for SUDs, self-harm thoughts, and childhood trauma, can feel intrusive and intimidating for patients. It is the APP's responsibility to create and sustain a safe environment for the patient. As APPs develop a therapeutic relationship with their patients, trust facilitates honest reporting of patient histories. When patients accurately report their histories, current symptoms, and use of substances, then collaborative treatment plans can be implemented, and outcomes can be measurably improved. The therapeutic relationship is also invaluable when evaluating whether a patient's complaints are due to malingering to avoid work, get disability benefits, or obtain drugs.

A mental health assessment should also include a physical assessment to rule out a medical cause for mental health issues (First, 2022). Lab tests, such as a thyroid panel, complete blood count, electrolytes, and vitamin B12 level, can eliminate physical conditions that may mimic mental health disorders, such as hypothyroidism, iron-deficiency anemia, or vitamin B12 deficiency. Medications used to treat general medical conditions, such as some antibiotics, stimulants, opioids, cannabis, Parkinson's disease medications, corticosteroids, anti-seizure medications, certain heart and blood pressure medications, and cough medications, can also cause mental health symptoms. Assessing medication adherence to mental health prescriptions can determine drug effectiveness.

Furthermore, an effective overall assessment contains information on other factors that can affect the treatment plan and the patient's ability to achieve optimal mental health. Thus, assessing social determinants of health, literacy, motivation, readiness to change, social support, and availability of resources (e.g., cooking equipment) is vital when formulating individualized treatment plans that include lifestyle changes.

APP Self-Reflection

APPs might consider the benefits of self-reflection about their own health behaviors before prescribing mental and physical health strategies for others. Self-reflection, or listening to self, is helpful for APPs to gain the skills required to effectively listen to their patients and facilitate and support health behavior change. Zuckoff (2012) provides self-reflective insight in his article on patient adherence to treatment. He poses a query that all APPs should ask themselves, "Why don't my patients do what is good for them or what I tell them to do?" The follow-up question should be, "Am I (the APP) doing the things I should be doing daily (e.g., drinking adequate water, exercising daily, and eating a healthy diet)?," to which the answer is often no. And yet healthcare providers often expect patients to do what they themselves are not willing to do. Regular personal and professional self-reflection can provide the APP insight into the challenges associated with health behavior changes. Additionally, an APP engaged in healthy behaviors is more likely to implement a person-centered, holistic healthcare model to assist patients, families, and communities in decision-making that promotes positive lifestyle changes and self-care.

Therapeutic Relationship: Initiating Healing Conversations

Establishing a therapeutic relationship is a critical and irreplaceable skill in assisting patients to address lifestyle practices that affect mental health. Active listening to develop an effective rapport should not be misconstrued as agreeing with the patient on maintaining unhealthy or unproductive strategies. Neither is it recommended to listen for the purpose of manipulating patients toward health behavior change. Conversely, listening for *understanding* is vital for establishing a therapeutic working relationship to facilitate behavior change and support optimal mental health.

The APP's listening skills are foundational to implementing motivational interviewing (MI), a counseling approach to treating mental health problems that optimizes conversations about change (Miller & Rollnick, 2013). MI enables the APP to move from frustrated thoughts like "What is the *matter with* this person?" to curiosity expressed as "I wonder *what matters to* this person?" This approach helps the patient discover a renewed source of personal motivation for change and will be instrumental in sustaining health behavior change.

MI helps APPs establish an effective, safe environment to conduct accurate mental health assessments and provide individualized treatment (Levounis et al., 2017). MI also helps APPs conduct difficult conversations about coping skills that hinder rather than help resolve unhealthy habits. As the therapeutic relationship is established, patients can share complicated feelings such as guilt, worthlessness, or preoccupation with perceived mistakes or past failures. These conversations can help remove perceived or actual obstacles to change.

Asking open-ended questions is another skill in the MI approach. It is important to ask open-ended questions that start with the words *what, when, where, why,* and *how* when assessing a patient's mental health status and discussing lifestyle changes. Close-ended questions requiring yes or no answers limit the depth of response a patient will provide. With practice, the skilled APP will know how to go between qualifying statements, open-ended questions, and closed-ended questions throughout the patient interview.

Scaling questions are Likert-style scale questions on the patient's sense of importance, confidence, readiness, willingness, or commitment to change behavior. The APP may ask the patient, "On a scale of 1 to 10, with 1 being not *important* and 10 being extremely *important*, how *important* is it to you to make [insert specific behavior change]?" The patient will respond with a number, giving the APP insight into the patient's motivation for change. The APP can repeat the scaling question, replacing the word *important* with *confidence, readiness, willingness,* or *commitment*. The importance, confidence, and readiness scale helps APPs to meet the patients where they are and to support them in identifying thoughts and habits they would like to change, replace, and possibly discard (Levounis et al., 2017; Miller & Rollnick, 2013).

Another effective MI strategy for approaching crucial and potentially complicated assessment areas is to use a technique known as normalizing statements. Normalizing communicates to the patients that their experience is not uncommon. For example, the APP could state, "Some people have told me that they sometimes get so down in the dumps that they have no energy to get up and get going. Then if things get worse, they may start having thoughts such as 'I just wish I wouldn't wake up tomorrow.' I am wondering if you ever feel that way and if you would feel comfortable enough to talk about such things?" This strategy also can be used to ask about other potentially sensitive topics and difficult questions, such as asking about weapons at home, serious threats to safety, and feelings associated with giving up an unhealthy habit.

As APPs increase their active listening and MI skills, they are more available to help their patients make behavior changes. MI dovetails nicely with the transtheoretical model of change, also known as the stages of change (Krebs et al., 2019). The stages of change model helps APPs organize their efforts into effective, pragmatic strategies appropriate to the patient's stage. Equally important, these strategies support APPs in overcoming feelings of frustration and burnout due to an inability to facilitate health behavior changes with patients.

Healthy Lifestyle Strategies for Mental Health

Interventions to improve mental health outcomes and prevent and treat physical issues share much in common. Various approaches have been developed to enhance and support healthy lifestyle changes, such as treatment algorithms (Driot et al., 2017), which hold promise. However, these do not identify the rich possibilities available in individualized care. Strategies such as nutritional guidance, stress management, physical activity, getting adequate sleep, and avoiding alcohol and tobacco serve as lifestyle pillars that will improve mental and physical health. This section describes a limited selection of these strategies, organized in the A-SMART framework, and offers some examples of prescriptions that an APP could provide to a patient when addressing mental health.

Adopt Healthy Eating

In nutritional psychiatry, new research emerges continually as the evidence builds on the links and effects between diet and mental health. Nutrition is likely a significant—if not *the most* significant—area of lifestyle improvements that hold promise for a healthy lifestyle change and optimal mental health outcomes. The International Society for Nutritional Psychiatry Research was launched in 2013, and the organization has continued to discover the connection between what people eat and how they feel.

New research also indicates an association between nutrition and mental health, though causality is unclear (Adan et al., 2019; Dimov et al., 2021). A plant-based diet with limited processed foods, oils, sugars, and processed flour has a strong correlation to positive mental health as a part of overall health (Bremner et al., 2020; Medawar et al., 2019). Consistent fruit and vegetable intake has been identified as a predictor of a health-promoting diet

(McMartin et al., 2013). Poor diet quality has been identified as including higher quantities of sugar, saturated fats, sodium, and alcohol than whole foods, such as nuts, legumes, fruits, and vegetables (Appelhans et al., 2012). Rather than assume that the APP's advice on diet and activity will be followed, it is advised that an empirically valid food intake tracking method be used. In this case, an excellent tool may be the assessment called the 4Leaf Survey, which can be found at http://4leafsurvey.com. This tool can help people become more aware of their intake of whole-plant foods.

Several studies have been conducted on food, mood, and nutrition. Findings include that people who engaged in plant-based diets experienced decreased depression and anxiety (Firth et al., 2019) and improved mental health (Hayhoe et al., 2021). Research on the possible biological influences of depression has shown that a positive impact can be made on mood through modifying dietary intake (Jacka et al., 2010, 2017; Li et al., 2017). Innovative programs such as Lettuce Be Happy found that eating more fruits and vegetables improved mental and physical health (Ocean et al., 2019). Plant foods contain minerals, vitamins, and fiber, which enhance the neurological pathways related to inflammation, oxidative stress, and depression (Firth et al., 2019). High fiber intake is also associated with decreased depressive symptoms (Xu et al., 2018).

An individual's relationship with food can be a very sensitive topic. Patients who do not have a healthy body mass index have usually made several attempts to decrease their weight, which provides an opportunity to use MI skills to listen for understanding rather than leaping into the conversation prematurely. The APP can make a stronger connection with a therapeutic relationship and maximize teachable moments by *lending patients hope* that they can successfully establish a healthy relationship with food and a health-promoting diet. The importance, confidence, and readiness scale questions can help keep patients focused on *what matters* to them and *why* they are making their choices, thus helping to cement healthy nutritional choices.

Neurochemistry and Nutrition

Food intake has been linked to the brain's production of certain neurotransmitters. There are a variety of nutrients that play a role in the synthesis of neurotransmitters, specifically vitamin D, essential polyunsaturated fatty acids omega-3 and omega-6, and folate. Many other nutrients and processes go into the development and functioning of neurotransmitters that play a role in developing healthy neuronal circuitry and preventing depression and anxiety symptoms. The aforementioned nutrients are a few that have been studied exclusively in the diagnoses discussed in this chapter.

Pharmaceutical interventions target dopamine, serotonin, histamine, acetylcholine, endogenous opioids, gamma-aminobutyric acid, and glutamate receptors. Each of these neurotransmitters has a different life cycle. With increasing data about possible nutritional connections to the prevention and treatment of mental health disorders, there is an opportunity to decrease dependence on pharmaceutical interventions or the use of polypharmacy. There is also the possibility of adjunctively treating depressive symptoms when an individual has suboptimal responses to current pharmaceutical approaches.

Serotonin is a neurotransmitter that influences an individual's affective state, satiety, and sleep regulation and can be influenced positively or negatively by an individual's diet and lifestyle (Shabbir et al., 2013). Many foods, including meats, cheeses, fruits, and vegetables, contain serotonin; however, it is not easily accessible to the central nervous system in this form due to the blood–brain barrier. The brain requires adequate amounts of serotonin's amino acid precursor, tryptophan, which can cross the blood–brain barrier and be converted in the presence of vitamin B6 for use within the central nervous system as serotonin (Shabbir

et al., 2013). Tryptophan production and bioavailability are stimulated through a complex carbohydrate-rich diet (Shabbir et al., 2013). Plant foods rich in vitamin B6 and tryptophan include lentils, beans, spinach, carrots, brown rice, bran, sunflower seeds, wheat germ, and whole-grain flour (Shabbir et al., 2013).

Folate, a water-soluble vitamin, also known as vitamin B9, is involved in neurotransmitter synthesis and is an essential cofactor in many metabolic processes required for the equilibrium of the central nervous system (Watanabe et al., 2012). Being a water-soluble vitamin, folate is an essential vitamin that must be consumed from the diet or be obtained via supplementation. The biologically active form of folate is L-methyl folate, which is directly involved in neurotransmitter synthesis as well as indirectly through the conversion process of homocysteine to the methyl donor for the synthesis of norepinephrine, dopamine, and serotonin (Watanabe et al., 2012). Folate levels and homocysteine levels can be measured via blood serum.

Long-chain omega-3 and omega-6 fatty acids play a significant role in overall neurological function and health status (Beezhold & Johnston, 2012; Farooqui et al., 2007). The essential fatty acids alpha-linolenic acid and linoleic acid must be consumed in the diet because the human body cannot produce them (Lucas et al., 2011). Dietary deficiencies of the omega-3 fatty acid alpha-linolenic acid have been linked with altered brain biochemistry in humans, affecting neuronal pathways, ion channels, and decreased protein transcription activity while in animal studies, decreased serotoninergic and dopaminergic neurotransmission in the frontal cortex has been observed (Lucas et al., 2011).

When prescribing dietary strategies that offer protective and beneficial effects on mental health, the APP should consider interventions that do not place individuals at higher risk for other illnesses, such as diabetes, heart disease, and obesity. Working with patients to increase dietary intake of specific vitamins and nutrients such as vitamin D, folate, and omega-3 and omega-6 fatty acids is easily achieved through recommending a balanced whole-foods diet (Bertone-Johnson et al., 2011; Watanabe et al., 2012).

Inflammation and Mental Health

Research reveals that the typical Western diet and chronic disease are linked to inflammation (Christ et al., 2019; Shi, 2019). An additional area of research into the role of food and nutrients is in exploring the link between inflammation and mental health. Inflammation in and of itself is a natural response by the immune system to protect the body from injury and stress. However, if the response is hyper- or hypo-inflammation, other diseases can be triggered (Yuan et al., 2019). Inflammation is an important factor in mood disorders. Research has suggested that inflammation is connected to many psychiatric disorders, including schizophrenia, bipolar disorder, the autism spectrum, major depression disorder, PTSD, sleeping disorders, thoughts of suicide, and OCD (Bauer & Teixeira, 2019; Yuan et al., 2019). Mechawar and Savitz (2016) found that those having increased inflammatory markers in cells and elevated plasma levels of cytokines experience more mood disorders. Clinical interest in the role of inflammation has led to the emerging field of immunopsychiatry, exploring the roles of the immune system and inflammation in major psychiatric disorders (Khandaker et al., 2017).

Recent evidence shows a strong relationship between inflammation and gut microbiota (Karl et al., 2018; Pickard et al., 2017). The gut microbiota is made up of fungi, bacteria, protozoa, and archaea and can be changed by diet, use of antibiotics, and host genetics (Pickard et al., 2017). Diets rich in high-fiber foods promote the growth of healthy intestinal microbiota, which reduces intestinal inflammation (Gentile & Weir, 2018; Tomova et al., 2019). Although diet is the factor most studied

in relation to the gut microbiota, other influences such as environmental stress, antibiotic use, sleep disturbance, psychological stress, and physical activity can also alter the makeup of the gut microbiota (Karl et al., 2018). The gut microbiota influences the absorption, metabolism, and storage of food eaten and therefore the body's physiology.

Several researchers demonstrated how the gut microbiome and the brain integrate with the central and enteric nervous systems, linking the emotional and cognitive centers of the brain (Martin et al., 2018; Noble et al., 2017). This gut–brain microbiome axis is a two-way system in which the gut influences the brain and vice versa. Three channels are involved: the nervous, gastrointestinal, and immune systems (Martin et al., 2018). Noble et al. (2017) reviewed research on the high saturated fat and sugar intake of the Western diet and its negative impact on cognitive function, noting evidence that the gut microbiome influences cognitive function through the gut–brain axis. The gut microbiota interacts with the central nervous system by regulating the brain chemistry and affecting the neuroendocrine systems, which are associated with anxiety, memory function, and the stress response (Foster & Neufeld, 2013).

The effect of impaired microbiota on cognitive function is noted across the life span. Shi (2019) studied 250,000 adolescents and found a correlation between soft drink consumption and aggressive behavior. Mangiola et al. (2016) found evidence suggesting an important role in the correlation between impaired microbiota of the gastrointestinal system and the development of autism, mood disorders, and other neuropsychiatric disorders.

The research linking the connection between inflammation and the gut microbiota on mental health is growing rapidly. APPs must understand this connection to advocate for healthy plant-based diet options for patients, including diets filled with fruits, vegetables, and other nutrient-rich high-fiber foods

(Evans et al., 2017). Encouraging patients to optimize a healthy gut microbiome through nutrition may significantly decrease inflammation and positively affect their mental health.

Stress Less

Numerous interventions exist to help patients to better manage stress and to promote mental health. Strategies such as mindfulness practices, meditation, and personal journaling show promise. Shankland et al. (2020) conducted an eight-week mindfulness program with 139 patients, which resulted in significant reductions in reported stress, anxiety, and depression and increased life satisfaction. A systematic review of mindfulness-based programs revealed that these programs are very popular and increase a sense of well-being in intervention patients compared to no intervention (Galante et al., 2021). Study results on the value of personal journaling show that participants enjoy a renewed sense of self, better mental health, and positive improvements in expressing themselves (Nurser et al., 2018; Wong et al., 2018).

Biofeedback

Biofeedback (also known as biofeedback training) is a noninvasive technique using interactive computer programs, mobile devices, or wearables for learning to control body functions, such as heart rate or breathing (Mayo Clinic, n.d.-b). Controlling the rate and depth of breathing during a stress response enables a person to be calmer and gain a sense of well-being. Biofeedback is an effective intervention that can reduce physiological and subjective stress and enhance performance (Kennedy & Parker, 2019). Alneyadi et al. (2021) reported that biofeedback could improve screening and management of anxiety. A meta-analysis (Pizzoli et al., 2021) on biofeedback training validated the usefulness of heart rate variability in improving symptoms of depression, suggesting that this strategy should be considered a vital addition to treatment plans. Biofeedback

training for heart rate variability also shows promise in children and adolescents to reduce physical and psychological stress symptoms and enhance well-being (Dormal et al., 2021).

Positive Social Strategies

It is essential for APPs to recognize and address social threats to mental health, including loneliness and isolation. An example of operationalizing social connectedness through clinical interventions is using social prescriptions. Social prescriptions have been defined as "a way of linking patients . . . with sources of support within the community to help improve their health and well-being" (Gray et al., 2020, p. 8). Social prescriptions promote social interactions in a positive manner that aligns with the patient's interests, goals, or concerns. Potential social interactions can occur in numerous venues, including sports events, zoos, parks, art events—anywhere groups of people gather for a specific cause or to explore. Examples of social prescriptions include the following:

- Attending religious events at a faith community
- Volunteering within the community
- Fundraising for a political agenda or cause
- Participating in a local gardening club, ballroom dancing, group hikes, or an art class

More research is needed to understand the impact of social prescribing on mental health (Bickerdike et al., 2017; Husk et al., 2019; Leavall et al., 2019). However, outcomes from Rx: Community, a pilot social prescription project in Ontario, included 12% of patients indicating an improvement in their mental health, 49% indicating a decrease in their isolation, and 19% noting an increase in their social activities (Alliance for Healthier Communities, n.d.). Another example of a successful social prescription intervention was initiated for American veterans. The nonprofit organization Vet Tix (www.vettix.org) secures tickets for family events, concerts, sporting events, and art shows throughout the United

States to redistribute to veterans and their loved ones. To date, this organization has distributed almost 2 million event tickets.

One pioneer in lifestyle medicine and positive psychology describes several important ways to grow social support networks (Lianov, 2021). These approaches can be impactful for patients and APPs:

- Identify the types of social support needed.
- Explore ways to deepen relationship bonds with family, friends, and community.
- Build new connections with those with similar interests.
- Recognize the value of even very brief positive social interactions with others.
- Attempt to have as many of these micro connections as possible.
- Choose high-quality social interactions whenever possible, including laughter, support, gratitude, kindness, and love.

Lianov (2021) cautions against promoting any types of social activities that include shopping. Retail shopping may lead to problematic overshopping and overspending to combat unpleasant feelings, ultimately leading to increased debt and minimal retirement savings. Yet careful spending for home improvement can lead to personal satisfaction and savvy investment. Interestingly, a tendency to overshop or become addicted to shopping emerges in adolescence, increases over time, then decreases in later years (Andreassen et al., 2015). While beyond the scope of this chapter, financial security certainly does have a relationship with mental health. APPs can help sustain healthy socialization by looking for opportunities to prescribe social activities where cost is not a factor.

While social media and virtual connectivity may be helpful at times, they are not a substitute for being with others in person. Evidence shows that the tendency to always be connected to electronic devices increases stress. Thomas et al. (2016) studied attitudes about unplugging devices across age groups and found more negativity about unplugging among young people. Yet in research by Twenge et al. (2018), a correlation was noted between the increased use of smartphones and social media and the rise of depression and suicide in youth. The positive effects of digital unplugging are well described by Syvertsen (2020), who reported that social media has changed how people eat, sleep, socialize, plan their lives, and break up/make up with friends—and not always for the best. Thus, supporting mental health and healthy lifestyles also includes a focus on determining the appropriate use of digital devices.

Move Often

A large and growing body of research demonstrates the benefits of multiple types of natural movement and exercise on mental health. This research includes the inverse relationship between physical activity and depression symptomology, which emphasizes the decrease in symptoms of depression with regular exercise (Schuch et al., 2018). It is hypothesized that there are multiple pathways in which physical activity improves mental health, including decreased inflammation, distraction from negative thoughts, and increased self-efficacy (Mikkelsen et al., 2017).

One of the challenges for APPs in the clinical setting is to help frame the value of physical movement and find ways for individuals seeking assistance to operationalize this movement within their life. Finding out what matters to the individuals and what they enjoy doing might be the first step. Once this information is established, it is critical to write an achievable exercise prescription that shows value to the recipient. While the list of activities known to boost mood and decrease symptoms of multiple mental health disorders is extensive, all physical movement should be encouraged for patients healthy enough to engage in it.

Tai Chi

Tai chi is a reasonably simple, easy-to-do exercise that may be especially appealing to those who are just getting started with increasing their level of physical activity. Its origin dates back to China hundreds of years ago and consists of gentle, flowing movements named after animals and their actions (Yeung et al., 2018). Multiple studies have demonstrated positive relationships between tai chi and mental health (Hu et al., 2021; Song et al., 2014; Yeung et al., 2018). Song et al. (2014) reported that after 45 days of treatment with tai chi exercise, there was a significant improvement in anxiety symptoms and a lower recurrence of anxiety disorder in elderly adults. In their review, Yeung et al. (2018) noted a significant improvement in psychological health with tai chi in patients diagnosed with anxiety and depression.

Yoga

Yoga involves multiple physical postures and exercises while emphasizing meditation, deep breathing, self-awareness, and relaxation (Büssing et al., 2012). A review of literature on yoga found it beneficial to mental health in various ways, including enhanced self-efficacy and self-confidence (Büssing et al., 2012). While there are inherent challenges to yoga research related to mental health, there appears to be evidence to suggest that yoga is beneficial for conditions such as anxiety, depression, and psychosis (Varambally & Gangadhar, 2016). While not fully substantiated in the literature, there is also encouraging evidence of the benefits of yoga as an intervention for the effects of trauma and trauma-informed yoga in addiction treatment (Esfeld et al., 2021; Macy et al., 2018).

Walking and Running

Growing evidence suggests that walking can improve mental health, especially depression. In a scoping review of the literature, Kelly et al. (2019) found growing evidence demonstrating a connection between mental health and walking, albeit with some caveats. The authors stated that the implications of the specific factors about walking (e.g., pace, setting, group, and solitary) are ill-defined. One study, called Happy Feet, demonstrated a small but significant improvement in mental health by those walking at least 10,000 steps per day for 100 days (Hallam et al., 2018). The evidence linking the positive effect of walking on older adult mental health (Han et al., 2021; Miller et al., 2020) has significant implications for APPs when considering pharmacotherapy because older patients may already be on multiple medications.

A scoping review of the literature on the relationship between running and mental health outcomes found consistent evidence that running bouts of variable lengths and intensities can improve mood and mental health (Oswald et al., 2020). While many patients may feel that running is beyond their ability, there are organizations and resources to help individuals get started. Almost every city has a runners' club that meets regularly to offer information and support. The November Project (https://november-project.com) is an example of a nonprofit organization with free exercise groups in multiple cities worldwide that provides accountability for people of all ages and fitness levels to engage in physical activity together.

Outdoor Activities

Multiple literature reviews have demonstrated a positive relationship between exposure to outdoor activities and mental health (Buckley et al., 2018). It appears that outdoor exercise can be particularly impactful for components of chronic disease, including depression (Frühauf et al., 2016). One randomized intercept model study demonstrated a significant association between depression and green space and physical activity, demonstrating the importance of outside activity to mental health (Cohen-Cline et al., 2015). Access to green space was also associated with mental well-being in children, improving attention and memory and moderating stress (McCormick, 2017). Walking with groups in natural settings, called green walking groups, enhances a sense of connection with others and promotes a sense of freedom among adults, with limited evidence to support improvement in mood and symptoms of depression (Swinson et al., 2020).

Whether it be the sunlight, clean air, open space, or mental diversion, outdoor physical activities seem, in general, to be quite beneficial. Unfortunately, a social determinant of health includes the outdoor environment surrounding one's residence. The APP should assess whether the patient's chosen outdoor surroundings are safe before encouraging outdoor activity. While strategies exist to promote safe physical activity despite barriers (Jarrett et al., 2011), outdoor exercise in some neighborhoods still might not be a viable option. Park Rx America (www.parkrxamerica.org) is a resource for healthcare professionals to write prescriptions for nature-based interventions (NBIs) at parks, which often have no charge for use or offer free/low-cost admission for seniors, veterans, and students. The Web platform offers resources for both providers and patients, including links to scientific articles, a database of parks nationwide, and text/email reminders.

Gardening. NBIs such as gardening require natural movement and can result in positive outcomes. In a recent qualitative study of 28 African Americans in Detroit, participants reported that gardening improved their mood and relieved stress (Beavers et al., 2022). A systematic review and meta-analysis found that gardening and other NBIs were effective for improving depressive mood and positive affect and reducing anxiety and negative affect (Coventry et al., 2021). The most effective NBIs lasted 8 to 12 weeks, with an optimal dose ranging from 20 to 90 minutes. Engaging in community gardens is also associated with mental health and well-being, providing an affordable option for patients who do not have garden space at home (Lampert et al., 2021).

Additional Activities

Other forms of physical movement not described in-depth for their mental health benefits but also worthy of attention include swimming, water aerobics, pickleball, tennis, and basketball (Teychenne et al., 2020). Mikkelsen et al. (2017) summarized the research demonstrating multiple ways in which the physiological and biochemical benefits of exercise can exert positive effects on mental health. The research overwhelmingly suggests that regular physical activity improves mental well-being and lessens stress, anxiety, and depression symptoms. The effect of physical activity is noted across the life span, with benefits noted in adolescents continuing into older adults (Bell et al., 2019; Callow et al., 2020). Positive effects of physical activity on mental health are noted globally, even among persons with severe mental illnesses (WHO, 2019).

Avoid Alcohol

As noted earlier, alcohol use and mental illness are closely linked. Engaging patients in discussion around strategies to decrease alcohol intake of any amount can minimize or eliminate mental and physical health risks and associated mental health implications. It may also be appropriate to address alcohol use as the primary problem if it causes clinically significant impairment or distress to the individual (Rani & Hemavathy, 2021). Refer to an alcohol counselor as needed to develop a structured recovery process.

Rest More

Adequate sleep and rest are critical to mental health and healthy lifestyles. Although this topic is covered in detail in another chapter, a brief overview is presented here to alert the APP of the implications of sleep and rest on mental health. The National Institutes of Health (2021) indicates that the amount of sleep people need varies by age. It is recommended that school-age children get about 9 hours of sleep per night, teens require 8 to 10 hours, and most adults should get 7 to 9 hours of sleep nightly.

A lack of sleep can interfere with making decisions, solving problems, controlling emotions, reacting, and focusing. People who lack the recommended sleep make more mistakes, have a slower reaction time, and take longer to finish projects. Children who do not have enough sleep can be overly active and have trouble paying attention. They may also be impulsive, experience mood swings, have decreased motivation, and feel sad or depressed (National Institutes of Health, 2021). The effects of sleep deprivation include poor balance, risk of heart disease, weight gain, lower sex drive, heart disease, risk of diabetes, weakened immune system, mood changes, memory issues, trouble thinking and concentrating, and accidents (Watson & Cherney, 2021).

Diet quality can affect sleep quality and adversely affect mental health. Ikonte et al. (2019) found that an inadequate intake of the micronutrients calcium and magnesium and vitamins A, C, D, E, and K was associated with sleep problems. In their review of studies on diet and sleep physiology, Frank et al. (2017) found that poor sleep outcomes were associated with the following diet components: low-fiber, high-saturated fat, and sugar intake; high-carbohydrate, low-fat diet; and protein and carbohydrate deficiencies. Consuming high simple-carbohydrate meals close to bedtime has been found to increase the number of nighttime awakenings and reduce the amount of deep sleep a person can achieve (St-Onge et al., 2016). On the other hand, the Dietary Approaches to Stop Hypertension (DASH) diet, which focuses on whole foods with high levels of potassium, fiber, and magnesium, tends to support high-quality sleep (Liang et al., 2020), thus improving mental health and functioning.

Other risk factors for poor sleep quality include obstructive sleep apnea, which causes frequent nighttime awakenings and impaired breathing. Alcohol ingestion can worsen obstructive sleep apnea and lead to upper airway blockage during sleep (St-Onge et al., 2016). Medications can also affect sleep quality. Selective serotonin reuptake inhibitor antidepressants, stimulants, nasal or oral decongestants, beta blockers, corticosteroids, statins, ACE inhibitors, cholinesterase inhibitors, thyroid hormone replacements, theophylline, and nicotine replacement medications can adversely affect sleep quality (Stahl, 2021).

Exercise can improve or jeopardize sleep quality and thus affect mental health. Moderate aerobic exercise increases slow-wave deep sleep, which rejuvenates the body, stabilizes the mood, and decompresses the mind. Exercise creates activity in the brain and may cause some people to stay awake. In addition, exercise raises body temperature, which leads to wakefulness. If this occurs, avoiding exercise for one to two hours before bed is recommended. Patients may need to experiment to discover the best timing and intensity to exercise to achieve their optimum level of sleep (Johns Hopkins Medicine, n.d.).

Treat Tobacco Use

Evidence shows a clear link between tobacco use and poor mental health outcomes (Smith et al., 2020). Therefore, preventing and treating tobacco use is a significant consideration in promoting the mental health of youth and adults (U.S. Preventive Services Task Force, 2020, 2021). There is a wealth of resources available to APPs who make it a priority to treat tobacco and nicotine use by employing evidence-informed strategies. Since 2008 when the U.S. Department of Health and Human Services published the *Clinical Practice Guideline 2008 Update* (Fiore et al., 2008), APPs have had access to a resource describing the most effective pharmacotherapies and counseling strategies. This source has not been fully translated into practice, and readers are encouraged to review this valuable resource. The CHEST Foundation published a tool kit that provides updated treatment information on the effective use of pharmacotherapy and counseling (Prezant et al., n.d.). The tool kit also includes valuable, accurate billing codes for reimbursement of care; clarity on the issue of electronic cigarette use; and links to useful resources for vulnerable populations. The American Psychiatric Nurses Association also provides open access to tobacco treatment education, links to training, and newly constructed nursing competencies for treating tobacco use and dependency (Essenmacher et al., 2021). APPs are encouraged to seek out these free resources for addressing tobacco use to positively impact the mental health of their patients.

Other Strategies for Supporting Mental Health

Many other strategies exist for supporting mental health, including acupuncture, Feldenkrais Method (FM), massage therapy, Healing Touch, and aromatherapy. These strategies are summarized in **Table 23.2**.

Acupuncture is the insertion of very thin specialized needles into the skin at specific points over the whole body or external ear structures (Mayo Clinic, n.d.-a). Acupuncture is used to alleviate adverse symptoms associated with physical conditions (e.g., cancer pain) and mental issues, such as PTSD (Grant et al., 2018), depression (Smith et al., 2018), and postpartum depression (Li et al., 2018). Results of studies are promising and generally acknowledge the lack of harm from the procedure, but the evidence is mixed as to the significance of the beneficial effects (Grant et al., 2018). Smith et al. (2018) found low-quality evidence supporting some reduction in depression when treated with acupuncture. The use of acupuncture to treat metabolic syndrome is also being studied. Li et al. (2021) examined 13 randomized controlled trials about the use of acupuncture to treat metabolic syndrome and noted improvements in hyperlipidemia indices and fasting blood sugars. These findings have implications for mental health because metabolic disorders can be induced as side effects of medication for mental health issues.

Not everyone is able to engage in physically rigorous exercise. However, the use of FM can be helpful for older people and persons with neurological disorders or chronic pain (Elgelid & Kresge, 2021). Brummer et al. (2018) described FM as gentle manipulation of the body limbs in a range of motion by a trained practitioner, which has been shown to treat pain effectively and to improve balance in older persons. In a review of the literature about FM, Stephens and Hillier (2020) found evidence supporting improved balance, reduced fear of falling, and effectiveness for chronic pain management. Ullmann et al. (2020) described a study protocol to measure improvements in cognitive executive function associated with FM. If successful, FM would be a promising low-cost intervention for older adults.

Massage therapy, the manipulation of muscle, connective tissue, and skin by a trained and certified massage therapist, has many therapeutic physical and mental health benefits (Mayo Clinic, n.d.-c). Studies show that massage therapies reduce stress and increase relaxation while improving immune function and treating pain (Mayo Clinic, n.d.-c). Rapaport et al. (2018) assessed the state of current knowledge of the usefulness and validity of massage therapy for psychiatric disorders. They found that massage may decrease hypothalamic-pituitary-adrenal activity, positively affect immune function, enhance parasympathetic tone, and modulate brain circuitry. They provided a detailed strategy for maximizing traditional psychiatric counseling with the concurrent use of massage therapy.

Minimal but valid studies support a technique related to massage known as Healing Touch (HT). HT is an energy-based complementary therapy that promotes relaxation, diminishes depression, eases anxiety, and increases the sense of well-being (Reeve et al., 2020).

Table 23.2 Other Strategies Supporting Mental Health

Strategy	Description	Useful Links
Acupuncture (whole body or auricular)	Technique in which trained, certified practitioners insert thin needles into the skin at specialized points; treats pain, mixed results with tobacco treatment and depression	https://www.nccaom.org https://acudetox.com https://www.nccih.nih.gov/health/acupuncture-in-depth
Aromatherapy	Centuries-old practice of using essential oils for therapeutic benefit; research on effectiveness is mixed but may improve symptoms of depression, anxiety, insomnia	https://naha.org/education/approved-schools https://www.aromaweb.com/articles/aromatherapypractitioners.asp https://courses.aromaticstudies.com/aromatic-scholars https://www.hopkinsmedicine.org/health/wellness-and-prevention/aromatherapy-do-essential-oils-really-work
Breathwork	Refers to breathing exercises or techniques to improve physical and mental health; very limited research	https://breathworkalliance.com/certified-schools
Feldenkrais Method	Somatic education uses movement and real-time awareness to guide positive changes (e.g., improved balance, pain reduction, flexibility, improved cognition).	https://feldenkrais.com
Massage therapy	Uses pressing, rubbing, and manipulation of skin, muscles, tendons, and ligaments; many different types; possible benefits include decreased anxiety, insomnia, and physical pain; research on effectiveness is mixed.	https://www.ncbtmb.org https://www.amtamassage.org/state-regulations/credentials-massage-therapy-profession https://www.nccih.nih.gov/health/providers/digest/massage-therapy-for-health-science

HT has been used to treat cancer pain, arthritis pain, and psychological distress. Reeve et al. (2020) studied the effects of using HT with patients who have PTSD and found a reduction in symptom severity. They recommended that HT, a low-cost and low-risk intervention, be implemented with the delivery of other PTSD care (Reeve et al., 2020).

Other lesser-known and less often used potentially helpful therapies include breathwork (methodical, mindful breathing techniques) and aromatherapy (various scents used to promote well-being). While more research is needed on the types and delivery methods of teaching patients about breathwork therapies, evidence shows that it is effective for anxiety, depression, and PTSD (Aideyan et al., 2020). Evidence shows that aromatherapy is effective at promoting relaxation and relieving stress and enhancing mood, balance, and well-being (Aćimović, 2021) and is an effective strategy to improve sleep quality (Lin et al., 2019), though further research is recommended.

Health Promotion Case Study Addressing Anxiety/Depression in a College-Age Female

Case Description: J.W., a 20-year-old female, presents to a primary care clinic with complaints of daily headaches once per week, disrupted sleep once per month, intermittent irritability, weight gain, and negative feedback from her work supervisor. She has been avoiding friends. She seeks help at the urging of her family and responds briefly to provider questions.

Psychiatric History: Separation anxiety as a child.

Medical History: Denied acute or chronic medical conditions.

Social History: She is a college senior taking 12 credit hours and lives with a roommate off campus. She recently ended a relationship with her boyfriend of six months. She is working at a coffee shop on campus.

Family History: The patient was raised by married biological parents. She has an older brother. Her father has been treated for panic attacks, and her mother has a history of postpartum depression.

Vital Signs: height 5'4", weight 102 pounds, blood pressure 130/84 mmHg left arm, heart rate 94 beats per minute, respiratory rate 18 beats per minute, temperature 97.2° F

Physical Exam: Unremarkable. No acute distress, well nourished. Appears stated age. Skin is warm, dry, and intact. Heart rate and rhythm are normal, with no murmurs, gallops, or rubs. There are no signs of respiratory distress. Lung sounds are clear in all lobes bilaterally without rales, rhonchi, or wheezes. Her gait is stable.

Lifestyle Vital Signs

- Adopt healthy eating: Skips breakfast and eats out for lunch and dinner
- Stress less: Recent breakup with boyfriend; negative feedback at work
- Move often: Not assessed
- Avoid alcohol: Not assessed
- Rest more: Delayed sleep onset and multiple nighttime awakenings
- Treat tobacco use: Nonsmoker

Critical Thinking Questions

- What additional subjective and objective data related to lifestyle behaviors do you want to assess and why?
- What mental health screening tools can you use to assess J.W.'s current level of anxiety and/or depression symptoms?
- What lifestyle management strategies would you consider for optimizing J.W.'s mental and physical health outcomes?
- What referrals to other providers and internet resources will you consider?

Additional Resource: Lee, J. S., Jaini, P. A., & Papa, F. (2020). An epigenetic perspective on lifestyle medicine for depression: Implications for primary care practice. *American Journal of Lifestyle Medicine, 16*(1), 76–88. https://doi.org/10.1177/1559827620954779

Health Promotion Activity: Labeling Feelings

Labeling feelings and emotional experiences demystifies the experience and empowers individuals to reflect on the cause-and-effect relationship between their behaviors and feelings, thus improving emotion regulation.

Complete a 24-hour Feelings Journal starting when you awake. Label your initial feeling of the day using feeling words (e.g., happy, nervous, sad, disappointed, stressed, content, cheerful, relieved). Capture your feelings throughout the day, before and after meals at least. Some individuals do best when they schedule an hourly self-check.

Resources

Center for Nonviolent Communication. (2005). Feelings inventory. https://www.cnvc.org/sites/default/files/2018-10/CNVC-feelings-inventory.pdf

Torre, J. B., & Lieberman, M. D. (2018). Putting feelings into words: Affect labeling as implicit emotion regulation. *Emotion Review, 10*(2), 116–124. https://doi.org/10.1177/175407391774

Interprofessional Approaches for Promoting Mental Health

APPs can engage professionals from many healthcare disciplines to collaboratively develop practical approaches to improve a patient's mental health, address risk factors for mental illness, and diagnose and treat severe mental illness. Interprofessional team members may include psychologists, psychiatrists, behavioral health specialists, addiction specialists, counselors, dietitians, nutritionists, exercise specialists, sleep specialists, social workers, and others.

Several community-based wellness programs are available to address mental health, such as local YMCAs and fitness facilities, healthcare facilities, and community colleges. Some of these programs are open to the public or available through membership or franchised well-being programs and may be beneficial in supporting optimal mental health and healthy lifestyles. Increased mental health awareness has led many schools and workplaces to offer resources and services to address mental health. Patients are encouraged to consider wellness programs near them, depending on affordability, needs, patient interests, and accessibility.

Summary

The reciprocal nature of mental and physical health is complex. Mental health affects physical health, and physical health affects mental health. Treatments for both mental and physical health issues cause and/or exacerbate both. It is not always clear how to assess for each disorder. These intricacies and implications are difficult for new APPs to grasp. It is also challenging for a busy, overwhelmed, established APP to keep up to date with the plethora of new evidence on supporting mental health and healthy lifestyles.

The primary purpose of this chapter is to provide APPs with evidence to understand the implications of morbidity and mortality of common mental health disorders that present in the primary care setting. The complex and correlative relationship between mental health and lifestyle has been discussed. Strategies to support optimal mental health and a healthy lifestyle have been reviewed. The information presented here is by no means comprehensive and is thus limited. There are likely many more strategies described herein, such as hypnosis or Reiki. Search parameters for the information for this chapter were mostly limited to the past five years, and as such older but valuable information may not have been included. Readers are strongly encouraged to network

TABLE 23.3	Evidence-Based Resources for Mental Health

Organization	URL
Anxiety and Depression Association of America	https://adaa.org
American Academy of Child and Adolescent Psychiatry	https://www.aacap.org
Child Mind Institute	https://childmind.org
Crisis Text Line	https://www.crisistextline.org
Food for the Brain	https://foodforthebrain.org
Life and Health Network	https://lifeandhealth.org/mindfulness
The Quell Foundation	https://thequellfoundation.org
National Alliance on Mental Illness	https://www.nami.org
National Center for Complementary and Integrative Health	https://www.nccih.nih.gov
NutritionFacts.org	https://nutritionfacts.org
Nedley Health (resources for depression)	https://www.nedleyhealth.com
PLANTSTRONG	https://plantstrong.com
Stay Safe Foundation (resources for PTSD)	https://staysafefoundation.org

with subject matter experts throughout their careers and stay up to date with healthy lifestyle strategies to achieve optimal mental health outcomes. See **Table 23.3** for additional mental health evidence-based resources.

The information in this chapter addresses established pillars to support overall health. Patients respond well to collaboratively formed plans to achieve healthy lifestyles. The A-SMART strategies provided in this chapter give APPs a framework for prescribing lifestyle change and collaboratively working with their patients to implement interventions to foster mental health. APPs should individualize the prescription to provide precise strategies that are the patient's expressed preferences because this will improve adherence. This chapter identified many opportunities to optimize lifestyles through prescriptive therapeutic interventions to improve mental and physical health.

Acronyms

ADAA: Anxiety and Depression Association of America

APP: advanced practice provider

A-SMART: adopt healthy eating, stress less, move often, avoid alcohol, rest more, and treat tobacco use

CDC: Centers for Disease Control and Prevention

FM: Feldenkrais Method

HT: Healing Touch

MI: motivational interviewing

MSE: mental status examination

NBI: nature-based intervention

NCBDDD: National Center on Birth Defects and Developmental Disabilities

NIMH: National Institute of Mental Health

OCD: obsessive–compulsive disorder

PTSD: post-traumatic stress disorder

SUD: substance use disorder.

References

Aćimović, M. (2021). Essential oils: Inhalation aromatherapy—a comprehensive review. *Journal of Agronomy, Technology and Engineering Management, 4*, 547–557.

Adan, R. A. H., van der Beek, E. M., Buitelaar, J. K., Cryan, J. F., Hebbrand, J., Higgs, S., Schellekens, H., & Dickson, S. L. (2019). Nutritional psychiatry: Towards improving mental health by what you eat. *European Neuropsychopharmacology, 28*(12), 1321–1332. https://doi.org/10.1016/j.euroneuro.2019.10.011

Aideyan, B., Martin, G. C., & Beeson, E. T. (2020). A practitioner's guide to breathwork in clinical mental health counseling. *Journal of Mental Health Counseling, 42*(1), 78–94. https://doi.org/10.17744/mehc.42.1.06

Allegrante, J. P., Wells, M. T., & Peterson, J. C. (2019). Interventions to support behavioral self-management of chronic diseases. *Annual Reviews, 40*, 120–146. https://doi.org/10.1146/annurev-publhealth-040218-044008

Alliance for Healthier Communities. (n.d.). *Rx: Community—Social prescribing in Ontario.* Retrieved May 15, 2022, from https://www.allianceon.org/Rx-Community-Social-Prescribing-In-Ontario

Alneyadi, M., Drissi, N., Almeqbaali, M., & Ouhbi, S. (2021). Biofeedback-based connected mental health interventions for anxiety: Systematic literature review. *JMIR mHealth and uHealth, 9*(4), e26038. https://doi.org/10.2196/26038

Andreassen, C. S., Griffiths, M. D., Pallesen, S., Bilder, R. M., Torsheim, T., & Aboujaoude, E. (2015). The Bergen Shopping Addiction Scale: Reliability and validity of a brief screening test. *Frontiers in Psychology, 6*, 1374. https://doi.org/10.3389/fpsyg.2015.01374

Anxiety and Depression Association of America. (n.d.-a). *Anxiety disorders—Facts and statistics.* Retrieved October 8, 2022, from https://adaa.org/understanding-anxiety/facts-statistics

Anxiety and Depression Association of America. (n.d.-b). *Depression facts and statistics.* Retrieved October 8, 2022, from https://adaa.org/understanding-anxiety/depression/facts-statistics

Anxiety and Depression Association of America. (n.d.-c). *Generalized anxiety disorder (GAD).* Retrieved October 8, 2022, from https://adaa.org/understanding-anxiety/generalized-anxiety-disorder-gad

Anxiety and Depression Association of America. (n.d.-d). *Post-traumatic stress disorder (PTSD).* Retrieved October 8, 2022, from https://adaa.org/understanding-anxiety/posttraumatic-stress-disorder-ptsd

Anxiety and Depression Association of America. (n.d.-e). *What is obsessive compulsive disorder (OCD)?* Retrieved October 8, 2022, from https://adaa.org/understanding-anxiety/co-occurring-disorders/obsessive-compulsive-disorder

Appelhans, B. M., Whited, M. C., Schneider, K. L., Ma, Y., Oleski, J. L., Merriam, P. A., Waring, M. E., Olendzki, B. C., Mann, D. M., Ockene, I. S., & Pagoto, S. L. (2012). Depression severity, diet quality, and physical activity in women with obesity and depression. *Journal of the Academy of Nutrition and Dietetics, 112*(5), 693–698. https://doi.org/10.1016/j.jand.2012.02.006

Ballou, S., Mitsuhashi, S., Sankin, L. S., Petersen, T. S., Zubiago, J., Lembo, C., Takazawa, E., Katon, J., Sommers, T., Hirsch, W., Rangan, V., & Jones, M. (2019). Emergency department visits for depression in the United States from 2006 to 2014. *General Hospital Psychiatry, 59*, 14–19. https://doi.org/10.1016/j.genhosppsych.2019.04.015

Bauer, M. E., & Teixeira, A. L. (2019). Inflammation in psychiatric disorders: What comes first? *Annals of the New York Academy of Sciences, 1437*(1), 57–67. https://doi.org/10.1111/nyas.13712

Beavers, A. W., Atkinson, A., Varvatos, L. M., Connolly, M., & Alaimo, K. (2022). How gardening in Detroit influences physical and mental health. *International Journal of Environmental Research and Public Health, 19*(13), 7899. https://doi.org/10.3390/ijerph19137899

Beezhold, B. L., & Johnston, C. S. (2012). Restriction of meat, fish, and poultry in omnivores improves mood: A pilot randomized controlled trial. *Nutrition Journal, 11*(9). https://doi.org/10.1186/1475-2891-11-9

Bell, S. L., Audrey, S., Gunnell, D., Cooper, A., & Campbell, R. (2019). The relationship between physical activity, mental wellbeing and symptoms of mental health disorder in adolescents: A cohort study. *International Journal of Behavior Nutrition and Physical Activity, 16*(138). https://doi.org/10.1186/s12966-019-0901-7

Bertone-Johnson, E. R., Powers, S. I., Spangler, L., Brunner, R. L., Michael, Y. L., Larson, J. C., Millen, A. E., Bueche, M. N., Salmoiro-Blotcher, E., Liu, S., Wassertheil-Smoller, S., Ockene, J. K., Ockene, I., & Manson, J. E. (2011). Vitamin D intake from foods and supplements and depressive symptoms in a diverse population of older women. *American Journal of Clinical Nutrition, 94*(94), 1104–1112. https://doi.org/10.3945/ajcn.111.017384

Beutel, M. E., Klein, E. M., Brähler, E., Reiner, I., Jünger, C., Michal, M., Wiltink, J., Wild, P. S., Münzel, T., Lackner, K. J., & Tibubos, A. N. (2017). Loneliness in the general population: Prevalence, determinants and relations to mental health. *BMC Psychiatry, 17*(1), 97. https://doi.org/10.1186/s12888-017-1262-x

Bickerdike, L., Booth, A., Wilson, P. M., Farley, K., & Wright, K. (2017). Social prescribing: Less rhetoric and more reality. A systematic review of the evidence. *BMJ Open, 7*(4), e013384. https://doi.org/10.1136/bmjopen-2016-013384

Bremner, J. D., Moazzami, K., Wittbrodt, M. T., Nye, J. A., Lima, B. B., Gillespie, C. F., Rappaport, M. H., Pearce, B. D., Shah, A. J., & Vaccarino, V. (2020). Diet, stress

and mental health. *Nutrients*, *12*(8), 2428. https://doi
.org/10.3390/nu12082428

Brummer, M., Walach, H., & Schmidt, S. (2018).
Feldenkrais "functional integration" increases
body contact surface in the supine position: A
randomized-controlled experimental study. *Frontiers in Psychology*, *9*, 2023. https://doi.org/10.3389
/fpsyg.2018.02023

Buckley, R. C., Brough, P., & Westaway, D. (2018).
Bringing outdoor therapies into mainstream mental
health. *Frontiers in Public Health*, *6*, 119. https://doi
.org/10.3389/fpubh.2018.00119

Büssing, A., Michalsen, A., Khalsa, S. B. S., Telles, S., &
Sherman, K. J. (2012). Effects of yoga on mental and
physical health: A short summary of reviews. *Evidence-
Based Complementary and Alternative Medicine*, *2012*,
165410. https://doi.org/10.1155/2012/165410

Cacioppo, J. T., & Cacioppo, S. (2018). Chapter three—
Loneliness in the modern age: An evolutionary theory
of loneliness (ETL). *Advances in Experimental Social
Psychology*, *58*, 127–197. https://doi.org/10.1016
/bs.aesp.2018.03.003

Callow, D. D., Arnold-Nedimala, N. A., Jordan, L. S., Pena,
G. S., Won, J., Woodard, J. L., & Smith, J. C. (2020).
The mental health benefits of physical activity in older
adults survive the COVID-19 pandemic. *American
Journal of Geriatric Psychiatry*, *28*(10), 1046–1057.
https://doi.org/10.1016/j.jagp.2020.06.024

Carlat, D. J. (2017). *The psychiatric interview* (4th ed.).
Wolters Kluwer.

Caroppo, E., Mazza, M., Sannella, A., Marano, G.,
Avallone, C., Claro, A. E., Janiri, D., Moccia, L., Janiri,
L., & Sani, G. (2021). Will nothing be the same again?
Changes in lifestyle during COVID-19 pandemic and
consequences on mental health. *International Journal
of Environmental Research and Public Health*, *18*(16),
8433. https://doi.org/10.3390/ijerph18168433

Center for Nonviolent Communication. (2005). *Feelings inventory*. https://www.cnvc.org/sites/default/files/2018
-10/CNVC-feelings-inventory.pdf

Christ, A., Lauterbach, M., & Latz, E. (2019). Western
diet and the immune system: An inflammatory
connection. *Immunity*, *51*(5), 794–811. https://doi
.org/10.1016/j.immuni.2019.09.020

Cohen-Cline, H., Turkheimer, E., & Duncan, G. E.
(2015). Access to green space, physical activity and
mental health: A twin study. *Journal of Epidemiology
and Community Health*, *69*(6), 523–529. https://doi
.org/10.1136/jech-2014-204667

Cohen Veterans Network and the National Council for
Behavioral Health. (2018, October 10). *America's
mentalhealth2018*. https://www.cohenveteransnetwork
.org/wp-content/uploads/2018/10/Research
-Summary-10-10-2018.pdf

Colton, C. W., & Manderscheid, R. W. (2006). Congruen-
cies in increased mortality rates, years of potential life
lost, and causes of death among public mental health clients in eight states. *Preventing Chronic Disease*, *3*(2), A42.

Conversano, C. (2019). Common psychological factors
in chronic diseases. *Frontiers in Psychology*, *10*, 2727.
https://doi.org/10.3389/fpsyg.2019.02727

Coventry, P. A., Brown, J. E., Pervin, J., Brabyn, S., Pateman,
R., Breedvelt, J., Gilbody, S., Stancliffe, R., McEachan,
R., & White, P. L. (2021). Nature-based outdoor activities for mental and physical health: Systematic
review and meta-analysis. *SSM Population Health*, *16*.
https://doi.org/10.1016/j.ssmph.2021.100934

Dikec, G., Arabaci, L. B., Uzunoglu, G. B., & Mizrak, S. D.
(2021). Metabolic side effect in patients using atypical antipsychotic medications during hospitalization.
Journal of Psychosocial Nursing and Mental Health, *56*(4).
https://doi.org/10.3928/02793695-20180108-05

Dimov, S., Mundy, L. K., Bayer, J. K., Jacka, F. N.,
Canterford, L., & Patton, G. C. (2021). Diet quality
and mental problems in late childhood. *Nutritional
Neuroscience*, *24*(1), 62–70. https://doi.org/10.1080
/1028415X.2019.1592288

Division of Population Health. (n.d.-a). *Data on excessive
drinking*. Centers for Disease Control and Prevention,
National Center for Chronic Disease Prevention and
Health Promotion. Retrieved May 15, 2022, from
https://www.cdc.gov/alcohol/data-stats.htm

Division of Population Health. (n.d.-b). *Dietary guidelines
for alcohol*. Centers for Disease Control and Prevention,
National Center for Chronic Disease Prevention and
Health Promotion. Retrieved May 15, 2022, from https://
www.cdc.gov/alcohol/fact-sheets/moderate-drinking.htm

Dormal, V., Vermeulen, N., & Mejias, S. (2021). Is heart
rate variability biofeedback useful in children and
adolescents? A systematic review. *Journal of Child
Psychology and Psychiatry*, *62*(12), 1379–1390. https://
doi.org/10.1111/jcpp.13463

Driot, D., Bismuth, M., Maurel, A., Soulie-Albouy, J.,
Birebent, J., Oustric, S., & Dupouy, J. (2017). Management of first depression or general anxiety disorder episode in adults in primary care: A systematic
metareview. *La Presse Médicale*, *46*(12), 1124–1138.
https://doi.org/10.1016/j.lpm.2017.10.010

Elgelid, S., & Kresge, C. (2021). *The Feldenkrais Method:
Learning through movement*. Handspring.

Esfeld, J., Pennings, K., Rooney, A., & Robinson, S.
(2021). Integrating trauma-informed yoga into addiction treatment. *Journal of Creativity in Mental Health*.
https://doi.org/10.1080/15401383.2021.1972067

Essenmacher, C., Baird, C., Houfek, J., Spielmann, M.
R., & Adams, S. (2021). Developing competency-
based nursing treatment for persons with tobacco
use disorder. *Journal of the American Psychiatric
Nurses Association*, *28*(1), 23–36. https://doi.org
/10.1177/10783903211058785

Evans, J., Magee, A., Dickman, K., Sutter, R., & Sutter,
C. (2017). A plant-based nutrition program. *American*

Journal of Nursing, *117*(3), 56–61. https://doi.org /10.1097/01.NAJ.0000513289.14377.0f

Farooqui, A. A., Horrocks, L. A., & Farooqui, T. (2007). Modulation of inflammation in brain: A matter of fat. *Journal of Neurochemistry*, *101*(3), 577–599. https:// doi.org/10.1111/j.1471-4159.2006.04371.x

Fiore, M. C., Jaén, C. R., Baker, T. B., Bailey, W. C., Benowitz, N. L., Curry, S. J., Dorfman, S. F., Froelicher, E. S., Goldstein, M. G., Healton, C. G., Henderson, P. N., Heyman, R. B., Koh, H. K., Kottke, T. E., Lando, H. A., Mecklenburg, R. E., Mermelstein, R. J., Mullen, P. D., Orleans, C. T., . . . Wewers, M. E. (2008). *Clinical practice guideline: Treating tobacco use and dependence: 2008 update*. U.S. Department of Health and Human Services, Public Health Service. https://www.ncbi .nlm.nih.gov/books/NBK63952

Firth, J., Marx, W., Dash, S., Carney, R., Teasdale, S. B., Solmi, M., Stubbs, B., Schurch, F. B., Carvalho, A. F., Jacka, F., & Sarris, J. (2019). The effects of dietary improvement on symptoms of depression and anxiety: A meta-analysis of randomized controlled trials. *Psychosomatic Medicine*, *81*(3), 265. https://dx.doi .org/10.1097%2FPSY.0000000000000673

First, M. B. (2022). Medical assessment of the patient with mental symptoms. *Merck Manual Professional Version*. https://www.merckmanuals.com/professional /psychiatric-disorders/approach-to-the-patient-with -mental-symptoms/medical-assessment-of-the-patient -with-mental-symptoms

Foster, J. A., & Neufeld, K. A. M. (2013). Gut-brain axis: How the microbiome influences anxiety and depression. *Trends in Neurosciences*, *36*(5), 305–312. https:// dx.doi.org/10.1016/j.tins.2013.01.005

Francis, H. M., Stevenson, R. J., Chambers, J. R., Gupta, D., Newey, B., & Lim, C. K. (2019). A brief diet intervention can reduce symptoms of depression in young adults: A randomized controlled trial. *PLoS One*, *14*(10), e0222768. https://doi.org/10.1371/journal .pone.0222768

Frank, S., Gonzalez, K., Lee-Ang, L., Young, M. C., Tamez, M., & Mattei, J. (2017). Diet and sleep physiology: Public health and clinical implications. *Frontiers in Neurology*, *8*, 393. https://doi.org/10.3389 /fneur.2017.00393

Frühauf, A., Niedermeier, M., Elliott, L. R., Ledochowski, L., Marksteiner, J., & Kopp, M. (2016). Acute effects of outdoor physical activity on affect and psychological well-being in depressed patients: A preliminary study. *Mental Health and Physical Activity*, *10*, 4–9. https://doi.org/10.1016/j.mhpa.2016.02.002

Fusar-Poli, P., Salazar de Pablo, G., DeMicheli, A., Nieman, D. H., Correll, C. U., Kessing, L. V., Pfennig, A., Bechdolf, A., Borgwardt, S., Arango, C., & van Amelsvoort, T. (2020). What is good mental health? A scoping review. *European Neuropsychopharmacology*, *31*, 33–46. https://doi.org/10.1016/j.euroneuro.2019.12.105

Galante, J., Friedrich, C., Dawson, A. F., Modrego-Alaron, M., Gebbing, P., Delgado-Suarez, I., Gupta, R., Dean, L., Dalgleish, T., White, I. R., & Jones, P. B. (2021). Mindfulness-based programs for mental health promotion in adults in nonclinical settings: A systematic review and meta-analysis of randomized controlled trials. *PLoS Medicine*, *18*(1), e1003481. https://doi .org/10.1371/journal.pmed.1003481

Gentile, C. L., & Weir, T. L. (2018). The gut microbiota at the intersection of diet and human health. *Science*, *362*(6416), 776–780. https://doi.org/10.1126/science .aau5812

Giuntella, O., Hyde, K., Saccardo, S., & Sadoff, S. (2021). Lifestyle and mental health disruptions during COVID-19. *Proceedings of the National Academy of Sciences of the United States of America*, *118*(9), e2016632118. https://doi.org/10.1073/pnas.2016632118

Grabbe, L. (2022). Trauma resiliency model therapy. In K. Wheeler (Ed.), *Psychotherapy for the advance practice psychiatric nurse: A how-to guide for evidence-based practice* (3rd ed., pp. 441–467). Springer.

Grant, S., Colaiaco, B., Motala, A., Shanman, R., Sorbero, M., & Hempel, S. (2018). Acupuncture for the treatment of adults with posttraumatic stress disorder: A systematic review and meta-analysis. *Journal of Trauma & Dissociation*, *19*(1), 39–58. https://doi.org /10.1080/15299732.2017.1289493

Gray, M., Adamo, G., Pitini, E., & Jani, A. (2020). Precision social prescriptions to promote active ageing in older people. *Journal of the Royal Society of Medicine*, *113*(4), 143–147. https://doi .org/10.1177/0141076819865888

Grossman, E. R., Benjamin-Neelon, S. E., & Sonnenschein, S. (2020). Alcohol consumption during the COVID-19 pandemic: A cross-sectional survey of US adults. *International Journal of Environmental Research and Public Health*, *17*(24), 9189. https://doi .org/10.3390/ijerph17249189

Hallam, K. T., Bilsborough, S., & de Courten, M. (2018). "Happy Feet": Evaluating the benefits of a 100-day 10,000 step challenge on mental health and wellbeing. *BMC Psychiatry*, *18*(1), 19. https://doi .org/10.1186/s12888-018-1609-y

Han, A., Kim, J., & Kim, J. (2021). A study of leisure walking intensity levels on mental health and health perception of older adults. *Gerontology & Geriatric Medicine*, *7*. https://doi.org/10.1177%2F2333721421999316

Hayhoe, R., Rechel, B., Clark, A. B., Gummerson, C. L., Smith, S. J., & Welch, A. A. (2021). Cross-sectional associations of schoolchildren's fruit and vegetable consumption, and meal choices, with their mental well-being: A cross-sectional study. *BMJ Nutrition, Prevention, & Health*, *4*. https://doi.org/10.1136/bmjnph-2020-000205

Herron, A. J., & Brennan, T. K. (2020). *The ASAM essentials of addiction medicine* (3rd ed.). American Society of Addiction Medicine & Wolters Kluwer.

Hu, L., Wang, Y., Liu, X., Ji, X., Ma, Y., Man, S., Hu, Z., Cheng, J., & Huang, F. (2021). Tai chi exercise can ameliorate physical and mental health of patients with knee osteoarthritis: Systematic review and meta-analysis. *Clinical Rehabilitation*, 35(1), 64–79. https://doi.org/10.1177/0269215520954343

Hunter, C. L., Goodie, J. L., Oordt, M. S., & Dobmeyer, A. C. (2017). *Integrated behavior health in primary care: Step-by-step guidance for assessment and intervention* (2nd ed.). American Psychological Association.

Husk, K., Elston, J., Gradinger, F., Callaghan, L., & Asthana, S. (2019). Social prescribing: Where is the evidence? *British Journal of General Practice*, 69(678), 6–7. https://doi.org/10.3399/bjgp19X700325

Ikonte, C. J., Mun, J. G., Reider, C. A., Grant, R. W., & Mitmesser, S. H. (2019). Micronutrient inadequacy in short sleep: Analysis of the NHANES 2005–2016. *Nutrients*, 11(10), 2335. https://doi.org/10.3390/nu11102335

Jacka, F. N., O'Neil, A., Opie, R., Itsiopoulos, C., Cotton, S., Mohebbi, M., Castle, D., Dash, S., Mihalopoulos, C., Chatterton, M. L., Brazionis, L., Dean, O. M., Hodge, A. M., & Berk, M. (2017). A randomised controlled trial of dietary improvement for adults with major depression (the "SMILES" Trial). *BMC Medicine*, 15(23). https://doi.org/10.1186/s12916-017-0791-y

Jacka, F. N., Pasco, J., Mykletun, A., Williams, L., Hodge, A., O'Reilly, S., Nicholson, G., Kotowicz, M., & Berk, M. (2010). Association of Western and traditional diets with depression and anxiety in women. *American Journal of Psychiatry*, 167(3), 305–311. https://doi.org/10.1176/appi.ajp.2009.09060881

Jarrett, R. L., Bahar, O. S., & Taylor, M. A. (2011). "Holler, run, be loud": Strategies for promoting child physical activity in a low-income, African American neighborhood. *Journal of Family Psychology*, 25(6), 825–836. https://doi.org/10.1037/a0026195

Johns Hopkins Medicine. (n.d.). *Exercising for better sleep*. Retrieved May 2, 2023, from https://www.hopkinsmedicine.org/health/wellness-and-prevention/exercising-for-better-sleep

Kalmakis, K. (2021). Integrating behavioral health in primary care: Time to shift paradigms. *Journal of the American Association of Nurse Practitioners*, 33(11), 847–848. https://doi.org/10.1097/JXX.0000000000000664

Karl, J. P., Hatch, A. M., Arcidiacono, S. M., Pearce, S. C., Pantoja-Feliciano, I. G., Doherty, L. A., & Soares, J. W. (2018). Effects of psychological, environmental and physical stressors on the gut microbiota. *Frontiers in Microbiology*, 9. https://doi.org/10.3389/fmicb.2018.02013

Kelly, P., Williamson, C., Niven, A. G., Hunter, R., Mutrie, N., & Richards, J. (2019). Walking on sunshine: Scoping review of the evidence for walking and mental health. *British Journal of Sports Medicine*, 52, 800–806. http://dx.doi.org/10.1136/bjsports-2017-098827

Kennedy, L., & Parker, S. H. (2019). Biofeedback as a stress management tool: A systematic review. *Cognition, Technology & Work*, 21, 161–190. https://doi.org/10.1007/s10111-018-0487-x

Khandaker, G. M., Dantzer, R., & Jones, P. B. (2017). Immunopsychiatry: Important facts. *Psychological Medicine*, 47(13), 2229–2237. https://doi.org/10.1017/S0033291717000745

Krebs, P., Norcross, J. C., Nicholson, J. M., & Prochaska, J. O. (2019). Stages of change. In J. C. Norcross & B. E. Wampold (Eds.), *Psychotherapy relationships that work: Evidence-based therapist responsiveness* (pp. 296–328). Oxford University Press.

Lam, J. A., Murray, E. R., Yu, K. E., Ramsey, M., Nguyen, T. T., Mishra, J., Martis, B., Thomas, M. L., & Lee, E. E. (2021). Neurobiology of loneliness: A systematic review. *Neuropsychopharmacology*, 46, 1873–1887. https://doi.org/10.1038/s41386-021-01058-7

Lampert, T., Costa, J., Santos, O., Sousa, J., Ribeiro, T., & Freire, E. (2021). Evidence on the contribution of community gardens to promote physical and mental health and well-being of non-institutionalized individuals: A systematic review. *PLoS One*, 16(8). https://doi.org/10.1371/journal.pone.0255621

Leavell, M. A., Leiferman, J. A., Gascon, M., Braddick, F., Gonzalez, J. C., & Litt, J. S. (2019). Nature-based social prescribing in urban settings to improve social connectedness and mental well-being: A review. *Current Environmental Health Reports*, 6, 297–308. https://doi.org/10.1007/s40572-019-00251-7

Lee, J. S., Jaini, P. A., & Papa, F. (2020). An epigenetic perspective on lifestyle medicine for depression: Implications for primary care practice. *American Journal of Lifestyle Medicine*, 16(1), 76–88. https://doi.org/10.1177/1559827620954779

Levounis, P., Arnaout, B., & Marienfeld, C. (2017). *Motivational interviewing for clinical practice*. American Psychiatric Association.

Li, S., Zhong, W., Peng, W., & Jiang, G. (2018). Effectiveness of acupuncture in postpartum depression: A systematic review and meta-analysis. *Acupuncture in Medicine*, 36(5), 295–301. https://doi.org/10.1136/acupmed-2017-011530

Li, X., Hong-Xiao, J., Dong-Qing, Y., & Zhang-Jin, Z. (2021). Acupuncture for metabolic syndrome: Systematic review and meta-analysis. *Acupuncture in Medicine*, 39(4), 253–263. https://doi.org/10.1177%2F0964528420960485

Li, Y., Lv, M.-R., Wei, Y.-J., Sun, L., Zhang, J.-X., Zhang, H.-G., & Li, B. (2017). Dietary patterns and depression risk: A meta-analysis. *Psychiatry Research*, 253, 373–382. https://doi.org/10.1016/j.psychres.2017.04.020

Liang, H., Beydoun, H. A., Hossain, S., Maldonado, A., Zonderman, A. B., Fanelli-Kuczmarski, M. T., & Beydoun, M. A. (2020). Dietary Approaches to Stop Hypertension (DASH) Score and its association with sleep quality in a national survey of middle-aged and older men and women. *Nutrients*, *12*(5), 1510. https://doi.org/10.3390/nu12051510

Lianov, L. (2021). *Strengths in the mirror: Thriving now and tomorrow.* New Degree Press.

Lin, P.-C., Lee, P.-H., Tseng, S.-J., Lin, Y.-M., Chen, S.-R., & Hou, W.-H. (2019). Effects of aromatherapy on sleep quality: A systematic review and meta-analysis. *Complementary Therapies in Medicine*, *45*, 156–166. https://doi.org/10.1016/j.ctim.2019.06.006

Lucas, M., Mirzaei, F., O'Reilly, E. J., Pan, A., Willett, W. C., Kawachi, I., Koenen, K., & Ascherio, A. (2011). Dietary intake of n-3 and n-6 fatty acids and the risk of clinical depression in women: A 10-y prospective follow-up study. *American Journal of Clinical Nutrition*, *93*(6), 1337–1343. https://doi.org/10.3945/ajcn.111.011817

Luhmann, M., & Hawkley, L. C. (2016). Age differences in loneliness from late adolescence to oldest old age. *Developmental Psychology*, *52*(6), 943–959. https://doi.org/10.1037/dev0000117

Macy, R. J., Jones, E., Graham, L. M., & Roach, L. (2018). Yoga for trauma and related mental health problems: A meta-review with clinical and service recommendations. *Trauma, Violence & Abuse*, *19*(1), 35–57. https://doi.org/10.1177/1524838015620834

Mangiola, F., Ianiro, G., Franceschi, F., Fagiuoli, S., Gasbarrini, G., & Gasbarrini, A. (2016). Gut microbiota in autism and mood disorders. *World Journal of Gastroenterology*, *22*(1), 361–368. https://doi.org/10.3748/wjg.v22.i1.361

Martin, C. R., Osadchiy, V., Kalani, A., & Mayer, E. A. (2018). The brain-gut-microbiome axis. *Cellular and Molecular Gastroenterology and Hepatology*, *6*(2), 133–148. https://doi.org/10.1016/j.jcmgh.2018.04.003

Mayo Clinic. (n.d.-a). *Acupuncture.* Retrieved May 15, 2022, from https://www.mayoclinic.org/tests-procedures/acupuncture/about/pac-20392763

Mayo Clinic. (n.d.-b). *Biofeedback.* Retrieved May 15, 2022, from https://www.mayoclinic.org/tests-procedures/biofeedback/about/pac-20384664

Mayo Clinic. (n.d.-c). *Massage therapy.* Retrieved May 15, 2022, from https://www.mayoclinic.org/tests-procedures/massage-therapy/about/pac-20384595

McCarron, R. M., Xiong, G. L., Rivelli, S., Muskin, P. R., Summergrad, P., & Suo, S. (2019). *Association of Medicine and Psychiatry: Primary care psychiatry* (2nd ed.). Wolters Kluwer.

McCormick, R. (2017). Does access to green space impact the mental well-being of children: A systematic review. *Journal of Pediatric Nursing*, *37*, 3–7. https://doi.org/10.1016/j.pedn.2017.08.027

McMartin, S., Jacka, F., & Colman, I. (2013). The association between fruit and vegetable consumption and mental health disorders: Evidence from five waves of a national survey of Canadians. *Preventive Medicine*, *56*(3–4), 225–230. https://doi.org/10.1016/j.ypmed.2012.12.016

Mechawar, N., & Savitz, J. (2016). Neuropathology of mood disorders: Do we see the stigmata of inflammation? *Translational Psychiatry*, *6*, e946. https://doi.org/10.1038/tp.2016.212

Medawar, E., Huhn, S., Villringer, A., & Witte, A. V. (2019). The effects of plant-based diets on the brain: A systematic review. *Translational Psychiatry*, *9*(226). https://doi.org/10.1038/s41398-019-0552-0

Melham, N. M., Porta, G., Oquendo, M. A., Zelazny, J., Keilp, J. G., Iyengar, S., Burke, A., Birmaher, B., Stanley, B., Mann, J. J., & Brent, D. A. (2019). Severity and variability of depression symptoms predicting suicide attempt in high-risk individuals. *JAMA Psychiatry*, *76*(6), 603–613. https://doi.org/10.1001/jamapsychiatry.2018.4513

Mikkelsen, K., Stojanovska, L., Polenakovic, M., Bosevski, M., & Apostolopoulos, V. (2017). Exercise and mental health. *Maturitas*, *106*, 48–56. https://doi.org/10.1016/j.maturitas.2017.09.003

Miller, K. J., Gonçalves-Bradley, D. C., Areerob, P., Hennessy, D., Messagno, C., & Grace, F. (2020). Comparative effectiveness of three exercise types to treat clinical depression in older adults: A systematic review and network meta-analysis of randomized controlled trials. *Ageing Research Reviews*, *58*, 100999. https://doi.org/10.1016/j.arr.2019.100999

Miller, W. R., & Rollnick, S. R. (2013). *Motivational interviewing: Helping people change* (3rd ed.). Guilford Press.

National Alliance on Mental Illness. (n.d.). *Mental health by the numbers.* Retrieved October 8, 2022, from https://www.nami.org/mhstats

National Center for Chronic Disease Prevention and Health Promotion. (n.d.). *Excessive alcohol use.* Centers for Disease Control and Prevention. Retrieved October 8, 2022, from https://www.cdc.gov/chronic-disease/pdf/factsheets/alcohol-use-factsheet-H.pdf

National Center for Health Statistics. (n.d.-a). *Depression.* Centers for Disease Control and Prevention. Retrieved May 15, 2022, from https://www.cdc.gov/nchs/fastats/depression.htm

National Center for Health Statistics. (n.d.-b). *Mental health.* Centers for Disease Control and Prevention. Retrieved May 15, 2022, from https://www.cdc.gov/nchs/fastats/mental-health.htm

National Center for Injury Prevention and Control. (n.d.-a). *Marijuana and public health: Data and statistics.* Centers for Disease Control and Prevention. Retrieved May 15, 2022, from https://www.cdc.gov/marijuana/data-statistics.htm

National Center for Injury Prevention and Control. (n.d.-b). *Opioid data analysis and resources.* Centers for Disease Control and Prevention. Retrieved May 15, 2022, from https://www.cdc.gov/opioids/data/analysis-resources.html

National Center on Birth Defects and Developmental Disabilities. (n.d.-a). *Anxiety and depression in children:*

Get the facts. Centers for Disease Control and Prevention. Retrieved May 15, 2022, from https://www.cdc.gov/childrensmentalhealth/features/anxiety-depression-children.html

National Center on Birth Defects and Developmental Disabilities. (n.d.-b). *Data and statistics on children's mental health.* Centers for Disease Control and Prevention. Retrieved May 15, 2022, from, https://www.cdc.gov/childrensmentalhealth/data.html

National Center on Birth Defects and Developmental Disabilities. (n.d.-c). *Post-traumatic stress disorder in children.* Centers for Disease Control and Prevention. Retrieved May 15, 2022, from https://www.cdc.gov/childrensmentalhealth/ptsd.html

National Institute of Mental Health. (n.d.-a). *Chronic illness and mental health: Recognizing and treating depression.* Department of Health and Human Services, National Institutes of Health. Retrieved May 2, 2023, from https://www.nimh.nih.gov/health/publications/chronic-illness-mental-health

National Institute of Mental Health. (n.d.-b). *Depression.* U.S. Department of Health and Human Services. Retrieved October 8, 2022, from https://www.nimh.nih.gov/health/topics/depression

National Institute of Mental Health. (n.d.-c). *Mental health information: Statistics.* Department of Health and Human Services, National Institutes of Health. Retrieved May 15, 2022, from https://www.nimh.nih.gov/health/statistics

National Institute of Mental Health. (n.d.-d). *Post-traumatic stress disorder.* Department of Health and Human Services, National Institutes of Health. Retrieved May 2, 2023, from https://www.nimh.nih.gov/health/publications/post-traumatic-stress-disorder-ptsd

National Institutes of Health. (2021, April). *Good sleep for good health: Get the rest you need.* U.S. Department of Health and Human Services. https://newsinhealth.nih.gov/sites/nihNIH/files/2021/April/NIHNiHApr2021.pdf

Nazarko, L., & Thorne, J. (2020). Providing holistic care to prevent hospital admission. *Journal of Prescribing Practice, 2*(2). https://doi.org/10.12968/jprp.2020.2.2.84

Noble, E. E., Hsu, T. M., & Kanoski, S. E. (2017). Gut to brain dysbiosis: Mechanisms linking Western diet consumption, the microbiome, and cognitive impairment. *Frontiers in Behavioral Neuroscience, 11*(9). https://doi.org/10.3389/fnbeh.2017.00009

Nurser, K. P., Rushworth, I., Shakespeare, T., & Williams, D. (2018). Personal storytelling in mental health recovery. *Mental Health Review Journal, 23*(1), 25–36. https://doi.org/10.1108/MHRJ-08-2017-0034

Ocean, N., Howley, P., & Ensor, J. (2019). Lettuce be happy: A longitudinal UK study on the relationship between fruit and vegetable consumption and well-being. *Social Science & Medicine, 222,* 335–345. https://doi.org/10.1016/j.socscimed.2018.12.017

Office of Disease Prevention and Health Promotion. (n.d.-a). *Increase the proportion of people with substance use and mental health disorders who get treatment for both—MHMD-07.* U.S. Department of Health and Human Services. Retrieved May 15, 2022, from https://health.gov/healthypeople/objectives-and-data/browse-objectives/mental-health-and-mental-disorders/increase-proportion-people-substance-use-and-mental-health-disorders-who-get-treatment-both-mhmd-07

Office of Disease Prevention and Health Promotion. (n.d.-b). *Increase the proportion of primary care visits where adolescents and adults are screened for depression—MHMD-08.* U.S. Department of Health and Human Services. Retrieved May 15, 2022, from https://health.gov/healthypeople/objectives-and-data/browse-objectives/mental-health-and-mental-disorders/increase-proportion-primary-care-visits-where-adolescents-and-adults-are-screened-depression-mhmd-08

Office of Disease Prevention and Health Promotion. (n.d.-c). *Mental health and mental disorders.* U.S. Department of Health and Human Services. Retrieved May 15, 2022, from https://health.gov/healthypeople/objectives-and-data/browse-objectives/mental-health-and-mental-disorders

Office of Disease Prevention and Health Promotion (ODPHP). (n.d.-d). *Mental health: Overview and impact.* U.S. Department of Health and Human Services. Retrieved May 15, 2022, from https://www.healthypeople.gov/2020/leading-health-indicators/2020-lhi-topics/Mental-Health

Office on Smoking and Health. (n.d.). *Smoking and tobacco use: Current cigarette smoking among adults in the United States.* Centers for Disease Control and Prevention, National Center for Chronic Disease Prevention and Health Promotion. Retrieved May 15, 2022, from https://cdc.gov/tobacco/data_statistics/fact_sheets/adult_data/cig_smoking/index.htm

Oswald, F., Campbell, J., Williamson, C., Richards, J., & Kelly, P. (2020). A scoping review of the relationship between running and mental health. *International Journal of Environmental Research and Public Health, 17*(21). https://doi.org/10.3390/ijerph17218059

Pearce, M., Garcia, L., Abbas, A., Strain, T., Schuch, F. B., Golubic, R., Kelly, P., Khan, S., Utukuri, M., Laird, Y., Mok, A., Smith, A., Tainio, M., Brage, S., & Woodcock, J. (2022). Association between physical activity and risk of depression: A systematic review and meta-analysis. *JAMA Psychiatry, 79*(6), 550–559. https://doi.org/10.1001/jamapsychiatry.2022.0609

Penninx, B. W. J. H., & Lange, S. M. M. (2018). Metabolic syndrome in psychiatric patients: Overview, mechanisms, and implications. *Dialogues in Clinical Neuroscience, 20*(1), 63–73. https://doi.org/10.31887%2FDCNS.2018.20.1%2Fbpenninx

Pickard, J. M., Zeng, M. Y., Caruso, R., & Nunez, G. (2017). Gut microbiota: Role in pathogen colonization, immune responses, and inflammatory disease. *Immunological Reviews*, 279(1), 70–89. https://doi.org/10.1111/imr.12567

Pizzoli, S. F. M., Marzorati, C., Gatti, D., Monzani, D., Mazzocco, K. M., & Pravettoni, G. (2021). A meta-analysis on heart rate variability biofeedback and depressive symptoms. *Scientific Reports*, 11, 6650. https://doi.org/10.1038/s41598-021-86149-7

Prezant, D., Farer, H., Bars, M., Tanner, N., Alexander, L. C., & Venkateshiah, S. (n.d.). *Tobacco dependence treatment toolkit*. CHEST Foundation. Retrieved May 2, 2023, from https://foundation.chestnet.org/wp-content/uploads/2021/06/Tobacco_Dependence_Treatment_Toolkit_CHEST_Foundation.pdf

Prochaska, J. J. (2011). Smoking and mental illness: Breaking the link. *New England Journal of Medicine*, 365(3), 196–198. https://doi.org/10.1056/NEJMp1105248

Protogerou C., McHugh, R. K., & Johnson, B. T. (2020). How best to reduce unhealthy risk-taking behaviours? A meta-review of evidence syntheses of interventions using self-regulation principles. *Health Psychology Review*, 14(1), 86–115. https://doi.org/10.1080/17437199.2019.1707104

Ramanuj, P., Ferenchik, E., Docherty, M., Spaeth-Rublee, B., & Pincus, H. A. (2019). Evolving models of integrated behavioral health and primary care. *Current Psychiatry Reports*, 21(4). https://doi.org/10.1007/s11920-019-0985-4

Rani, R. A. N., & Hemavathy, V. (2021). Counseling for alcoholism. *Natural Volatiles & Essential Oils*, 8(4), 1714–1718.

Rapaport, M. H., Schettler, P. J., Larson, E. R., Carroll, D., Sharenko, M., Nettles, J., & Kinkead, B. (2018). Massage therapy for psychiatric disorders. *Complementary and Integrative Medicine*, 16(1), 24–31. https://doi.org/10.1176/appi.focus.20170043

Reeve, K., Black, P. A., & Huang, J. (2020). Examining the impact of a healing touch intervention to reduce post-traumatic stress disorder symptoms in combat veterans. *Psychological Trauma: Theory, Research, Practice, and Policy*, 12(8), 897–903. https://doi.org/10.1037/tra0000591

Schroeder, S. A., Clark, B., Cheng, C., & Saucedo, C. B. (2017). Helping smokers quit: The Smoking Cessation Leadership Center engages behavior health by challenging old myths and traditions. *Journal of Psychoactive Drugs*, 50(2), 151–158. https://doi.org/10.1080/02791072.2017.1412547

Schuch, F. B., Vancampfort, D., Firth, J., Rosenbaum, S., Ward, P. B., Silva, E. S., Hallgren, M., Ponce de Leon, A., Dunn, A. L., Deslandes, A. C., Fleck, M. P., Carvalho, A. F., & Stubbs, B. (2018). Physical activity and incident depression: A meta-analysis of prospective cohort studies. *American Journal of Psychiatry*, 175(7), 631–648. https://doi.org/10.1176/appi.ajp.2018.17111194

Shabbir, F., Patel, A., Mattison, C., Bose, S., Krishnamohan, R., Sweeney, E., Sandhu, S., Nel, W., Rais, A., Sandhu, R., Mgu, N., & Sharma, S. (2013). Effect of diet on serotonergic neurotransmission in depression. *Neurochemistry International*, 62(3), 324–329. https://doi.org/10.1016/j.neuint.2012.12.014

Shankland, R., Tessier, D., Strub, L., Gauchet, A., & Baeyens, C. (2020). Improving mental health and well-being through informal mindfulness practice: An intervention study. *Applied Psychology Health and Well-Being*, 13(1), 63–83. https://doi.org/10.1111/aphw.12216

Shi, Z. (2019). Gut microbiota: An important link between Western diet and chronic diseases. *Nutrients*, 11(10), 2287. https://doi.org/10.3390/nu11102287

Smith, C. A., Armour, M., Myeong, S. L., Wang, L.-Q., & Hay, P. J. (2018). Acupuncture for depression. *Cochrane Database of Systematic Reviews*, 2018(3). https://doi.org/10.1002/14651858.CD004046.pub4

Smith, P. H., Chhipa, M., Bystrik, J., Roy, R., Goodwin, R. D., & McKee, S. A. (2020). Cigarette smoking among those with mental disorders in the U.S. population: 2012–2013 update. *Tobacco Control*, 29, 29–35. http://doi.org/10.1136/tobaccocontrol-2018-054268

Smoking Cessation Leadership Center. (2022). *Drug interactions with tobacco smoke*. https://smokingcessationleadership.ucsf.edu/sites/smokingcessationleadership.ucsf.edu/files/Documents/FactSheets/376701_CABHWI_Drug%20Interactions_2022_PRINT.pdf

Song, Q.-H., Shen, G.-Q., Xu, R.-M., Zhang, Q.-H., Ma, M., Guo, Y.-H., Zhao, X.-P., & Han, Y.-B. (2014). Effect of tai chi exercise on the physical and mental health of the elder patients suffered from anxiety disorder. *International Journal of Physiology, Pathophysiology and Pharmacology*, 6(1), 55–60.

Stahl, S. M. (2021). *Stahl's psychopharmacology: Neuroscientific basis and practical applications* (5th ed.). Cambridge University Press.

Stephens, J., & Hillier, S. (2020). Evidence for the effectiveness of the Feldenkrais Method. *Kinesiology Review*, 9(3), 228–235. https://doi.org/10.1123/kr.2020-0022

Stickley, A., & Koyanagi, A. (2016). Loneliness, common mental disorders and suicidal behavior: Findings from a general population survey. *Journal of Affective Disorders*, 197, 81–87. https://doi.org/10.1016/j.jad.2016.02.054

St-Onge, M. P., Mikic, A., & Pietrolungo, C. E. (2016). Effects of diet on sleep quality. *Advances in Nutrition*, 7(5), 938–949. https://doi.org/10.3945/an.116.012336

Substance Abuse and Mental Health Services Administration. (2020). *Key substance use and mental health indicators in the United States: Results from the 2019 National Survey on Drug Use and Health*. Center for Behavioral

Health Statistics and Quality. https://www.samhsa.gov/data/sites/default/files/reports/rpt29393/2019NSDUHFFRPDFWHTML/2019NSDUHFFR090120.htm

Swinson, T., Wenborn, J., & Sugarhood, P. (2020). Green walking groups: A mixed-methods review of the mental health outcomes for adults with mental health problems. *British Journal of Occupational Therapy, 83*(3), 162–171. https://doi.org/10.1177%2F0308022619888880

Syvertsen, T. (2020). *Digital detox: The politics of disconnecting.* Emerald.

Terziev, V. (2019). Social activity and human resources as social development factors. *International E-Journal of Advances in Social Sciences, 5*(13), 283–289. https://doi.org/10.18769/ijasos.531329

Teychenne, M., White, R. L., Richards, J., Schuch, F. B., Rosenbaum, S., & Bennie, J. A. (2020). Do we need physical activity guidelines for mental health: What does the evidence tell us? *Mental Health and Physical Activity, 18*, 100315. https://doi.org/10.1016/j.mhpa.2019.100315

Thomas, V., Azmitia, M., & Whittaker, S. (2016). Unplugged: Exploring the costs and benefits of constant connection. *Computers in Human Behavior, 63*, 540–548. https://doi.org/10.1016/j.chb.2016.05.078

Tomova, A., Bukovsky, I., Rembert, E., Yonas, W., Alwarith, J., Barnard, N. D., & Kahleova, H. (2019). The effects of vegetarian and vegan diets on gut microbiota. *Frontiers in Nutrition, 6*, 47. https://doi.org/10.3389/fnut.2019.00047

Torre, J. B., & Lieberman, M. D. (2018). Putting feelings into words: Affect labeling as implicit emotion regulation. *Emotion Review, 10*(2), 116–124. https://doi.org/10.1177/175407391774

Twenge, J. M., Joiner, T. E., Rogers, M. L., & Martin, G. N. (2018). Increases in depressive symptoms, suicide-related outcomes, and suicide rates among U.S. adolescents after 2010 and links to increased new media screen time. *Clinical Psychological Science, 6*(1). https://doi.org/10.1177/2167702617723376

Ullmann, G., Li, Y., Ray, M. A., & Lee, S. T. (2020). Study protocol of a randomized intervention study to explore effects of a pure physical training and a mind-body exercise on cognitive executive function in independent living adults age 65–85. *Aging Clinical and Experimental Research, 33*, 1259–1266. https://doi.org/10.1007/s40520-020-01633-w

U.S. Preventive Services Task Force. (2020). Primary care interventions for prevention and cessation of tobacco use in children and adolescents: U.S. Prevention Services Task Force recommendation statement. *JAMA, 323*(16), 1590–1598. https://doi.org/0.1001/jama.2020.4679

U.S. Preventive Services Task Force. (2021, January 19). *Final recommendation statement: Tobacco smoking cessation in adults, including pregnant persons: Interventions.* https://www.uspreventiveservicestaskforce.org/uspstf/recommendation/tobacco-use-in-adults-and-pregnant-women-counseling-and-interventions#fullrecommendationstart

Varambally, S., & Gangadhar, B. N. (2016). Current status of yoga in mental health services. *International Review of Psychiatry, 28*(3), 233–235. https://doi.org/10.3109/09540261.2016.1159950

Villarroel, M. A., & Terlizzi, E. P. (2020). *Symptoms of depression among adults: United States, 2019.* Centers for Disease Control and Prevention, National Center for Health Statistics. https://www.cdc.gov/nchs/products/databriefs/db379.htm

Watanabe, H., Ishida, S., Konno, Y., Matsumoto, M., Nomachi, S., Masaki, K., Okayama, H., & Nagai, Y. (2012). Impact of dietary folate intake on depressive symptoms in young women of reproductive age. *Journal of Midwifery & Women's Health, 57*(1), 43–48. http://doi.org/ 10.1111/j.1542-2011.2011.00073.x

Watson, J. (2021, December 22). Last call? Moderate alcohol's health benefits look increasingly doubtful. *Medscape Medical News.* https://www.medscape.com/viewarticle/965387

Watson, S., & Cherney, K. (2021, December 15). *Effects of sleep deprivation on the body.* Healthline. https://www.healthline.com/health/sleep-deprivation/effects-on-body

Wong, Y. J., Owen, J., Gabana, N. T., Brown, J. W., McInnis, S., Toth, P., & Gilman, L. (2018). Does gratitude writing improve the mental health of psychotherapy clients? Evidence from a randomized controlled trial. *Psychotherapy Research, 28*(2), 192–202. https://doi.org/10.1080/10503307.2016.1169332

Woodward, J. J. (2020). The pharmacology of alcohol. In A. J. Herron & T. K. Brennan (Eds.), *The ASAM essentials of addiction medicine* (3rd ed., pp. 44–49). Wolters Kluwer.

World Health Organization. (2019). *Motion for your mind: Physical activity for mental health promotion, protection, and care.* https://apps.who.int/iris/bitstream/handle/10665/346405/WHO-EURO-2019-3637-43396-60933-eng.pdf?sequence=1&isAllowed=y

World Health Organization. (2022, June 17). *Mental health: Strengthening our response.* https://www.who.int/news-room/fact-sheets/detail/mental-health-strengthening-our-response

Xu, H., Li, S., Song, X., Li, Z., & Zhang, D. (2018). Exploration of the association between dietary fiber intake and depressive symptoms in adults. *Nutrition, 54*, 48–53. https://doi.org/10.1016/j.nut.2018.03.009

Yeung, A., Chang, J. S. M., Cheung, J. C., & Zou, L. (2018). Qigong and tai-chi for mood regulation. *Complementary and Integrative Medicine, 16*(1), 40–47. https://doi.org/10.1176/appi.focus.20170042

Yuan, N., Chen, Y., & Xia, Y. (2019). Inflammation-related biomarkers in major psychiatric disorders: A cross-disorder assessment of reproducibility and specificity in 43 meta-analyses. *Translational Psychiatry, 9,* 233. https://doi.org/10.1038/s41398-019-0570-y

Zablotsky, B., & Terlizzi, E. P. (2020). *Mental health treatment among children aged 5–17 years: United States, 2019.* Centers for Disease Control and Prevention, National Center for Health Statistics. https://www.cdc.gov/nchs/data/databriefs/db381-H.pdf

Zimmerman, M., Balling, C., Chelminski, I., & Dalrymple, K. (2018). Understanding the severity of depression: Which symptoms of depression are the best indicators of depression severity? *Comprehensive Psychiatry, 87,* 84–88. https://doi.org/10.1016/j.comppsych.2018.09.006

Zuckoff, A. (2012). "Why won't my patients do what's good for them?" Motivational interviewing and treatment adherence. *Surgery for Obesity and Related Diseases, 8*(5), 514–521. https://doi.org/10.1016/j.soard.2012.05.002

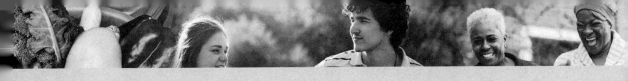

Index

Note: Locators followed by '*f*' and '*t*' refer to figures and tables, respectively.

© Kathleen Gail/Shutterstock; © StoryTime Studio/Shutterstock; © kali9/Getty Images